CLINICAL INTEGRATION:
MEDICINE

Student reviewers

Our medical textbooks are assessed and reviewed by the following medical students:

University of Aberdeen School of Medicine and Dentistry: Dylan McClurg
Barts and The London School of Medicine and Dentistry: Jay Singh
University of Birmingham College of Medical and Dental Sciences: Hannah Morgan
Cardiff University School of Medicine: Chloe Chia
The University of Edinburgh Medical School: Tanith Bain
University of Exeter Medical School: Zoe Foster
Hull York Medical School: Maalik Imtiaz
King's College London GKT School of Medical Education: Karan Sagoo
University of Liverpool School of Medicine: Sophie Gunter
University of Manchester Medical School: Holly Egan
Norwich Medical School: Aneesa Khan
University of Nottingham School of Medicine: Tom Charles
University of Sheffield Medical School: Rebecca Nutt
St George's, University of London: Nawshin Basit
Swansea University Medical School: Jack Bartlett
University of Central Lancashire School of Medicine: Katie Chi Kei Cheung
University College London Medical School: Camila Nicklewicz

We are grateful for their essential feedback.

Additional student reviewers wanted

We are keen to recruit more student reviewers, particularly at UK medical schools where we don't currently have anyone in post. If you would like to apply for the position, please contact Simon Watkins (simon.watkins@scionpublishing.com) and explain why you would be suitable for the role.

Errors, omissions (and any other feedback)

We've worked really hard with the authors to ensure that everything in the book is correct. However, errors and ambiguities can still slip through in books as complex as this. If you spot anything you think might be wrong, please email info@scionpublishing.com and we will look into it straight away. If an error has occurred, we will correct it for future printings and post a note about it on our website so that other readers of the book are alerted to this. Please also use this email address if you have more general feedback about the book.

Thank you for your help.

Hx Ex Ix Rx

CLINICAL INTEGRATION:

MEDICINE

Edited by

Nicholas Law (MBBS)

Manda Raz (MBBS (Hons))

Sharmayne Brady (MBBS (Hons), BMedSc (Hons), FRACP)

Ar Kar Aung (BMedSci, MBBS, FRACP, MPHTM)

Scion

© Scion Publishing Ltd, 2021

First published 2021

All rights reserved. No part of this book may be reproduced or transmitted, in any form or by any means, without permission.

A CIP catalogue record for this book is available from the British Library.

ISBN 9781911510727

Scion Publishing Limited

The Old Hayloft, Vantage Business Park, Bloxham Road, Banbury OX16 9UX, UK

www.scionpublishing.com

Important Note from the Publisher

The information contained within this book was obtained by Scion Publishing Ltd from sources believed by us to be reliable. However, while every effort has been made to ensure its accuracy, no responsibility for loss or injury whatsoever occasioned to any person acting or refraining from action as a result of information contained herein can be accepted by the authors or publishers.

Readers are reminded that medicine is a constantly evolving science and while the authors and publishers have ensured that all dosages, applications and practices are based on current indications, there may be specific practices which differ between communities. You should always follow the guidelines laid down by the manufacturers of specific products and the relevant authorities in the country in which you are practising.

Although every effort has been made to ensure that all owners of copyright material have been acknowledged in this publication, we would be pleased to acknowledge in subsequent reprints or editions any omissions brought to our attention.

Registered names, trademarks, etc. used in this book, even when not marked as such, are not to be considered unprotected by law.

Typeset by Evolution Design & Digital Ltd, Kent, UK

Printed in the UK

Last digit is the print number: 10 9 8 7 6 5 4 3 2 1

CONTENTS

ABOUT THE EDITORS

Dr Nicholas Law

MBBS

Nicholas Law is a junior doctor with a keen interest in medical oncology and general medicine. He studied undergraduate medicine at Monash University, Australia. Nicholas is also involved in improving medical education and junior doctor welfare at his local institution.

Dr Manda Raz

MBBS (Hons)

Manda Raz is an Australian doctor affiliated with Peninsula Health in Melbourne, with a broad interest in academia, research and acute care medicine. He completed his MBBS from Monash University, Australia. Dr Raz is the recipient of several scholarships, awards and medals for his academic achievements and contribution to empirical research and clinical governance. He is also the author and editor of multiple books and reference works spanning a number of clinical, legal and administrative specialties, and is currently studying for his MBioethics.

Dr Sharmayne Brady

MBBS (Hons), BMedSc (Hons), FRACP

Sharmayne Brady is a senior staff specialist in Rheumatology at Alfred Health and also works in private practice. She is also an NHMRC-supported PhD scholar. She studied undergraduate medicine and completed a Bachelor of Medical Science at Monash University, Australia. Dr Brady completed physician training at the Alfred Hospital in Melbourne and completed her rheumatology specialist training at both the Alfred and Western Hospitals in Melbourne. Sharmayne has published fifteen papers in leading peer-reviewed journals and has presented her research at several leading international and national conferences over the past ten years. She has also worked as a specialist at Box Hill and Cabrini Hospitals in Melbourne and worked as a sub-investigator for several randomised controlled clinical trials with the Musculoskeletal Research Unit at Monash University.

Dr Ar Kar Aung

BMedSci, MBBS, FRACP, MPHTM

Ar Kar Aung is currently a consultant physician in General Medicine and Infectious Diseases at Alfred Hospital, Melbourne, Australia, and is also an adjunct senior research fellow at Monash University. He was the previous Director of Physician Education at Alfred Health. He has served in key leadership positions as the Chair of Advance Training Committee in General and Acute Care Medicine at the Royal Australasian College of Physicians and as a Director on the Board of Internal Medicine Society of Australia and New Zealand.

LIST OF CONTRIBUTORS

Cindy Bach
Cases 81, 82, 86, 88 and 89

Kathryn Connelly
Cases 91–100

Jessica Deitch
Cases 13, 17 and 18

Mauli Govinna
Cases 11, 12, 16 and 19

Thushan Hettige
Cases 71–80

Qinyuan Hu
Cases 51–60

Rohan Khanal
Cases 83–85, 87 and 90

Nathan Kuk
Cases 21–30

John Lee
Cases 2, 5, 6, 8 and 10

Elisabeth Ng
Cases 14, 15 and 20

Briony Shaw
Cases 31–40

Udit Thakur
Cases 1, 3, 4, 7 and 9

Naomi Whyler
Cases 41–50

Kate Williams
Cases 61–70

PREFACE

Medicine is hard. We all know that. There are a million things to read up and a million things to remember. But what if there is a better method to learn about medicine? What if you could go through cases and think about and discuss relevant information pertaining to the clinical condition? We believe that a patient-centred method allows the reader to consolidate relevant clinical information to diagnose and manage clinical conditions.

This book therefore helps readers link basic medical science with clinical context and build an appreciation of how pathophysiology manifests as recognisable clues. The book shows readers the logical connections between patient history, examination findings, investigation results, management rationale and their underlying mechanisms. By working through complete cases, readers learn to understand the 'why and how' behind the diagnosis, investigation and management of common clinical problems.

We wrote the book for students in their clinical years of medical school trying to make sense of the overwhelming medical world. However, this book is also suitable for foundation year doctors and internal medicine trainees sitting their MRCP (Membership of Royal College of Physicians UK) examinations.

Nicholas Law
Manda Raz
Sharmayne Brady
Ar Kar Aung

ABBREVIATIONS

ABG	arterial blood gas		BMS	bare metal stent
ABI	ankle brachial index		BNP	brain natriuretic peptide
ACEi	angiotensin-converting enzyme inhibitor		BOHB	beta-hydroxybutyrate
ACR	albumin–creatinine ratio		BP	blood pressure
ACS	acute coronary syndrome		BPH	benign prostatic hyperplasia
ACTH	adrenocorticotrophic hormone		bpm	beats per minute
ADH	antidiuretic hormone		bvFTD	behavioural variant frontotemporal dementia
ADT	androgen deprivation therapy		CABG	coronary artery bypass graft
AF	atrial fibrillation		CAD	coronary artery disease
AFP	alpha-fetoprotein		CAUTI	catheter-associated urinary tract infection
AIDP	acute inflammatory demyelinating polyradiculoneuropathy		CCB	calcium channel blocker
AIDS	acquired immune deficiency syndrome		CCP	cyclic citrullinated peptide
AIHA	autoimmune haemolytic anaemia		CCU	coronary care unit
AKI	acute kidney injury		CD	Crohn's disease
ALL	acute lymphoblastic leukaemia		CEA	carcinoembryonic antigen
ALP	alkaline phosphatase		CF	cystic fibrosis
ALS	amyotrophic lateral sclerosis		CFTR	cystic fibrosis transmembrane conductance regulator
ALT	alanine aminotransferase		CK	creatine kinase
AML	acute myeloid leukaemia		CKD	chronic kidney disease
ANA	antinuclear antibody		CLL	chronic lymphocytic leukaemia
ANCA	antineutrophil cytoplasmic antibody		CML	chronic myeloid leukaemia
APLS	antiphospholipid syndrome		CMP	calcium, magnesium and phosphate
APML	acute promyelocytic leukaemia		CMV	cytomegalovirus
aPTT	activated partial thromboplastin time		CNS	central nervous system
ARB	angiotensin receptor blocker		COPD	chronic obstructive pulmonary disease
ARDS	acute respiratory distress syndrome		COX	cyclooxygenase
ARNI	angiotensin receptor-neprilysin inhibitor		CPAP	continuous positive airway pressure
ARR	aldosterone to renin ratio		CPP	cerebral perfusion pressure
ARV	antiretroviral		CPR	cardiopulmonary resuscitation
AST	aspartate aminotransferase		CRH	corticotrophin-releasing hormone
ATP	anti-tachycardia pacing		CRP	C-reactive protein
ATRA	all-trans retinoic acid		CSF	cerebrospinal fluid
AV	atrioventricular		CT	computed tomography
BAL	bronchoalveolar lavage		CT CAP	CT chest/abdomen/pelvis
BGL	blood glucose level		CTE	CT enterography
BMD	bone mineral density			
BMI	body mass index			

CTPA	computed tomography pulmonary angiography		ESRD	end-stage renal disease
CTSI	CT severity index		EUS	endoscopic ultrasound/ultrasonography
CVAD	central venous access device		EVD	external ventricular drain
CVD	cardiovascular disease		FAEE	fatty acid ethyl ester
CXR	chest X-ray		FBE	full blood examination
DAT	direct antiglobulin test		FEV_1	forced expiratory volume
DCIS	ductal carcinoma *in situ*		FHH	familial hypocalciuric hypercalcaemia
DES	drug-eluting stent		FISH	fluorescence *in situ* hybridisation
DEXA	dual energy X-ray absorptiometry		FNA	fine needle aspiration/aspirate
DHEA	dehydroepiandrosterone		FODMAP	fermentable oligo-, di-, mono-saccharides and polyols
DIC	disseminated intravascular coagulation		FP	ferroportin
DIPJ	distal interphalangeal joint		FTD	frontotemporal dementia
DKA	diabetic ketoacidosis		FVC	forced vital capacity
DLB	dementia with Lewy bodies		G6PD	glucose-6-phosphate dehydrogenase
DLBCL	diffuse large B cell lymphoma		GABA	gamma-aminobutyric acid
DLCO	diffusing capacity for carbon monoxide		GBM	glomerular basement membrane
DMARD	disease-modifying antirheumatic drug		GCA	giant cell arteritis
DNE	diabetes nurse educator		GCS	Glasgow Coma Scale
DOAC	direct oral anticoagulant		GCSF	granulocyte colony-stimulating factor
DSA	donor-specific antibody		GCT	germ cell tumour
DVT	deep venous thrombosis		GFR	glomerular filtration rate
EBV	Epstein–Barr virus		GGT	gamma-glutamyl transpeptidase
ECF	extracellular fluid		GI	gastrointestinal
ECG	electrocardiogram		GMC	giant migrating contraction
ED	Emergency Department		GnRH	gonadotrophin-releasing hormone
EEG	electroencephalogram		GORD	gastro-oesophageal reflux disease
eGFR	estimated GFR		GP	general practitioner
EGFR	epidermal growth factor receptor		GPA	granulomatosis with polyangiitis
EGPA	eosinophilic granulomatosis with polyangiitis		GTN	glyceryl trinitrate
ELISA	enzyme-linked immunosorbent assay		GVHD	graft-versus-host disease
EMA	endomysial		HAV	hepatitis A virus
EMG	electromyography		HBV	hepatitis B virus
ENA	extractible nuclear antigen		HCC	hepatocellular carcinoma
ePASP	estimated pulmonary artery systolic pressure		hCG	human chorionic gonadotrophin
EPO	erythropoietin		HCV	hepatitis C virus
ER	oestrogen receptor		HDL	high density lipoprotein
ERA	endothelin receptor antagonist		HDU	high dependency unit
ERCP	endoscopic retrograde cholangiopancreatography		HFrEF	heart failure with reduced ejection fraction
ESR	erythrocyte sedimentation rate		HHS	hyperosmolar hyperglycaemic state
			HIT	heparin-induced thrombocytopenia

HIV	human immunodeficiency virus	LVH	left ventricular hypertrophy
HLA	human leucocyte antigen	LVOT	left ventricular outflow tract
HNPCC	hereditary non-polyposis colon cancer	MACE	major adverse cardiac events
HOCM	hypertrophic obstructive cardiomyopathy	MCHC	mean corpuscular haemoglobin concentration
HPV	human papillomavirus	MCPJ	metacarpophalangeal joint
HR	heart rate	MCS	microscopy, culture and sensitivity
HRCT	high resolution CT	MCV	mean corpuscular volume
HRT	hormone replacement therapy	MDT	multidisciplinary team
HSV	herpes simplex virus	MEN	multiple endocrine neoplasia
HTN	hypertension	MFI	median fluorescence intensity
IBD	inflammatory bowel disease	MGUS	monoclonal gammopathy of unknown significance
IBS	irritable bowel syndrome	MI	myocardial infarction
ICD	implanted cardioverter-defibrillator	MMSE	mini mental state examination
ICP	intracranial pressure	MND	motor neurone disease
ICS	inhaled corticosteroid	MPA	microscopic polyangiitis
ICU	intensive care unit	MPN	myeloproliferative neoplasm
IDA	iron-deficiency anaemia	MR	magnetic resonance
Ig	immunoglobulin	MRA	mineralocorticoid receptor antagonist
ILD	interstitial lung disease	MRCP	magnetic resonance cholangiopancreatography
INR	international normalised ratio	MRI	magnetic resonance imaging
IPF	idiopathic pulmonary fibrosis	MRSA	methicillin-resistant *Staphylococcus aureus*
IPH	idiopathic pulmonary hypertension	MSCC	metastatic spinal cord compression
IRIS	immune reconstitution inflammatory syndrome	MSH	melanocyte-stimulating hormone
ITP	idiopathic thrombocytopenic purpura	MTPJ	metatarsophalangeal joint
IV	intravenous	NADH	nicotinamide adenine dinucleotide (NAD) + hydrogen (H)
IVC	intravenous cannula	NADPH	nicotinamide adenine dinucleotide phosphate
IVIg	intravenous immunoglobulin	NAFLD	non-alcoholic fatty liver disease
JVP	jugular venous pressure	NASH	non-alcoholic steatohepatitis
KUB	kidneys, ureter, bladder	NCS	nerve conduction studies
LABA	long-acting beta-agonist	NIV	non-invasive ventilation
LAD	left anterior descending	NSAID	non-steroidal anti-inflammatory drug
LBBB	left bundle branch block	NSCLC	non-small cell lung cancer
LDH	lactate dehydrogenase	NSGCT	non-seminomatous germ cell tumour
LDL	low density lipoprotein	NSTEMI	non-ST elevation MI
LFT	liver function test	NYHA	New York Heart Association
LHRH	luteinising hormone-releasing hormone	OA	osteoarthritis
LMWH	low molecular weight heparin	OGD	oesophagogastroduodenoscopy
LOS	lower oesophageal sphincter		
LV	left ventricular		
LVEF	left ventricular ejection fraction		

ONJ	osteonecrosis of the jaw
PAC	plasma aldosterone concentration
PCI	percutaneous coronary intervention
PCR	polymerase chain reaction
PE	pulmonary embolism
PEFR	peak expiratory flow rate
PEG	percutaneous endoscopic gastrostomy
PEP	post-exposure prophylaxis
PET	positron emission tomography
PICC	peripherally inserted central catheter
PIPJ	proximal interphalangeal joint
PJP	*Pneumocystis jirovecii* pneumonia
pMDI	pressurised metered dose inhaler
PMR	polymyalgia rheumatica
PND	paroxysmal nocturnal dyspnoea
PPI	proton pump inhibitor
PR	per rectum
PRA	plasma renin activity
PRBC	packed red blood cells
PRC	plasma renin concentration
PrEP	pre-exposure prophylaxis
PRN	pro re nata (as required)
PSA	prostate-specific antigen
PT	prothrombin time
PTH	parathyroid hormone
PTHrP	parathyroid hormone-related protein
PTU	propylthiouracil
PUD	peptic ulcer disease
PVE	prosthetic valve endocarditis
RA	rheumatoid arthritis
RAAS	renin–angiotensin–aldosterone system
RANK(L)	receptor activator of nuclear kappa-B (ligand)
RBBB	right bundle branch block
RBC	red blood cell
RCC	renal cell carcinoma
REM	rapid eye movement
RF	rheumatoid factor
RGC	retrograde giant contraction
ROSC	return of spontaneous circulation
RPC	rhythmic phasic contraction
RR	resting rate

RUQ	right upper quadrant
RV	right ventricular
RVH	right ventricular hypertrophy
SBP	spontaneous bacterial peritonitis
SCD	sudden cardiac death
SCLC	small cell lung cancer
SCT	stem cell transplant
SIADH	syndrome of inappropriate antidiuretic hormone secretion
SIRS	severe inflammatory response syndrome
SLE	systemic lupus erythematosus
SLL	small lymphocytic lymphoma
SMBG	self-monitoring of blood glucose
STEMI	ST elevation MI
sTfR	soluble transferrin receptor assay
STI	sexually transmitted infection
SVC	superior vena cava
T1DM	type 1 diabetes mellitus
T2DM	type 2 diabetes mellitus
TAVR	transcatheter aortic valve replacement
TCR	T-cell receptor
TFT	thyroid function test
TIBC	total iron-binding capacity
TIPS	transjugular intrahepatic portosystemic shunt
TKI	tyrosine kinase inhibitor
TLS	tumour lysis syndrome
TNF	tumour necrosis factor
TNM	tumour, node, metastasis
TPMT	thiopurine methyltransferase
TPO	thyroid peroxidase
TRAb	thyrotrophin receptor antibody
TRUS	transrectal ultrasonography
TRV	tricuspid regurgitant jet velocity
TSH	thyroid-stimulating hormone
TTE	transthoracic echocardiogram
tTG	transglutaminase
TTP	thrombotic thrombocytopenic purpura
U&E	urea and electrolytes
UC	ulcerative colitis
UEC	urea, electrolytes and creatinine
USDA	ursodeoxycholic acid

UTI	urinary tract infection
UV	ultraviolet
VATS	video-assisted thoracic surgery
VBG	venous blood gas
VEGF	vascular endothelial growth factor
VEGFR	vascular endothelial growth factor receptor
VF	ventricular fibrillation
VT	ventricular tachycardia
VTE	venous thromboembolism
VZV	varicella zoster virus
WCC	white blood cell count
WHO	World Health Organization

CASE 1: Aortic dissection

History

- A **47-year-old** [1] male presents with sudden onset **severe tearing central chest** [2] pain **radiating to his back** [3] . He reports it started thirty minutes after he had a tablet of **cocaine**.
- He reports a history of **poorly treated hypertension** [4] for which he has never taken medications.
- The patient states his father was a **tall man like himself** [5] with some **"issues with his heart valves"** [5] , but was unable to provide further detail.
- However, he has **never been tested** [6] since he is estranged from his family and **doesn't like visiting doctors** [6] .
- He has never had **similar chest pain** [7] to this previously.
- He is a **current smoker** [8] with a 40 pack year history but reports **nil illicit drug use** [8] .
- He has no history of **previous cardiac surgery or chest trauma** [9] .
- He is previously opioid naive and has already received **10mg morphine and 50mcg of fentanyl** [10] by the ambulance officers.
- The patient reports feeling **light-headed** [11] in the last few minutes and appears to be **becoming increasingly unwell** [11] .

[1] Typically advanced age is a risk factor for Stanford classification type B aortic dissection with other associated risk factors such as hypertension. A young or middle-aged patient presenting with features of aortic dissection is epidemiologically more likely to be presenting with type A aortic dissection.

[2] Central chest pain with radiation to the back is the most common symptom occurring in over 90% of patients presenting with aortic dissection. Pain described as 'tearing, sharp or ripping' in nature is particularly concerning for dissection. Abrupt onset thoracic or abdominal chest pain with a tearing quality forms one of the clinical features in the triad suggestive of aortic dissection. Furthermore, pain predominantly located in the chest, more so than the back or abdomen, is suggestive of ascending aorta involvement.

[3] Typically in descending aortic dissections, the pain is located primarily in the posterior chest/upper back. However, as most type A aortic dissections also include a distal extent of dissection, descending aortic manifestations may be present as well. This suggests that the aortic dissection likely extends beyond the aortic arch into the descending aorta.

[4] Systemic hypertension is one of the most important predisposing factors of acute aortic dissection. Hypertension is more common in type B aortic dissection but nonetheless is also associated with type A dissection. Untreated hypertension in a patient presenting with sudden onset tearing chest pain is concerning for aortic dissection.

[5] Aortic dissection is associated with genetically mediated collagen disorders such as Marfan syndrome and Ehlers–

Danlos syndrome. The patient's family history is concerning for a genetic collagen disorder that is likely Marfan syndrome. Marfan syndrome is typically present in up to 50% of those presenting with aortic dissection below the age of 40. Most patients with Marfan syndrome and aortic dissection have a family history of aortic dissection or aortic root dilation. Marfan syndrome follows an autosomal dominant inheritance pattern.

[6] This patient could have had aortic root dilation since birth which has not been monitored or treated with beta blockers to attenuate aortic root dilation. Additionally, with poorly controlled hypertension his risk for type A aortic dissection is high. Risk of cardiovascular death is very high in such individuals and they require close monitoring and optimisation.

[7] The chest pain is new; having never experienced such pain before excludes other differentials including gastritis and angina. The quality and intensity of the chest pain associated with aortic dissection is typically unlike any previous chest pain experienced by the patient.

[8] Smoking is another risk factor associated with aortic dissection as it can cause weakening of aortic walls. Cocaine use is also associated with aortic dissection as it produces an abrupt severe increase in blood pressure (BP) due to catecholamine release.

[9] Previous cardiac surgery or catheterisation for coronary or valvular disease can be complicated by aortic dissection. While trauma rarely leads to classic aortic dissection, it can result in a localised tear in the aortic isthmus. Motor vehicle

related chest trauma can, however, result in aortic rupture or transection.

10 The patient has received significant amounts of opioid analgesia and still remains in pain. In a patient that is previously opioid naive, high amounts of analgesia is concerning for the severity of the underlying aetiology causing the pain. Such a patient should warrant thorough investigation even if the aetiology isn't apparent initially.

11 Light-headedness in this presentation is suggestive of the patient becoming increasingly haemodynamically unstable. It warrants urgent stabilisation of the patient and identification of the aetiology, in order that appropriate therapy can be provided to prevent multi-organ failure and death.

Examination

- On examination the patient appears **pale** [1] and **presyncopal** [1].
- He is a **tall man** [2] with a **bulging chest** [2].
- He is still **speaking in full sentences** [3] but can be seen holding his central chest and epigastric region.
- **Resting rate (RR) is 22** [4], he is saturating at **94% on air and is afebrile** [5].
- There is also a **30mmHg difference in systolic blood pressure between both arms** [6], with the right arm blood pressure measurement reading of 60/45 and left arm 90/55.

- Pulse is **125bpm and regular** [7].
- When assessing radial pulses, he is noted to have a **weak right radial pulse** [8] compared to his left.
- Jugular venous pressure (JVP) is **elevated to 4–5cm** [9] with the patient positioned at 45 degrees.
- Upon auscultation of the heart, an **early diastolic murmur** [10] is appreciated at left upper sternal border.
- Auscultation of the **lungs was unremarkable** [11].
- **Nil neurological deficits** [12] such as hemiplegia, dysphasia, dysarthria or sensory loss are observed.

1 The patient appearing pale and presyncopal on general examination is concerning for insufficient cardiac output and a reduced mean arterial pressure. These features are once again suggestive of haemodynamic instability in this patient.

2 A bulging chest appearance is concerning for pectus carinatum, which is often a phenotypic characteristic of Marfan syndrome. Furthermore, individuals with Marfan syndrome are usually tall. These features are consistent with the patient having an underlying genetic predisposition. Other physical features include pectus excavatum, increased arm span to height ratio, scoliosis, elbow extension greater than 170 degrees/joint hypermobility, high arched palate, flattened cornea/displacement of the ocular lens and pes planus.

3 Given that the patient is still speaking in full sentences, at this point the patient is still maintaining his airway. Throughout this initial assessment period, the airway, breathing and circulation need to be monitored very closely and managed as appropriate if any issues are identified. The patient appears to be in peri-arrest and is deteriorating in the setting of the likely type A aortic dissection.

4 The patient is only mildly tachypnoeic which is likely in keeping with the shock presentation. However, underlying causes of respiratory distress should be excluded, such as haemothorax resulting from the aortic dissection.

5 Absence of hypoxia and the patient being afebrile reduces the likelihood of an infective process and septic

shock precipitating the presentation. Moreover, the absence of hypoxia also makes primary respiratory complications or a primary respiratory aetiology less likely.

6 A difference in blood pressure between arms is a very concerning feature suggesting type A aortic dissection with involvement of the aortic arch. With a reduced blood pressure in the right arm, the concern is that the dissection of aorta is causing impaired blood flow into the brachiocephalic artery. The brachiocephalic artery provides circulation to the right upper limb through the right subclavian artery.

7 Tachycardia is an indicator of the patient's state of likely hypovolaemic shock; currently the patient is trying to compensate for hypotension by increasing the heart rate. Regularity of the pulse is indicative that the patient isn't in atrial fibrillation.

8 A weak right radial pulse is another sign for extension of the aortic dissection to at least the arch of the aorta. This is a marker of severity in type A aortic dissection and is associated with increased mortality. Variation of pulse and/or variation of blood pressure between limbs is another high risk feature that is part of the clinical triad suggesting acute aortic dissection.

9 An elevated JVP is often a marker of either hypervolaemia or right heart dysfunction. In this scenario, it is unlikely that the patient is clinically overloaded, given the blood pressure and overall clinical scenario. However, an elevated JVP can also suggest the presence of a large pericardial effusion, preventing right heart filling, that causes distension of neck veins. Pericardial effusion leading to cardiac tamponade is a common consequence of this presentation.

10 An early diastolic murmur at the left sternal border is consistent with aortic regurgitation. This may be pre-existing in a patient with likely an underlying genetic predisposition to aortic root dilation. However, acute dissection into the aortic valvular annulus leading to severe aortic regurgitation is a known complication.

11 Lungs being clear on auscultation is further reassuring that the aortic dissection hasn't ruptured or leaked into the pleural space. Typically you will hear left basal dullness of auscultation if an effusion has accumulated due to acute aortic dissection.

12 Neurological deficits can result from aortic dissection due to carotid artery dissection or compression, which can produce a hemiplegia along with other neurological features. Additionally, spinal occlusion due to dissection may produce paraplegia with sensory loss.

Investigations

- A 12-lead ECG reveals **non-specific anterior-lateral T wave inversion and ST depression** [1].
- Chest X-ray demonstrates **normal lung fields** [2] but an **abnormally large cardiac silhouette** [3] as well as **mediastinal widening** [4].
- An **urgent bedside transthoracic echocardiogram (TTE)** [5] is completed which reveals a **large pericardial effusion** [6] with **moderate ventricular compression and interdependence** [6].
- A dilated aortic root with **dissection flap prolapse and evidence of severe aortic regurgitation is visualised** [7].
- Furthermore, on imaging of the aorta a **linear echodensity** [8] is visualised with **false lumen flow** [8] to at least the **mid-distal ascending aorta on TTE** [9].
- Urgent bloods are completed including **X-match and group and hold of 10 units of packed red blood cells (PRBC)** [10].
- The patient's haemoglobin was **115g/L** [11] with a normal renal function **(estimated glomerular filtration rate (eGFR) >90ml/min/1.73m^2)** [11] and normal coagulation profile.

1 Non-specific ischaemic electrocardiogram (ECG) changes are suggestive of insufficient blood flow through the coronary arteries. A potential differential remains an acute myocardial infarction and this should be excluded appropriate with investigations. However, aortic dissection can also produce non-specific ECG changes if it leads to coronary ischaemia through involvement of the coronary arteries.

2 A normal lung field is reassuring, as this implies that the patient is not having a large tension pneumothorax, which could also cause the patient to develop life-threatening shock. Additionally, the absence of pleural effusions is reassuring that the dissection hasn't ruptured or leaked into the pleural cavity.

3 A large cardiac silhouette is a non-specific sign which could represent underlying cardiomegaly due to dilated cardiomyopathy. However, in this presentation it further raises questions regarding the possibility of an underlying pericardial effusion.

4 Mediastinal widening is in keeping with the diagnosis of acute aortic dissection. Mediastinal widening and/or aortic widening is the third feature in the clinical triad for acute aortic dissection, especially type A.

5 In a haemodynamically unstable patient, the ideal modality of investigation is transoesophageal echocardiography as it is a portable procedure that can yield the diagnosis within minutes and is easily performed in the emergency cubicle. However, it is a procedure that can only be performed by senior members of the cardiology team. In contrast, a transthoracic echocardiogram is even more readily available and most emergency physicians and cardiology trainees can perform this imaging modality. It is particularly good at identifying ascending aortic dissection and coexistent aortic valve disruption, and providing assessment of pericardial effusions.

6 The large pericardial effusion is likely contributing to the patient's shock and hypotension. The presence of ventricular compression and interdependence is suggestive of tamponade physiology resulting from this effusion. This patient requires urgent intervention given these findings.

7 The presence of a dissection flap prolapse leading to aortic regurgitation is suggestive of acute aortic regurgitation resulting from aortic dissection. Given that the patient likely has Marfan syndrome, it is unlikely that he will have an intrinsically normal valve. In such scenarios, aortic valve replacement is warranted. In people with intrinsically normal valves who have aortic regurgitation due to a correctable aortic valve complication, repair is feasible.

8 A linear echodensity in the ascending aorta likely represents the dissection flap. False lumen blood flow is further suggestive of the presence of type A acute aortic dissection on the TTE.

9 A major limitation in TTE imaging of the aorta is the inability to adequately visualise past the mid-distal ascending aorta. The transverse and descending aorta are typically not visualised through this imaging modality. While TTE certainly provides the diagnosis, the extent of the dissection is not known exactly in this patient.

10 Given the imaging findings and haemodynamic instability, this patient requires urgent surgical intervention.

He will most definitely require significant blood products, given the significant blood loss that has already occurred and will occur intra-operatively. Preoperative bloods are warranted as well and should be sent off now.

11 The patient is mildly anaemic, likely secondary to extensive intrathoracic bleeding. Because the baseline haemoglobin is not available it is hard to quantify how much blood has been lost based on this result. Normal renal function and clotting factors are reassuring and positive prognostic factors suggesting the absence of involvement of other systems at this stage.

Management

Immediate

The patient must be **transferred to a resuscitation cubicle** [1] in the emergency department as this is a medical emergency. With any medical emergency it is essential to ensure the **airway, breathing and circulation (ABC)** [2] is optimised first. **Two large-bore intravenous cannulas** (IVCs) [3] should be inserted immediately. An **arterial line** [4] can also be considered. Given hypotension secondary to hypovolaemia from intrathoracic bleeding, **intravenous fluid** [5] should be given to the patient as a bolus. Providing blood pressure support through vasoactive agents such as **metaraminol, adrenaline or noradrenaline** [6] should be avoided. PRBC should be available urgently due to ongoing blood loss. Once the patient is optimised with regard to the ABCs, definitive treatment can be provided.

Surgical management

This patient is **not a candidate for sole medical management** [7] of his aortic dissection. Acute type A aortic dissection is **a surgical emergency** [8]. The **absence of significant comorbidities** and **neurological symptoms** [9] suggestive of stroke are positive prognostic factors. The patient appears to be a suitable surgical candidate hence urgent cardiothoracic referral and transfer to the operating theatre should be arranged.

An **open repair of the dissection** [10] with aortic valve replacement and drainage of the large pericardial effusion is required and would provide definitive management.

Long-term

There are three main long-term management strategies in patients who survive the initial dissection and in this case operative repair:

Anti-impulse therapy

Aggressive antihypertensive therapy is required long-term to **reduce systemic blood pressure and the rate of rise in systolic blood pressure** [11]. **Patient education regarding this is imperative** [12].

Identification of associated genetic conditions

Formal screening for underlying genetic conditions [13] should be completed in this patient. **Screening first-degree family members** [14] with TTE can also be considered.

Surveillance imaging

Baseline **computed tomographic (CT) angiography** [15] or thoracic magnetic resonance (MR) should be performed prior to discharge. Follow-up imaging with either modality at 3, 6 and 12 months, and annually thereafter is suggested, **even if the patient remains asymptomatic** [16].

1 Transfer to a resuscitation cubicle is required as the patient is very unwell and can deteriorate very rapidly. Hence, full resuscitation facilities should be available. If they are not available, urgent transfer is required.

2 Ensure the patient is maintaining their airway; if there are concerns, endotracheal intubation or airway adjuncts should be implemented. Since the patient is still speaking, this is not required at this point. Continue to monitor saturations and respiratory rate as a measure of breathing. Finally, circulation support is likely needed in this individual, given the hypovolaemic state.

3 Given the poor circulatory state, two large IVCs are required in order to support the circulation. These can be used to provide fluids, blood and medications in order to stabilise the patient haemodynamically.

4 An arterial line will be useful for continual blood pressure monitoring and frequent blood sampling in this patient.

5 Intravenous fluid therapy will replace some of the lost intravascular volume and support the blood pressure and circulation.

6 These are vasoactive agents and inotropes that can be used in the acute setting to support blood pressure in most instances. However, they should be avoided in acute aortic dissection to prevent hypertension. Metaraminol causes peripheral vasoconstriction through its α1-adrenergic agonist action, consequently increasing systolic blood pressure. Noradrenaline also stimulates α1 and α2 adrenergic receptors to increase peripheral vascular resistance and hence blood pressure. Adrenaline primarily has β1 agonistic actions that increase heart rate and contractility. Adrenaline also has adrenergic actions to a lesser extent, while noradrenaline has β-agonist actions to a lesser extent.

7 Indicators for medical management of aortic dissection are uncomplicated type B dissection, stable isolated arch dissection or chronic stable type B dissection. This patient does not meet any of these criteria. When medically managing a patient, the aim is reduce the systemic blood pressure and myocardial contractility in order to prevent further spread of intramural haematoma and rupture.

8 Time is very important in type A aortic dissections, with the rate of mortality increasing with every hour without surgical intervention. Surgery is the only definitive management, especially in a patient with apparent complications from the acute aortic dissection such as aortic regurgitation and the development of a large pericardial effusion with tamponade physiology. There is also likely involvement of the coronary arteries given the non-specific anterior–lateral ECG changes.

9 The absence of other medical comorbidities, such as advanced age, malignancy and dementia, that may limit survival of the patient to less than one year makes the patient an appropriate surgical candidate. Haemorrhagic stroke is also a relative contraindication to surgical intervention due to intraoperative heparinisation for induction onto coronary artery bypass. The absence of any neurology is reassuring in this patient.

10 An open repair will involve evacuation of the pericardial effusion, excision of the intimal tear, reconstitution of the aorta with a synthetic graft followed by replacement of the aortic valve with either bio-prosthetic or metallic valve. A metallic valve in this patient, although it provides superior longevity, would consign the patient to lifelong warfarin therapy, which may not be suitable due to previous compliance issues.

11 Aggressive blood pressure control will reduce aortic wall stress and prevent further dissections in the long term. Beta blockers are typically first-line agents but other antihypertensive agents will usually be required to achieve sufficient blood pressure control. The target blood pressure should be less than 120/80.

12 Patient education is very important in all patients especially if there is a history of poor medical attendance and adherence. Close follow-up with multiple members of the medical profession and family education can assist in improving long-term management.

13 It is highly likely this patient has Marfan syndrome that has predisposed this presentation. Screening for this needs to occur so relevant investigations and treatments can be provided regarding any associated genetic conditions. As a general rule, patients with Marfan syndrome should only participate in low to moderate intensity exercise. They should avoid exercising to exhaustion and especially activities which involve the Valsalva manoeuvre.

14 Given the likely genetic predisposition, TTE of first-degree relatives to assess for aortic aneurysm, dilated aortic root or bicuspid aortic valve is reasonable.

15 CT angiography of the aorta is more readily available but it does expose the patient to considerable ionising radiation which should be avoided if possible. CT angiography also requires iodine-based contrast which can cause nephrotoxicity. Ideally, MR angiography should be used in young patients but understandably this is not always feasible.

16 Serial imaging aims to detect the following abnormalities: recurrence of the dissection, aneurysm formation or leakage at the surgical anastomosis. In the early stages, the patient will often be asymptomatic despite the presence of these abnormalities on imaging.

CASE 2: Aortic stenosis

History

- A **67-year-old** [1] female presents to her general practitioner (GP) with **5 months of dyspnoea** [2].
- She originally ascribed this to just getting older, but now **she becomes dyspnoeic when mobilising around the shops** [3] and is unable to walk the dogs without stopping frequently. **This was never an issue before** [4].
- When inquiring about syncope, she reports not having any syncopal events but on **one hot day, she felt like she was going to faint** [5] when she was cleaning the house and had to sit down.
- She also recalls feeling **dyspnoeic with only mild exertion when she had a viral chest infection** [6] a few months ago but did not seek medical attention as the dyspnoea resolved with the resolution of the infection.
- She reports **no associated chest pain or palpitations** [7].
- She reports **no orthopnoea, paroxysmal nocturnal dyspnoea or peripheral oedema** [8].
- She is an **ex-smoker of 30 pack years** [9], but quit 10 years ago.
- Otherwise her **past medical history** [10] and family history are unremarkable.

[1] The two most common valvular pathologies (myxomatous mitral regurgitation and calcific aortic stenosis) are degenerative in their pathophysiology and thus their incidence increases with age. 10% of people older than 85 years will have aortic stenosis.

[2] This patient has presented with chronic, progressive dyspnoea. The differentials for this presentation include more than just cardiological diagnoses. One should also think of respiratory system disorders such as chronic obstructive pulmonary disease and interstitial lung disease.

[3] When someone presents with dyspnoea, it is useful to identify their current exercise tolerance. Mobilising around the shops would most likely be less than a kilometre's worth of walking. This information is also useful as it identifies that this dyspnoea is limiting the patient's usual activities of daily living.

[4] Her current exercise tolerance is significantly decreased compared to her premorbid exercise tolerance. It's important to compare baselines. You wouldn't know unless you remembered to ask!

[5] The classical triad of symptoms in aortic stenosis is syncope, angina and dyspnoea, remembered by the mnemonic **SAD**. These three symptoms should always be attained and quantified on history as their presence carries prognostic significance. Patients presenting with angina have a 5-year mean survival. Patients presenting with syncope have a 3-year mean survival and patients with dyspnoea from congestive heart failure have a 2-year mean survival. This patient has not had syncope, but has had an episode of presyncope. Aortic stenosis results in a fixed cardiac output state and in periods of stress or hypovolaemia, patients may experience presyncope or syncope. In this case it was dehydration on a hot day that resulted in the presyncopal episode.

[6] Here is another clue. Degenerative calcific aortic stenosis is asymptomatic for a long period of time; approximately 10 years. In periods of physiological stress, however, the symptoms may become apparent.

[7] Patients with aortic stenosis may present with angina. Around half of the patients would have concomitant coronary artery disease and the other half have angina due to increased oxygen demand in the hypertrophied myocardium and altered coronary flow.

[8] The patient does not have any other signs of left heart failure apart from exertional dyspnoea.

[9] Smoking is an independent risk factor that increases the progression of aortic stenosis. Calcific aortic stenosis occurs from a combination of degenerative and inflammatory processes. Smoking causes an inflammatory state, promoting calcium deposition which in turn stiffens the leaflets and reduces the valve area.

[10] Complete your cardiovascular history by ascertaining all traditional risk factors for ischaemic heart disease such as hypertension, dyslipidaemia, diabetes and family history of ischaemic heart disease. Additionally, it is worthwhile asking for a past history of rheumatic fever. Prior to the advent of antibiotics, rheumatic fever was the most common cause of aortic stenosis. It causes commissural fusion, fibrosis and stiffening of the aortic cusps, resulting in a stenotic valve.

Examination

- The patient appears well with **no signs of increased work of breathing** [1]. She is not obese.
- Her heart rate is 70bpm and is regular. Her blood pressure is 150/95mmHg. Her respiratory rate is 16 and her saturations are 97% on air. She is afebrile.
- Examination of the hands revealed **no clubbing or nicotine stains** [2].
- There was an **anacrotic carotid pulse** [3]. The JVP is not elevated.
- The apex beat is displaced to the **6th intercostal space, just lateral to the mid-clavicular line and is pressure loaded** [4].

- Auscultation of the chest reveals a **harsh crescendo–decrescendo ejection systolic murmur loudest in the right upper sternal edge** [5], with the murmur **radiating to the carotids** [6].
- This murmur is accentuated with the patient **breathing out, leaning forward and squatting** [7].
- The murmur did not change in intensity with **Valsalva manoeuvre** [8].
- Auscultation of the lungs reveal **clear air entry** [9], with no dullness to percussion.
- She does not have any peripheral stigmata of **infective endocarditis** [10] such as Janeway lesions, Osler nodes or splinter haemorrhages.
- There was **no peripheral oedema** [11].

[1] As always, the initial assessment of patient is the observation. Here she looks well, which largely rules out an acute pathology. No increased work of breathing shows that there is no respiratory compromise at rest.

[2] The patient presents with dyspnoea, which should indicate to the doctor to look for peripheral signs of respiratory disease as well as cardiovascular disease. Clubbing would indicate interstitial lung disease, and nicotine stains would indicate chronic obstructive pulmonary disease.

[3] Characterising the pulse helps in differentiating between aortic stenosis and regurgitation. This is best done at the carotid or brachial artery. The radial pulse is weak and not the best for characterisation. If the stenosis is severe, there may be a slow upstroke (anacrotic pulse), or the peak of the pulse may be late (*tardus*) or have decreased amplitude (*parvus*). If the pulse has a delayed peak and a small volume it is called *pulsus parvus et tardus*.

[4] The apex beat is displaced inferolaterally from its original position at the 5th intercostal space, mid-axillary line due to left ventricular hypertrophy. The apex beat can be characterised as pressure loaded if it is sustained or forceful. This occurs in concentric hypertrophy. In eccentric hypertrophy you may have a volume loaded apex beat which is diffuse and non-sustained.

[5] The classical description of the murmur of aortic stenosis is a crescendo–decrescendo mid-systolic ejection murmur best heard at the right upper sternal border (aortic region) that radiates to the carotids. It is a mid-systolic murmur as the left ventricular pressure only exceeds the systemic pressure and the pressure gradient of the aortic valve during mid-systole. A2 may also be softened or absent due to an immobile aortic valve. As the severity of the aortic stenosis worsens, the murmur also changes. A2 becomes delayed, which may merge with P2, resulting in a single S2. If A2

becomes even more delayed you may have paradoxical splitting, where the aortic valve closes later than the pulmonic valve. Additionally, for patients with a congenital bicuspid valve, there may be an ejection systolic click early after S1; and for patients who have developed a stiff and non-compliant left ventricle, an S4 may be heard.

[6] Radiation of the murmur to the carotids excludes pulmonic stenosis, aortic sclerosis and hypertrophic obstructive cardiomyopathy as the cause of the ejection systolic murmur.

[7] Dynamic manoeuvres are performed to confirm your suspicion of aortic stenosis compared to other valvular pathologies. First step is to differentiate between left-sided murmurs and right-sided murmurs by listening to the murmur in both expiration and inspiration. Expiration promotes venous return from the pulmonary veins into the left side of the heart, thereby increasing left ventricular end diastolic volume. This corresponds to more stroke volume (as per Frank Starling's Law), which in turn results in an increased turbulent flow across the mitral and aortic valves. Conversely, inspiration decreases the intrathoracic pressure, which increases venous return to the right side of the heart. This then increases the right ventricular end diastolic volume, the right ventricular stroke volume and the turbulent flow across the tricuspid and pulmonary valves. Once the murmur has been localised to a left-sided lesion best heard in the aortic region, you can accentuate the murmur by having the patient lean forward. This brings the aortic valve closer to the chest wall so that it is heard more easily. Then you can differentiate between aortic stenosis and hypertrophic obstructive cardiomyopathy (HOCM) with further manoeuvres. The murmur of aortic stenosis will increase with manoeuvres that increase preload, such as squatting and passive leg raising. These same manoeuvres decrease the murmur of HOCM, as increased preload improves the left ventricular outflow

tract (LVOT) obstruction. Manoeuvres that will increase the murmur of HOCM are the Valsalva manoeuvre and isometric handgrip, as it increases the afterload and worsens the LVOT obstruction.

8 Valsalva is a forced expiration against a closed glottis. This increases the intrathoracic pressure, which dramatically reduces the venous return to the left side of the heart. The decreased left ventricular end diastolic volume results in worsened LVOT obstruction in HOCM and thus the murmur is worse. This is pathognomonic of HOCM.

9 Clear air entry leans against interstitial lung disease, where you would expect to hear fine inspiratory bibasal crepitations, and chronic obstructive airways disease where

you have a prolonged expiratory phase and expiratory wheeze.

10 Infective endocarditis is a common differential when patients present with valvular abnormalities. Bear in mind, it is more common to cause aortic regurgitation than stenosis. Peripheral stigmata of infective endocarditis include splinter haemorrhages, Osler nodes (erythematous tender nodules on fingers or toes), Janeway lesions (non-tender erythematous maculopapular lesions in palms of hands or soles of feet) or Roth spots (retinal haemorrhages with clear centres).

11 The lack of peripheral oedema demonstrates that there is no biventricular failure from the aortic stenosis.

Investigations

- Her 12-lead ECG shows sinus rhythm with a heart rate of 74 beats per minute (bpm), marked **left axis deviation** [1] and **severe left ventricular hypertrophy** [2] with the sum of the S wave in V1 and R wave in V6 being 40mm.
- There is also a mildly **prolonged QRS complex** [3] with a duration of 0.1 seconds and **T-wave inversion and concave 2mm (0.2mV) ST segment depression in the lateral leads** [4].
- Chest X-ray demonstrates a **normal cardiac silhouette** [5] but **post-stenotic dilatation of the aorta** [6].

- Basic serology is **unremarkable** [7].
- Transthoracic echocardiogram was performed as an outpatient and showed **severe aortic stenosis** [8] with a mean pressure gradient of 60mmHg and an aortic valve area of $0.7cm^2$.
- There was also **moderate left ventricular concentric hypertrophy** [9].
- The left ventricular ejection fraction (LVEF) was 45%. She also underwent **cardiac angiography** [10] to rule out concomitant coronary artery disease.

1 The mean electrical axis of the heart has shifted to the left, indicating left-sided predominance of myocardium; this may indicate a degree of left ventricular hypertrophy.

2 Left ventricular hypertrophy is the most common ECG finding in aortic stenosis. The heart has adapted to the pathological stress placed upon it from aortic stenosis. The fact that the heart has had time to remodel shows that this process has been occurring for a long time. Concentric left ventricular remodelling occurs from sarcomeres being laid down in parallel, which aids the left ventricle in ejecting against a higher pressure load. This also increases myocardial oxygen demand and makes the heart more susceptible to ischaemia.

3 Aortic stenosis can affect the conductive system of the heart. When extensive, the calcification of the aortic valve can also extend into the conduction system into the atrioventricular node, causing AV nodal block or even intraventricular block. Here, the patient has slightly delayed intraventricular conduction, as described by the mildly prolonged QRS.

4 These ECG findings indicate an LV strain pattern that is common in hypertensive heart disease or aortic stenosis. Classically the lateral leads have T wave inversion and concaved ST segment depression. This is differentiated from an ischaemic change as there is usually horizontal ST segment depression or elevation in NSTEMIs or STEMIs.

5 Despite the concentric hypertrophy, you can have a normal cardiac silhouette on chest X-ray. There may be rounding of the LV border and apex if there is severe concentric hypertrophy.

6 Post-stenotic dilatation of aorta is the most common X-ray finding in aortic stenosis. In a lateral view, you may see aortic valve calcification, but it is not always present.

7 Serology is commonly unremarkable in aortic stenosis.

8 Transthoracic echocardiogram is the investigation of choice in diagnosis of aortic stenosis. It provides information about the leaflet morphology and can also grade the severity of the stenosis. It can also assess for the sequelae of aortic stenosis such as degree of hypertrophy, any concomitant functional mitral regurgitation and increased pulmonary artery pressures. Leaflet morphology helps distinguish the cause of aortic stenosis. If there are two leaflets, then congenital bicuspid aortic stenosis is diagnosed. Bicuspid valves are unequal in size and progressively thicken and calcify, usually necessitating replacement earlier on in life. Patients become symptomatic in middle age. Aortic stenosis is graded with three parameters: jet velocity, pressure gradient and valve area. For reference, the normal aortic valve area is 2–4cm².

 i Mild aortic stenosis has a jet velocity of <3 metres/second, a pressure gradient of <25mmHg and an aortic valve area of >1.5cm²
 ii Moderate aortic stenosis has a jet velocity of 3–4 metres/second, a pressure gradient of 25–40mmHg and an aortic valve area of 1–1.5cm²
 iii Severe aortic stenosis has a jet velocity of >4 metres/second, a pressure gradient of >40mmHg and an aortic valve area of <1cm².

9 ECG findings of left ventricular hypertrophy may not all correlate to echocardiographic findings of hypertrophy. In this case there is a slight discrepancy between the ECG and echocardiographic severity of left ventricular hypertrophy.

10 Cardiac angiography serves multiple purposes. It serves to determine the peri-operative risk for an aortic valve replacement and if severe coronary lesions are present, it can determine if any bypass grafting needs to be done at the time of the aortic valve replacement. Furthermore, in the case where the patient presents with angina, it can delineate whether or not the angina is from myocardial oxygen demand or from coronary disease. Finally, it can accurately measure the degree of stenosis in patients who have discrepant clinical and echocardiographic findings.

Management

Acute

It is uncommon for patients with aortic stenosis to have **emergency presentations** [1] and they can usually be managed on an outpatient basis. Those with acute symptoms can present with angina pectoris, cardiogenic syncope or acute pulmonary oedema. The specific management of these patients is outlined in *Cases 9, 6* and *4*, respectively. This patient presented with progressive dyspnoea without signs of decompensation and thus she would be suitable for an urgent referral to a cardiothoracic clinic for consideration of surgical aortic valve repair.

Monitoring

Patients who do not meet **criteria for surgery** [2] require **regular surveillance** [3] with serial echocardiograms. The aortic valve area on average decreases by around 0.1cm² per year, which increases the pressure gradient to around 7mmHg per year. Therefore even if patients do not require an aortic valve replacement, they will require intervention later.

Medical treatment

Medical treatment in patients with aortic stenosis is limited, as no medications are known to have prognostic benefit or delay disease progression. Medical treatment, when indicated, is for symptom management:

1. For angina, **beta blockers** [4] can be used.
2. For heart failure, **loop diuretics** [5] are used.
3. **Digoxin** [6] could also be used for patients in heart failure.

Intervention

The choice of intervention depends on the age, level of function and the patient's comorbidities. For children, very young adults with congenital aortic stenosis or those who are unfit for surgical replacement, balloon valvuloplasty can be considered. For others who are elderly (>75 years old) with inoperable aortic stenosis, transcatheter aortic valve replacement can be an option. Otherwise, surgical aortic valve replacement is the surgery of choice.

Surgical aortic valve replacement

Surgical replacement would be the recommended treatment [7] for this patient, as she presented with symptomatic aortic stenosis and is fit enough to undergo the surgery. It is the only definitive treatment for severe aortic stenosis. Aortic valve replacement requires median sternotomy and all of its associated **morbidities** [8]. **Bioprosthetic valves do not last as long as mechanical valves** [9], but also do not carry with them the systemic thromboembolic risk that mechanical valves do. Patients require **follow-up** [10] on discharge to assess for late complications and valve function.

Transcatheter aortic valve replacement (TAVR)

This is a relatively new non-surgical intervention where a bioprosthetic valve is implanted within the native aortic valve. This is done mostly via **femoral arterial access**[11], but in patients with difficult anatomy, a direct transaortic or transapical approach may be required. It improves effective aortic valve orifice area and haemodynamics; and has better survival rates than medical management. The **evidence for this procedure is emerging**[12], but it is a good alternative for patients who are deemed too high risk for surgical aortic valve replacement.

Percutaneous balloon aortic valvuloplasty

This is a **non-surgical, palliative treatment**[13] option for patients with aortic stenosis. It has a percutaneous approach, where a catheter with a balloon is threaded through the aortic valve and inflated, opening the stenotic valve. It does not alter prognosis and there is a **high rate of restenosis**[14].

1 Aortic stenosis is usually picked up incidentally via auscultation. When it isn't, it can present with either of the triad of symptoms. Thankfully, most patients have not acutely decompensated and can be referred to the cardiothoracic surgeon and cardiologist in a timely matter.

2 Indications for surgery include symptomatic patients with severe aortic stenosis. For those who are asymptomatic, surgery is indicated if their LVEF is <50%, they have severe hypertrophy (>15mm wall thickness) or have significant ventricular arrhythmias. Patients should be under the age of 75 and be fit to undergo major cardiovascular surgery.

3 Regular surveillance is most commonly for patients who are asymptomatic with mild to moderate aortic stenosis. These patients are re-evaluated every 6 months as their aortic stenosis will continue to progress and patients may develop symptoms, worsening exercise tolerance or LV systolic dysfunction.

4 Beta blockers slow the heart and decrease the overall oxygen use. They are only used if angina is the predominant symptom.

5 Loop diuretics decrease the preload to prevent exacerbation of heart failure that develops in aortic stenosis. This needs to be balanced with the risk of hypovolaemia, as patients can tip into hypotension and develop syncope.

6 Digoxin can help with dyspnoea in patients with heart failure.

7 Surgical replacement is the only definitive therapy and it is recommended for all patients with severe aortic stenosis who can safely undergo surgery. Timing is important to maximise the benefit and minimise the risk for the patient. Patients who may not be deemed suitable for surgery include the elderly (>75 years), those who are frail (poor functional status) and medically comorbid.

8 Aortic valve replacement requires median sternotomy, cardiopulmonary bypass, aortic cannulation and a post-operative ICU stay. This is safe for many patients, but patients need to be well selected for the procedure and complications should be prevented vigilantly to ensure an uncomplicated postoperative course.

9 Choice of valve depends on the expected lifespan for the patient. Bioprosthetic valves are not as durable but have less systemic thromboembolic risk and do not need lifelong anticoagulation (they do, however, need 3–6 months of anticoagulation postoperatively). Mechanical valves are much more durable, but patients need to remain on warfarin with an international normalised ratio (INR) of 2.5–3.5 due to high risk of systemic thromboembolic events.

10 Patients should be routinely followed up post-surgery to ensure adequate valvular function and to assess for complications such as prosthetic valve thrombosis, conduction disorders and paravalvular leaks.

11 Femoral arterial access is needed so that a catheter can be placed up into the aorta and through the aortic valve to ensure appropriate implantation of the aortic valve. Specific complications associated with femoral arterial access are noted in *Case 8*.

12 Current evidence demonstrates that it improves the prognosis for patients who traditionally have no treatment options for their inoperable severe aortic stenosis. In high risk patients, survival rates are similar with transcatheter aortic valve replacements (TAVRs) and surgical aortic valve replacements. There are some important differences in periprocedural risks. TAVR patients were demonstrated to have more major vascular complications and strokes. Patients undergoing surgical aortic valve replacement were demonstrated to have more major bleeding complications and new-onset atrial fibrillation.

13 Balloon valvuloplasty does not change the disease process and therefore does not change the disease progression. It is used only to improve the symptoms of aortic stenosis or as a bridging therapy to transcatheter aortic valve replacement or surgical aortic valve replacement.

14 Restenosis of aortic valve and clinical deterioration usually occur within 6–12 months and long-term outcomes mimic those of untreated aortic stenosis. It is worth noting that quality of life was noted to have improved in patients with balloon valvuloplasty vs. no treatment at short term (30 days and 6 months) but not at 12 months.

CASE 3: Atrial fibrillation

History

- A **61-year-old man** [1] presents to the Emergency Department (ED) because of palpitations.
- The **palpitations began 2 hours ago** [2] while watching television.
- He describes the **palpitations as uncomfortable and fast** [3].
- He says he may have had **similar episodes in the past** [4] but they never lasted this long.
- He has **no chest pain** [5] or **dyspnoea** [6] at the time of presentation.
- He has an **exercise tolerance in excess of 3km** [7].
- He reports **no orthopnoea or paroxysmal nocturnal dyspnoea** [8].
- He has otherwise **been well over the past few days and reports no infective symptoms** [9].
- He has a background of **alcohol abuse** [10] and can drink up to 14 units of alcohol per night.
- He also has a history of **type 2 diabetes mellitus** [11], **hypertension** [12], **asthma** [13] and **obesity** [14].

[1] The incidence of atrial fibrillation (AF) increases with age. A patient in their 30s presenting with palpitations is far more likely to have some other type of supraventricular tachycardia. The risk of AF also increases with the presence of other medical comorbidities such as diabetes, heart failure, coronary artery disease, hypertension, chronic kidney disease, etc.

[2] This patient has a clear onset of symptoms that is likely to coincide with the commencement of a possible arrhythmia. AF is usually asymptomatic and can present with a wide spectrum of symptoms; these may be cardiac.

[3] Palpitations are a common complaint in symptomatic AF. The fact that the patient describes them as fast raises the concern that the patient is also tachycardic, likely with rapid ventricular rate.

[4] Intermittent episodes of palpitations in the past are consistent with arrhythmias. In the case of AF, it is likely to be paroxysmal rather than permanent. It may be helpful to get the patient to tap out the palpitations to establish whether the rhythm is irregular, regular, fast or slow. If the patient reports the ability to self-terminate the palpitations, then this would be suggest of supraventricular tachycardia such as atrioventricular nodal tachycardia.

[5] Coronary artery disease is not very commonly associated with AF. AF can occur transiently in 6–21% patients presenting an acute myocardial infarction and hence the presence of chest pain must be explored. It is postulated that atrial ischaemia due to the myocardial infarction leads to AF.

[6] AF and heart failure commonly occur together. Often an acute exacerbation of heart failure can precipitate AF. Each of them can predispose to each other and must be screened

for in the history. Heart failure can lead to atrial stretching that predisposes to AF (which is often quite difficult to treat in the setting of underlying structural changes). AF causes a reduction in cardiac output, which may result in hypotension and acute heart failure.

[7] The patient has reasonable exercise tolerance, suggesting that overall cardiac function is not greatly impaired. It is important to get an understanding of current exercise tolerance in all patients presenting with cardiac symptoms. Exercise tolerance is also a significant prognostic factor.

[8] These are signs of pulmonary congestion and left-sided cardiac failure, which is common in patients presenting with palpitations.

[9] Infection is known to cause acute presentations of heart failure or any arrhythmia such as AF. The risk of AF increases after infection with the influenza virus and pneumonia, hence it is important to screen for infection in patients presenting with palpitations and suspected AF.

[10] Alcohol consumption is a significant risk factor for developing AF. AF occurs in around 60% of heavy drinkers with or without an underlying alcoholic cardiomyopathy. Often, episodes of AF occur post periods of increased alcohol intake such as weekends or holidays.

[11] Hypoglycaemia in the setting of diabetes can also predispose patients to palpitations. It is important to take a detailed medication history and check blood glucose levels (BGLs). Diabetes is also associated with the development of AF; it is postulated that increased left ventricular mass and arterial stiffness may be mechanisms for the development of AF in diabetic patients.

12 Hypertension is also associated with an increased risk of AF. If hypertension is aggressively treated, patients might be tachycardic and have palpitations (which can mimic atrial fibrillation) to compensate for hypotension.

13 Chronic airways disease can predispose patients to developing pulmonary hypertension which may lead to remodelling of the heart. This remodelling can be linked to the presence of arrhythmias.

14 Obesity is also linked with complications such as obstructive sleep apnoea and right-sided heart failure. Once again the remodelling of the heart can lead to disruption of conduction pathways and arrhythmias. Furthermore, obesity is linked with an increased size of the left atrium, increased left atrial pressure and diastolic dysfunction, which increases the risk of developing AF.

Examination

- On examination the patient appears **mildly uncomfortable but is otherwise alert** [1].
- He smells **strongly of alcohol** [2].
- There is no evidence of **diaphoresis and he appears well perfused** [3].
- His blood pressure is currently **120/75mmHg** [4]; his heart rate is **155bpm and is irregularly irregular** [5].
- He is not **febrile or hypoxic, and has normal respiratory rate** [6].

- His **jugular venous pressure is not elevated** [7] but on close inspection **A waves are absent** [8].
- There is an appreciable **apical–radial pulse deficit** [9].
- **Heart sounds are dual** [10] with **no added sounds** [11].
- **Breath sounds are normal** [12] with no added sounds.
- There is **no hemiplegia, weakness, speech disturbances** [13], **nystagmus or vertigo** [14].

1 The patient is likely distressed by the palpitations but appears to be otherwise well. In patients presenting with more acutely life-threatening arrhythmias such as ventricular tachycardia, cardiac output is commonly compromised leading to haemodynamic instability.

2 Alcohol is strongly associated with AF. This suggests a significant history of alcohol abuse and poor self-care. The patient must be assessed for signs and symptoms of alcoholic cardiomyopathy.

3 Diaphoresis may be a sign of acute haemodynamic instability in the setting of underlying myocardial ischaemia or life-threatening arrhythmia. Assessment of haemodynamic stability is paramount regardless of the underlying arrhythmia, as it will guide management.

4 Most of the medications used in AF will also cause hypotension and hence it is very important to monitor this. AF reduces cardiac output due to impaired diastolic filling, leading to a reduction in stroke volume. This leads to some degree of hypotension in the patient. Nonetheless, this patient appears haemodynamically stable and normotensive at this stage.

5 This is highly suggestive of AF with rapid ventricular rate. It is due to rapid and irregular beating of the atria, typically coming from ectopic foci outside of the sinus node. These impulses are conducted irregularly, leading to this rhythm.

6 The patient is not in any respiratory distress. Patients presenting with heart failure or a lower respiratory tract infection may trigger AF in a patient with an underlying predisposition for AF. There does not seem to be any respiratory decompensation in this patient.

7 Elevated JVP is a sign for right heart failure or tricuspid regurgitation; both can be mechanisms that predispose to arrhythmias such as AF. Fluid status is very important in the assessment of a patient presenting with AF with rapid ventricular rate. If the patient is also in acute heart failure then the treatment will need to be tailored accordingly and beta blockers should be avoided.

8 Since atrial contraction is lost in AF, A waves in the JVP are no longer visualised. This is a very difficult sign to appreciate but is nearly always pathognomonic with AF.

9 The apex beat can be difficult to palpate, especially in obese patients. An apical radial pulse deficit is seen in AF where the radial heart rate is less than the apical heart rate. Since the heart rate is irregular, some contraction will occur with insufficient filling of the left ventricle and results in beats with insufficient stroke volume to transmit the pressure wave to the arm.

10 The presence of an S3 heart sound may be a sign of systolic heart failure in the setting of an overly compliant myocardium (because S3 is produced when a large amount of blood strikes a 'stretchable' left ventricle), whereas an S4 heart sound can be a sign of diastolic heart failure or active ischaemia. The absence of both is reassuring.

11 Valvular heart disease, particularly mitral regurgitation, can lead to myocardial remodelling, left atrial enlargement and hence AF. It is especially important to exclude a mitral stenosis murmur (mid-diastolic rumble at the apex with presystolic accentuation). AF with moderate to severe mitral stenosis is considered valvular AF and is very high risk for thromboembolic complications, particularly stroke.

12 The patient has no signs of acute pulmonary congestion which might be a sign of acute heart failure. Auscultation of the chest forms a significant part of the patient's volume assessment. This patient appears to be relatively euvolaemic. There are also no apparent unilateral crepitations or wheeze that may be concerning for infection.

13 Often patients presenting with signs of acute ischaemic stroke may be found to be in AF. Weakness, speech disturbances and hemiplegia are some of the many features of anterior circulation stroke.

14 Nystagmus and vertigo are signs of a posterior circulation stroke. In an embolic stroke secondary to AF, patients can have multi-territory deficits. AF is a major risk factor for future ischaemic strokes and hence clinicians must make sure to exclude stroke in these patients.

Investigations

- A 12-lead ECG reveals **an irregularly irregular rhythm with an absence of P waves** [1].
- It is a **narrow complex tachycardia** [2] with a rate of around **150bpm** [3]. Bloods are performed which reveal a **potassium of 3.5mmol/L** [4] but normal full **blood examination, renal function** [5] and **thyroid function** [6].
- The chest X-ray shows **normal cardiac silhouette** [7] and **nil overt signs of fluid overload** [8].

- A bedside echocardiogram reveals a **left ventricular ejection fraction of 55% with mild hypertrophic changes** [9] and **normal valvular function** [10].
- There is **bilateral mild–moderate atrial enlargement** [11].
- **No thrombus is seen in the left atrium** [12] on transthoracic echocardiogram (TTE).

1 This is in keeping with AF on ECG and represents irregular beating of the atria. Sometimes fibrillation waves can also be seen along the baseline of the ECG, which is further suggestive of AF. Be mindful, however, that fibrillatory waves may mimic P waves and lead to misdiagnosis. Other features of AF include an absence of an isoelectric baseline.

2 Typically, the ECG in AF will be narrow complex unless there is an underlying bundle branch block, accessory pathway or rate-related aberrant conduction.

3 This is suggestive of AF with rapid ventricular rate; the irregular atrial beats from ectopic foci are being conducted and leading to frequent ventricular contraction. This is leading to regular contractions without sufficient filling time and reduced cardiac output.

4 Hypokalaemia increases the risk of AF compared to normokalaemia. Any patients with low potassium should be treated with IV or oral treatment to replete serum potassium.

5 Renal function and full blood exam should be done with all patients. Renal failure and infection can be identified on these investigations. Furthermore, these bloods provide a baseline for the patient at admission.

6 Clinical or subclinical hyperthyroidism is present in less than 5% of patients with AF. Thyroid function tests should be obtained in all patients with first episode AF or those with frequent exacerbation, as this might be an exacerbating cause.

7 Cardiomegaly is a sign of heart failure or cardiomyopathy which may be seen in AF. Flattening of the left atrial border can also be seen on chest X-ray in patients with severe left atrial dilatation.

8 The absence of pulmonary congestion and pleural effusions on chest X-ray further confirms the euvolaemic status of this patient. If this patient were overloaded and given beta blockers acutely, it could send them into acute cardiogenic shock.

9 This patient has normal left ventricular ejection fraction, hence systolic function is maintained. In patients with reduced ejection fraction, cardioselective beta blockers would be indicated. Systolic dysfunction on echocardiogram independently predicts an increased risk of stroke in patients with AF. The presence of underlying conditions such as left ventricular hypertrophy and focal wall motion abnormalities may also be found through this. An echocardiogram can also be used when the patient is in sinus rhythm to evaluate the relative atrial contribution to left ventricular filling.

10 This is significant as occult mitral stenosis may present with AF. The absence of mitral valve pathology influences the risk of thrombus formation. Long-term sinus rhythm is often very difficult in patients with mitral stenosis unless they have procedural repair.

11 Normal left atrial dimension is less than 4cm and enlargement is common in AF. Hypertension and mitral valve disease are common causes for left atrial dilatation. Left atrial enlargement is prognostically important and decreases the probability of long-term maintenance of sinus rhythm.

12 While TTE can be used to identify left atrial thrombus, it has poor sensitivity. It is unable to sufficiently visualise the left atrial appendage, a common side for thrombi. Ideally, a transoesophageal echocardiogram should be used if thrombus needs to be excluded with greater accuracy.

Management

Acute

In patients with new onset AF with a rapid ventricular rate, an assessment needs to be made regarding the **need for urgent cardioversion** [1]. If the patient does not require cardioversion, **rate control is recommended** [2] to improve symptoms and reduce the risk of **tachycardia-mediated cardiomyopathy** [3]. Patients with heart failure with reduced ejection fraction **can be difficult to rate control** [4].

Given that this patient has had symptoms for <48 hours, they **should be considered for cardioversion** [5] to revert back to sinus rhythm. These patients **do not require maintenance antiarrhythmics** [6]. **In patients in AF for > 48 hours** [7], cardioversion cannot be done acutely without a transoesophageal echocardiogram to exclude atrial thrombi.

Anticoagulation

All patients with **non-valvular atrial fibrillation** [8] should be assessed for stroke risk using the **CHA_2DS_2-VASc risk tool** [9]. **Bleeding risk** [10] should also be assessed in these patients. Patients with **valvular AF** [11] should be anticoagulated with warfarin regardless of their other comorbidities.

Long-term

Long-term management revolves around **managing the underlying aetiology** [12]. Furthermore, adequate **long-term rate and rhythm control** [13] needs to evaluated. If AF is recurrent, **catheter ablation can be explored** [14] to ensure better long-term maintenance of sinus rhythm. In patients with heart failure with reduced ejection fraction, **AF ablation is associated with a significant benefit** [15].

1 Urgent cardioversion is indicated in patients presenting with acute ischaemia, significant hypotension such that they won't tolerate pharmacological treatment, severe heart failure or the presence of a pre-excitation syndrome leading to rapid conduction, classically through an accessory pathway. Urgent cardioversion can only be considered when the onset of atrial fibrillation appears to clearly be within the last 48 hours.

2 First-line rate control agents include beta blockers or centrally acting calcium channel blockers. A goal acutely of ≤100bpm is sufficient for a patient who is otherwise asymptomatic and has normal systolic function. Digoxin is typically avoided in patients for rate control.

3 Chronic tachycardia leads to significant structural changes in the heart such as ventricular dilatation. Often the tachycardia cardiomyopathy predisposes to further arrhythmias of the heart.

4 Patients with acutely decompensated heart failure and reduced ejection fraction should be treated with IV amiodarone or digoxin to acutely control heart rate. Beta blocker therapy should only be commenced or increased once the patient has been stabilised from the heart failure perspective. It is rare to need cardioversion for acute heart failure unless they are becoming haemodynamically unstable. The mainstay for treatment is managing fluid overload with diuretics and vasodilators. Initial attempts of rate reduction should be to achieve a rate <120bpm in this setting.

5 The decision to offer patients cardioversion if they are otherwise haemodynamically stable is dependent on multiple factors. Cardioversion in very elderly patients or patients with large left atrial dimensions above 5cm are normally excluded; if needed, cardioversion is carefully considered on a case-by-case basis. Patients with a reversible underlying disorder such as thyroid disease, pericarditis and postoperative AF should be offered cardioversion. These patients should ideally be young (<65 years) and have normal left ventricular systolic function. The absence of hypertension is also preferred. Patients with acute heart failure presenting with new onset AF can be offered cardioversion as it will improve the cardiac output. Finally, patients who have only developed atrial fibrillation recently and where it appears to be early in its natural history should ideally be offered cardioversion.

6 Patients with first presentation AF who have been cardioverted do not require antiarrhythmics such as amiodarone, flecainide or sotalol, in the first instance at least.

7 For patients with AF >48 hours in duration, 4 weeks of anticoagulation prior to cardioversion and another 4 weeks post cardioversion is required. This is to prevent any atrial thrombi causing acute stroke from embolisation. Transoesophageal echocardiography can be used to screen patients for the presence of thrombus if cardioversion is required before 4 weeks. Long-term anticoagulation following the completion of 4 weeks post cardioversion is dependent on the patient's thromboembolic risk profile.

8 Please note that CHA_2DS_2-VASc is only valid in patients with non-valvular AF.

9 The CHA_2DS_2-VASc risk tool stands for the following:
C – congestive heart failure (1 point)
H – hypertension (1 point)
A_2 – age ≥75 (2 points)
D – diabetes (1 point)
S_2 – history of stroke, TIA or thromboembolism (2 points)
V – vascular disease: history of MI, peripheral arterial disease, aortic atherosclerosis (1 point)
A – age between 65 and 74 (1 point)
Sc – sex category; i.e. female sex (1 point).

A patient with non-valvular AF and a score of ≥2 should be anticoagulated from a stroke prevention perspective. A CHA_2DS_2-VASc score of 2 represents an approximate 2% annual risk of stroke, and a score of 6 represents a 10% stroke risk. Patients with a score of 1 are borderline and should be anticoagulated on clinical judgement. The current recommendation is for the use of direct oral anticoagulants (DOACs) for AF anticoagulation, rather than warfarin. However, patients already on warfarin and maintaining a therapeutic INR can be kept on warfarin. Furthermore, patients who have mechanical heart valves should only be anticoagulated with warfarin. Patients with severe chronic kidney disease should be treated with warfarin; however, there is growing evidence of DOACs in this patient subgroup.

10 Bleeding risk should also be assessed in all these patients and if the bleeding risk outweighs the stroke risk, anticoagulation should not be commenced. The HAS-BLED score can be used to evaluate the bleeding risk but unfortunately, this remains somewhat imprecise in estimating individual bleeding risk.
The HAS-BLED score stands for the following:
H – hypertension (1 point)
A – abnormal renal and liver function (1 point each)
S – stroke (1 point)
B – bleeding (1 point)
L – labile INRs (1 point)
E – elderly (1 point)
D – drugs or alcohol (1 point each).

A score of 2 equates to a risk of 1.88 bleeds per 100 patient years and a score of 4 equates to 8.7 bleeds per 100 patient years.
In patients who are at a very high bleeding risk or have a contraindication to anticoagulation, left atrial appendage occlusion devices can be considered. The mesh device epithelialises over the atrial appendage and prevents it from acting as a source of thrombus for strokes. The risks associated with this procedure include iatrogenic stroke and cardiac tamponade.

11 Patients with valvular AF, which is defined as them having underlying moderate or severe mitral stenosis, have a far higher stroke risk profile and require warfarin with an INR target of at least 2.5.

12 Patients need to be optimised from a risk factor perspective long-term for hypertension, diabetes, coronary artery disease, heart failure, etc. to prevent further remodelling of the heart that may lead to the AF becoming permanent. In patients with AF, the presence of heart failure, intraventricular conduction delay on ECG and previous myocardial infarction are the greatest indicators for mortality.

13 Follow-up post acute AF is required to ensure adequate control of the heart rate and/or rhythm. The rate control agents may be titrated up if required. Typically patients post first episode of AF that has been cardioverted will not be on any pharmacological therapy. Another important factor that needs to be followed up is the compliance with anticoagulant therapy in patients and also the continual need for anticoagulation. If there are concerns regarding compliance, then clotting factor 10a levels can be tested for compliance with apixaban and rivaroxaban. Blood dabigatran levels can also be measured if required.

14 Catheter ablation of atrial fibrillation has been shown to be an effective method of maintaining sinus rhythm and reducing symptoms. However, the mortality and stroke data in patients who have had ablation are not convincing at this stage. Thus, the primary benefit for catheter ablation of patients remains for symptomatic control at this point. In patients with no significant structural heart disease but drug-resistant atrial fibrillation, sinus rhythm is maintained effectively with catheter ablation. AF ablation is not without risks, and these include cardiac tamponade, stroke, vascular trauma and nerve damage.

15 Patients with symptomatic AF who have heart failure with reduced ejection fraction have higher rates of mortality and morbidity. If these patients have failed attempts with anti-arrhythmic drugs, they should be considered for AF ablation as this has been shown to reduce mortality.

CASE 4: Heart failure with reduced ejection fraction

History

- A **74-year-old Caucasian male** [1] presents with **a 2-month history of progressive shortness of breath** [2].
- He reports **marked limitation of physical activity**; he is **unable to walk to the bathroom without stopping** [3]. He remains **symptom-free at rest** [4], however.
- He also **reports his legs becoming swollen** [5] over this period but puts this down to having spent more time sitting on the couch.
- He hasn't **noticed any palpitations** [6].
- He has also noticed **difficulty sleeping at night because of a dry cough** [7].

- The **patient reports using 3 pillows overnight** [8] over the past month.
- He doesn't report any **abdominal pain** [9], **chest pain** [10], **wheeze or fevers** [11]. However, he does report feeling **very tired** [12] over this period.
- He has a past history of **hypertension, type 2 diabetes mellitus** [13] and a previous acute myocardial infarction with **one stent** *in situ* [14].
- He reports **poor compliance** [15] with his medications.
- He is a **non-smoker** [16] and **drinks socially** [17].

1 The incidence of heart failure increases with age; around 6–10% of the population above 65 will have congestive heart failure. Heart failure is one of the leading causes of hospitalisations in patients >65 years. Older age is associated with increased likelihood of heart failure in a patient presenting with dyspnoea.

2 Progressive dyspnoea is a common presenting complaint for patients presenting with decompensated cardiac failure. Dyspnoea is a symptom with high sensitivity for heart failure but poor specificity. Dyspnoea is a symptom of central fluid accumulation in the lungs. This occurs due to a reduction in cardiac output that is most apparent on exertion.

3 The patient has a significant level of debilitation on physical activity. It is likely he has New York Heart Association (NYHA) Class III of Heart Failure. While symptoms alone can be used to classify the severity of congestive heart failure, the link between symptoms and the degree of left ventricle dysfunction is weak.

4 Being symptomatic at different levels of exertion would be concerning for severity of heart failure. It would be consistent with NYHA Class IV if the patient was symptomatic at rest.

5 This almost certainly represents peripheral oedema. Peripheral oedema is a sign of right-sided heart failure, and typically accumulates gradually. The presence of right heart failure may also contribute to the prognosis in patients with heart failure, with increasing severity linked with worse clinical outcomes.

6 Palpitations must be screened for as arrhythmias are a significant cause of heart failure. Additionally, the presence of atrial fibrillation in patients with heart failure is associated with poorer outcomes. Atrial fibrillation may worsen symptoms in patients with heart failure. The current consensus in heart failure patients with AF is that any reversible causes for AF should be identified and corrected if possible. Patients with significantly reduced ejection fraction with AF not responding to medical therapy should be considered for ablation.

7 This likely represents paroxysmal nocturnal dyspnoea (PND), a common feature of pulmonary congestion and left-sided cardiac failure. The patient typically has attacks of shortness of breath and coughing overnight.

8 This represents worsening orthopnoea which is another sign of pulmonary congestion. The inability to lie flat limits the ability of patients to sleep without extra pillows. In acutely decompensated heart failure with severe pulmonary oedema, patients may want to sit upright and sleep in the chair.

9 Abdominal pain may be present in patients with significant right heart failure. Right upper quadrant pain can be secondary to congestive hepatomegaly, ascites, reduced bowel perfusion and intestinal oedema.

10 The presence of chest pain may indicate significant coronary ischaemia that is causing the ischaemic heart disease. Symptoms of acute coronary syndrome need to be assessed, as acute cardiogenic shock may be the result of ischaemia.

11 It is important to exclude a primary pulmonary aetiology causing shortness of breath and cough. The presence of fever may suggest an acute pneumonia or infective process. Wheeze can indicate chronic obstructive pulmonary disease or asthma. The absence of both is reassuring that it is likely due to decompensated heart failure.

12 Fatigue is a common symptom in chronic heart failure. This is due to the patient being in a low output state for an extended period of time. However, it is essential to investigate for anaemia in all patients with heart failure, particularly if fatigue is reported. Several studies have demonstrated increased mortality in patients with anaemia and heart failure.

13 Hypertension and type 2 diabetes mellitus (T2DM) are risk factors for ischaemic heart disease, which is the most common cause of heart failure in the developed world. In addition to age and LVEF, the presence of diabetes is the most powerful independent predictor of mortality and heart failure hospitalisations.

14 This patient likely has ischaemic cardiomyopathy, with ischaemic heart disease being the underlying aetiology.

Ischaemic heart disease accounts for 40–70% of patients with heart failure in the developed world.

15 Post myocardial infarction (MI), poor compliance with medications, particularly beta blockers and angiotensin receptor enzyme inhibitors, can lead to LV remodelling and a higher incidence of heart failure. Patients with hypertension prior to MI are even more likely to have LV remodelling after MI, and have a greater incidence of hospitalisation from heart failure.

16 Smoking is a risk factor for vascular disease and particularly ischaemic heart disease. All patients who are current smokers need to be educated regarding smoking cessation. Healthy lifestyle is associated with lower incidence of both coronary artery disease and lifetime risk of heart failure.

17 Alcoholic cardiomyopathy is another cause that must be considered in patients. Especially if the underlying aetiology isn't apparent, a detailed social history with regard to alcohol and illicit substances must be completed. Illicit substances such as methamphetamines are also associated with cardiomyopathy.

Examination

- The patient is sitting **upright in the chair** [1] and appears to **be short of breath in between sentences** [2] with use of accessory muscles.
- The peripheries appear **slightly pale but not overly cool** [3].
- His blood pressure is **172/94mmHg** [4], pulse is **96bpm** [5] and **respiratory rate 22**.
- **Oxygen saturation is 91% on air** [6] by pulse oximetry and **temperature is 36.1°C** [7].
- A **prominent jugular vein is noted at 5cm** [8] above the sternal angle.
- **Pulsus alternans** [9] is not appreciated.
- **A displaced apical beat** [10] is noted on chest examination.
- On auscultation of the heart, there are **no murmurs** [11] but an **S3 gallop** [12] is heard.
- There is no **loud P2 or parasternal heave** [13].
- Examination of the lungs reveals **coarse crepitations bilaterally** [14] to the mid-zone and **dullness at the bases** [14].
- Abdominal examination is unremarkable; there is **no hepatomegaly** [15].
- **Pitting oedema to mid-shin** [16] is appreciated bilaterally.

1 Patients with acute pulmonary oedema will often be seated upright to help reduce dyspnoea. They are unable to tolerate a supine position as it leads to increased airway resistance, bronchial obstruction and expiratory flow limitation.

2 These are signs of respiratory distress with insufficient oxygen transfer occurring, which contributes to the symptoms. These are compensatory mechanisms by the body to help increase the oxygenation levels of blood.

3 Pale peripheries can be a sign of decreased perfusion and increased oxygen extraction. It can represent advanced heart failure if extremities are pale, cool and sometimes

cyanotic. Peripheral vasoconstriction may not be apparent in patients being treated with vasodilators.

4 Hypertension in this patient is a sign of poorly controlled risk factors. However, in advanced heart failure patients often become hypotensive due to poor cardiac output. It also means heart failure medications need to be commenced and up-titrated. The blood pressure needs to be reduced significantly for prognostic benefit.

5 Resting tachycardia is a feature of the severity of heart failure. This patient clearly is not optimised from a heart failure perspective and the heart rate should be far slower. In any patient who is tachycardic it is vital to exclude an underlying arrhythmia, as this can be contributing to/causing the cardiac failure.

6 The patient is hypoxic and mildly tachypnoeic, which suggests that there is likely an element of left heart failure leading to pulmonary congestion. This patient certainly requires hospitalisation to stabilise their respiratory status and optimise heart failure management.

7 The patient does not appear to have any features of active infection that might be leading to his acute hypoxia. It is also important to establish if he has had any fevers over the preceding days.

8 The JVP must be assessed with the patient sitting at 45° to get an estimate of the jugular venous pressure. Elevated JVP is generally present if peripheral oedema is due to heart failure. High intracapillary pressure is responsible for fluid movement into the interstitium. Be mindful that superior vena cava (SVC) obstruction, tricuspid stenosis, pulmonary hypertension, constrictive pericarditis and pericardial effusion will also raise the JVP.

9 Pulsus alternans is characterised by evenly spaced alternating strong and weak peripheral pulses. This phenomenon is strongly suggestive of severe left ventricular systolic failure and should be assessed in all patients presenting with new heart failure. The exact pathophysiology behind this is not clear, but it may be associated with contractility variations secondary to shifts in preload and afterload.

10 A displaced apex is usually indicative of left ventricular enlargement and it can sometimes be accompanied by a parasternal heave. This is another sign of left ventricular dysfunction.

11 Valvular heart disease is another common cause of heart failure and could be precipitating this presentation. Valvular disease accounts for roughly 10% of patients with heart failure.

12 An S3 gallop is associated with increased left ventricular end diastolic pressures and left atrial pressure exceeding 20mmHg. The presence of an S3 has low sensitivity but high specificity for the clinical diagnosis of heart failure.

13 Loud P2 and parasternal heave are signs of pulmonary hypertension. Patients may also develop a pulmonary regurgitation murmur secondary to pulmonary hypertension. Patients with chronic heart failure often develop pulmonary hypertension which can contribute to dyspnoea, as pulmonary pressures rise with exertion.

14 Coarse crepitations to the mid-zone are in keeping with the overall picture of congestive cardiac failure in this patient. There is clearly an element of systolic dysfunction that has led to accumulation of fluid in the lungs. Furthermore, dullness at the bases is suggestive of bilateral pleural effusions, likely secondary to cardiac failure. Both these findings are contributing to the symptoms of dyspnoea, orthopnoea and PND in this patient.

15 Hepatomegaly and abdominal pain are signs of severe right-sided cardiac failure. Patients may also develop ascites and abdominal oedema as a result of this. In patients with intestinal oedema, there may be altered intestinal absorption of oral loop diuretics and usually IV diuresis is indicated.

16 The finding of peripheral oedema is in keeping with the elevated JVP; it suggests an element of right heart failure. Due to higher pressures in the right heart, fluid has been shifting out from the intravascular space to the interstitium peripherally.

Investigations

- An **ECG is completed** [1] on arrival at the ED which shows **sinus rhythm** [2] with **left bundle branch block morphology** [3] (old) but otherwise **nil acute ischaemic changes** [4].
- An initial panel of blood is sent which reveals **normal FBE** [5], **liver function tests** [6] and **iron studies** [7].
- Serum electrolytes and creatinine reveals a **mildly raised creatinine of 106mmol/L** [8] and an eGFR of 64ml/min/1.73m².
- Chest X-ray reveals **cardiomegaly, pulmonary congestion and small bilateral pleural effusions** [9].
- An **inpatient transthoracic echocardiogram** [10] is completed which reveals a **reduced ejection fraction of 35% with left anterior descending artery territory hypokinesis** [11].
- Some **hypertrophic changes are observed** [12] but otherwise the **valvular function is normal** [13].

1 Most patients with heart failure with reduced ejection fraction have a significant abnormality on ECG. An ECG is also important for identifying evidence of acute myocardial infarction or ischaemia, as that may be the precipitant for decompensated heart failure.

2 Cardiac arrhythmias can precipitate or cause heart failure. The patient being in sinus rhythm, while reassuring, does not completely exclude arrhythmia; they could be having paroxysmal atrial fibrillation, for example.

3 Among patients with heart failure, a widened QRS such as the one seen on left bundle branch block (LBBB) is associated with increased mortality. The reason for this is partly due to a conduction defect causing ventricular desynchrony and worsening systolic function over time. A new LBBB with symptoms of chest pain is also considered a STEMI equivalent finding.

4 In the setting of an LBBB, it is difficult to appreciate traditional ischaemic changes on ECG. In LBBB the baseline ST segments and T waves tend to be shifted in a discordant direction and hence the Sgarbossa criteria need to be applied in this setting.

5 A full blood examination is sent to assess mainly for anaemia or infection as it may exacerbate pre-existing heart failure.

6 Liver function tests may be deranged in the setting of right heart failure and hepatic congestion. In the setting of derangement, it can provide a baseline value for ongoing monitoring.

7 Patients with heart failure should be investigated for iron deficiency, especially in the setting of anaemia. Iron depletion may contribute to patients' symptoms of fatigue in the setting of heart failure.

8 Baseline electrolytes and creatinine is necessary when commencing inpatient diuresis and/or renally excreted medications such as angiotensin-converting enzyme inhibitors (ACEi). Renal impairment may be caused by the heart failure exacerbation or might contribute to it. Hyponatremia generally indicates severe heart failure due to a state of hypervolaemia that the body is unable to compensate for.

9 The findings of this chest X-ray are likely secondary to heart failure. Chest X-rays are useful for differentiating heart failure from primary pulmonary disease. Other findings that might be suggestive of heart failure include Kerley B lines and upper lobe diversion. A cardiac to thoracic width ratio above 50% on a posterior–anterior projection is in keeping with cardiomegaly.

10 This patient did not have a brain natriuretic peptide (BNP) test done and proceeded straight to echocardiogram, as the suspicion for heart failure is very high. In this case, the patient needs an echocardiogram regardless so a BNP will not add much more. A BNP is typically suggested in patients where the diagnosis of heart failure is uncertain and a negative test will negate the need for an echocardiogram. The echocardiogram in this case is used to identify findings consistent with heart failure to help stratify it (systolic vs. diastolic dysfunction, valve dysfunction, etc).

11 The echocardiogram findings are consistent with heart failure with reduced ejection fraction (HFrEF). Given that there are hypokinetic segments in the left anterior descending artery territory and a known history of coronary artery disease, this patient most likely has ischaemic cardiomyopathy. Sometimes segmental abnormalities can also occur in dilated cardiomyopathy but there is no evidence of this on echocardiogram.

12 The presence of hypertrophic changes is likely secondary to long-standing poorly controlled hypertension. This will lead to diastolic dysfunction, hence this patient likely has features of both systolic and diastolic dysfunction.

13 Valvular disease should always be assessed on echocardiography when investigating for heart failure. Valvular disease can be the primary cause of heart failure. In particular, if there is a degree of mitral regurgitation that is important, as it may provide a falsely elevated left ventricular ejection fraction due to blood flowing errantly retrograde through the mitral valve. If aortic stenosis was present it could have also been attributed to the hypertrophic changes in the left ventricle.

Management

Short-term

The initial approach to patients presenting with acute dyspnoea from acute decompensated heart failure is as follows:

1. **Airway assessment and continuous pulse oximetry** [1]
2. **Supplemental O$_2$ and ventilatory support** [2]
3. **Vital signs assessment** [3] – especially blood pressure
4. **Continuous cardiac monitoring** [4] included a full 12-lead ECG
5. **Intravenous access** [5]
6. **Upright position** [6]
7. **Diuretic therapy** [7]
8. **Vasodilator therapy** [8]
9. **Strict fluid balance, daily weights and fluid restriction** [9]

Long-term

Management of HFrEF includes management of **contributing factors and associated conditions** [10], **lifestyle modification** [11], pharmacological therapy and device therapy if indicated.

Pharmacological therapy

The following agents should be considered initially in all patients with HFrEF:
- **Diuretics** [12]
- **ACEi** [13], **angiotensin receptor-neprilysin inhibitor (ARNI)** [14] or **angiotensin receptor blocker (ARB)** [15]
- **Beta blocker** [16]

Additional therapy that can be considered if suitable:
- **Mineralocorticoid receptor antagonist** [17]
- **Ivabradine** [18]

Device therapy

Patients with advanced heart failure with reduced ejection fraction may have evidence of abnormal ventricular conduction. These patients are at increased risk of mortality and may be candidates for **cardiac resynchronisation therapy with defibrillator** [19]. These patients are usually candidates for implantable cardioverter-defibrillators as well and this can be done at the same time.

1 Airway assessment forms a part of all resuscitative protocols. Airway assessment and continuous pulse oximetry will guide oxygenation and ventilation. Assess the patient's voice and breath sounds. Suction or airway manoeuvres may be required to optimise this.

2 Supplemental oxygen and assisted ventilation should be provided on an as-needed basis to treat hypoxaemia (SpO$_2$ <90%). Consideration of non-invasive ventilation and intubation should be made. Oxygen is not required in patients without hypoxaemia as it may cause vasocontraction and reduction in cardiac output.

3 Blood pressure is extremely important as it will dictate the amount of diuresis and vasodilator therapy the patient will tolerate. If the patient has severe decompensated heart failure, a high dependency unit bed should be considered as they will require regular observations and interventions.

4 A full 12-lead ECG should always be obtained in such patients. In the case of significant decompensation, cardiac monitoring should be initiated as the patient will undergo significant electrolyte and fluid shifts that could result in ECG changes. Furthermore, underlying conduction abnormalities that may be precipitating the presentation will be more easily identified.

5 Intravenous access should be obtained and blood sent off at the same time. IV access is important to deliver medications such as diuretics.

6 Upright positioning assists in reducing airway resistance and reduces the patient's work of breathing.

7 While diuretics provide no mortality benefit in patients with chronic heart failure, they are essential in effectively relieving congestive symptoms. They form the mainstay for successful treatment in acute decompensated heart failure. Typically loop diuretics such as furosemide or bumetanide are first line. In patients previously naive to diuretics with normal renal function, the initial dose of furosemide should be 20–40mg IV. If there is little or no response, the dose can be doubled at 2-hourly intervals up to the maximum dose. A continuous insulin infusion can also be considered.

8 Vasodilators are required to correct elevated filling pressures and/or LV afterload in patients with acute decompensated heart failure. Nitrates are commonly used as they cause predominantly venous vasodilation and reduce LV filling pressure. Nitroglycerin can be given as sublingual, topical or IV infusion. The benefit of intravenous nitrates is that they allow for closer titration according to clinical benefit and blood pressure. Nitroprusside or nesiritide are vasodilators that primarily decrease arterial tone and are recommended in patients who need urgent afterload reduction (usually in the setting of severe hypertension).

9 Strict fluid balance should include urine output monitoring (consider insertion of indwelling catheter). Fluid balance and daily weights help clinicians titrate the patient's heart failure therapy accordingly. A fluid restriction should be considered in all patients with refractory heart failure and should be used in most patients being actively treated for acute heart failure.

10 Treatment should address contributing factors such as hypertension, myocardial infarction, valvular heart disease, arrhythmias, diabetes mellitus, thyroid dysfunction and infection.

11 The following lifestyle modifications should be suggested to all patients presenting with HFrEF: cessation of smoking, restriction or abstinence from alcohol consumption, consumption of a low sodium diet (limit to 3g/day of sodium intake), fluid restriction to 1.5–2L per day initially, reduction of weight and daily weight monitoring to detect fluid accumulation.

12 Diuretics should be used to reduce fluid overload both in the acute and chronic settings. While there is no apparent mortality benefit to this treatment at present, it provides symptomatic relief. Loop diuretics (furosemide and bumetanide) can be used in all stages of congestive cardiac failure and are useful in primary pulmonary oedema and refractory heart failure.

13 ACEi improve survival in patients with left ventricular systolic dysfunction. They reduce preload and afterload, improve cardiac output and inhibit tissue renin–angiotensin systems, consequently improving symptoms and reducing mortality. Usually for patients presenting with acutely decompensated cardiac failure, ACEi are initiated before beta blockers, since ACEi provide rapid haemodynamic benefit and will not exacerbate heart failure during that initial phase.

14 ARNI is only for patients with established HFrEF (with ejection fraction ≤40%) who are tolerating target dose of ACEi or ARB. Patients must have an eGFR >30ml/min/1.73m^2, systolic blood pressure >100 and no history of angioedema prior to starting. For those already on ACEi, a 36-hour washout of ACEi is required before starting an ARNI. ARNIs have shown a greater mortality benefit over traditional ACEi/ARB treatment.

15 Patients who cannot tolerate ACEi or ARNI due to angioedema or other side-effects should be commenced on a single-agent ARB instead. Hyperkalaemia or renal insufficiency on ACEi is not a reason to commence ARB, however.

16 All patients with HFrEF with no or minimal evidence of fluid overload should be treated with cardioselective beta blockers such as carvediol, bisoprolol, nebivolol or metoprolol extended release. Beta blockers improve overall and event-free survival in patients with NYHA class II–III heart failure. Beta blockers can reduce the sympathetic tone and cardiac muscle remodelling associated with chronic heart failure.

17 If the patient has tolerated the above treatment and has sufficient blood pressure, eGFR >30ml/min/1.73m^2 and baseline serum potassium <5.0mEq/L, they should be commenced on mineralocorticoid receptor antagonist (MRA) – spironolactone or eplerenone. It is indicated in patients with NYHA class II–IV heart failure and ejection fraction ≤40% and it also reduces mortality. Patients on this medication must be monitored closely for serum potassium and renal function.

18 Ivabradine is a selective sinus node inhibitor for patients with HFrEF in sinus rhythm with a heart rate >70 despite maximal beta blocker therapy or contraindication to beta blocker use. Ivabradine also reduces the risk of hospitalisation in patients with chronic HFrEF.

19 Patients with NYHA class II–IV with QRS duration >120ms and LVEF ≤35% who have been on maximal medical therapy for at least 3 months should be considered for cardiac resynchronisation therapy. The longer the QRS and/or presence of LBBB morphology, the stronger the indicator for device therapy. Cardiac resynchronisation therapy involves insertion of a biventricular pacemaker to promote synchronous contraction of both the right and left ventricles. In the above population, an implantable cardioverter-defibrillator for primary prevention of sudden cardiac death is also indicated. Hence, typically a cardiac resynchronisation therapy with defibrillator (CRT-D) device is inserted.

CASE 5: Mitral regurgitation

History

- A 62-year-old female presents to her GP with **three months of worsening fatigue and intermittent palpitations** [1].
- Associated with this is decreased **exercise tolerance** [2]. She reports being able to carry her groceries from her local grocer to her house (a distance of around 1km) relatively easily, but is finding she needs to **take a few breaks** [3] on the way, which concerns her.
- On further questioning she also reveals she has noticed some **ankle swelling** [4] over the past couple of weeks and woke up **last night short of breath** [5].
- Otherwise she has **no chest pain, no presyncopal episodes or syncope** [5].
- She has been **recently well** [6] and her past medical history is only significant **for hypertension which is well controlled on her usual ramipril** [7].
- She has **not commenced any new medications of late** [8].
- In terms of her family history, the patient's mother died from a stroke aged 83.

[1] Often, the initial symptom of left-sided valvular disease such as mitral regurgitation may be non-specific. In this case, the initial symptom was fatigue. Here the long-standing nature of the patient's symptoms shows that this has been a chronic issue and it is likely that there has been a period of being asymptomatic prior to developing symptoms. The chronicity of symptoms has diagnostic significance and primary degenerative causes of mitral regurgitation become more likely than ischaemic causes. The history of palpitations here should raise suspicion for either tachycardia or irregular heart rhythms such as atrial fibrillation.

[2] Compared to the patient's baseline, there is a degree of compromised left ventricular output.

[3] Most people are able to walk on the flat at a leisurely pace for 1km even if they lead sedentary lifestyles. Needing to take breaks due to dyspnoea should raise concern in the treating doctor and a detailed cardiovascular assessment should ensue.

[4] Peripheral oedema is a sign of right heart failure, as is a pulsatile liver, congestive hepatomegaly and raised JVP. There are many causes of right heart failure, but in this case it will be due to left heart failure from mitral regurgitation. The cardiovascular system is a closed circuit where the output from the right ventricle should equal the output in the left ventricle. A deficiency in one side of the cardiovascular system will compromise the other and in time, result in biventricular failure.

[5] What the patient is describing here is PND. This is a sign of severe left heart failure and patients may have had orthopnoea in the lead up to this. Always complete your cardiovascular systems review if a patient's chief complaint is cardiovascular in nature. The lack of chest pain in the history also leans against an ischaemic process.

[6] At this stage of assessing the patient, without an echocardiogram, the only thing that is apparent is that the patient is in heart failure. Knowing that the patient has been previously well, with no preceding infective symptoms, helps in that infective/inflammatory aetiologies such as viral-induced cardiomyopathy and infective endocarditis become less likely.

[7] Uncontrolled hypertension is a risk factor for heart failure with preserved ejection fraction and had the patient's blood pressure been high and untreated, may have been a confounding factor in her presentation.

[8] In an elderly patient with cardiovascular history, it is important to take a good drug history. Recently commenced drugs such as non-steroidal anti-inflammatory drugs (NSAIDs), calcium channel blockers, antidepressants, PDE-5 inhibitors and chemotherapy agents have the ability to tip the patient over to heart failure.

Examination

- From the end of the bed, the patient **appears well** [1]. She has a slim body habitus.
- She does not appear dyspnoeic but displays **mildly increased work of breathing** [2] with mild sternocleidomastoid use.
- Her heart rate is **123bpm and is irregularly irregular** [3].
- Blood pressure is **160/80mmHg** [4].
- **RR is 26 and saturations are 88% on air** [5]. She is afebrile. The **JVP is 5cm** [6].
- Auscultation of the heart reveals a harsh **pansystolic murmur** [7] loudest in the **apex, radiating to the axillae** [8].

- This murmur is accentuated when she is **in deep expiration, gripping her hands and in the left lateral decubitus position** [9].
- The apex beat is **displaced to the mid-axillary line** [10] of the 6th intercostal space.
- Auscultation of the lungs reveals **bibasal crepitations and dullness to percussion in the bases** [11].
- There was **peripheral oedema to knees** [12] on examination.
- The patient was referred to the emergency department after review at her GP.

1 Again, the initial assessment of the patient should be observation. One can quickly assess the urgency of the situation by how unwell a patient looks.

2 There is mildly increased work of breathing. The history of biventricular failure (with predominance of left-sided symptoms) suggests that there will be a degree of pulmonary oedema on examination. Respiratory compromise can be assessed in work of breathing. Increased use of the sternocleidomastoid muscles, intercostal and subcostal recession and tripoding are all signs of increased work of breathing. In adults, a tracheal tug is suggestive of severe increased work of breathing.

3 Irregularly irregular pulse is most suggestive of AF, but without a confirmatory ECG, an irregular pulse may be misconstrued for a regularly irregular pulse. Irregularly irregular pulse could also mean a variety of other rhythms such as frequent premature ventricular complexes, focal or multifocal atrial tachycardia, sinus node dysfunction or atrial flutter with variable block.

4 The patient is tachycardic, but does not have blood pressure compromise.

5 Tachypnoea with associated hypoxia depict type 1 respiratory failure. Given the history of heart failure symptoms with lack of infective symptoms, it is most likely due to acute pulmonary oedema.

6 JVP of 5cm with peripheral oedema to knees is a sign of right heart failure.

7 A murmur occurs when there is turbulent flow across a valve. Pansystolic murmurs occur when there is regurgitation across an atrioventricular valve (mitral vs. tricuspid) from the ventricle into its atria. One can localise these lesions to either the left lower sternal edge (tricuspid) or the apex (mitral).

8 The mitral valve is best heard at the apex with the bell of the stethoscope, and mitral regurgitation classically radiates to the axillae. Severe regurgitation/valvular pathology may radiate throughout the precordium.

9 There are numerous dynamic manoeuvres that can accentuate left-sided and right-sided murmurs. Left-sided regurgitant murmurs can be accentuated by exercises that increase the afterload of the heart, such as isometric hand grip, transient arterial occlusion (by placing blood pressure cuffs on both arms and inflating to ~20–40mmHg). Laying the patient in the left lateral decubitus position places the apex of the heart closer to the surface in the thoracic cavity, making it easier to hear the murmur. Aortic murmurs can be accentuated by having the patient lean forward. Left-sided lesions are also heard better during expiration, where there is decreased intrathoracic pressure and increased venous return, promoting further turbulent flow through valves due to the increased volume being run through the heart.

10 A displaced apex beat is indicative of cardiomegaly of any cause. In the overall picture here, there has been some chronic remodelling of the heart to compensate for the valvular pathology. If an apex beat is displaced, it can be further characterised as a pressure-loaded or volume-loaded apex beat.

11 Bibasal crepitations are more often than not due to a hypervolaemic state such as pulmonary oedema. It is possible to have bibasal pneumonia, but this is uncommon. Associated with the bibasal crepitations are dullness to percussion, suggestive of fluid in the bases of the lungs, i.e. bibasal pleural effusions.

12 Peripheral oedema suggests that there is a degree of biventricular failure in this patient.

Investigations

- 12-lead ECG shows **left axis deviation** [1], heart rate of 103bpm with **no discernible P waves and an irregularly irregular R–R interval** [2].
- There is also marked **left ventricular hypertrophy** [3].
- Chest X-ray revealed an increased **cardiothoracic ratio of 0.6** [4], with **bilateral blunting of the costodiaphragmatic angles and upper lobe diversion of blood vessels** [5].
- FBE and urea, electrolytes and creatinine are normal. TTE was performed as an inpatient which revealed **severe mitral regurgitation** [6] secondary to a **flail segment of the posterior mitral valve leaflet** [7]. **The mitral valve leaflets were 6mm in width** [7].
- **There were no vegetations seen** [8].
- The **vena contracta width was 0.73cm, the regurgitant fraction was 53% and the ERO was 0.45cm² ** [9].
- There was also **moderate left atrial enlargement** [10] and moderate **eccentric left ventricular hypertrophy** [11] with **LVEF of 40%** [12].
- The estimated **pulmonary artery pressure was 35mmHg** [13].
- **Transoesophageal echocardiography** [14] was also performed pre- and postoperatively for peri-operative planning and to assess the valve post mitral valve repair.

1 The mean electrical axis of the heart has shifted to the left, indicating left-sided predominance of myocardium which may indicate a degree of left ventricular hypertrophy.

2 This is the definition of atrial fibrillation on ECG. There may also be a wandering isoelectric line or if there is rapid ventricular response, rate-related ischaemic changes such as T wave inversion or ST segment depression/elevation.

3 We can correlate the clinical findings of displaced apex beat and pansystolic murmur in the apex to the electrocardiographic findings here. The left ventricle has had to remodel and hypertrophy in order to keep up the systemic cardiac output with the regurgitation back into the left atrium.

4 The cut-off for cardiomegaly on chest X-ray is a cardiothoracic ratio of >0.5.

5 There is also radiographic evidence of heart failure. The inability of the left heart to eject all of the venous return it receives has resulted in backlog into the pulmonary venous system. Radiographically it is represented by upper lobe diversion (increased prominence of upper lobe pulmonary veins), increased interstitial markings and Kerley B lines and bilateral pleural effusions, which when mild appear as blunting of the costodiaphragmatic angles.

6 The key investigation here would be an echocardiogram. It is the best non-invasive means of assessing the valvular morphology to show the aetiology behind the mitral regurgitation, quantify the severity of the mitral regurgitation, see the associated changes within the left ventricle and left atrium and also assess for sequelae of the primary valvular pathology such as raised pulmonary artery pressure.

7 The mitral valve apparatus is a complex and dynamic 3-dimensional structure with multiple components. The valve itself, which is named after a bishop's mitre, has a ring-shaped fibrous annulus and from this annulus, two main leaflets which close over the valve during systole. There is a large anterior leaflet and a smaller posterior leaflet. These leaflets have chordae tendineae that are themselves attached to papillary muscles which anchor the leaflets to the left ventricular wall to prevent prolapse into the left atrium during systole. Mitral regurgitation occurs when the mitral valve fails to close during systole, allowing regurgitation from the left ventricle back into the left atrium. This can occur from pathology of the mitral valve apparatus or from distortion of the left ventricular geometry preventing leaflet coaptation/apposition during systole. The main aetiologies of mitral regurgitation are listed below.

Primary mitral regurgitation (primarily a valvular pathology):
- mitral valve prolapse
- papillary muscle rupture
- chordae tendineae rupture
- leaflet perforation, i.e. infective endocarditis.

Secondary mitral regurgitation (primarily a myocardial pathology, also known as functional regurgitation):
- regional wall motion abnormality from previous infarcts
- dilated cardiomyopathy
- myocarditis
- left ventricular dysfunction of any cause.

In this specific case the thickened valve leaflets and the flail segment of the posterior mitral valve leaflet suggest that mitral valve prolapse is the cause of mitral regurgitation. Mitral valve prolapse most commonly occurs from myxomatous degeneration where the fibrous layer of the valve thins, allowing mucoid material to accumulate. Over time it elongates and thins the chordae tendineae, predisposing them to rupture. It also causes the valve leaflets to become floppier, impairing the coaptation of the leaflets in systole. Other rarer causes of mitral valve prolapse are connective tissue disorders such as Marfan syndrome, Ehlers–

Danlos syndrome, pseudoxanthoma elasticum, osteogenesis imperfecta and systemic lupus erythematosus. Although not heard in this case, the classical auscultation finding in mitral valve prolapse is a crisp mid-systolic click (due to abruptly tightened chordae tendineae in systole) with a late systolic murmur.

8 While the history is not suggestive of an infectious aetiology, there is a need to exclude infectious endocarditis as a cause of mitral regurgitation, as the treatment vastly differs to that for other causes of mitral regurgitation.

9 Quantifying mitral regurgitation has prognostic significance. When comparing two patients who are asymptomatic, the patient with severe mitral regurgitation will have much lower life expectancy than the patient with mild mitral regurgitation. This is because the patient with severe mitral regurgitation will have less cardiovascular reserve and will be more prone to developing heart failure. The current guidelines suggest that severe mitral regurgitation is indicated by a vena contracta (regurgitant jet) maximal width of ≥0.7cm, regurgitant fraction of ≥50% and effective regurgitant orifice of ≥0.4cm^2.

10 Mitral regurgitation results in blood regurgitating back into the left atrium, resulting in increased left atrial end-diastolic volume. Over time, the volumetric overload of the left atrium causes it to dilate. This dilatation of the left atrium results in progressive fibrous remodelling of the left atrium as well, resulting in increased risk of developing AF and other atrial arrhythmias. You may also see ECG signs of left atrial enlargement in patients with chronic mitral regurgitation with prolongation of the P wave duration (>120ms) or P-mitrale, which is when the P wave has a bifid morphology in lead II; this may also be seen in V1–6.

11 The heart can undergo hypertrophy due to increased haemodynamic load. In this case where there is chronic volume overload, the cardiomyocyte lays down further sarcomeres *in series*. This results in elongation of the cardiomyocyte and thus an increased left ventricular chamber radius and an overall increased volume of the left ventricle. This is called eccentric hypertrophy. Conversely, when there is chronic pressure overload, the cardiomyocyte lays down further sarcomeres *in parallel*, which thickens the cardiomyocyte and does not greatly change the left ventricular chamber radius. Instead it allows the left ventricle to create higher systolic pressures to pump against the pressure. This is called concentric hypertrophy. Unfortunately with excess concentric hypertrophy, the compliance of the left ventricle will be reduced, making the ventricle stiff and unable to relax. This results in diastolic dysfunction.

12 It is clear from the decreased left ventricular ejection fraction that the left ventricle is unable to pump out a normal volume of blood into the system, despite the compensatory eccentric hypertrophy. The inability of the left ventricle to pump out all of its received venous return has resulted in backlog into the pulmonary arterial system and systemic venous system. This decompensation is obvious upon history and examination as the patient has symptoms and signs of biventricular failure. LVEF values are classified as follows:

- 55–70%: normal
- 40–54%: mildly reduced
- 35–39%: moderately reduced
- <35%: severely reduced

13 Any cause of left-sided heart failure can eventually cause pulmonary arterial hypertension. Chronic backlog of fluid into the left atrium increases pulmonary venous pressure and in turn, pulmonary arterial pressure. In cases of chronic mitral regurgitation, however, pulmonary hypertension is relatively rare and thus signs of right ventricular hypertrophy are usually absent.

14 Transoesophageal echocardiograms provide a 3-dimensional view of the valvular apparatus as opposed to the 2-dimensional view obtained in its corresponding transthoracic study. This makes it an invaluable peri-operative investigation that helps in planning out a surgery.

Management

Supportive

Patients need to be admitted under the **cardiology team in the coronary care unit** [1] initially. If they are presenting with pulmonary oedema, provide supportive therapy and aim for euvolaemia.

- **Supplemental oxygen** [2] via nasal prongs should be administered to maintain saturations above 92%
- Then obtain intravenous access
- Administer **IV furosemide** [3] to offload the fluid
- Further supportive therapy for this will be

commencement of a **1.5 litre fluid restriction, a strict fluid balance chart and daily weights** [4] to monitor diuresis and fluid loss.

Manage the rapid ventricular response of the AF with **oral metoprolol** [5]. Patients with AF should have their CHA_2DS_2-VASc score calculated and be appropriately anticoagulated. Usually patients will require oral anticoagulation via warfarin, or a direct oral anticoagulant (i.e. apixaban, rivaroxaban or dabigatran). For those undergoing procedures, however, **low** molecular weight heparin such as enoxaparin [6] may be used for its shorter half-life.

Surgical

The only definitive management for mitral valve regurgitation is surgery and a referral to the cardiothoracic team will be made for consideration of the type of surgery. As a general rule **surgical treatment** [7] only really has a role in patients with primary mitral regurgitation. Surgical intervention has only a limited role in secondary mitral regurgitation as the problem is not with the valve itself, rather the myocardium; thus, fixing the valvular pathology will not carry any significant prognostic benefit. Furthermore, surgical intervention in primary mitral regurgitation is aimed at mimicking the native valve as much as possible. Thus mitral valve repair is preferred over mitral valve replacement and if mitral valve replacement is needed, chordal preservation is preferred over removal of the chordae.

Postoperative care

Patients need to be monitored in **HDU/ICU with cardiac monitoring** [8] for the first few days postoperatively. Mitral valve surgery requires median sternotomy and cardiopulmonary bypass and patients are prone to many **complications** [9] in the immediate postoperative period.

Follow-up

Post mitral valve repair, patients require follow-up in the cardiothoracic clinic, initially 6 weeks post repair to ensure adequate wound healing and that no late complications of the valve repair occur. From there patients can be reviewed 6–12 monthly until discharge from clinic. Parallel to this, patients should be followed up in **cardiology clinic** [10] with serial echocardiograms to assess resolution of the hypertrophy and to manage the AF.

---

1 Patients with acute valvular pathology are usually admitted under cardiology to a coronary care unit. The cardiothoracic surgical team may be involved early if there are indications for urgent valvular surgery.

2 The patient is dyspnoeic and hypoxic. Supplemental oxygen should be given to correct hypoxia as a first-line measure. Failing nasal prongs/cannulae, you can use a Hudson mask or if needed, a non-rebreather reservoir mask. In cases where the saturations are still <92% despite a non-rebreather mask, continuous positive airway pressure (CPAP) can be given. It has been shown to have a mortality benefit and reduce the need for intubation. If the patient is hypotensive, CPAP should not be given as it can further worsen the hypotension. This is because CPAP increases the intrathoracic pressure, which lessens the natural pressure gradient that allows for venous return. The decreased venous return reduces the preload of the heart and as per Frank Starling's law, decreases stroke volume and cardiac output.

3 IV furosemide is needed to correct the hypervolaemic state in acute pulmonary oedema. For patients who are furosemide naive, a stat dose of 40–80mg may be administered. For patients who are already on furosemide in the community, a higher dose may be needed to achieve adequate diuresis.

4 For patients in heart failure, after the acute management, supportive therapy is needed to prevent further occurrences of acute pulmonary oedema. A fluid restriction is important to prevent hypervolaemia. A strict fluid balance chart will assess the volume of diuresis. Daily weights are the best measure of fluid loss on a day-to-day basis.

5 This patient has a rapid rate. In this instance, metoprolol is a good means of attaining rate control. Digoxin can be considered, but is not as effective as metoprolol for rate control.

6 Therapeutic enoxaparin is the choice of anticoagulation in patients with AF who are awaiting a procedure. This is because enoxaparin's action is relatively short-lived when compared to warfarin or DOACs and can be withheld 12 to 24 hours prior to a procedure with minimal increased bleeding risk. Comparatively, warfarin requires INR correction with vitamin K or prothrombin complex concentrate and DOACs require a minimum of 48 hours to be renally excreted. Of the DOACs, only dabigatran has a reversal agent (idarucizumab).

7 This patient requires surgical intervention as she has chronic primary mitral regurgitation with features of decompensation (signs of biventricular failure and new onset AF). Indications for mitral valve surgery in primary mitral regurgitation are as follows.
In symptomatic patients:
- chronic severe primary mitral regurgitation, with LVEF >30%
- severe left ventricular systolic dysfunction, with LVEF <30%
- acute mitral regurgitation from either papillary muscle rupture in a STEMI or infective endocarditis.

In asymptomatic patients:
- severe mitral regurgitation with preserved LV function and:
  - new onset of either AF or pulmonary hypertension
  - high likelihood of durable repair, low surgical risk and flail leaflet and LV end systolic dimension ≥40mm
- severe mitral regurgitation with severe LV dysfunction refractory to medical therapy and high likelihood of durable repair and low comorbidities.

Further benefits to mitral valve repair compared to mitral valve replacement are that patients need not have lifelong anticoagulation with warfarin, the repair lasts longer than replacements and there is an overall mortality benefit with mitral valve repair. With regard to mitral valve replacement, mechanical prostheses are preferred over the bioprosthetic valves for their better durability. These patients require lifelong anticoagulation with warfarin, aiming for an INR of 2.5–3.5.

8 Patients who have undergone major cardiothoracic surgery are at risk of developing a low cardiac output state, which can quickly result in deterioration and death. Monitoring in a high dependency unit (HDU) or intensive care unit (ICU) environment allows the team to promptly recognise deterioration and treat the patient appropriately. Reasons for developing a low cardiac output include haemorrhage, tamponade, arrhythmias, hypoxia and myocardial stunning post surgery.

9 Complications can occur either from the median sternotomy or the valve surgery itself. Major complications include:

- Wound:
  - superficial wound infections
  - deep sternal wound infection
  - wound dehiscence
  - sternal instability
  - massive sternal haemorrhage
- Valve:
  - prosthetic endocarditis
  - repair failure
  - prosthetic thrombosis
  - paravalvular leak
- Cardiac:
  - dysrhythmias
  - tamponade
- Stroke
- Brachial plexus injury from sternal wound retraction.

Late complications of mitral valve repair are a failure of repair. Late complications of mitral valve replacement are paravalvular leak, prosthetic endocarditis and thrombosis. These are horrible complications.

10 Concomitant cardiology follow-up is important. The patient will require serial echocardiograms to assess for resolution of eccentric left ventricular hypertrophy, any residual left ventricular dysfunction, improvement in left atrial volume index (if the atria are noted to be large prior to surgery secondary to the regurgitation) and pulmonary hypertension. Additionally, if the patient has had significant AF, or has received a prosthetic valve (valvular AF), they will need cardiology input to optimise their treatment.

CASE 6: Mobitz 2 second-degree heart block

History

- You review a 61-year-old male whom the ED has referred to you with **syncope for investigation** [1].
- He had an **unwitnessed sudden onset syncope** [2] with **headstrike** [3] earlier today whilst gardening.
- He has no **prodromal symptoms** [4] and his family says he **could not have been out for more than 5 seconds** [5] as his family noted he collapsed soon after turning on the hose. **The patient reports recovering quickly after the event** [5].
- **He has no tongue biting, bladder or bowel incontinence or frothing at the mouth that his family had noticed** [6].
- **Prior to the syncope** [7], he had no tinnitus, nausea, feeling of being faint, visual disturbances or a painful/emotional trigger.
- He reported **occasionally feeling faint and dizzy** [8] whilst walking during the past couple of weeks, but never had a syncope. Otherwise he has no chest pain, palpitations, shortness of breath, orthopnoea or PND.
- His past medical history was significant for a **recent anterior STEMI** [9] with successful percutaneous coronary intervention (PCI) to proximal LAD 4 months earlier, **hypertension** [10] and a 20 pack year smoking history.
- He has no previous history of **epilepsy or stroke** [11].

[1] Throughout your clinical practice, you will develop a 'classical clinical vignette' or the pathognomonic presentation for each pathology. Conversely, you will then be able to create a differential diagnosis list based on each presentation. Broadly speaking, syncope has three main differential diagnoses. It is cardiogenic syncope (valvular, ischaemic, arrhythmic syncope), neurocardiogenic syncope (vasovagal syncope) or seizures.

[2] For syncopal events it is always best to obtain a collateral history from a witness. The clarity of the history may differ for patients recalling their own syncope. A sudden onset syncope should raise concern for seizure or cardiogenic syncope.

[3] Beyond the syncope, patients will often present with injuries related to losing consciousness. Always ask about headstrike and injuries. Repeated headstrike can result in traumatic brain injury and recurrent haemorrhages, which carry a large burden of morbidity.

[4] This is the 'presyncope' part of the history. Ask for visual aura, sensory hallucinations, chest pain, shortness of breath or palpitations. Having no prodromal symptoms is suspicious for a cardiogenic syncope.

[5] This is the 'syncope' part of the history. Ask for the duration of syncope. Syncope longer than a minute leans away from cardiogenic syncope and other causes of syncope such as vasovagal syncope or seizure. Cardiogenic syncope is classically of short duration and rapid recovery with the restoration of cardiac output.

[6] During the 'syncope' part of the history look for features of seizure as described.

[7] This is the completion of the 'presyncope' portion of the history. Patients with vasovagal syncope may have triggers such as heat, emotional distress, fear or pain and may experience nausea, vomiting, tunnel vision or sounds getting more distant. Patients with seizure may have a preceding visual aura.

[8] Asking the patient if they were well previous to the event will occasionally yield very important information. Here we gain more information on the mechanism behind the syncope. Feeling presyncopal on mobilisation raises concern for insufficient cardiac output during exertion that may be well compensated when the patient is resting.

[9] This is significant as an anterior STEMI can result in necrosis and fibrosis of not only the myocardium, but also the underlying conductive system. Namely, the atrioventricular node and the fascicles/bundle branches can be affected. Patients post anterior STEMI can commonly have left bundle branch blocks because of this. Further information is needed here regarding past medical history of T2DM, dyslipidaemia and family history of cardiovascular disease, to complete the cardiovascular risk stratification of the patient.

[10] Unchecked hypertension can also cause fibrous remodelling of the heart, resulting in conductive disturbances.

[11] The patient does not have previous history of stroke or epilepsy, which also leans the clinician away from seizures as the cause of syncope.

Examination

- From the end of the bed, the patient **appears well** [1] . They have a normal body habitus.
- The patient has a **fresh graze on the left forehead** [2] and multiple bruises on the left side, presumably from the syncope.
- They do not have any **bony tenderness** [3] along the head, spine or joints.
- The heart rate is **54bpm and regularly irregular** [4] .

- The blood pressure is **110/80mmHg** [5] . The respiratory rate is 16 and saturations are 97% on air. The patient is afebrile.
- Auscultation reveals **dual heart sounds with no murmurs** [6] .
- Clinically they are **euvolaemic** [7] with a JVP of 2cm, clear air entry bilaterally throughout the lungs, normal central capillary refill time and no peripheral oedema.

[1] The patient with asymptomatic second-degree AV block may appear well.

[2] Remember to actively look for injurious sequelae to the syncope. These require investigations to exclude fracture and bleeding. If there was fresh bleeding from the head, you would also want to assess clinically for signs of base of skull fracture such as Battle sign (mastoid ecchymosis), peri-orbital ecchymoses (raccoon eyes), haematotympanium and cerebrospinal fluid (CSF) in nose/ear discharge (otorrhoea/ rhinorrhoea), as there could be a fistula between the dura and skull base.

[3] Clinically the patient does not seem to have any fractures. Fractures are rarely ever asymptomatic. The bony cortex is richly innervated with nerve fibres and patients will always present with pain that will be elicited on palpation. When assessing for fractures remember to palpate all the major joints and bones in the body: suture lines of the cranium, midline tenderness along the length of the spine, wrists, forearm, elbow, shoulder (acromioclavicular joint), hips, knees and ankles.

[4] Regularly irregular pulses place us in the realm of bigeminy, AF with slow ventricular response, type 2 Mobitz block and potentially sinoatrial exit block as differentials. The heart rate is only mildly bradycardic and does not raise concern.

[5] The patient is normotensive, but beware normotension in the previously hypertensive patient. In these instances, the change in blood pressure is clinically significant. This may indicate a decreased output or hypovolaemic state for the patient.

[6] The cardiovascular examination would not be complete without assessment of valvular lesions. Mitral valve lesions in particular are known to predispose for atrial arrhythmias.

[7] Always assess the volume status of the cardiovascular patient. If they were clinically overloaded or dry, that would require correction with either diuresis or volume repletion.

Investigations

- 12-lead ECG shows left axis deviation, a heart rate of 50bpm with regular **P waves** [1] .
- **Every 2nd or 3rd P wave is not followed by a QRS complex** [2] .
- The **PR interval stays consistent** [3] throughout.
- The **QRS complex is narrow** [4] .
- Otherwise there are no ventricular escape rhythms on the ECG, **no ST segment elevation or T wave inversion** [5] .
- Serology shows a normal full blood examination

with urea, electrolytes and creatinine revealing a **K of 6.3 with normal renal function** [6] .
- Calcium, magnesium, phosphate panel is normal; specifically the **magnesium is 1.1mmol/L** [7] .
- **Thyroid-stimulating hormone (TSH) is normal** [8] .
- **Venous blood gas (VBG) shows no elevated lactate** [9] .
- A CT brain reveals no **intracranial haemorrhage** [10] and X-rays of the left shoulder and left knee show **no fracture** [11] .

[1] The key investigation here is the ECG. Regular P waves are important to note as this indicates no sinus node dysfunction – any cause of symptomatic sinus node dysfunction is an indication for permanent pacemaker

implantation. Elderly patients with past history of cardiovascular disease and diabetes are at higher risk of sinus node dysfunction. Sinus node dysfunction is a spectrum of disease that includes:

- inappropriate sinus bradycardia
- bradycardia–tachycardia syndrome
- sinus pause or sinus arrest
- sinoatrial exit block, where the conduction of P waves to the atrial tissue is impaired.

2 P wave and QRS dissociation indicates atrioventricular block. We can distinguish between the subtypes of atrioventricular block by assessing the PR interval.

3 A consistently prolonged PR interval with a drop in QRS complex indicates Mobitz type 2 block. This carries clinical significance. Mobitz type 2 is a higher degree of AV block and more commonly progresses to complete heart block. The classical ECG findings are a consistent PR interval, consistent P–P intervals and the R–R interval surrounding the dropped beat being a multiple of preceding R–R intervals. Our patient here has a non-conducted P wave every 2nd or 3rd P wave, which essentially thirds or halves their cardiac output. The conduction abnormality here in Mobitz type 2 AV nodal block is commonly below the level of the AV node. It can be in the His bundle, in one of the two bundle branches or one of the three fascicles.

- The reason Mobitz type 2 progresses to complete heart block is not because of progressive fatigue in AV nodal cells; rather it is because they unexpectedly fail to conduct the P wave to the ventricles. The common causes of this are structural deficits such as a previous anterior myocardial infarct or fibrosis of the heart from systemic diseases (autoimmune processes or infiltrative diseases).
- Progressive prolongation of the PR interval prior to dropping of the QRS complex indicates Mobitz type 1 block. Mobitz type 1 AV block, otherwise known as Wenckebach, results from a reversible conduction abnormality at the level of the AV node. In Wenckebach, AV nodal cells progressively fatigue until they fail to conduct a QRS complex. Common causes of this are reversible ischaemia, myocarditis, increased vagal tone, electrolyte abnormalities and medications that slow conduction through the AV node, such as calcium channel blockers or beta blockers. The treatment of Mobitz type 1 is therefore relatively simple: you just need to treat the underlying pathology. Progression to complete heart block is rare and invasive means of pacing are not usually required.

4 Mobitz type 2 block is commonly associated with wide QRS complex if the conduction disturbance is below the level of the His bundle.

5 Assess for ischaemic changes when a conduction abnormality is present as they usually go hand in hand.

6 Although it may not be the principal cause of the Mobitz type 2 block, hyperkalaemia will surely aggravate and complicate the clinical scenario and hinder conduction through the AV node. Management of hyperkalaemia depends on the presence of ECG changes. Features of hyperkalaemia on ECG include:
- peaked T waves, which is usually the first sign
- PR interval prolongation
- widening of the QRS complex
- AV block, bundle branch block, fascicular blocks
- sine wave appearance – which is a preterminal rhythm to asystole or ventricular fibrillation.

In terms of management, if there are features of hyperkalaemia you would give:
- IV 10% of 10mmol of calcium gluconate for stabilisation of the cardiac membrane potential, to prevent fatal arrhythmias
- 50ml of 50% dextrose and 10 units of Actrapid (short-acting insulin) IV, to push the potassium into the cells
- Resonium to bind the potassium in the serum
- furosemide to encourage loss of total body potassium.

7 In cardiology, a K of ≥4mmol/L and Mg ≥1mmol/L is ideal and any electrolyte deficiencies should be corrected to this level.

8 It is not the most common cause, but severe hypothyroidism can result in bradyarrhythmias.

9 The lactate on the VBG assesses for poor end-organ perfusion and, if elevated, is suggestive of heart failure that requires prompt correction.

10 As stated previously, ensure to investigate the injuries to exclude further sequelae. A CT brain is indicated in patients with headstrike to rule out an intracranial haemorrhage.

11 X-rays confirm your clinical suspicion of no fracture.

Management

A patient with high degree AV block should be admitted to the **coronary care unit and placed on continuous cardiac monitoring** [1] with a view to inpatient permanent pacemaker implantation. For supportive therapy, **Resonium should be administered for their hyperkalaemia** [2] and **their regular metoprolol withheld** [2].

If the patient remains asymptomatic and has no further syncopal episodes or progression to complete heart block, there is no need for urgent resuscitation. If they do, however, become syncopal or develop complete heart block, it is important to do the following.

Acute

Resuscitation

Assess the patient via the ABCD approach. Ensure the patient is alert, maintaining their airway and has appropriate saturations. Correct these prior to progressing onto circulation. If the patient is alert and bradycardic, assess for hypotension and end-organ hypoperfusion. Obtain an urgent ECG. If the **ECG shows complete heart block, you may see ventricular escape rhythms** [3]. Clinically patients will most commonly be hypotensive.

Chronotropy

Obtain IV access and administer **IV atropine 0.5mg stat. Assess for response and repeat in 5 minutes** [4]. Failing this, the patient will need to be commenced on **IV isoprenaline or adrenaline** [5] for positive chronotropy.

Pacing

As patients are receiving isoprenaline or adrenaline, ensure you have the equipment set up for pacing. **Transcutaneous pacing** [6] is a great non-invasive means of pacing as it does not take long to set up. Transcutaneous pacing is when external pacing impulses are delivered to cause myocardial depolarisation and cardiac contraction to maintain cardiac output. It is delivered by the use of an external defibrillator (in pacing mode) and defibrillator pads. It is important to place the pads in an antero-posterior position, with the anterior pad in the left lower part of the sternum near the apex and the posterior pad over the left scapula.

Failing this, patients will require urgent **transvenous cardiac pacing wire** [7] placement. This is an invasive means of pacing where a pacing lead is placed through the tricuspid valve and into the right ventricle. The pacing impulses are then delivered directly into the right ventricle. In order to do this you require central venous access (i.e. internal jugular vein, subclavian vein and femoral vein). Due to the need for central venous access, it cannot be implemented as quickly as transcutaneous pacing and so commonly transcutaneous pacing is trialled first, then if unsuccessful, urgent preparation for transvenous pacing is made. When advancing the pacing lead, its proper placement is confirmed via fluoroscopic guidance, but in the absence of fluoroscopy, it can be done with echocardiography and continuous cardiac monitoring. Once transvenous pacing is established, the isoprenaline or adrenaline infusion can be weaned and the patient can undergo **permanent pacemaker implantation** [8].

Long-term

Long-term follow-up

The patient was discharged home with follow-up through the **pacemaker clinic** [9] for optimisation of the pacemaker function and to troubleshoot any problems that may arise.

---

[1] In addition to considering what sort of acute medical therapy you will give to the patient, it is equally important to consider the right place the patient should be nursed. A coronary care unit (CCU) is the right place for this patient. The nursing staff there are experienced and trained in reading ECGs and see cardiology presentations every day. They also have a greater capacity for continuous cardiac monitoring, which is indicated for the patient with symptomatic bradyarrhythmia who is at risk of developing complete heart block.

[2] For any emergency or non-emergency cases of bradyarrhythmia, do not forget supportive therapy. In this case, correcting the hyperkalaemia and withholding their beta blocker would improve conduction through the AV node.

[3] In the case of a deteriorating patient, having the patient in the CCU is beneficial. Cardiac deteriorations may not be easily detected in a normal 4-bed ward that does not have cardiac monitoring or cardiac nurses who see these issues every day. Ventricular escape rhythms occur when the heart rate drops below 40, allowing the intrinsic automaticity of the ventricular myocytes to depolarise.

[4] Atropine is an anticholinergic drug that inhibits parasympathetic nervous system action on the AV node and is the first-line medication of choice for bradycardia due to either sinus node dysfunction or AV nodal block.

[5] Isoprenaline and adrenaline are positive chronotropic and inotropic agents that mainly act as a bridging tool to adequate pacing. Isoprenaline is a more selective beta agonist than adrenaline and is safe for peripheral infusion. Certain patients who have failed to respond to adrenaline may respond to isoprenaline. Adrenaline is the agent of choice in patients with severe hypotension (systolic BP

<80mmHg) and it also has potent alpha-adrenoreceptor agonist effects. Note that both these agents can cause atrial and ventricular arrhythmias due to sympathomimetic effects.

6 Transcutaneous pacing is used in an emergency setting to manage temporary bradyarrhythmias or as a bridge for long-term pacemaker therapy. Ensure that you have good mechanical capture (not just electrical capture!) by ensuring the pulse oximetry waveform corresponds with the transcutaneous pacing; and ensuring that distal pulses (radial, dorsalis pedis) are present, with the pulses corresponding to each QRS on the monitor. Aim for heart rates between 60 and 120bpm. Transcutaneous pacing can be uncomfortable for the patient as it essentially delivers shocks and may cause skeletal muscle contractions and mild skin burns. It is worthwhile prescribing some analgesia for patients to tolerate transcutaneous pacing; some patients may need sedation which should be performed with guidance from ICU or anaesthetics. In cases where transcutaneous pacing is prolonged, change pad placement every 5 hours to reduce skin burns and discomfort. If there is failure to capture, you may need to turn up the current (measured in milliamperes) or change the application of the pads.

7 The benefits of transvenous pacing over transcutaneous pacing are that it has a higher success rate in terms of capture, it can be used for longer and is not as uncomfortable to the patient. The downsides are that complications from venous access are relatively common. There is a risk of pneumothorax and haemothorax from subclavian vein access. Infection and thrombus formation most often occur with femoral access, and pulmonary emboli can also occur. Due to infection risk, temporary pacing wires should not be used for longer than 24 hours.

8 Complete heart block and symptomatic second-degree heart block are all indications for permanent pacing. This patient in particular requires a pacemaker as he was syncopal with second-degree heart block and is at high risk of developing complete heart block. Other indications for a permanent pacemaker insertion are:
- sinus node dysfunction: from frequent sinus pauses or symptomatic chronotropic incompetence
- acquired high-degree atrioventricular block
- chronic bifascicular block, either being an advanced second-degree AV block or intermittent third-degree AV block
- post MI if there is persistent AV block or bradycardia

- hypersensitive carotid sinus syndrome
- for symptomatic or inappropriate bradycardia post cardiac transplantation
- hypertrophic cardiomyopathy with sinus node dysfunction and AV block
- for patients who require pacing to prevent pause-dependent ventricular tachycardia (VT).

Pacemaker generators are placed in the subcutaneous tissue in the left infraclavicular region with the pacing leads placed into the right side of heart via subclavian venous access. The pacemaker has two basic functions. First, sensing, which is to sense atrial or ventricular depolarisation, and secondly, pacing, which is to depolarise the atria or ventricles. Identifying the basic pacing system of a pacemaker can be done by an international three-letter identification code. The first letter is the chamber that is paced and the second letter is the chambers that are sensed. The letters used to identify the chambers are V = ventricle, A = atria and D = dual (atria and ventricle). The third letter is what the device does in response to a sensed event. I = inhibits a pacing stimulus, T = triggers a pacing stimulus, D here is restricted to dual chamber systems, but D here (in the third letter) means atrial inhibition and ventricular triggering. If the pulse generator senses a ventricular event, however, the pacemaker will inhibit its ventricular trigger. Finally, O = nothing. Pacemaker implantation can be performed under sedation with local anaesthesia and is usually free of complications. Pocket-related complications include a pocket haematoma or local infection. Lead-related complications include a haemothorax or pneumothorax when attaining subclavian access, arrhythmias, chamber perforation resulting in tamponade, access vein thrombosis and infection of pacer lead causing endocarditis. Complications related to pacemaker generator include infection, malfunction, pacemaker-mediated tachycardia and pacemaker syndrome. Batteries last between 5 and 10 years.

9 Pacemaker clinic follow-up is very important in all patients who have received a pacemaker. All patients should have early surveillance within 6 weeks of a pacemaker insertion. At each follow-up, a history is taken for fatigue, chest pain, dyspnoea, palpitations and presyncope or syncope. A full medication review and cardiovascular exam is conducted. Then the device is interrogated. All of this information is obtained to ensure optimisation of the device and to prevent complications. If the device is working well, follow-up can be extended to a yearly basis.

CASE 7: Pericarditis

History

- A **43-year-old Caucasian female** [1] presents with a **two-day history** [2] of acute **sharp central chest pain** [3].
- She complains of **concomitant shortness of breath** [4], with the pain particularly **worse upon deep inspiration** [5].
- There is **no associated nausea, vomiting or diaphoresis** [6].
- Upon further questioning she reveals that **the pain is worst when lying flat, it is relieved by sitting forward** [7] and she has been **struggling to sleep at night** [8].

- However, she reports **no paroxysmal nocturnal dyspnoea or orthopnoea** [9].
- She reports having had a **recent viral illness around 3 weeks ago** [10] but otherwise has been well.
- She reports **nil trauma** [11] to the chest.
- She has **not travelled overseas** [12] in the last few years.
- She has **no history of any cardiac issues** [13].
- She has no known **renal disease** [14] that she is aware of.
- She describes **no unintentional weight loss, night sweats or rigors** [15].

[1] Pericarditis in young patients is typically idiopathic or secondary to infection. Increased age raises concern for more sinister causes such as malignancy. Furthermore, females are more commonly associated with autoimmune conditions and that must be considered as well. This could be the first presentation of a rheumatological condition.

[2] One-day history of chest pain suggests an acute aetiology. While it is unlikely to be acute coronary syndrome (ACS) if the patient has continued to have pain for two days, this still needs to be excluded. A thorough chest pain history will often help distinguish the underlying aetiology. It is important to assess if the chest pain is exertional and if there is any radiation. Pericarditis pain typically radiates to the trapezius ridge. Chest pain from pericarditis is typically fairly sudden in onset.

[3] Sharp central chest pain is a feature of pericarditis. However, it is important to distinguish it from pulmonary embolism, aortic dissection and more common causes such as musculoskeletal pain and gastro-oesophageal pain, which all can present with sharp central chest pain.

[4] Pericarditis often presents with an element of shortness of breath. This can be the result of the patient's inability to take deep breaths. However, dyspnoea does not form the major clinical manifestation of acute pericarditis. It is important to exclude other respiratory and cardiac causes of dyspnoea in such patients.

[5] Pleuritic chest pain is very classic for pericarditis. More than 95% of patients present with chest pain which is classically pleuritic. It can also be exacerbated when coughing; often it is good to ask the patient to take a deep breath in and ask if the intensity of the pain changes.

[6] Nausea, vomiting or diaphoresis raise concerns for ACS or a gastrointestinal (GI) aetiology. The absence of this in the setting of pleuritic chest pain is reassuring. The patient may have nausea, vomiting or infective symptoms in the days or weeks preceding which would be consistent with a viral aetiology.

[7] This is another very classical feature of chest pain consistent with acute pericarditis. Leaning forwards tends to reduce pressure on the parietal pericardium, particularly with inspiration, which is why patients experience relief in this position.

[8] Often due to positional chest pain, patients may struggle to sleep. It is important to ensure that there are no features of heart failure or obstructive airways disease contributing to the poor sleep.

[9] The absence of PND and orthopnoea is reassuring that there is no feature of heart failure and pulmonary oedema. This is important to exclude, given the history of breathlessness presented in the vignette.

[10] A viral prodrome with flu-like respiratory or GI symptoms is typical in viral aetiology. Nonetheless, it is important to screen for other causes of pericarditis so that a major underlying condition is not missed. This is consistent with the diagnosis of acute pericarditis and often patients will have had a recent viral illness.

11 Trauma must be excluded in all patients presenting with pericarditis or any pleuritic chest pain. It is estimated that 12% of large symptomatic pericardial effusions are caused by trauma. In the setting of acute trauma, the patient might need urgent intervention to prevent haemodynamic compromise.

12 Recent long-haul travel is a risk factor for pulmonary embolism in a patient presenting with pleuritic chest pain. Additionally, tuberculous pericarditis is an important complication of tuberculosis (TB). TB is extremely uncommon in developed countries unless the patient has had exposure to someone with it or recently travelled abroad to a TB-endemic area. The diagnosis can be difficult to establish and is often delayed or missed, leading to constrictive pericarditis along with increased mortality. Hence, recent travel is a screening question for tuberculous pericarditis as well.

13 It is important to screen for known cardiac disease. Even a past history of pericarditis is vital, as often these patients have failed first-line management of pericarditis. Constrictive pericarditis is a chronic disease which is the result of scarring and loss of normal elasticity of the pericardial sac. Constrictive pericarditis is typically chronic and this is essential information to know.

14 Patients with end-stage renal disease may develop pericarditis and/or pericardial effusions. Occasionally it may even result in constrictive pericarditis. Two forms of pericarditis in renal failure have been previously described: uraemic pericarditis and dialysis-associated pericarditis. Uraemic pericarditis results from inflammation of the membranes of the pericardial sac. Dialysis pericarditis is observed in patients on maintenance dialysis who have insufficient dialysis and/or fluid overload.

15 It is important to screen for underlying causes for pericarditis in a patient. Causes such as malignancy, metabolic (uraemia-, myxoedema- and dialysis-associated), secondary to radiation, drugs, toxins, autoimmune or infectious, need to be briefly screened for.

Examination

- The patient **doesn't appear generally unwell** [1] and is sitting in bed relatively comfortably.
- There is no evidence of **increased work of breathing** [2] or **diaphoresis** [3] on general examination. The patient is **tachycardic** [4] with a heart rate of 110bpm and **tachypnoeic** [4] with a RR of 24.
- She is **saturating 96% on air** [5] and **BP is 105/65mmHg** [6].
- The patient is **afebrile** [7] with a temperature of 36.7°C.
- There is **no radio-radio delay** and **strong peripheral pulses are palpated** [8].
- The **JVP is not elevated** [9].

- **Kussmaul's sign** [10] is absent.
- **Pulsus paradoxus** [11] is not observed upon inspiration.
- On auscultation of the heart, a superficial scratchy sound, likely representing a **pericardial rub** [12], is heard loudest at the left lower sternal border.
- On auscultation of the lungs, **reduced air entry is heard bibasally** [13] but otherwise **vesicular breathing** [13] is heard.
- The abdominal examination is unremarkable, with **no hepatomegaly or ascites** [14].
- There are **no signs of peripheral oedema** [15].

1 The patient appears systemically well and not haemodynamically unwell. This is reassuring that the patient does not have a significant pericardial effusion resulting in reduced cardiac output. The likelihood is a large pulmonary embolism and aortic dissection is also reduced.

2 Increased work of breathing is commonly a sign of the condition having a respiratory component such as asthma, chronic obstructive pulmonary disease (COPD), pulmonary oedema, pneumothorax and pulmonary embolism. Patients typically have normal work of breathing, if not shallow breathing to reduce the pain.

3 Diaphoresis is typically not seen during pericarditis unless the underlying aetiology is acute infection. Diaphoresis may be seen during ACS, an important chest pain differential that needs to be considered throughout.

4 Tachycardia can often be seen in patients with pericarditis, often secondary to pain. This needs to be monitored closely, especially if the patient starts becoming hypotensive. Mild tachypnoea is also commonly seen in patients with pericarditis due to the pleuritic nature of the pain, with patients only taking shallow breaths in.

5 Normal saturations are reassuring in this patient, suggesting there isn't a perfusion mismatch or a primary aetiology leading to hypoxia. Hypoxia is very uncommon in patients with pericarditis unless it leads to significant pericardial effusion or poor cardiac output leading to pulmonary oedema.

6 The patient is not hypotensive; since they are young this is likely to be their normal blood pressure. Hypotension would be concerning for the presence of a large pericardial effusion, leading to impaired cardiac output.

7 Fever in a patient with pleuritic chest pain warrants the exclusion of pneumonia, pleurisy, spontaneous bacterial pleuritis, hepatic or pulmonary abscess, myocarditis, infective exacerbation of COPD, etc. It is rare for patients with pericarditis to present with a primary infection at the same time.

8 It is imperative to exclude aortic dissection in any patients presenting with sharp pleuritic chest pain. It is a life-threatening diagnosis and the absence of the above features is reassuring that this is more consistent with pericarditis.

9 An elevated JVP is found on the vast majority of patients with constrictive pericarditis – this is due to impaired right ventricular filling. The abnormal pericardium does not expand to accommodate increased venous return to the right heart during inspiration, leading to a raised JVP. A normal JVP is suggestive that there is no significant component, if any, of constrictive pericarditis present.

10 Kussmaul's sign is another sign present in patients with constrictive pericarditis, but it does not distinguish constrictive pericarditis from right heart failure or severe tricuspid regurgitation.

11 Pulsus paradoxus is also a sign of constrictive pericarditis but occurs in fewer than 20% of cases. It is a rare sign in which there is an exaggerated drop in systolic blood pressure during inspiration. It may be seen more commonly in patients with concomitant pericardial effusion of coexisting pulmonary disease.

12 A pericardial rub is a highly specific sign for acute pericarditis. Pericardial friction rubs are typically triphasic with a superficial scratchy quality. The rub may be localised or widespread but is typically best heard over the left sternal border. Manoeuvres to assist auscultation include application of firm pressure with the diaphragm, auscultating during suspended respiration and with the patient leaning forward. Nevertheless, pericardial friction rub is a major clinical manifestation of acute pericarditis.

13 Reduced air entry at the bases may suggest atelectasis at the base of the lungs. This may be due to the patient's inability to take deep breaths in due to the pain. Nil additional breath sounds are heard, suggestive of infective changes. However, it may also represent pleural effusions secondary to aortic dissection or tamponade.

14 Hepatomegaly or ascites would represent significant right heart failure or constrictive pericarditis. The absence of these suggests this is likely an acute pericarditis presentation, as opposed to chronic. Other differentials would include an intrahepatic pathology with irritation of the diaphragm causing chest/shoulder tip pain.

15 Once again peripheral oedema would be suggestive of right heart failure. This would not typically be expected in acute pericarditis, given the majority of pericarditis is usually transient and self-limiting.

Investigations

- A 12-lead ECG shows **diffuse ST elevation** [1] with **reciprocal ST segment depression in leads aVR and V1** [2].
- Mild **PR segment elevation** [3] is noted in lead aVR with **PR depression** [3] in V6.
- **No Q waves** [4] are observed.
- There is **no AV block or bundle branch block morphology** [5].
- A chest X-ray is requested, which shows a **normal cardiac silhouette** [6] and **normal lung fields** [7].
- Formal laboratory bloods are requested: the full blood count reveals an elevated **white blood cell count** [8] of 13.4 x 10^9 cells per litre.
- **Serial troponins** [9] are negative and the patient has a **normal UEC** [10].
- An elevated **C-reactive protein** level (65mg/L) and **ESR** (45mm/hr) is observed [11].
- **ANA titres, rheumatoid factor and complement levels** [12] are negative.
- **HIV serology** and **QuantiFERON TB assay** [13] are both negative.
- A bedside echocardiogram reveals a **trivial pericardial effusion** [14] with **normal systolic and valvular function** [15]. **Pericardial thickness is normal**, with **normal filling during early diastole** [15].

1 The causes of ST elevation are numerous, including acute myocardial infarction, coronary vasospasm, LBBB morphology, left ventricular hypertrophy, ventricular aneurysm, raised intracranial pressure, takotsubo cardiomyopathy, benign early repolarisation and finally pericarditis. Global ST segment elevation is typically seen in pericarditis with the typical concave/saddleback ST elevation.

Typically in STEMI patients, the ST elevation is convex as opposed to concave in the case of pericarditis.

2 You do not typically get reciprocal ST depression in pericarditis; however, there is typically ST depression in aVR and occasionally V1 in acute pericarditis. ST elevation in an acute STEMI is normally limited to anatomical groupings with reciprocal ST changes seen.

3 PR elevation in aVR and PR depression in other leads is seen frequently in pericarditis due to concomitant atrial current of injury. These findings are rarely seen in acute STEMI and it is a way to help differentiate the two entities.

4 The progression of ST elevation to Q waves would be suggestive of acute myocardial infarction with completion of infarct. This would be highly concerning for AMI as opposed to pericarditis.

5 The presence of AV block, bundle branch block pathology or QT prolongation would raise concerns regarding acute MI as opposed to pericarditis. These are complications that may result in myocardial ischaemia and should not typically be seen in pericarditis.

6 An enlarged cardiac silhouette could suggest cardiac myopathy or the presence of the pericardial effusion. For the cardiac silhouette to be enlarged, at least 200ml of pericardial fluid must accumulate. This would be unusual for it to be secondary acute pericarditis.

7 Normal lung space is consistent with acute pericarditis. Acute pulmonary oedema or consolidation can often be seen on CXR in patients presenting with acute chest pain.

8 An elevated white blood cell count (WCC) is commonly seen in pericarditis, as it represents a localised inflammatory process. It is important to evaluate the differential count and ensure it is primarily neutrophilia. A raised WCC can also represent acute infection, so it is important to screen for this in the overall assessment of the patient.

9 Troponins are completed to exclude acute myocardial infarction. However, acute pericarditis may be associated with increased cardiac biomarkers such as troponin. Such patients typically have myopericarditis; however, distinguishing acutely from a STEMI may be difficult, especially if there is a large troponin leak.

10 Uraemic pericarditis is a common cause in patients with chronic kidney disease. A normal urea, electrolytes and creatinine (UEC) is reassuring that the pericarditis is not secondary to renal disease.

11 CRP and ESR are typically elevated in acute pericarditis as they are markers of inflammation. The levels will usually rise proportionate to the intensity of the disease. While an elevation in these markers supports the diagnosis, they are not sensitive or specific for acute pericarditis. Furthermore, in the initial phase of acute pericarditis they may remain normal.

12 A basic rheumatological screen is often completed in young women who are otherwise well. Acute pericarditis is very rarely the initial presentation of systemic lupus erythematosus. Additionally, even if the antinuclear antibody (ANA) level is positive it is a non-specific test and it is important to evaluate how strongly positive it is by assessing the titres.

13 HIV and TB can very rarely present with acute pericarditis. Testing for TB is most helpful in immunocompromised or HIV-positive patients, in areas where TB is endemic or if they have had recent exposure.

14 A trivial or small pericardial effusion is very common in acute pericarditis. However, the absence of pericardial effusion does not exclude the diagnosis. It is also useful in excluding large pericardial effusion causing cardiac tamponade, particularly in hypotensive patients.

15 Normal systolic and valvular function is reassuring in this patient. In patients with constrictive pericarditis, echocardiography can reveal increased pericardial thickness along with bilateral enlargement, septal bounce, dilatation of the inferior vena cava and hypermobile atrioventricular valves. Furthermore, echocardiography can be useful if purulent pericarditis is suspected or if there are concerns regarding myocarditis. Finally, it is also important for the assessment of cardiomegaly to assess the patient for cardiomyopathy.

Management

Short-term

The likely diagnosis in this patient is **idiopathic or viral pericarditis** [1]. The patient is commenced on combination **NSAIDs** [2] and **colchicine** [3]. **Glucocorticoids are not indicated** [4] in this patient initially, but if the pain does not settle, this might be required. **Pericardiocentesis is not indicated** [5] in this patient. The patient was **observed for a short period** [6] to monitor for response to treatment and to **ensure no complications** [6]. A **proton pump inhibitor** [7] can be considered to minimise side-effects. Education should be provided to **avoid strenuous physical activity** [8].

Follow-up and ongoing treatment

Since the patient **does not exhibit any high risk features** [9], they would be suitable for discharge with **tapering of treatment** [10] monitored by their GP. Education is provided to the patient regarding **reasons to re-present** [11] to hospital and the resolution of symptoms as per the natural course of the disease. The **overall prognosis** [12] is quite good in the setting of acute idiopathic or viral pericarditis.

1 When treating pericarditis it is important to establish what the underlying diagnosis is. The diagnosis helps the treatment to be tailored accordingly. The most common cause is idiopathic or viral and this is usually treated symptomatically.

2 For all patients with idiopathic or viral pericarditis, NSAIDs are the mainstay of initial treatment. NSAIDs alone appear to be effective in 70–80% of pericarditis cases presumed to be of this aetiology. Ibuprofen, aspirin or indomethacin are the typical NSAIDs used to both reduce inflammation and relieve pain in most patients. However, there is no evidence that NSAIDs actually alter the natural history of acute pericarditis.

3 Colchicine is typically offered initially in conjunction with NSAIDs in the absence of any contraindication for patients with idiopathic or viral pericarditis. Colchicine, when used in conjunction with NSAIDs, reduces symptoms and the rate of recurrent pericarditis. Colchicine should be administered for a total of 3 months for patients with first episode acute pericarditis. Interestingly, colchicine can also be efficacious for pericarditis caused by systemic inflammatory disease or post cardiac injury syndromes.

4 As a general rule, glucocorticoids should be used for initial treatment of acute pericarditis in patients with contraindications to NSAIDs in this setting. Steroids can also be considered in certain aetiologies such as systemic inflammatory disease, pregnancy and renal failure. When glucocorticoids are used, they should be at the lowest dose possible due to long-term side-effects. Steroids may also be considered in patients who failed initial therapy with NSAID plus colchicine, which suggests refractory pericarditis.

5 Pericardiocentesis is only considered for significant pericardial effusion or if there are signs of cardiac tamponade. Most patients with uncomplicated low risk acute pericarditis are managed effectively with medical therapy alone. Other indications for drainage may be if there is suspicion of a malignancy or bacterial aetiology causing moderate–large effusion, frequent/highly symptomatic recurrences of pericarditis with effusion or if there is evidence of constrictive pericarditis.

6 Given the patient has a clear history of a recent viral prodrome, acute onset of chest pain and convincing ECG changes, they can safely be treated on an outpatient basis once the initial evaluation is complete. NSAIDs and colchicine should be commenced in the ED, with most patients responding to this to some degree within the department.

7 NSAIDs can cause GI side-effects such as gastritis and ulcers, particularly when used for a long period or at high doses. Hence, any patient with other patient risk factors for GI toxicity (such as history of peptic ulcer disease, age >65 or concurrent use of aspirin, corticosteroids or anticoagulants) should be provided gastroprotection in the form of proton pump inhibitors.

8 Strenuous activity may trigger recurrence of symptoms. Such activity should be avoided until symptom resolution and normalisation of biomarkers. In the case of myopericarditis, withdrawal from competitive sport is recommended for 6 months and return only after normalisation of inflammatory markers, ECG and echocardiogram.

9 High risk patients with pericarditis should be admitted to hospital and evaluated thoroughly. Features of high risk pericarditis include: fever, subacute course, features of cardiac tamponade or large pericardial effusion, immunosuppressed patients, acute trauma, anticoagulation therapy, failure to improve with NSAID and colchicine therapy after 7 days, or elevated cardiac troponin.

10 Duration of treatment is based on resolution of symptoms and normalisation of the CRP. An approach to tapering can be weekly monitoring of CRP using high dose NSAIDs until resolution of symptoms occurs (typically around 2 weeks) and normalisation of CRP, at which point the tapering begins. Colchicine should continue for 3 months.

11 If the use of NSAIDs and colchicine for one week has not resulted in an improvement in symptoms or leads to clinical deterioration, this suggests that a cause other than idiopathic or viral pericarditis is present. In this case it is suggested that the patient presents to the hospital. Furthermore, if progression or change in the nature of chest pain or associated symptoms occur then the patient should also present urgently for further evaluation.

12 Patients with idiopathic or viral pericarditis have a good long-term prognosis. These are rarely complicated by cardiac tamponade. Approximately 1% of patients with acute idiopathic pericarditis develop constrictive pericarditis. It is estimated that 15–30% of patients not treated with colchicine develop recurrent or incessant disease. Finally, female gender is also associated with increased risk of complications, possibly due to the higher frequency of underlying autoimmune aetiologies.

CASE 8: ST elevation myocardial infarction

History

- A **56-year-old Caucasian male** [1] is brought in by ambulance to the ED with **sudden onset central crushing chest pain radiating to his jaw whilst gardening** [2].
- He reports associated **dyspnoea, diaphoresis and palpitations** [3].
- The pain has been mildly relieved with **paracetamol, IV morphine and sublingual GTN** [4] administered by the paramedics.

- The patient has a significant past medical history of **T2DM on insulin, hypercholesterolaemia, hypertension, morbid obesity with a BMI of 46 and a 30 pack year smoking history** [5].
- The **patient's father** [6] had multiple coronary artery bypass surgeries in the past and died from an AMI at the age of 70.
- On further questioning the patient reports having had **worsening chest pain in the past couple of months when walking the dog** [7].

[1] Increasing age and male gender are non-modifiable risk factors for coronary artery disease. Note that ST elevation myocardial infarction (STEMI) can occur in people who are relatively young as well.

[2] This is a history of typical chest pain. Typical features are of sudden or acute onset, central location, pain that is pressure-like in nature, radiates to the arms and the jaw, aggravated by emotional stress or exertion and relieved with rest or nitroglycerin. Atypical features of chest pain may include radiation through to the back, no association with emotional stress or exertion, no relief with nitrates, pleuritic chest pain, positional chest pain or pain that is reproducible on palpation and slow onset over hours; an alternative diagnosis should be considered. It is wise to note, however, that patients can present with STEMIs despite an atypical history.

[3] Commonly patients with STEMIs will have associated symptoms with their chest pain. Diaphoresis occurs from the hyperadrenergic drive. Dyspnoea can occur either from acute pulmonary oedema resultant from the decreased left ventricular ejection fraction or from hypoxaemia due to decreased cardiac output. Palpitations can occur either from palpitations from other arrhythmias that may occur in the setting of myocardial ischaemia, e.g. supraventricular tachycardia, atrial fibrillation, or more concerningly, conscious ventricular tachycardia. Other associated symptoms include nausea or vomiting.

[4] Pain from STEMIs is more severe than with stable angina. At this stage, the patient would have already received a loading dose of dual antiplatelets, paracetamol, glyceryl trinitrate (GTN) and intravenous opioids. This pain regime would be enough to appease most cases of stable angina.

[5] It is important to elicit on history the presence of cardiovascular risk factors, as originally described by the seminal Framingham study. This not only raises the clinical suspicion of a cardiovascular event, but also provides the doctor with risk factors to optimise in the long term for aggressive secondary prevention. This patient has a high risk profile for acute MI. He has advanced diabetes (on insulin), has a high body mass index (BMI) and is a smoker. Smoking not only accelerates plaque deposition, but encourages a pro-inflammatory state which promotes plaque rupture.

[6] Again, family history is a staple part of the cardiovascular history. Ischaemic heart disease is a complex phenotype that has strong genetic components. The patient's father had severe ischaemic heart disease warranting multiple bypass grafts and ultimately succumbed to his illness. It is obvious here that ischaemic heart disease is also this patient's most prognostically significant illness.

[7] It is useful to see if the patient has had ischaemic-sounding chest pain in the past. In this particular case, the patient has had crescendo angina in the lead up to his presentation which indicates that he has had symptomatic obstructive coronary artery disease for a while, and it should raise suspicion of more than one stenosis in his coronaries.

Examination

- **From the end of the bed** [1], the patient has a large body habitus and looks **unwell** [2].
- He is alert and oriented. He is also **diaphoretic, clammy and has mildly increased work of breathing** [3].
- His heart rate is **110bpm** [4] and regular.
- Blood pressure is **160/70mmHg** [5].

- Respiratory rate is 24, O_2 saturation is **90% on air** [6] and he is afebrile. JVP is 4cm. The apex beat is not displaced.
- Heart sounds are **dual with no murmurs** [7] and the **lungs reveal bibasal crepitations** [8].
- There is no evidence of **peripheral oedema** [9].

[1] Throughout clinical practice you will get a good sense of whether a patient is sick via the proverbial 'end-of-the-bed-o-gram'. Be sure not to underestimate the power of observation, as simple observation will give you lots of information in a short space of time.

[2] A patient with typical chest pain who looks unwell should immediately raise the concern of ACS. Patients with stable angina rarely look unwell.

[3] Although it is easy to overstate one's pain, it is impossible to fake autonomic signs such as diaphoresis and clamminess. These are objective signs of ACS that you should always look for when assessing patients from the end of the bed.

[4] The approach here, in this critical care situation, would be to assess the patient from A-B-C to D. Here, the most deranged vital sign is the tachycardia. This is secondary to sympathetic nervous system activation in the setting of severe chest pain. It will be pertinent to obtain an ECG to assess the cardiac rhythm.

[5] The patient is hypertensive. This is helpful on two counts. First, we can deduce that the patient has adequate end-organ perfusion with this blood pressure (meaning there is no haemodynamic compromise). Secondly, the patient has adrenergic activation either from pain or as a compensatory mechanism to increase cardiac output. For any patient presenting with a STEMI you should look for signs of acute cardiogenic shock, which would be hypotension (sBP <90mmHg), signs of end-organ hypoperfusion (worsening mentation, cyanosis, oliguria or acute kidney injury (AKI), ischaemic hepatitis and rising lactate).

[6] Hypoxia can either occur from pulmonary oedema or from decreased cardiac output to the tissues. Hypoxia is not a feature of stable angina or unstable angina. A cardiorespiratory examination should be performed on any patient with hypoxia in the emergency department.

[7] There are different murmurs and additional heart sounds that can occur in the context of an ST elevation myocardial infarction. In terms of murmurs, you can have acute mitral regurgitation with STEMIs due to ischaemic papillary muscle dysfunction or partial rupture. This is classically seen 2–10 days post STEMI and is associated more with inferior STEMIs than anterior STEMIs. The presentation may range from silent to volume overload. With regard to additional heart sounds, you may hear an S4 gallop. This occurs when a non-compliant and stiffened left ventricle receives blood from the atrial contraction. Recall that diastole is a metabolically active phase of the cardiac cycle and left ventricular relaxation is impaired in the ischaemic muscle.

[8] Bibasal crepitations are features of left heart failure which would be classical of anterolateral STEMIs (as they affect the left ventricle). With decreased cardiac output, there is increased left ventricular end-diastolic volume which corresponds to an increased left ventricular end-diastolic pressure. This in turn results in increased pressure in the pulmonary veins and the pulmonary vasculature that causes pulmonary oedema. This is what is causing dyspnoea and bibasal crepitations in our patient.

[9] With no peripheral oedema, we can deduce that the patient does not have features of right heart failure. To be more thorough, you can check for a pulsatile liver, hepatomegaly suggestive of congestive hepatopathy and an elevated JVP.

Investigations

- 12-lead ECG shows 5mm horizontal **ST segment elevation in leads V1 through to V4** [1] and 3mm **ST segment depression in leads II, III, aVF** [2].
- Serial troponins revealed a **troponin peak of 8236ng/L and CK of 923mmol/L** [3].

- A **chest X-ray** [4] showed a normal cardiothoracic ratio, mildly increased interstitial markings with mild bilateral blunting of the costodiaphragmatic angles.
- Full blood examination revealed an **Hb of 130g/L, WCC of 15 x 10^9 cells per litre, and platelet count of 350 x 10^9 per litre** [5].

- Urea, electrolytes and creatinine were **normal** [6] , K is 4.3mmol/L.
- Fasting lipids on the following morning revealed total cholesterol of **4.5mmol/L, triglycerides of 2.4mmol/L, LDL of 2.4mmol/L, HDL of 1mmol/L and LDL:HDL ratio of 2.4** [7] .
- HbA1c is **9.2%** [8] .
- Upon arrival at the ED, the patient was wheeled urgently to the **angiography lab** [9] .
- **Right-sided radial arterial access was obtained**

on first pass [10] and the coronary angiogram revealed a **90% stenosis of the mid-distal left anterior descending (LAD) artery** [11] and other mild disease in the left circumflex (LCx) and right coronary artery (RCA).

- A transthoracic echocardiogram four weeks after the ST elevation myocardial infarction demonstrated **moderate hypokinesis of the anterior wall** [12] and an **LVEF of 45–50%** [13] . The estimated pulmonary artery pressure was normal.

[1] The ECG is the single most helpful investigation in this situation. It is point of care, quick and gives you information regarding the vascular territories of the heart. You will also gain an insight into any history of heart disease such as PR depression suggestive of atrial infarction, pathological Q waves indicative of prior infarctions, T wave inversion, left ventricular hypertrophy (from hypertension or from valvular pathology), left axis deviation, LBBB, other atrial or ventricular arrhythmias and of course, the heart rate. Here, a horizontal ST segment elevation in the anterior leads suggests a lesion in either the left main or the LAD artery. If there is corresponding ST elevation in aVR as well, think of a left main coronary artery lesion.

[2] In a STEMI, you will have reciprocal changes. If there is an infarction in the anterior leads, expect reciprocal changes in the inferior leads. This is evident here with depression in leads II, III and aVF. A good mnemonic to remember which STEMI causes which reciprocal ST depression is **PAILS:**

Posterior STEMI – anterior reciprocal ST depression
Anterior STEMI – inferior reciprocal ST depression
Inferior STEMI – lateral reciprocal ST depression
Lateral STEMI – inferior or septal reciprocal ST depression
Septal STEMI – posterior reciprocal ST depression

[3] A portable chest X-ray may or may not get done acutely as the acute goal is reperfusion. In this patient, there are signs of fluid overload. There is increased interstitial marking and blunting of the costodiaphragmatic angles suggestive of fluid in the diaphragmatic recesses. This is a poor prognostic sign in a STEMI and is demonstrative of not only an infarcted heart, but a poorly functioning, compromised left ventricle. You may have some ancillary signs here such as increased cardiothoracic ratio suggestive of cardiomegaly, and some concomitant signs of chronic obstructive airways disease; patients who have STEMIs often have significant smoking histories or other incidentalomas.

[4] The troponin and creatine kinase is obviously very elevated, suggestive of an MI. Troponin is very sensitive and can rise in any cause of myocardial insult, e.g. right ventricular strain from a saddle pulmonary embolus or pericarditis. A troponin level this high, however, is usually only indicative of infarction.

[5] You can have an elevated white cell count (predominantly neutrophilia) in the setting of an acute STEMI. This would be a sign of generalised inflammation in the body from ischaemic damage, as opposed to an infection. The haemoglobin is normal; frequently anaemia may be a contributing factor to an ACS. It is also important to check for thrombocytopenia as the patient will need an invasive procedure (angiogram) and can help stratify bleeding risk.

[6] UECs are another important investigation as angiograms, like any other fluoroscopic procedure, require the use of radio-opaque contrast. Contrast is renally cleared and even though the risk of contrast-induced nephropathy, subsequent acute tubular necrosis and acute renal failure in a normal kidney is low, the risk is not zero. If a patient has chronic kidney disease, the decision for angiogram would only be made if they would also be supported by a form of renal replacement therapy such as haemodialysis. This would require urgent liaising with the consulting renal team.

[7] You should perform fasting lipids and an HbA1c on all patients presenting with a STEMI. There is a direct stepwise increased risk of major adverse cardiac events (MACE) between a patient's lipid and HbA1c status. The patient is hyperlipidaemic, which will require optimisation of his lipid-lowering therapy.

[8] The patient's HbA1c is 9.2%. He has a past history of T2DM on insulin and oral hypoglycaemics. Whenever someone is on insulin for type 2 diabetes, one should understand that their underlying pathology is advanced. It is obvious that their glycaemic control is suboptimal and that their glycaemic control will have to be optimised during their inpatient stay. It is not uncommon to unveil a diagnosis of diabetes during a cardiology admission for a myocardial infarction. The cut-off for diagnosing diabetes is an HbA1c >6.5%. Otherwise the traditional oral glucose tolerance test can be performed.

[9] After initial stabilisation, the catheterisation lab staff should be notified and the patient be wheeled to the angiography lab urgently. Time is muscle!

10 For an angiogram you can attain arterial access via the radial artery or the femoral artery. Here a transradial approach was attained on first pass. Each access has its benefits and downsides. With the transradial approach, there is reduced bleeding risk, smaller haematomas, decreased hospitalisation and lower rates of vascular complications. Additionally, patients usually prefer the radial approach. The downside to the transradial approach is that it requires more contrast and is harder to cannulate. The classical transfemoral approach is being used less because of the advantages of the transradial approach, but it is still much easier to access, the patient receives less radiation time and less contrast is needed for adequate opacification of the coronary arteries. There is, however, a need for bed rest, increased risk of vascular complications such as haematoma, pseudoaneurysm/arterial dissection and the need to screen for relative contraindications. There are no true absolute contraindications, but a transradial approach should be considered in patients with:

- peripheral vascular disease
- active groin infection
- prior surgery or radiation therapy to the groin

- morbid obesity
- presence of iliac or aortoiliac aneurysms
- previous vascular complications such as arteriovenous fistulae, dissection or ischaemic limb from femoral arterial access.

11 Once access has been attained and the catheter is near the coronary ostia, contrast can be injected to investigate for the culprit lesion. The electrocardiogram already gave a clue as to where the culprit lesion may be. Here it was the mid-distal LAD artery. It is important to assess the other coronary arteries, especially in the diabetic patient, to proactively look for stenoses that may result in further infarcts down the track.

12 After the acute inciting myocardial infarction, the patient now has a regional wall motion abnormality. This is because the infarcted muscle has been replaced by fibrotic tissue.

13 The regional wall motion abnormality has now mildly affected the ejection fraction of the left ventricle. Although mild, without further aggressive secondary prevention the patient may be at risk of developing heart failure in the future.

Management

Immediate

Resuscitation

The immediate priority in management of a STEMI is to assess the patient and ensure they are **adequately resuscitated** [1]. The patient requires no airway adjuncts, and no airway manoeuvres were necessary as they are maintaining their airway. They should be administered oxygen via a Hudson mask to aim for saturations above 94%. Given that the patient was only mildly tachycardic and there was no hypotension, fluid challenge does not need to be considered. Rather, given the pulmonary oedema, a stat IV furosemide dose should be administered and an indwelling catheter inserted for accurate fluid balance assessment. Prior to being wheeled to the catheterisation lab, patients need to be placed on **cardiac monitoring** [2].

Analgesia

For analgesia the patient requires multiple sublingual GTN sprays, paracetamol 1g stat and 5mg of IV morphine to start. It is important to assess the patient ongoing as they may require more opiate analgesia.

Activation of catheterisation lab

The on-call cardiology registrar needs to be notified and the **catheterisation lab activated** [3]. There is no revascularisation without a catheterisation team. Usually the team consists of the cardiology registrar, interventional cardiology fellow, the interventional cardiologist and other ancillary staff. They will consent the patient and take them to the catheterisation lab.

Revascularisation

Rapid reperfusion is the cornerstone of STEMI management. This can be achieved either by **thrombolysis** [4], **percutaneous coronary intervention (PCI)** [5] with either drug-eluting stents (DES) or bare metal stents (BMS) or with **emergency coronary artery bypass graft (CABG) surgery** [6]. Whilst they are on the way to hospital, they should receive a loading dose of **dual antiplatelets** [7] (aspirin 300mg and either ticagrelor 180mg or clopidogrel 300mg). If the time frame from diagnosis to STEMI is less than 90 minutes, fibrinolysis is not advised as revascularisation will be attained promptly. Fibrinolysis is indicated if there is no access to a catheterisation lab or there are significant delays to PCI. If PCI is attained, it is important to note the degree of flow via a **TIMI score and the door to balloon time** [8].

Post STEMI care

Routine post STEMI care is bed rest until the next day and continuation of dual antiplatelets. In the time post STEMI, the patient needs to remain on continuous cardiac monitoring and at each review, be assessed for **complications from arterial access and myocardial ischaemia** [9].

Long-term

Risk factor modification

This patient requires optimisation of their lipid-lowering regime, hypertension and glycaemic control. With regard to **lipid-lowering therapy** [10], they should be commenced on a medium to high dose statin.

Hypertension [11] should be managed with an ACEi or ARB as first-line agents. **Glycaemic control** [12] can be improved by reinforcing the importance of lifestyle modifications, up-titrating existing oral hypoglycaemic agents and insulin regimes. If the patient is an **active smoker** [13], give them advice on smoking cessation and have ongoing follow-up with the GP.

Chronic remodelling

In addition to an ACEi/ARB, the patient should also be commenced on a beta blocker. These prevent chronic fibrous remodelling of the heart post STEMI and improve mortality.

Cardiac rehabilitation

Finally, the patient should be referred to **cardiac rehabilitation** [14] on discharge, with ongoing outpatient follow-up with the cardiology department.

---

1 Ideally, resuscitation should occur simultaneously as the patient is heading to the catheterisation lab. The approach to the STEMI patient is the same approach you would have for any critically ill patient, via the ABCD approach. Assess the airway for patency and the patient's overall mentation. In this case, the airway was well protected and patent. With regard to breathing, oxygen saturations were aimed at 94% (too high an oxygen level can result in hyperoxygenation reperfusion injury of the myocardium) with a Hudson mask. With regard to circulation, the patient received furosemide for volume correction in the acute instance.

2 Due to risk of atrial and ventricular arrhythmias in STEMIs, all patients receive continuous cardiac monitoring for the first 24–48 hours post STEMI.

3 Notifying the STEMI team is paramount in minimising the door to stent time. Each health network will have its own means of activating the catheterisation lab. It may be a 'code STEMI' or calling the on-call cardiology registrar. If the patient is located in a rural environment, the paramedics will transfer the patient to the most appropriate medical centre and pre-notify them prior to arrival.

4 Thrombolysis is the dissolution of a thrombus/embolus. It is utilised for treatment of a STEMI when there is no feasible means of attaining a primary PCI in a timely manner. Common agents are streptokinase, alteplase and tenecteplase. The choice of which thrombolytic agent to use will depend on local protocol. Success of thrombolysis increases the sooner it is given, with success rates varying between 50 and 70% for patients who present within 4 hours. Success of thrombolysis will be characterised by resolution

of the ST segments. There are absolute contraindications to thrombolysis:

- active internal bleeding
- previous ischaemic stroke within 1 year
- previous haemorrhagic stroke at any time
- suspected aortic dissection
- any previous trauma or surgery in the past 2 weeks
- recent head trauma
- intracranial neoplasm.

5 Percutaneous coronary intervention is where a small catheter is placed across the culprit plaque lesion. From here, usually a balloon tip covered with a stent is also threaded through the plaque and inflated. This compresses the plaque and ensures stent expansion and apposition to the vessel wall. DES are most commonly used as they have lower in-stent restenosis rates than BMS. This does not correlate to any improved mortality rates, however. Most patients are suitable for primary PCI. Furthermore, rescue PCI can be performed in patients who have failed to respond to thrombolytic therapy. Overall it has better outcomes than thrombolysis: better left ventricular function, higher patency rate and less recurrent ischaemia. This is because thrombolysis does not affect the stenosis from the atheroma, only the thrombosis.

6 Emergency CABG is relatively uncommon. The general indications are for persistent pain despite primary PCI, high risk coronary anatomy (left main coronary artery or LAD ostial disease) and patients who have had previous CABGs that have now been occluded. Given the high morbidity, CABG is contraindicated in patients who are beyond 6 hours from the onset of their chest pain, due to risk of haemorrhage into their infarcted areas.

7 Dual antiplatelets are needed for their antithrombotic effects and are administered at their loading dose to enhance pharmacologic reperfusion and for subsequent secondary prevention post STEMI. Aspirin and either clopidogrel/ticagrelor have significant mortality and morbidity benefits in acute STEMIs.

8 The TIMI Coronary Grade Flow is a standardised grading system for coronary angiography. Grade 0 means no perfusion, grade 1 means penetration of obstructive lesion without perfusion, grade 2 means partial perfusion and grade 3 means complete perfusion. Most patients receiving PCI will attain TIMI grade 3 flow. There is a 'golden hour' within the door to balloon time where the potential for salvaging myocardium is the greatest. Nationally, we aim for a door to balloon time <90 minutes.

9 There are certain complications in the STEMI patient which we as clinicians need to look out for. Patients can develop multiple complications:
- Cardiogenic shock: which may require intra-aortic balloon counter-pulsation and left ventricular assist device insertion.
- Left ventricular aneurysm: most commonly affects the apex of the heart. The four usual concerns regarding a ventricular aneurysm are heart failure (as the aneurysmal segment is dyskinetic), left ventricular thrombus formation (placing the patient at increased risk of systemic thromboembolic events such as ischaemic limb and stroke), ventricular tachycardia (the ischaemic scar is a focus for ventricular arrhythmias) and ongoing angina.
- AF: can occur indirectly from a hyperadrenergic state or from direct atrial infarction.
- Ventricular fibrillation or tachycardia: which requires prompt direct current cardioversion.
- Ventricular septal defect: from infarction of the interventricular septum. The characteristic murmur in this instance would be a pansystolic murmur at the left lower sternal edge.
- Acute mitral regurgitation: from ischaemic rupture of the papillary muscles, most commonly after an inferior STEMI.
- Left ventricular free wall rupture: a fatal complication, which can occur when the left ventricular wall ruptures due to thinning during chronic remodelling.
- Right ventricular failure: leading to acute right heart failure resulting in hypotension and cardiogenic shock.
- Pericarditis or Dressler's syndrome: typical pericarditis can occur a few days after the initial infarction whilst Dressler's syndrome is an autoimmune pericarditis that can occur 3–4 weeks after the initial infarction.

10 Statins have pleiotropic effects in ischaemic heart disease. Not only do they serve as secondary prevention (or primary prevention) as part of lipid-lowering therapy, they have a role in plaque stabilisation and decreased rupture of an atherosclerotic plaque. Statins should be prescribed in all patients who have had a STEMI regardless of their initial lipid profile. For further lipid-lowering therapy one could consider ezetimibe, proprotein convertase subtilisin/kexin type 9 inhibitors (PCSK9 inhibitors) and fenofibrates. Targets for lipid therapy include low density lipoprotein (LDL) <1.8mmol/L, high density lipoprotein (HDL) >1mmol/L, total cholesterol <4mmol/L and triglycerides <2.0mmol/L.

11 Perindopril has a dual role: not only is it the medication of choice for control of hypertension, it also prevents chronic fibrous remodelling of the heart. Blood pressure aims are a systolic blood pressure of <140mmHg and diastolic blood pressure of <90mmHg. Other pharmacotherapy options include ARBs, dihydropyridine calcium channel blockers (CCBs), thiazides and moxonidine.

12 Glycaemic control is paramount in preventing further acceleration of the patient's ischaemic heart disease. As a general principle, reinforce lifestyle modification first, then seek to increase the oral hypoglycaemic regimen (metformin, sulfonylureas, etc.) prior to increasing insulin. If glycaemic control is difficult, a referral to the consulting endocrinology service may be made. Patients should be followed up with their GP or an endocrinologist.

13 Smoking cessation and lifestyle modification are much more important than pharmacotherapy; however, this is very hard to implement. National guidelines suggest 150 minutes of moderate intensity exercise a week, but this is hard to fulfil, especially if the patient has a busy job, children to look after and is generally unmotivated. Having a good GP will improve adherence to therapy and develop a positive therapeutic relationship that will change outcomes for the patient.

14 Finally, on discharge the patient will need cardiac rehabilitation to help them receive further education regarding their cardiovascular health, help assist in return to work and other occupational activities and promote lifestyle modification.

CASE 9: Stable angina

History

- A **60-year-old male** [1] **accountant** [2] of **Indian descent** [3] complains of **central crushing chest pain** [4] radiating down both arms **after running** [5] to the train station.
- There were **no other associated symptoms** [6].
- He reports the pain was **relieved with rest** [7].
- His past medical history includes **hypertension**[8] and **diabetes mellitus** [8], both of which are treated with oral medications.

- The patient also has a significant **family history of cardiovascular disease** [9], from which his mother passed away at the **age of 63 years** [9].
- On further questioning, the patient reveals he has previously had **similar chest pain** [10] while walking, forcing him to stop for a short period of time, but attributes this to his poor fitness level.

[1] Increasing age and male gender are non-modifiable risk factors for coronary artery disease (CAD). It is estimated that from the age of 40 onwards, each additional decade of life is associated with an approximate doubling of the risk of all vascular disease. Females are thought to have an approximately 20% lower risk than males for all MACE.

[2] Accountants typically have a desk-based job which can lead to an overall sedentary lifestyle. This places them at risk of cardiovascular disease. Weekly exercise and activity should be explored further in the history.

[3] The prevalence of CAD is higher in patients originating from sub-continental populations. Compared with Caucasians, patients from the Indian sub-continent have a higher prevalence of CAD, MI and associated cardiovascular mortality. Hence, the suspicion for cardiac-related chest pain is raised.

[4] This is one of three features of classical cardiac chest pain; it is suggestive of ischaemic heart disease. Angina is typically described more as a discomfort rather than pain – other terms that can be used include squeezing, tightness, pressure, constriction, heavy weight on chest, etc. It is generally not described as sharp or stabbing and should not change with respiration or position. Other features more typical of non-ischaemic chest pain are the primary pain location in the mid- or lower abdomen, any discomfort reproducible by palpation or movement, fleeting pains lasting for a few seconds or less and pain radiating into the lower extremities or above the mandible.

[5] Angina is typically elicited by exercise or physical activities that increase myocardial oxygen demand. Recreational drugs such as cocaine can also trigger myocardial ischaemia, and patients should be questioned about their use. Precipitation of chest pain by physical activity is another traditional feature of angina.

[6] Other features associated with ACS include diaphoresis, nausea, vomiting, light-headedness, clamminess and fatigue. Sometimes angina may be associated with shortness of breath or wheezing, which reflects mild pulmonary congestion. Left ventricular end diastolic pressures may be increased due to myocardia failing to relax normally in diastole (as this is energy-dependent) and thus this can lead to pulmonary congestion.

[7] Improvement with rest or glyceryl trinitrate (GTN) is another cardinal feature of anginal pain, which lends to the underlying aetiology being CAD.

[8] Hypertension and diabetes are both modifiable risk factors for CAD. The lifetime risk of developing cardiovascular disease (CVD) is significantly higher among patients with hypertension. The target blood pressure for patients with diabetes is 125–130/80mmHg as per the latest guidelines, but the exact target still remains a slightly contentious topic. Furthermore, insulin resistance, hyperinsulinaemia and elevated blood glucose are all associated with atherosclerotic CVD. Diabetic patients will typically have a greater burden of other CVD risk factors such as hypertension, obesity, increased LDL cholesterol and hypertriglyceridaemia.

[9] Family history is another independent risk factor for the development of CAD. Generally, a positive family history is considered death from CVD in a first-degree relative before the age of 55 in males and before the age of 65 in female relatives.

[10] Chest pain that is reproducible with exertion is consistent with underlying ischaemic heart disease. It is important to question whether the nature of the pain has changed at all or the level of exertion required to induce it. Given that it occurs with a similar level of exertion as previously, this makes ACS less likely and is more consistent with stable angina.

Examination

- The patient appears **comfortable and pain-free** [1] at rest.
- There is no evidence of **increased work of breathing** [2] or **diaphoresis** [2] on general examination.
- He appears to have a **large body habitus** [3] with a BMI likely in excess of 30.
- RR is 16 and **BP 155/90mmHg** [4] . Pulse is **80bpm** [4] **and regular** [5] .

- O_2 saturations are **96% on air** [6] and the patient is **afebrile** [7] .
- **JVP is not elevated** [8] and **Kussmaul's sign is negative** [9] . The apex beat is not displaced or dyskinetic.
- **Heart sounds are dual** [10] with **no murmurs auscultated** [11] ; there is no paradoxical **splitting of the** second **heart sound** [12] .
- Auscultation of the lungs reveals a **clear chest** [13] .
- There is no evidence of **peripheral oedema** [14] .

[1] The patient appears well and haemodynamically stable, which would be more consistent with stable angina as opposed to ACS. The fact that the patient is pain-free at rest is another reassuring feature.

[2] Increased work of breathing may reflect pulmonary congestion. It can also be a sign of increased severity of the underlying aetiology. Diaphoresis is a sign that would be more concerning for ACS and would warrant urgent work-up and referral to cardiology if appropriate.

[3] Obesity is a modifiable risk factor for CVD. Obesity further strengthens the case for likely underlying CAD. This is an important feature that should be addressed in the management of this patient. Lifestyle modifications are essential in preventing disease progression. Reduction of weight will also assist in reducing blood pressure and optimising glycaemic control in diabetes.

[4] Haemodynamic stability is an important measure in any patient presenting with chest pain. If the patient is stable it allows time for a thorough work-up. Bradycardia and/or hypotension is seen in up to 50% of inferior infarcts secondary to parasympathetic hyperactivity. Hypotension is also a measure of poor cardiac output and is concerning for a large territory infarct or other aetiology presenting with chest pain, such as aortic dissection or cardiac tamponade.

[5] Arrhythmias such as AF may be present from atrial infarction and this is reassuring. In AF you would expect an irregular heart rate. Furthermore, the presence of AF with rapid ventricular response may also precipitate chest pain in patients with pre-existing CAD. Ventricular tachycardia can also result from acute myocardial infarction which would present with a far higher rate.

[6] The patient is not hypoxic which is also reassuring that there is no significant pulmonary congestion. Moreover, it makes a primary lung aetiology less likely.

[7] CVD does not typically cause fevers unless it is secondary to infective endocarditis. If the patient was febrile, other causes of chest pain such as community-acquired pneumonia would need to be excluded for the cause of the fever.

[8] JVP is typically increased with right ventricular infarction, leading to hypokinesis and poor contraction. This leads to poor right ventricular filling and a raised JVP. The JVP being non-elevated is in keeping with a stable angina aetiology.

[9] Kussmaul's sign is a paradoxical rise in JVP on inspiration or a failure in the appropriate fall of the JVP with inspiration. It is both a specific and sensitive sign of right ventricular infarction in patients with suspected inferior infarction. It is also associated with constrictive pericarditis.

[10] In severe coronary artery disease an S3 or S4 may be auscultated. While an S3 can be heard in healthy young children and adults, it is typically pathological in patients >40 years and suggests a high left atrial pressure and increased left ventricular end diastolic pressures. Myocardial ischaemia can lead to decreased myocardial relaxation and hence decreased LV distensibility, which can produce the S4 heart sound.

[11] In any patient with suspected ischaemia, a new ventricular septal defect and mitral regurgitation murmur must be excluded. Mitral regurgitation results from papillary muscle dysfunction secondary to ischaemia. Ventricular septal defect murmurs are concerning for ventricular septal rupture secondary to ischaemia. It is once again reassuring that neither of these are present.

[12] Severe myocardial ischaemia can lead to the second heart sound being paradoxically split due to delayed relaxation of the left ventricular myocardium and delayed closure of the aortic valve.

[13] Listening to the lungs is imperative with any patient with chest pain or cardiac aetiology. It provides vital information with regard to the fluid status and if there is any pulmonary congestion. Additionally, other respiratory aetiologies can be included or excluded through a thorough chest examination including auscultation of the lungs.

14 The presence of peripheral oedema would suggest that the patient is fluid overloaded. The causes of fluid overload are numerous but in this case, you would want to exclude decompensated cardiac failure, which would be concerning for a large territory infarct.

Investigations

- 12-lead ECG shows nil **ST segment elevation or depression or new LBBB** [1]; there is **no T wave flattening or inversion** [2].
- There is, however, **marked LVH** [3] meeting the **Sokolow–Lyon criteria** [4], S wave depth in V1 + R wave height in V5 = 40mm.
- **Serial troponins** [5] are performed, which are both within normal limits.
- Chest X-ray demonstrates **nil increased interstitial markings** [6] or **overt consolidation** [7].
- The **cardiac silhouette** [8] is within normal limits.
- UEC results reveal a mildly raised creatinine of 101mmol/L and an **eGFR of 69ml/min/1.73m^2** [9]. HbA1c for the patient was 6.7%.
- The patient consequently undergoes stress echocardiography testing which was limited by poor exercise tolerance and was non-definitive. There were some concerns regarding the anterior wall and anterior septum wall but this wasn't confirmed; the study did not show any severe **regional wall motion hypokinesis** [10] during stress.
- No **significant valvular disease** [11] was seen and a **left ventricular ejection fraction of 60%** [12] was estimated.
- Based on the findings from the non-invasive testing, the **patient** underwent coronary angiography with an estimated **65–70% stenosis of the mid LAD** [13] disease and mild disease in the first obtuse marginal branch.
- A decision for **medical management** [14] was made for the treatment of this stable CAD.

1 An ECG is definitely the most essential investigation that should be performed on all patients with chest pain. It is quick and non-invasive; it should be completed as a priority. The absence of ST segment changes or new LBBB (which is also treated as a STEMI) is reassuring that the patient is not having a STEMI.

2 Dynamic T wave flattening or inversion usually signifies myocardial ischaemia and may be present in non-ST elevation myocardial infarction (NSTEMI). ST segment depression is another finding associated with NSTEMI. With any patient with ST depression on ECG, it is important to closely examine for ST elevation in other leads and consider a posterior lead ECG to exclude a posterior STEMI.

3 Left ventricular hypertrophy (LVH) in this patient is likely due to poorly managed hypertension, leading to remodelling of the left ventricle. Poorly managed hypertension greatly increases the risk of underlying CVD.

4 The Sokolow–Lyon criteria are the most commonly used criteria for diagnosing LVH on ECG. To meet the Sokolow–Lyon criteria the following condition must be met: S wave depth in V1 + tallest R wave height in V5–V6 >35mm.

5 Serial troponins should be done in all patients presenting with chest pain that is likely cardiac. They help delineate between an acute cardiac syndrome and stable angina, particularly in the absence of ECG changes suggestive of ischaemia.

6 Increased interstitial markings can sometimes be referred to as a fine reticular pattern and acutely are representative of pulmonary oedema or interstitial pneumonitis. This CXR excludes significant pulmonary oedema.

7 Consolidation is any process that fills the alveoli with fluid, blood or other substances. Usually patients with pneumonia have lobar consolidation. Diffuse consolidation is generally the result of heart failure or overt fluid overload from other causes. Typically in congestive heart failure you will find bilateral perihilar consolidation with air bronchograms with increased interstitial markings.

8 Typically in patients with cardiogenic oedema, there will also be an increased heart size on chest X-ray; this is by no means a definitive relationship.

9 An eGFR of 69ml/min/1.73m^2 indicates chronic kidney disease (CKD) stage II which, given the other comorbidities, is likely due to diabetic nephropathy. This indicates imperfect glycaemic control, predisposing the patient to the development of atherosclerotic plaque within the coronary vessels.

10 With stress the normal left ventricle becomes hypercontractile. Cavity size is small and ejection fraction increases. The presence of new or worsening segmental wall motion with stress is suggestive of the presence of haemodynamically significant coronary artery stenosis supplying those segments. Based on the location of the hypokinetic or akinetic ventricular wall (in severe CAD), the obstructive CAD can be localised. In this case, the results were non-definitive and given the strongly suggestive history, the decision was made to proceed straight to angiography.

11 During stress echocardiography, a baseline resting echocardiogram is obtained for comparison. This baseline echocardiogram also assesses gross valvular structure and function along with ventricular function, chamber sizes, wall thickness and assessment of all segments of the heart. Aortic stenosis can also cause angina and since there is normal valvular function, it can be reasonably excluded.

12 This is a normal left ventricular ejection fraction; typically anything >55% is considered normal. This is indicative that the patient does not have left ventricular systolic dysfunction which can result from severe CAD and ischaemic cardiomyopathy.

13 Coronary angiography is completed through radial or femoral arterial access, where a catheter is introduced into the heart to visualise the coronary arteries. A 65–70% stenosis in the mid left anterior descending along with mild disease in the obtuse marginal is generally not considered significant enough for percutaneous coronary intervention (PCI). The only reason for PCI with the current findings would be failed medical management and ongoing symptoms interrupting the patient's lifestyle.

14 Medical management entails pharmacological-based therapies to reduce progression and treat symptoms. This will be discussed in detail below.

Management

Immediate

Acute symptom management involves **cessation of physical activity** [1] during the episode. Furthermore, to shorten the episode of angina **GTN** [2] in the form of a sublingual preparation is first-line therapy. While taking GTN, patients should be **advised to sit down** [3]. GTN can be taken every 5 minutes up to a total of 15 minutes. If the pain persists past 10 minutes despite two doses of GTN, the patient should take a third dose and call an ambulance for **urgent presentation** [4] to the ED.

Lifestyle

Risk factor reduction is a central component of managing patients with stable angina. An emphasis needs to be placed on reducing modifiable risk factors. Patients should be educated regarding **cessation of smoking** [5] if they smoke and **weight reduction** [6]. Education should be provided regarding **increasing exercise and implementation of healthy eating** [7]. Help patients **set up clear goals** [8] and targets for managing risk factors. Finally, patients should be advised to avoid heavy, sudden and unaccustomed exertion and acute emotional stress.

All patients with CAD should receive **annual influenza vaccines** [9].

Long-term

Long-term management of stable angina is based on two core principles: anti-anginal therapy and prevention of disease progression.

Anti-anginal therapy

For a patient with stable angina, **beta blockers** [10] are usually used first-line to prevent episodes of angina. For patients with left ventricular dysfunction (LVEF <40%) use a **cardioselective beta blocker** [11]. **Non-dihydropyridine calcium channel blockers** [12] can be used as an alternative if beta blocker therapy is contraindicated.

A dihydropyridine calcium channel blocker (CCB) such as amlodipine can be added to a beta blocker if angina persists. A **long-acting nitrate** [13] can also be added either to a beta blocker, or to a non-dihydropyridine CCB. If a combination of two anti-anginal medications does not provide sufficient symptomatic relief, referral to a cardiologist is recommended. Nicorandil is another option for patients with refractory angina despite optimal therapy.

Prevention of disease progression

The following pharmacological regimen should be considered in all patients with stable ischaemic heart disease:

1. **Antiplatelet therapy** [14] – low dose aspirin
2. **High dose statin** [15] therapy
3. **Antihypertensive optimisation** [16] with strict targets in hypertensive patients
4. **Glycaemic control optimisation** [17] in diabetic patients.

Patients should also be referred to a **cardiac rehabilitation programme** [18]. Patients with chronic stable angina require follow-up on a regular basis; **6–12-monthly follow-up** [19] is suggested.

1 Stopping any precipitating factor such as physical activity will shorten the episode of angina and improve oxygen delivery to myocardium.

2 GTN dilates the coronary vessels, allowing for greater flow through the stenosis and relieving symptoms. This will be not effective in STEMI which typically presents with total coronary occlusion.

3 A side-effect of the use of GTN is hypotension and orthostatic hypotension. Therefore, patients need to be educated regarding the importance of sitting down while taking their GTN, to prevent a fall resulting from orthostatic hypotension. A trial of a single dose of GTN under supervision while the patient is asymptomatic can be considered so that they are able to recognise its effect.

4 If the pain is unresponsive to GTN after two doses, it is concerning for ACS or other pathology causing chest pain. In this case, urgent presentation to the ED is required for detailed investigation and management.

5 Smoking is a modifiable risk factor for atherosclerosis in both coronary and non-coronary arteries. The incidence of myocardial infarction is increased sixfold in women and threefold in men who smoke at least 20 cigarettes a day. Smoking cessation leads to a decrease in cardiac event range between 7 and 47% , which is quite substantial.

6 Obesity is associated with a number of CAD risk factors such as hypertension, insulin resistance, elevated LDL cholesterol and triglycerides. Reduction in weight has been shown to reduce the annual cardiovascular event rate.

7 Diet factors that lead to increased CVD risk include: high glycaemic index, low consumption of fruit and vegetables, high consumption of red meat, high consumption of trans fatty acids and low consumption of fibre. Furthermore, exercise of even moderate degree has a protective effect against CVD and all-cause mortality.

8 Providing advice can be very easy for patients but it is important to set reasonable goals so that the patient stays motivated. Education about the improvement in CVD outcomes by management of risk factors can be motivating for patients. One particular method of effective goal setting that can be utilised is setting up SMART goals. The goals set up should be **S**pecific, **M**easurable, **A**chievable, **R**ealistic and **T**ime-related.

9 There is substantial evidence that providing an influenza vaccine to patients with CVD has benefit. Patients with CVD have an increased risk for complications from influenza.

10 Beta blockers reduce the heart's chronotropy and inotropy. By doing so, beta blockers reduce the myocardial oxygen demand and hence delay the ischaemic threshold and thus enhance exercise tolerance. In addition, for patients who have had an MI, beta blockers have been shown to prevent re-infarction.

11 Cardioselective beta blockers include carvedilol, bisoprolol, nebivolol or metoprolol succinate. They have been shown to have a mortality benefit in patients with HFrEF.

12 Diltiazem or verapamil can be used as an alternative to beta blockers. Never use diltiazem or verapamil in combination with a beta blocker, as it can cause severe bradycardia and lead to heart failure.

13 Long-acting nitrates include transdermal glyceryl trinitrate and modified-release isosorbide mononitrate. However, caution must be taken with these as tolerance to nitrates develops quickly. To avoid this, ensure a period free from nitrates each day; this can be done by wearing the patch for 14 hours each day or using isosorbide mononitrate once daily. Long-acting nitrates do not improve overall survival.

14 If no contraindication, all patients should be treated with low dose aspirin to reduce disease progression. Clopidogrel is an alternative in patients who are allergic to aspirin.

15 All patients regardless of their baseline LDL cholesterol should be treated with high dose statin therapy if they have proven stable ischaemic heart disease. Statin therapy reduces cardiovascular morbidity and mortality in patients with established CVD. If LDL cholesterol targets are not met, additional lipid-modifying medications may be required.

16 Hypertension is an important modifiable risk factor that should be managed to stringent targets of 125–130/80mmHg in patients with ischaemic heart disease. In this case, given the patient has a history of type 2 diabetes, they should be commenced on an ACEi or ARB if they aren't already on it.

17 The first-line medication for the management of type 2 diabetes is metformin. As discussed previously, it is important to maintain strict glycaemic control to prevent further atherosclerosis in the coronary arteries. Patients with stable ischaemic heart disease who cannot tolerate metformin should be trialled on a glucagon-like peptide-1 (GLP-1) receptor agonist (liraglutide, semaglutide, dulaglutide) or sodium-glucose co-transporter 2 (SGLT2) inhibitor (empagliflozin, canagliflozin), since they have proven mortality benefit. The only issue with GLP-1 receptor agonists is that they are administered subcutaneously, which can be an issue with some patients. Furthermore, if the patient has known HFrEF, an SGLT2 inhibitor should be strongly considered as it poses a significant mortality benefit on current evidence.

18 Cardiac rehabilitation is an effective means of educating the patient about a graded programme of regular moderate exercise. It is also an avenue for providing advice regarding other supports and services and assists in lifestyle modification.

19 Follow-up is required to establish if there has been declining exercise tolerance, change in the nature of the angina, medication compliance and new adverse events; and to assess if sufficient effort is being made to modify risk factors. These are all red flags and need to be monitored closely in all patients with stable angina.

CASE 10: Ventricular tachycardia

History

- A 66-year-old gentleman is brought in by ambulance to the **resuscitation bay of the emergency department** [1] post cardioversion by paramedics in the community.
- He was out at dinner with friends when he reported sudden onset palpitations, dizziness and fatigue. He then describes **promptly losing consciousness** [2].
- He does not recall any preceding **chest pain or dyspnoea** [3]. He has never had any episodes like this previously.
- **Collateral history** [4] from friends reveals that bystander **cardiopulmonary resuscitation** [5] was commenced and the paramedics were called. After 15 minutes, paramedics arrived on the scene.

- Cardiac monitoring revealed **monomorphic ventricular tachycardia** [6].
- Given the patient had no pulse, one shock of **unsynchronised cardioversion was delivered** [7] and the patient regained consciousness; **total downtime was 18 minutes** [8].
- His past medical history is significant for **two STEMIs** [9], one anterior STEMI 2 years prior and one lateral STEMI 4 years prior, both treated with PCI and drug-eluting stents. He also has T2DM on insulin and well controlled hypertension and dyslipidaemia.
- When asked about family history, he reveals **both of his parents had ischaemic heart disease and his father died in his sleep at the age of 60** [10].

[1] As you progress through your medical career, you will receive more and more referrals from the ED. The resuscitation bay contains the most unwell patients in the department due to severe derangements in their ABCDs or due to high risk of deterioration. In this case, the patient is in the resuscitation bay due to high risk of developing pulseless sustained ventricular tachycardia (VT) and may need prompt cardioversion and advanced life support.

[2] The classical history for VT will be progression of symptoms from palpitations and dizziness to presyncope and finally syncope. VT is commonly haemodynamically unstable due to inefficient pumping of blood and thus patients will most often be syncopal. Other common associated symptoms may be fatigue, malaise and feeling of impending doom.

[3] It is important to ask for chest pain and dyspnoea. Chest pain is important because it screens for acute MI. In this case the patient may have a silent infarct due to his advanced diabetes and so this will have to be corroborated with ECG findings and troponins post resuscitation. Acute MI and previous ischaemic heart disease is the leading cause for malignant ventricular arrhythmias, i.e. ventricular fibrillation (VF) or VT. Furthermore, it is important to look for dyspnoea in the history, as patients with left ventricular dysfunction or HFrEF with a left ventricular ejection fraction (LVEF) <35% are at higher risk of malignant ventricular arrhythmias.

[4] Being a doctor is like being a detective. You must strive always to obtain information from all the available sources.

When reviewing patients in the ED, talk to the patient and also obtain collateral history from the ambulance officers, bystanders and friends. This will give you the clinical information you need to make the best decision possible. Collateral history is especially key in a syncope history – the patient would not be able to give you any reliable information as they had lost consciousness!

[5] Prompt cardiopulmonary resuscitation (CPR) as a bridge to cardioversion saves lives. The statistics on out-of-hospital CPR survival rates are grim, but when it is started early and effectively delivered, it is life-sustaining treatment that buys time until medical services arrive. It is paramount to notify medical services as soon as possible, as every minute carries poorer prognosis.

[6] The ideal outcome for this case would have been locating the nearest automated external defibrillator to minimise downtime. The next best thing is waiting for the ambulance officers to arrive with their cardiac monitor to delineate between VT and VF. In this case, the rhythm captured was pulseless monomorphic ventricular tachycardia. The differential diagnoses for the causes of VT are:
- most commonly acute myocardial infarction and ischaemic cardiomyopathy subsequent to infarction
- structural heart disease such as dilated cardiomyopathy, hypertrophic cardiomyopathy, arrhythmogenic right ventricular cardiomyopathy
- electrolyte deficiencies
- systemic diseases that also manifest in the heart (systemic lupus erythematosus, sarcoidosis,

haemochromatosis, amyloidosis and rheumatoid arthritis)
- medications causing prolongation of the QTc.

7 There is a difference in indications for synchronised and unsynchronised cardioversion. Synchronised cardioversion is when a low energy shock delivery is synchronised to the peak of the R wave. This prevents a shock being delivered during cardiac repolarisation (during the T wave) as this would precipitate VF. This is generally preserved for AF, atrial flutter, atrial tachycardia and other supraventricular tachycardias that have failed anti-arrhythmic drug therapy as well as haemodynamically stable VT. Unsynchronised cardioversion is defibrillation. It is when a high energy shock is delivered anywhere within the cardiac cycle. This is indicated when there is no coordinated intrinsic cardiac activity within the heart, such as pulseless VT (in this case) or in VF.

8 Downtime is defined as the total time between syncope and return of spontaneous circulation (ROSC). Ideally you would like a downtime of <20 minutes (or even none at all) to ensure favourable outcomes.

9 The most important component of the past medical history is ascertaining the presence of previous myocardial infarcts. Scarred myocardium from previous infarcts provides a region of slowed conduction that allows a re-entrant circuit to develop. Once this is present, VT can occur spontaneously or form triggers such as electrolyte depletion, acute ischaemia or decompensated heart failure. Our patient here has had two previous infarcts and although both were managed with emergency primary PCI, undoubtedly there would have been some fibrosis that occurred, which promotes the development of VT.

10 The family history here caps off the risk stratification for the patient. He is obviously high risk for VT/VF. Both of the patient's parents had ischaemic heart disease, with one who died in his sleep. Sudden death is often described as sudden cardiac death (SCD) as >90% of sudden death is from VT or VF.

Examination

- From the end of the bed, the patient is on **continuous cardiac monitoring** [1] (which reveals sinus normocardia) and **looks well** [2].
- There is some **mild bruising over the chest wall** [3] from CPR.
- He is **alert and oriented** [4] with a heart rate of 78bpm, blood pressure of 132/75mmHg, respiratory rate of 16 and SpO$_2$ of 97% on air.
- At time of review in the ED, the patient did **not appear pale, had warm peripheries, a strong carotid and femoral pulse** [5] and no murmurs on auscultation.
- There are **no cannon A waves** [6]. He is euvolaemic.
- From the ambulance handover notes, the patient at the time of CPR **appeared pale, had no response to pain and no carotid or femoral pulse** [7].

1 Continuous cardiac monitoring is very important in managing patients with VT/VF. Although he has attained ROSC, he may deteriorate yet again from sinus rhythm to VT, VF or asystole. If the VT was part of an acute coronary syndrome, you may also detect other comorbid arrhythmias with monitoring. Another benefit of cardiac monitoring as opposed to telemetry is that you can capture and print out arrhythmias onto a 12-lead ECG.

2 It is always important to observe whether or not a patient looks well.

3 CPR, when done correctly, should be traumatic. The bony thoracic cage protects the heart and the only way to compress the heart correctly is to compress the thoracic cage to the point where it will also compress the heart. This commonly results in broken ribs and subcutaneous bruising. If the patient is finding it difficult to breathe due to pain, ensure appropriate analgesia and obtain a chest X-ray to assess the number and severity of rib fractures.

4 Orientation and alertness denote adequate cerebral perfusion from restored heart rhythm and suggest that there has not been severe hypoxic ischaemic brain injury from the downtime. All in all, the fact that the patient is alert and oriented means that there is good neurological prognosis following this episode of cardiac arrest. It is not uncommon for patients who have had prolonged CPR to not be alert or oriented despite ROSC. Around 80% of patients who are admitted to ICU post out-of-hospital cardiac arrests are comatose. Poor neurological outcomes can be predicted in patients who exhibit signs of hypoxic ischaemic brain injury within 72 hours, such as no motor response to pain and bilateral absence of corneal and pupillary reflexes. If investigating for poor neurological outcome, one could also assess for malignant patterns on electroencephalogram (EEG), e.g. status epilepticus and unreactive burst-suppression and signs of diffuse ischaemic brain injury on CT brain.

5 Overall these signs indicate adequate perfusion of the body. When assessing for pulse, a central pulse (carotid or femoral) should be palpated.

6 Cannon A waves occur when the right atrium and right ventricle contract simultaneously instead of one after the other. The contraction of the right ventricle closes the tricuspid valve to prevent regurgitant flow. When the tricuspid valve closes, the blood in the right atrium, despite its contraction, can only flow back into the jugular vein, resulting in a large pulsation called a cannon A wave. Cannon A waves are not always present in VT and are not always specific for VT. They can also occur in other dysrhythmias that cause atrioventricular dissociation, such as complete heart block.

7 The ambulance handover notes reveal objective signs of hypoperfusion. The lack of response to pain indicates cerebral hypoperfusion, and the lack of carotid and femoral pulses would explain the patient's pallor, indicating peripheral hypoperfusion.

Investigations

- 12-lead ECG from the ambulance showed **monomorphic ventricular tachycardia** [1] at a rate of around 160bpm. There was QRS prolongation of 160ms, atrioventricular dissociation, extreme mean electrical axis deviation and a fusion beat.
- 12-lead ECG from the resuscitation bay showed a normal **QTc interval of 390ms** [2].
- FBE showed a Hb of 13.4g/dl with a normal WCC and platelet count.
- UEC and calcium, magnesium and phosphate (CMP) showed a **K of 3.4mmol/L, Mg of 0.84mmol/L and Ca of 2.3mmol/L** [3].

- There were **no elevated troponins** [4].
- A transthoracic echocardiogram performed as an **inpatient revealed an LVEF of 30% resultant from severe hypokinesis of the anteroseptal and lateral left ventricular wall** [5]. The pulmonary artery pressure was normal.
- The decision was made not to proceed to **left heart catheterisation** [6] due to the absence of chest pain and normal troponins.
- Given clear cause of VT, **cardiac MRI was also not pursued** [7].

1 Monomorphic ventricular tachycardia is when the QRS complex looks consistent beat-by-beat. If the QRS morphology is not consistent, consider polymorphic VT or VF. VT has numerous ECG features, but by definition you need to have a heart rate of >100bpm (tachycardia) and QRS broadening, meaning QRS complex of >120ms (supraventricular conduction will result in a narrow QRS unless there is pre-existing bundle branch block). Very commonly you will also have extreme axis deviation to the northwest. This is achieved by a positive QRS in aVR and negative QRS in leads I and aVF. Other signs that may or may not be present on ECG include:
- atrioventricular dissociation – when P waves conduct at their own individual rate and the ventricles conduct at their own rate with no association between the two. Most commonly this is seen in complete heart block. Look for buried P waves within the broad QRS complexes and map them out.
- capture beats – a narrow complex QRS that occurs when the sinoatrial node is able to conduct one uninterrupted impulse to the ventricles. The capture beat's QRS morphology should be very similar to the patient's usual QRS complex during sinus rhythm.
- fusion beats – a hybrid QRS complex that occurs when a sinus and ventricular impulse coincide.
- Brugada's sign – when the duration from the start of the QRS to the nadir (or bottom) of the S wave is >100ms.
- Josephson's sign – the notching that can occur near the nadir of the S wave.
- RSR complexes with a 'taller left rabbit ear'. This is in contrast to a right bundle branch block (RBBB) where the 'right rabbit ear' is taller.

- negative or positive concordance – there is commonly no 'RS' morphology to monomorphic VT in the precordial leads. In leads V1–6, positive concordance occurs from a dominant R wave and entirely positive complexes. Negative concordance will have a dominant S wave and entirely negative complexes.

A classic clinical scenario is the differentiation of VT from SVT with aberrancy. For clues regarding VT, look for all the signs listed above, but most pertinently the extreme axis deviation, presence of AV dissociation and capture/fusion beats. Non-ECG factors that may increase suspicion of VT are an age >35, presence of structural heart disease, heart failure or previous ischaemic heart disease. ECG features that increase the suspicion for SVT with aberrant conduction are features suggestive of Wolff–Parkinson–White syndrome and the presence of the same bundle branch block in previous ECGs.

2 It is important to check for the QTc interval. Although impossible in the acute VT episode, assess the QTc in the ECGs taken before and after the VT. A prolonged QTc is defined as a QTc >440ms in males and >460ms in females. Prolonged QTc is associated with torsades de pointes (means 'twisting of the points' in French) which is a type of polymorphic VT. The risk of precipitating torsades de pointes is highest when the QTc is >500ms. There are congenital prolonged QT syndromes, but in clinical practice torsades de pointes is most associated with medications. Examples of QTc-prolonging medications include class III anti-arrhythmics (sotalol, amiodarone), azoles, macrolides, fluoroquinolones and various psychotropic drugs.

3 As previously stated, the most common cause of VT is either previous ischaemic infarcts allowing for re-entrant VTs. Other causes of VT include severe hypokalaemia, hypocalcaemia and hypomagnesaemia, which can all prolong the QT interval and cause polymorphic VT. In monomorphic VT, it is also important to optimise electrolytes, so obtaining a baseline level can help guide in repletion of electrolytes. Aim for K >4mmol/L and Mg >1mmol/L.

4 Troponins are a key serological investigation in acute VT. If there are severely elevated troponin levels suggestive of acute myocardial infarction, they would undergo urgent left heart catheterisation to look for the culprit lesion for the VT.

5 Transthoracic echocardiogram here serves two purposes. First, it can help in quantifying the LVEF to see if the patient meets criteria for implanted cardioverter-defibrillator (ICD) implantation for secondary prevention of VT/VF for HFrEF and secondly, it helps to assess for the presence of structural heart disease that may be complicating the VT.

6 Left heart catheterisation is done to assess the coronary arteries. When a patient presents with an out-of-hospital cardiac arrest with elevated troponin or with features of acute myocardial infarction on ECG, the VT is secondary to the infarct and thus an urgent angiogram should be performed. If you cardioverted in that situation, the patient would just deteriorate into VT/VF again as the ischaemia has not resolved. A particularly high risk lesion for VT/VF is a left main coronary artery occlusion and patients can suffer VT even after reperfusion due to transient electrical instability.

7 Cardiac magnetic resonance imaging (MRI) is the gold standard for imaging the structural VT substrate. It is performed for diagnostic clarity to differentiate further between ischaemic and non-ischaemic cardiomyopathy by characterising scar distribution and extent of scar transmurality. Furthermore it is able to detect subtle structural abnormalities to assess for myocarditis, sarcoid and amyloid cardiomyopathies.

Management

Inpatient

Patients with VT need to be admitted to the **coronary care unit and placed on continuous cardiac monitoring** [1]. Their **electrolytes should be replaced** [2]. Management of ventricular tachycardia differs depending on whether or not it is non-sustained VT or sustained VT.

Non-sustained ventricular tachycardia

Non-sustained VT is when an episode of VT lasts longer than 3 beats but less than 30 seconds. Treatment for non-sustained VT is rarely indicated and is only in cases of haemodynamic compromise or if patients have significant symptoms associated with the episode of non-sustained VT. Prior to pharmacological management, one should manage electrolyte depletion or treat the underlying cause. Treatment can include **beta blockers, verapamil, flecainide or amiodarone** [3].

Sustained ventricular tachycardia

Sustained VT is when an episode of VT lasts longer than 30 seconds. It can be further divided up into haemodynamically stable and haemodynamically unstable sustained VT. Haemodynamically unstable VT is more common. For patients with **haemodynamically unstable VT** [4], call a code blue and aim for immediate

direct current unsynchronised cardioversion and management as per the Advanced Life Support algorithm. For haemodynamically stable VT, there is time, so patients can be trialled with chemical cardioversion instead of direct cardioversion first. Chemical cardioversion can be achieved by IV infusion of lignocaine or amiodarone. Failing this, or if haemodynamic compromise ensues, cardioversion will be required.

Torsades de pointes

Torsades de pointes is a polymorphic VT associated with prolonged QTc intervals, typically with QTc intervals that are >500ms. It can occur due to congenital long QT syndrome or from medications or electrolyte depletion. Treatment for congenital long QT syndrome would be beta blockers such as metoprolol or propranolol. Otherwise you would aim for immediate unsynchronised cardioversion in episodes of torsades de pointes and then replete the electrolytes and withhold any QTC-prolonging medication.

ICD implantation

All patients with VT should have an early referral to the inpatient cardiology service. There they can have a review by an electrophysiologist for consideration of an **implanted cardioverter-defibrillator** [5]. There are two main ways in which ICDs treat VT: **anti-tachycardia pacing (ATP) or overdrive pacing** [6] and defibrillation.

Long-term

Anti-arrhythmic therapy

Amiodarone [7] is most commonly used for treatment of ongoing sustained ventricular tachycardia. There are other anti-arrhythmics that may be used, but these should all be under specialist guidance.

Risk factor modification

No changes need be made to the **patient's antihypertensive treatment or lipid-lowering regime** [7]. The patient's **HbA1c was found to be 8.6%** [8] and his oral hypoglycaemic and insulin regime should be appropriately up-titrated. He should also be referred to the **diabetes clinic for ongoing follow-up** [9].

The patient was discharged home with follow-up in the **cardiac device clinic** [10].

---

1 It is important to consider not only which medical care to provide to the patient, but which nursing care would be best for the patient. This patient requires specialised cardiac nursing care with nurses who can recognise ventricular arrhythmias on cardiac monitoring and know the importance of calling code blues and notifying the treating medical team promptly.

2 Electrolyte repletion is a key staple of the supportive treatment in cardiac arrhythmias. If this was a case of polymorphic VT, it would also be important to perform a medication review to assess for the burden of QTc-prolonging medication and to adjust their medications accordingly.

3 One can use atenolol or metoprolol. For patients with contraindications to beta blockers (such as asthma), verapamil or flecainide can be suitable alternatives, but there needs to be caution with the use of flecainide in the case of CAD or structural heart disease.

4 In haemodynamically unstable VT, you opt for the treatment course with the quickest outcome. This would be cardioversion. The code blue should be called as patients can lose their ability to protect their airway due to cerebral hypoperfusion. Anaesthetics are present at each code blue and will be able to provide expert airway support and intubation, should the need arise.

5 Implanted cardioverter-defibrillators (ICDs) are devices for patients who are at high risk of SCD and for certain indications, carrying a substantial mortality benefit. They are implanted in the same way as permanent pacemakers (refer to *Case 6*) and have similar complications. There are hybrid devices available that are both ICDs and pacemakers. The patient here has two indications for ICD implantation: an episode of haemodynamically significant VT in the absence of reversible conditions, and ischaemic cardiomyopathy with LVEF <35%. Indications for primary prevention of SCD include:
- patients with structural heart disease and sustained VT
- previous AMI (>40 days) with LVEF ≤35% with NYHA II–III symptoms
- previous AMI (>40 days) with LVEF ≤30% with NYHA I symptoms

- LVEF ≤40% due to prior AMI and positive VT stimulation study
- non-ischaemic cardiomyopathy with LVEF ≤35% and NYHA II–III symptoms
- patients with history of AMI with inducible VF/VT in electrophysiology study
- unexplained syncope in a patient with non-ischaemic cardiomyopathy with significant LV dysfunction.

Indications for secondary prevention of SCD include:
- survivors of cardiac arrest from VT or VF
- sustained VT and significant structural heart disease.

6 Anti-tachycardia pacing is when the ICD delivers a burst of ventricular pacing at a rate faster than the intrinsic rate of the tachycardia. The pacing successfully interrupts and terminates the re-entrant cycle of the arrhythmia, allowing normal intrinsic conduction of the heart to take over. ATP can effectively terminate VT in 90% of cases; however, it carries a small risk (~1–5%) of accelerating the arrhythmia into a faster cycle VT or VF. In this instance, the ICD would deliver a high energy shock to defibrillate.

ATP is more beneficial to the patient as it is a painless means of terminating VT and it doesn't consume as much battery life as defibrillation, enhancing ICD longevity. If the ICD detects the patient is in a very fast heart rate (commonly >200bpm), or the VT fails to terminate with multiple bouts of ATP, the ICD will defibrillate the patient.

Note that ICDs do not prevent, but rather treat VT and VF. Hence, there is a need for patients to remain on anti-arrhythmic drugs even though they have an ICD.

7 In conjunction with the anti-arrhythmic therapy and ICD, the physician should treat the underlying disease that predisposed the patient to the VT. In this case, it would be the optimisation of CAD risk factors to prevent further infarctions and worsening of the patient's ischaemic cardiomyopathy.

8 An HbA1c of 8.6% corresponds with mean blood sugar levels of 11mmol/L. Ideally, an HbA1c of <7% should be achieved for a patient with known ischaemic heart disease.

9 Diabetes is the patient's main unoptimised risk factor for ischaemic heart disease. Having ongoing specialist input for the patient's diabetes management will be crucial in preventing further acceleration of his underlying ischaemic heart disease.

10 ICDs require interrogation with early surveillance 6 weeks after implantation and then if no issues arise, every 6–12 months in a cardiac device clinic. At each appointment, physicians take a history to assess for inappropriate shocks, adherence to medications and complications of ICD implantation. They will also check the battery life and lead parameters, review the arrhythmia log and adjust medications accordingly. Some health networks have the infrastructure to follow up patients remotely, where patients can upload their arrhythmia log online, which physicians assess every day. If any actionable items arise, then the health service calls the patient in for clinic follow-up for a formal review.

CASE 11: Addison's disease

History

- A 44-year-old **man** [1] presents with a **3-month history** [2] of **fatigue** [3] and **anorexia** [4].
- He reports that the fatigue has gradually **worsened over time** [5].
- The patient has also noted a 4kg **loss of weight** [6].
- His wife reports that the patient's **skin colour** [7] appears to have changed recently.
- The patient denies any **nausea, vomiting** [8], **dizziness, syncopal episodes** [9] or **loss of consciousness** [10].
- There is no **arthralgia or myalgia** [11].
- There have been no **recent illnesses** [12] or **trauma** [13].
- He is otherwise healthy with no significant **past medical history** [14].
- He does not take any **regular medications** [15] besides occasional over-the-counter multivitamin capsules.
- He lives at home with his wife and is **working happily as a primary school teacher** [16].

[1] The most common cause of primary adrenal insufficiency, or Addison's disease, is the destruction of the adrenal cortex by an autoimmune process (autoimmune adrenalitis). Isolated autoimmune adrenal insufficiency is more common in males, whilst it is more common for females to have multiple endocrine organ involvement.

[2] The onset of Addison's disease can be subtle with gradual development of symptoms, which can delay the diagnosis.

[3] In primary adrenal insufficiency, the symptoms relate to glucocorticoid and mineralocorticoid deficiency. Fatigue is a common symptom present in 84–95% of patients. Patients may describe it as weakness or tiredness.

[4] Some patients may also present with salt craving, or report large amounts of salt ingestion. Although not a common symptom, it is more specific to primary adrenal insufficiency.

[5] The severity of signs and symptoms depends on the rate of loss of adrenal function. While some patients may present with vague and non-specific symptoms, for others primary adrenal insufficiency may remain undetected until a stress or illness precipitates an adrenal crisis.

[6] Weight loss is seen in most patients. It is mainly due to anorexia. However, it is also important to consider the contributing role of dehydration. In patients presenting with weight loss, malignancy should also be considered as a differential diagnosis. Metastatic cancer infiltration is also another cause of primary adrenal insufficiency.

[7] Skin hyperpigmentation occurs due to cortisol deficiency. There is an increased production of a prohormone (proopiomelanocortin) which, when cleaved, produces

active hormones including adrenocorticotrophic hormone (ACTH) and melanocyte-stimulating hormone (MSH). It is the MSH that is responsible for melanin synthesis. In elevated levels, MSH causes increased melanin synthesis and leads to hyperpigmentation.

[8] Some patients can present with abdominal symptoms such as nausea, vomiting and abdominal pain. They may report diarrhoea that alternates with constipation. This can at times lead clinicians to pursue incorrect differential diagnoses and delay correct management. Abdominal pain and vomiting should also alert clinicians to the possibility of an adrenal crisis. Loss of fluid through the GI tract through diarrhoea or vomiting can precipitate an adrenal crisis.

[9] Cardiovascular symptoms such as dizziness and syncope are due to volume depletion secondary to aldosterone deficiency.

[10] The first presentation in a patient with previously undiagnosed primary adrenal insufficiency can be adrenal crisis. Adrenal crisis can present as shock and with non-specific symptoms such as nausea, vomiting, fever, lethargy, weakness, confusion or even coma.

[11] Patients can report musculoskeletal symptoms including diffuse arthralgia and myalgia. In some, these may be the predominant symptom.

[12] Infections including TB, HIV and fungal infections can lead to primary adrenal insufficiency (infectious adrenalitis). Serious infection or an acute stress can also precipitate an adrenal crisis.

[13] Blunt trauma can have the potential complication of adrenal insufficiency. This is more relevant in patients

presenting with abdominal pain, back pain or flank pain, and following motor vehicle accidents.

14 A substantial proportion of patients (50–65%) with autoimmune adrenal insufficiency can also have other autoimmune endocrine disorders such as coeliac disease, type 1 diabetes mellitus and Graves' disease.

15 For patients with known primary or secondary adrenal insufficiency who are on replacement glucocorticoids and mineralocorticoids, insufficient daily doses can trigger an adrenal crisis. Additionally, as discussed, in the event of an acute illness, absorption of medication may be reduced (e.g. due to vomiting or diarrhoea in the setting of viral gastroenteritis). Anticoagulant therapy is a major risk factor for adrenal haemorrhage or infarction leading to adrenal crisis in patients with no pre-existing adrenal insufficiency. There are medications which may cause primary adrenal insufficiency. These can include, but are not limited to, drugs that inhibit cortisol synthesis (e.g. ketoconazole, fluconazole and etomidate – an anaesthetic-sedative) and drugs that accelerate the metabolism of cortisol (e.g. phenytoin, barbiturates and rifampicin).

16 Patients with long-standing untreated primary adrenal insufficiency may present with psychiatric symptoms. Patients or family can report symptoms consistent with depression, psychosis (social withdrawal, irritability, agitation, delusions or hallucinations), mania and anxiety, amongst others.

Examination

- The patient's blood pressure is 110/80mmHg with a **drop to 94/60mmHg upon standing** [1].
- The remaining vital signs are within normal range and the patient is **afebrile** [2].
- The patient's **BMI** [3] is within the normal range.
- His skin is diffusely **hyperpigmented** [4], with the most prominent hyperpigmentation present on his knuckles and palmar creases.
- There is also hyperpigmentation in the **oral mucosa** [5].
- There are no areas of **vitiligo** [6].
- The neck examination is unremarkable, with no **goitre** [7] present.
- The abdomen is **soft and non-tender** [8].
- The remainder of the **physical examination is normal** [9].
- A bedside fingerprick test reveals a **BSL** [10] of 5.5mmol/L.

1 Due to the deficiency of mineralocorticoids (aldosterone), patients with primary adrenal insufficiency can have a postural hypotension and/or a low resting blood pressure.

2 As discussed previously, infection can be the precipitant for a patient presenting in adrenal crisis. Fever can be exaggerated due to the hypocortisolaemia. A febrile patient should prompt further investigation.

3 In a patient presenting with a history of weight loss, calculate the BMI as an aid in monitoring nutritional status and guiding further management.

4 Hyperpigmentation is characteristic of patients with primary adrenal insufficiency. It is generalised but may be more pronounced in sun-exposed areas and extensor regions such as back, neck, face, elbows and knuckles. However, sometimes vaginal and perianal mucosa can be affected as well.

5 Areas such as shoulders, knuckles, elbows, spine and knees, which are more prone to friction and pressure, can show more prominent hyperpigmentation. The waist, midriff and areas where there is friction from a bra strap can also be affected. This also applied to body areas with normally increased pigmentation, such as the axilla and perineum.

6 In dark-skinned patients, palmar creases may naturally be darker than the remainder of their skin. It is important to compare with other family members' and determine the presence of any additional pigmentation. Nails can also show darkening with longitudinal bands. Also observe and ask patients about any scars which may be pigmented, new freckles and darkening of pre-existing freckles.

7 Mucosal hyperpigmentation is generally seen in the inner surface of the lips and buccal mucosa. It may be more pronounced along the denture line where teeth pinch the mucous membrane when eating. Hyperpigmentation may be seen under the tongue and along the outer border of the lips.

8 Vitiligo can be a sign of underlying autoimmune disease and represents immune-mediated destruction of dermal melanocytes. In some patients with autoimmune primary adrenal insufficiency small areas of depigmentation, usually bilateral and symmetrical, can occur.

9 Examine for evidence of other coexisting autoimmune conditions such as autoimmune thyroiditis and Graves' disease.

10 Patients presenting in adrenal crisis with primary adrenal insufficiency can have generalised abdominal tenderness on deep palpation. The exact cause of this physical finding is unclear. In such an instance, where patients are likely to present with nausea and vomiting as well, clinicians may be led to consider surgical causes.

11 It is common in women to note decreased axillary and pubic hair as a result of the loss of adrenal androgen

production. This is rare in men as most of their androgen production occurs in the testes.

12 Patients presenting in adrenal crisis may be significantly hypoglycaemic.

Investigations

- **Laboratory testing** [1] is performed.
- Testing reveals a low **early-morning serum cortisol level** [2] and an elevated **serum adrenocorticotrophic hormone (ACTH) level** [3].
- **Serum electrolyte results** [4] reveal a **hyponatraemia** [5] and **hyperkalaemia** [6].
- The **calcium, magnesium and phosphate levels** [7] are all within the normal range.
- Haematological testing shows a **mild anaemia and eosinophilia** [8].

- An **ACTH stimulation test** [9] is performed, which confirms the diagnosis of **primary adrenal insufficiency** [10] in this patient.
- Following this a **CT scan** [11] of the abdomen is performed, which is largely unremarkable, and no **further imaging studies** [12] are deemed necessary.
- The patient is tested for **21-hydroxylase (21-OH) antibodies** [13], which returns a positive result.

1 In the absence of classic symptoms and signs, the diagnosis of chronic primary adrenal insufficiency can be difficult. Further investigations are required to determine the aetiology of the adrenal insufficiency.

2 The diagnosis of adrenal insufficiency, regardless of the aetiology, requires the patient to have inappropriately low serum cortisol level. Generally, the serum cortisol levels are highest in the early hours (6–8am). If a patient has an early-morning cortisol level of <3mcg/dl (80nmol/L), this suggests a diagnosis of adrenal insufficiency. Urinary cortisol can also be measured; however, it can be normal in patients with partial adrenal insufficiency and therefore cannot be used as a screening tool.

3 The ACTH level is helpful in determining whether the patient has a primary, secondary or tertiary adrenal insufficiency. ACTH is produced by the anterior pituitary gland and is responsible for stimulating the release of cortisol from the adrenal cortex. In primary adrenal insufficiency, the ACTH level is expected to be high, as this indicates that the abnormality is at the level of the adrenal gland (not responding appropriately to the stimulation by ACTH). There is a lack of negative feedback to regulate the amount of ACTH produced due to the lack of glucocorticoids, thereby causing an increased production of ACTH. If the ACTH level is low, this indicates that the pathology is either at the level of the pituitary gland (secondary) or the hypothalamus (tertiary). In these situations, the cortisol levels are low which is a reflection of the reduced levels of ACTH or lack of ACTH production.

4 Reduced secretion of cortisol and aldosterone in Addison's disease causes typical electrolyte abnormalities; however, in an urgent situation treatment should not be delayed whilst awaiting formal serum electrolyte results. A typical pattern involves hyponatraemia, hyperkalaemia and

metabolic acidosis. Blood should be obtained for random cortisol level testing and treatment commenced immediately.

5 When plasma cortisol levels are low, antidiuretic hormone (ADH) levels in the body increase. The reduced systemic blood pressure (due to lack of cortisol) can also stimulate hypersecretion of ADH. ADH causes water retention and can thereby cause a reduction in plasma sodium concentration. Aldosterone deficiency can also contribute to hyponatraemia by causing renal sodium wasting and therefore causing volume depletion. In response, ADH hypersecretion can occur. This is because the hypovolaemia reduces the osmotic threshold for ADH release in the hypothalamus.

6 One of the main functions of aldosterone is to increase urinary potassium excretion. Therefore, when there is hypoaldosteronism, there is decreased excretion of potassium, causing hyperkalaemia.

7 Rarely, there may be a hypercalcaemia, associated with acute renal insufficiency.

8 Presence of eosinophilia suggests adrenal insufficiency in the right context. Normocytic anaemia can be seen in some patients.

9 The ACTH stimulation test (also known as the Synacthen test) can be performed using either high or low dose synthetic ACTH. The principle of the test is to assess the cortisol level in response to stimulation with ACTH. In a person with intact pituitary–adrenal axis, the serum cortisol level should rise within 30–60 minutes (depending on the dose used) in response to the ACTH. A positive test (where there is an absence or inappropriately low plasma cortisol response) alongside elevated plasma renin and elevated ACTH is required for the diagnosis of primary adrenal insufficiency.

10 It is important to determine the type of adrenal insufficiency as, depending on the aetiology, underlying causes need to be managed (e.g. treatment of TB as the cause of primary adrenal insufficiency).

11 A CT scan is useful in narrowing down the list of potential aetiologies of primary adrenal insufficiency. Enlarged or calcified adrenal glands on CT can suggest malignancy, infection or a haemorrhagic cause. Although the above findings on a CT can be helpful in excluding autoimmune adrenal insufficiency as a cause, a normal CT scan does not exclude TB as a cause. Further testing including a CXR, acid-fast bacilli, polymerase chain reaction (PCR) and mycobacterial culture on specimens (e.g. sputum) can be used if active TB is suspected in high risk populations.

12 Further scans such as a positron emission tomography (PET) scan can be performed in instances where malignancy is suspected. This reduces the need for other more invasive measures, such as CT-guided needle aspiration of the adrenal gland.

13 Measurement of serum 21-OH antibodies can be performed to investigate a clinical suspicion of autoimmune primary adrenal insufficiency, and where no other clear cause is evident. These antibodies are directed against an enzyme which is required for the production of cortisol. In these patients, it is important to investigate for any other autoimmune conditions and endocrine pathologies.

Management

Immediate

As this patient is presenting with chronic adrenal insufficiency, not complicated by **adrenal crisis** [1], no immediate steps are required in this situation.

Short-term

A discussion is held with the patient and his family about the new **diagnosis of Addison's disease** [2]. He is informed about the need for **commencing medication** [3]. The patient is started on **oral hydrocortisone** [4] 12mg in the morning and 8mg in the **afternoon** [5]. He is also commenced on **fludrocortisone** [6] 100mcg orally daily. A **sick day management plan** [7] is also established together with the patient and his family. They are also informed of the **modification of glucocorticoid doses** [8] during minor illnesses.

Long-term

The patient is scheduled for a **dual energy X-ray absorptiometry (DEXA) scan** [9]. A **follow-up clinic appointment** [10] is organised in the outpatient department to review results and monitor his **response to the replacement therapy** [11]. His **progress** [12] is assessed and the patient is reviewed for any complications.

1 Adrenal crisis is a medical emergency that requires immediate management. If clinical suspicion is high, waiting for investigation results should never delay commencement of treatment.
Patients should be promptly started on IV glucocorticoid therapy. The recommended treatment for an adult is 100mg IV hydrocortisone as a stat dose initially, followed by 50mg every 6 hours until patient is stable. In the event of IV access not being available, an oral alternative of prednisolone 40mg can be used.
Patients will also require IV fluid therapy. As hyperkalaemia usually resolves with IV therapy, IV insulin should not be used. If there is hypoglycaemia present, this should also be corrected.

2 Patient education is vital in the management of Addison's disease. There should be a thorough understanding of the disease. This should include an explanation of the hormone deficiency, the importance of adherence to replacement therapy and the severe consequences of non-compliance.

3 Primary adrenal insufficiency requires lifelong treatment with glucocorticoid replacement. The aim of the treatment is to mimic the pattern of natural cortisol synthesis by the adrenal glands. Generally, patients should be started on the lowest dose possible to relieve symptoms.

4 Hydrocortisone is commonly used in the management of adrenal insufficiency. As prednisolone can cause growth suppression, it should be avoided in children. In adults, particularly if there are concerns around adherence, prednisolone can be used for maintenance therapy as it has a longer duration of action and can be given as a once-daily dose. Dexamethasone is another long-acting glucocorticoid; however, it is not commonly used for replacement therapy as the dosing can be difficult to predict and patients may be overtreated.

5 Twice-daily dosing is the recommended starting regimen for most adults. As there are adverse effects associated with glucocorticoid administration in the evening, dosing should be done in the morning and mid-afternoon. Adjustments to the dose should be done slowly and in small increments. It is important that when patients are unwell or are undergoing procedures/surgery, the glucocorticoid dose is adjusted accordingly, to reflect the normal increase in secretion of cortisol in our body that occurs in response to acute stress. This is vital to prevent an adrenal crisis.

6 Mineralocorticoids are generally eventually required for maintaining a normal blood pressure in patients with adrenal insufficiency. Therapy with mineralocorticoids aims to maintain normal levels of plasma sodium, potassium and plasma renin concentrations. Unlike glucocorticoids, the dose of mineralocorticoids does not need to be adjusted acutely when there is an acute illness or stress. However, for some patients with excessive sweating in warm weather, increased loss of salt in perspiration may be an indication for a dose increase.

7 Patients with primary adrenal insufficiency do not have a normal renin–angiotensin– aldosterone response to hypovolaemia. They also lack a normal response to stress. This poses a risk for the patients at home as they must learn to recognise these conditions and adjust their therapy accordingly. When discharging patients home, ensure that they are provided with take-home injectable short-acting glucocorticoid (e.g. hydrocortisone) for use in an emergency, as well as normal saline and syringes. Educate the patient and a family member or carer on correct injection techniques. Generally, the circumstances under which this should be administered, in addition to seeking immediate medical attention, include any event of large fluid loss (i.e. significant blood loss, vomiting or diarrhoea) and symptoms of an adrenal crisis, including unresponsiveness. Additionally, patients should be provided with a medical emergency document summarising their medical condition, medications and contact physician details. It is also helpful to arrange for patients to have an emergency alert bracelet or necklace.

8 In the event of a minor illness, patients can self-increase the dose of glucocorticoid. The recommendations are variable, but in general the dose can be increased by 2–3 times the usual dose. However, caution should be taken if a patient is suffering from nausea or vomiting, as the absorption of the oral replacement may be compromised. For patients who are planned for elective surgery, a preoperative consultation should be carried out to create a modified dosing plan for glucocorticoid replacement therapy. The additional dose is variable and depends on the level of stress that is expected to be induced by the surgery (minor vs. major surgical procedures). Generally, patients should be able to resume their usual maintenance replacement dose day two or three postoperatively.

9 Long-term treatment with glucocorticoids carries its own set of risks. One of the most prominent side-effects is that of lowering bone mineral density (BMD) and of osteoporosis. Therefore, these patients require a baseline measurement of BMD and an assessment of fracture risk at the time of diagnosis. Following this, BMD should be assessed every 2 years. If there is a notable reduction in BMD, adjustment of glucocorticoid therapy may be required. It may also be necessary to revisit the possibility of other endocrine conditions such as thyroid disease or coeliac disease. Other side-effects of long-term glucocorticoid therapy can include diabetes, weight gain, bruising and thinning of the skin.

10 Treatment should be led by a specialist clinician with ongoing monitoring. Once the patient is stable on a treatment regimen, the frequency of follow-up clinic appointments can be reduced to once a year. Ongoing monitoring for other autoimmune diseases (e.g. type 1 diabetes) should be performed. Laboratory testing can be used as a screening tool.

11 Some patients may remain symptomatic despite glucocorticoid and mineralocorticoid therapy. Although not routinely recommended, some of these patients may benefit from androgen replacement therapy with dehydroepiandrosterone (DHEA). Reported benefits of DHEA replacement include improved general wellbeing in patients, improved sexual function in women, increased bone density and lean body mass.

12 The efficacy of the treatment can be objectively measured using serum sodium, potassium and renin concentration measurements at clinic visits. The aim is to maintain plasma renin in the upper to normal range. This indicates optimal mineralocorticoid replacement.

CASE 12: Conn's disease

History

- A 38-year-old male is found to be **hypertensive** [1] during a routine blood pressure measurement taken at a new GP clinic.
- He is unsure of his **previous blood pressure readings** [2].
- On further history taking, he reports a history of **nocturia** [3] (3–4 times per night), intermittent **headaches** [4] and **lethargy** [5]. He states the duration of symptoms as possibly 'years'.
- He reports his **weight** [6] has been stable over the last few years. He denies any **weakness or muscle cramping** [6].

- The patient denies **palpitations, sweating or heat intolerance** [7].
- There is no history of **visual changes** [8].
- There is no significant **past medical history** [9].
- The patient does not take any **regular medications** [10].
- He is **otherwise well** [11] and is currently working as an IT technician.
- There is a **family history of hypertension** [12], with the patient's mother being diagnosed with hypertension at the age of 55.
- There is no **family history of stroke** [13].

1 Hypertension (HTN) is the main clinical feature of primary hyperaldosteronism; a condition of aldosterone hypersecretion which is autonomous or relatively independent to the renin–angiotensin system. Aldosterone production is also not suppressed by salt-loading. Excess aldosterone increases sodium reabsorption, and sometimes potassium wasting, in the distal nephron, leading to water retention and an increase in the circulatory volume. Hypervolaemia increases systemic vascular resistance, leading to HTN.

2 For patients presenting with HTN, the diagnosis should be confirmed with consecutive readings. If confirmed, a range of differential diagnoses should be considered. The causes of HTN can be broadly classified into essential hypertension and secondary hypertension. The majority of cases of HTN are due to essential hypertension, the incidence of which increases with age. HTN in a young patient should prompt consideration for causes of secondary hypertension, including endocrine abnormalities (such as primary aldosteronism, Cushing's syndrome and phaeochromocytoma), renal parenchymal or vascular diseases (e.g. renal artery stenosis) and coarctation of the aorta.

3 Ask about symptoms of nocturia and polyuria in patients. This can occur as a result of the volume overload in primary aldosteronism. Long-standing hypokalaemia can lead to nephrogenic diabetes insipidus, due to impaired urine-concentrating ability, which would present with these symptoms.

4 Headaches can occur with severe HTN but if associated with sweating and tachycardia, they can suggest phaeochromocytoma (catecholamine-secreting tumour). Although rare, this differential diagnosis can be difficult to exclude based on history alone.

5 Lethargy is a fairly non-specific symptom that needs to be considered within the clinical context.

6 Weight gain can occur in Cushing's syndrome, which is a differential for secondary hypertension. A history of weight loss associated with lethargy or fatigue should trigger further assessment to exclude malignancy.

7 Less commonly, patients may present with muscle cramps, weakness, paraesthesia and palpitations, related to hypokalaemia.

8 Visual changes, particularly bilateral temporal hemianopia, may indicate a pituitary macroadenoma and may offer an alternative cause of secondary hypertension such as Cushing's syndrome.

9 Patients with primary aldosteronism can be at a higher risk of T2DM and metabolic syndrome.

10 Enquire about medication use including diuretics. In patients with primary aldosteronism, the plasma potassium levels can eventually reach a steady state. However, progressive hypokalaemia can occur in the context of diuretic use. Additionally, common drugs such as NSAIDs and certain antihypertensive medications can affect the aldosterone to renin ratio (refer to Investigations section).

11 Some patients may report symptoms of depression, anxiety, difficulty concentrating and irritability, which could affect their quality of life.

12 Patients with primary aldosteronism are at increased risk of cardiovascular morbidity and mortality. Assess any additional cardiovascular risk factors for the patient, including a family history of cardiac events.

13 Risk factors for the development of primary aldosteronism include a family history of primary aldosteronism, family history of HTN and stroke. There can be early onset HTN (at <40 years of age) in familial primary aldosteronism type I and III.

Examination

- The patient's vital signs are normal apart from a **blood pressure of 168/100mmHg** [1]. A repeated measurement using the other arm reveals a similar result.
- **BMI** [2] is calculated at 24kg/m^2.
- On general inspection, the patient does not have **moon-like facies, bruising, evidence of thinning skin or abdominal striae** [3].
- The pulse is **regular** [4] with no **radio-femoral delay** [5].
- There are no **cardiac murmurs** [6] present and auscultation of the chest is clear.
- Abdomen is soft and non-tender on examination. There are no **palpable masses** [7] or **renal bruit** [8].
- **Fundoscopy** [9] is performed as part of the physical examination, which reveals mild opacification of the arterial wall, consistent with **hypertensive retinopathy** [10].
- A bedside ECG is also done, showing sinus pattern with changes consistent with **left ventricular hypertrophy** [11].

1 As discussed earlier, HTN is the main clinical feature of this condition, and blood pressure readings are generally substantially elevated. Generally clinical examination is targeted towards ruling out other causes of secondary hypertension. Coexisting tachycardia may point toward phaeochromocytoma.

2 As these patients are also at a higher risk of metabolic syndrome, assess for contributing risk factors including a high BMI.

3 Examination should further explore some differential diagnoses. Look for features consistent with Cushing's syndrome. Other features include central obesity and proximal muscle weakness. In women, signs of excessive androgen may be present. This can include hirsutism (excess facial hair), oily skin and acne.

4 Assess for an irregular pulse: patients with primary aldosteronism may have higher rates of AF due to electrolyte derangement, as well as MI and stroke.

5 Coarctation of the aorta can cause a radio-femoral delay. Another classic feature is low or undetectable blood pressure in the lower extremities. HTN can be the first presentation of this condition in previously undiagnosed adults.

6 A systolic murmur may be heard in the infraclavicular area, associated with coarctation of the aorta.

7 A mass associated with phaeochromocytoma may be palpable in some cases.

8 A renal bruit may be heard in patients with renal artery stenosis. Renovascular disease is a cause of secondary hypertension.

9 Fundoscopy should be part of the physical examination of patients with newly diagnosed HTN.

10 Sustained hypertension may lead to retinal microvascular changes. Mild changes include arteriovenous nicking, narrowing of retinal artery and arterial wall thickening. In more advanced stages, fundoscopy may reveal retinal haemorrhages, cotton-wool spots or exudates. Papilloedema may be seen in severe cases, and requires prompt management.

11 Left ventricular hypertrophy can reflect long-standing HTN, where pressure overload results in the hypertrophy. ECG changes include increased R wave amplitude in left-sided leads (I, aVL, V4–V6) and increased S wave amplitude in right-sided leads (III, aVR, V1–V3). Delayed repolarisation due to the thickened left ventricular wall can lead to ST segment and T wave abnormalities in the lateral leads.

Investigations

- The full blood examination is unremarkable. Electrolyte testing reveals **hypokalaemia** [1].
- Calcium, **magnesium** [2] and phosphate levels are within the normal range.
- **Renal function** [3] is normal.
- **Urinary catecholamines** [4] are also normal. Further laboratory tests are requested to assess plasma renin and aldosterone.
- The results show a low **plasma renin activity (PRA)** [5] with a **high plasma aldosterone concentration (PAC)** [6, 7].

- The **aldosterone to renin ratio (ARR)** [8] is high, suggestive of primary aldosteronism.
- An **oral sodium loading test** [9] is performed to confirm the diagnosis.
- Following this, an **adrenal CT scan** [10] is performed; this shows a **left adrenal mass measuring 2.5cm in diameter** [11].
- **Adrenal venous sampling** [12] shows lateralisation of aldosterone production to the left adrenal gland.
- **Dexamethasone suppression testing** [13] reveals a normal result.

[1] Hypokalaemia occurs as a result of the loss of K⁺ ions in exchange for sodium in the distal nephron. There is also urinary loss of hydrogen, which if prolonged can result in a metabolic alkalosis. However, this is an inconsistent finding and is not present in all cases of primary aldosteronism. Diagnosis of primary hyperaldosteronism should thus still be considered in patients presenting with normokalaemic HTN. Hypokalaemia can also be seen in Cushing's syndrome – correlation with clinical findings on history and examination is needed.

[2] Rarely, patients with an excess of aldosterone can have mild hypomagnesaemia, thought to be secondary to urinary magnesium wasting.

[3] A normal renal function deems renal disease unlikely in this patient as a cause of HTN. Urinalysis is useful in detecting red cell casts and active sediments of glomerulonephritis. If renal artery stenosis is suspected, a renal artery Doppler could be performed.

[4] This test is performed as the first test in patients where there is a low clinical suspicion for phaeochromocytoma.

[5] Sodium reabsorption and the resultant increased circulating volume acts to suppress the release of renin. This causes low plasma renin activity and subsequently a low concentration of plasma renin. In clinical practice, plasma renin may be measured either as PRA, direct active renin (DAR) concentration or plasma renin concentration (PRC).

[6] PAC is inappropriately elevated in aldosteronism. It is important to note that in practice, PRC and PAC should be measured in the morning with the patient sitting upright, as these results can be impacted by the time of day and posture of the patient.

[7] If both plasma renin and plasma aldosterone are elevated, consider renovascular disease as a cause of secondary aldosteronism. The mechanism is: increased renin production → an increase in angiotensin II production → increased aldosterone secretion.

On the other hand, if plasma renin and aldosterone are both reduced, this can suggest an excess of a mineralocorticoid other than aldosterone, such as the mineralocorticoid deoxycorticosterone, produced in certain types of congenital adrenal hyperplasia.

[8] An excess of aldosterone provides negative feedback on the production of renin. This causes a decrease in renin production, subsequently resulting in a high ARR (also written as PAC/PRA ratio). As discussed previously, some medications can impact the result; consideration can be given to modifying antihypertensive medications (changing to alternative antihypertensives with less effect on the ARR – examples include verapamil, diltiazem, prazosin and hydralazine) prior to the blood test. However, the risks of this should be carefully weighed. If the ARR is performed whilst the patient is on certain medications that can impact on the result, expert input should be sought in interpreting the outcome. An ARR ratio of >20 is indicative of primary aldosteronism. The ARR is primarily a screening tool only and does not confirm the diagnosis.

[9] The patient is given a high sodium diet for 3 days. Following this, serum electrolytes are measured and a 24-hour urine sample is collected. If the urine aldosterone excretion within the 24-hour period exceeds 12mcg, the diagnosis of primary aldosteronism is confirmed. This test requires accurate and complete collection of urine. Other tests that can be used to confirm the diagnosis of primary aldosteronism include fludrocortisone suppression test (where fludrocortisone acetate and slow release normal saline is given – failure of plasma aldosterone to be appropriately suppressed confirms the diagnosis) and saline infusion test (this involves measurement of plasma aldosterone following administration of 0.9% intravenous saline). Prior to commencing these tests, hypokalaemia should be corrected and potassium levels maintained at a close to normal level.

[10] Once the diagnosis of primary aldosteronism has been confirmed, the aetiology has to be established. In general, Conn's disease (aldosterone-secreting adrenal

adenoma) presents with more severe HTN and more marked hyperkalaemia with higher levels of plasma aldosterone compared with bilateral hyperplasia. Clear distinction requires further imaging studies. A CT scan can be used to assist in distinguishing between bilateral hyperplasia, unilateral aldosterone-producing adenoma or adrenal carcinoma. CT is a suitable modality for initial imaging of the adrenal glands.

11 This finding is consistent with Conn's syndrome (unilateral, hypodense mass with a normal contralateral adrenal gland). Some adenomas can warrant surgical removal, usually due to their malignant potential. A unilateral mass can raise suspicion for adrenal carcinoma, although typically of larger size (>4cm). In patients with hyperplasia, CT may show adrenal gland thickening or micronodular changes bilaterally – in some cases they may appear normal in CT.

12 Adrenal venous sampling can be performed if a patient is considered for surgical management, where confirmation of unilateral disease is needed (if CT inconclusive and to avoid unnecessary/inappropriate surgical measures based on CT findings alone). It is also recommended if CT confirms unilateral disease but the patient is over the age of 35. The adrenal veins are sampled using cannulas inserted into bilateral veins, with cortisol and aldosterone levels measured. Unilateral disease is confirmed if the plasma aldosterone concentration is significantly higher on the affected side, compared with the contralateral gland.

13 There is a possibility of cortisol co-secretion in some aldosterone-producing adenomas. This can be assessed by measuring baseline serum cortisol and ACTH, followed by administration of dexamethasone overnight. Serum cortisol and ACTH can be remeasured in the morning. Where there is concurrent and autonomous adrenal cortisol production, there will be a low baseline ACTH with failure of cortisol levels to be appropriately suppressed following dexamethasone.

Management

- **Management options** [1] are surgical or pharmacological.
- In this patient, **surgical management** [2] is appropriate.
- The diagnosis of **primary aldosteronism and its implications** [3] are discussed with the patient and family.
- An in-depth conversation is held with the patient detailing the proposed management plan and **expected outcome** [4].
- He is assessed for **operative suitability** [5] in the pre-operative clinic.
- His **potassium levels** [6] are optimised and he is commenced on medication to control HTN.
- He undergoes a left **laparoscopic**

adrenalectomy [7]. The operation is successfully completed without any immediate complications.
- Following a period of **monitoring in hospital** [8], the patient is discharged with **instructions for home** [9].
- Follow-up in a **postoperative review** [10] clinic is organised.
- The patient is asked to attend for **further blood tests** [11] prior to presenting to the clinic appointment.
- His blood pressure in the clinic is **155/85mmHg** [12].
- He is commenced on **spironolactone 25mg orally daily** [13].
- The patient is booked for further follow-up visits to continue **monitoring his progress** [14].

1 The main aim of management in patients with primary aldosteronism is to control the excessive production of aldosterone, thereby preventing the side-effects and complications associated with sustained hypertension, including renal and cardiovascular complications. For patients with hypokalaemia, the goal of treatment is to normalise the potassium and maintain it.

2 Identifying the aetiology of the aldosteronism is vital, as management varies depending on the cause. Surgical management is appropriate in patients with unilateral aldosterone-secreting adenoma or unilateral hyperplasia. Patients with bilateral hyperplasia may benefit from pharmacological therapy with mineralocorticoid receptor antagonists (MRAs). Spironolactone can be offered – discuss with the patient the potential side-effects of gynaecomastia,

impotence, decreased libido (in men), breast tenderness and menstrual irregularities (in women). The potassium-sparing diuretic amiloride is another option for those intolerant of spironolactone. Adrenalectomy is rarely appropriate in bilateral adrenal hyperplasia (increased risk associated with bilateral adrenalectomy – need for lifelong replacement of glucocorticoids and mineralocorticoids).

3 Increased awareness of primary aldosteronism is required to improve screening amongst the family members. Primary care providers should be aware of the indications for screening. This could allow earlier diagnosis and reduce the prevalence of end-organ damage.

4 In some patients, HTN can persist despite treatment. Although the severity may be significantly improved, it may only be cured in approximately 50–60% of patients. This is an important point to be discussed and made clear to the patient when considering surgical management. All treatment options, their risks, benefits and expected outcomes should be carefully explored with the patient and family.

5 Assessment of operative candidates should focus on comorbid conditions that may increase risk of anaesthetic and recovery complications. Ask patients about airway disease, heart disease, renal disease, previous anaesthetic complications and allergies. Physical fitness including BMI and exercise tolerance should be assessed. If a patient is deemed unsuitable for surgery or a patient declines surgery, they can be managed with aldosterone antagonists or MRAs.

6 In the period leading up to the surgery, patients with hypokalaemia should be commenced on potassium supplementation. They can also be commenced on a mineralocorticoid antagonist such as spironolactone. Repletion of potassium and optimisation of blood pressure can minimise operative risk by improving cardiovascular function.

7 Total adrenalectomy is performed rather than a partial adrenalectomy (removing only the adenoma; the adrenal gland remains intact). This avoids the risk of resecting a non-secreting nodule and leaving behind a smaller but hyperfunctioning nodule which may not be visualised but is actually the cause of the symptoms. Note that adrenal venous sampling can only indicate the side of the abnormality, not the exact nodule or location on the gland. A laparoscopic approach is associated with fewer operative and postoperative complications and tends to lead to a shorter duration of stay in hospital compared to an open approach. These complications can include wound infections, haemorrhage, pulmonary embolism, deep vein thrombus, urinary infections and atelectasis.

8 Treat the patient with isotonic saline (avoid potassium unless patient remains hypokalaemic) at an 8- or 12-hourly rate postoperatively. As part of the postoperative management, monitor closely for hyperkalaemia. Potassium supplementation should be discontinued. Withhold any potassium-sparing diuretics. If commenced, discontinue mineralocorticoid antagonists and decrease antihypertensives. Importantly, check plasma aldosterone levels on day one postoperatively. Undetectable levels indicate a long-term cure. Transient hypokalaemia in the immediate postoperative period can occur. This is a reflection of a combination of the cessation of potassium supplements, cessation of aldosterone antagonists and supplementation with potassium-free IV fluid.

9 Patients should be advised on continuing a salt-rich diet following discharge. As for any postoperative patient, advise them on appropriate wound care, provide additional waterproof dressings and caution against heavy lifting or vigorous activity. Inform patient and family of how and when to contact a medical professional or attend the ED.

10 In routine postop review, assess the patient's progress, examine the wounds to ensure proper healing and ask about any complications. Enquire about quality of life following surgery to determine whether they need any extra services in place during the period of recovery.

11 Biochemical testing provides an objective indication of improvement. Following surgery, hypokalaemia should be corrected (if present pre-operatively); continue to monitor serum potassium to ensure the patient does not become hyperkalaemic. The risk of hyperkalaemia is due to the chronic suppression of the renin–aldosterone mechanism. This means that there is suppression of aldosterone production in the contralateral gland. Therefore, once the hypersecreting gland has been removed, there are very low levels of aldosterone in the body. Aldosterone levels gradually normalise over a few weeks.

If a patient is found to be hypokalaemic, they should be re-evaluated for recurrent primary aldosteronism. Generally, patients report improvement in symptoms regardless of whether they were hypokalaemic or normokalaemic prior to the surgery. In patients who had preoperative renal impairment, serum creatinine levels should be checked.

12 HTN is cured in many patients, whilst a mild degree can persist in some patients. Certain patient factors have been found to be associated with a higher likelihood of complete resolution of HTN following surgical management, including younger age, absence of a family history of HTN and a shorter duration of HTN prior to management. Patients who were using fewer than two antihypertensive agents pre-operatively are also more likely to be responsive to surgery.

13 In persistent HTN, patients should be commenced on an aldosterone antagonist as first-line treatment. If patients experience bothersome side-effects with spironolactone, they can be commenced on amiloride 5mg twice daily as an alternative. Eplerenone is another highly selective mineralocorticoid antagonist with a better side-effect profile than spironolactone; however, it is significantly more expensive.

14 The dose of spironolactone should be adjusted based on the subsequent blood pressure readings. Patients on spironolactone should have serum potassium and creatinine measured periodically, particularly within the first 4–6 weeks of treatment. This is especially important in patients with pre-existing renal insufficiency or diabetes. Caution the patient against the use of NSAIDs as these can interfere with the efficacy of spironolactone. Subsequent antihypertensive agents may need to be added if HTN persists. Low doses of a thiazide drug may be appropriate (e.g. hydrochlorothiazide). Patients should be closely monitored for volume contraction when on multiple aldosterone antagonist agents as there is a risk of prerenal failure and severe hyperkalaemia. Take particular care in patients who have pre-existing low glomerular filtration rates.

CASE 13: Cushing's syndrome

History

- A **35-year-old female** [1] presents with increasing weight gain over 6 months, not in keeping with her diet and activity level.
- Her **weight has suddenly increased** [2] and she now has significant abdominal obesity as well as increased weight around the face, neck and upper back.
- She reports increasing **irregularity in her menstrual cycle** [3] over the last 4 months.
- She has also noticed increasing central **lower back pain** [4] over the past month, although denies history of falls or trauma and has no complicating sensory changes in her lower limbs or incontinence.
- She remains active with gentle walking; however, she has noticed **difficulty getting out of chairs** [5] in the last few months.

- She reports recent difficulties with **anxiety and irritability** [6].
- Of note, she has no history of **headaches nor vision changes** [7].
- She does not have concerns of **hirsutism or acne** [8].
- She has been well recently, with no history of **infections** [9].
- She has no known medical history, in particular no previous **hypertension nor diabetes** [10].
- She takes no regular **medications and denies exogenous steroid use** [11].
- She is a **non-smoker** [12] and has no family history of lung cancer.
- She drinks **alcohol occasionally, denies low mood or history of depression and denies current pregnancy** [13].

[1] Cushing's syndrome is a state of chronic hypercortisolism, aetiologies of which can be classified as adrenocorticotrophic hormone (ACTH)-independent or ACTH-dependent. Cortisol is a hormone secreted by the adrenal cortex in response to ACTH, which is produced by the pituitary gland. ACTH is secreted in response to corticotrophin-releasing hormone (CRH) which is produced by the hypothalamus. Cortisol acts to inhibit the secretion of CRH and ACTH through negative feedback. Loss of this hypothalamic–pituitary–adrenal regulation leads to inappropriately high cortisol levels in Cushing's syndrome. The duration and degree of elevation of cortisol levels correlate with disease severity. The most common endogenous cause of Cushing's syndrome is Cushing's disease, making up approximately two-thirds of endogenous Cushing's syndrome cases. Cushing's disease is an ACTH-dependent condition where hypercortisolism occurs due to excessive secretion of ACTH by a pituitary tumour. Cushing's disease most commonly presents in females between the ages of 25 and 45 years. Aside from a list of very rare causes, endogenous Cushing's syndrome can also be caused by ectopic ACTH-secreting tumours and primary adrenal neoplasms.

[2] Cushing's syndrome most commonly presents with sudden onset weight gain. The weight gain shows a predilection for the abdomen, face, neck and upper back.

[3] Menstrual irregularities, including oliguria, amenorrhoea and variable menses, are common features of Cushing's syndrome in females of this age. Menstrual irregularities are due to low luteinising hormone and follicle-stimulating hormone, which is a result of suppression of gonadotrophin-releasing hormone by excess cortisol. These hormone changes in male patients with Cushing's syndrome commonly result in erectile dysfunction and decreased libido.

[4] Back pain is common in Cushing's syndrome and can be multifactorial in nature: increasing obesity, decreased physical activity, osteoporosis and associated increased fracture risk. Osteopenia and osteoporosis, most commonly affecting the vertebrae and ribs, can be part of the presentation of Cushing's syndrome. Bone loss occurs due to chronic excessive glucocorticoid levels, causing decreased intestinal calcium absorption, decreased bone formation, increased bone resorption and decreased renal calcium absorption. In the context of osteoporosis, vertebral compression fractures can occur secondary to low impact trauma or from usual activities that involve twisting and bending. These fractures may be asymptomatic or cause localised mid-line pain over the affected region. Assessing neurological function is important in ruling out neurological complications from a potential vertebral osteoporotic fracture.

[5] Proximal myopathy is a common symptom of Cushing's syndrome and is a risk factor for falls, which particularly presents an issue in a patient with osteoporosis.

6 Psychological symptoms are common in Cushing's syndrome and include emotional lability, irritability, depression and anxiety. Paranoia and manic symptoms are less common.

7 Most commonly Cushing's disease is caused by a pituitary microadenoma (an adenoma with a diameter of ≤10mm) which generally do not cause symptoms secondary to mass effect on local structures. Macroadenomas are uncommon in Cushing's disease; however, if present, these tumours can result in headaches or visual changes from compression on cranial nerves II, III, IV or VI, the optic chiasm or the cavernous sinus, and panhypopituitarism from local mass effect.

8 Clinical features of androgen excess include hirsutism, oily skin and acne. Androgen excess is seen in cases of Cushing's syndrome in women caused by adrenal carcinomas, as these tumours are inefficient at converting cholesterols to cortisol which results in the secretion of large amounts of androgen precursors. This does not occur in males with Cushing's syndrome as the testes are the major source of androgens, rather than the adrenal glands.

9 A complication of Cushing's syndrome is increased frequency of infections secondary to corticosteroid-related immunosuppression. Patients with severe hypercortisolism, as seen with exogenous high dose glucocorticoid use or ectopic ACTH syndrome, have increased risk of opportunistic infections.

10 It is important to assess for hypertension as well as hyperglycaemia, which commonly occurs with uncontrolled Cushing's syndrome. Dyslipidaemia is also common in this group of patients.

11 Iatrogenic exogenous glucocorticoid use, including use of long-term prednisolone and other similar medications, is the most common cause of Cushing's syndrome.

12 Ectopic ACTH secretion from a tumour can result in Cushing's syndrome. The most commonly associated tumour is small cell lung cancer.

13 It is important in history taking with a patient with some evidence of hypercortisolism to consider the potential for pseudo-Cushing's syndrome. Patients with pseudo-Cushing's syndrome present with some or all of the clinical features that resemble true Cushing's syndrome and have some evidence of hypercortisolism. However, the Cushing's-like state resolves if the underlying primary condition resolves. Pseudo-Cushing's syndrome can occur with severe depression, chronic alcohol excess, pregnancy, severe obesity and physical stress such as illness or surgery.

Examination

- The patient does not appear unwell. Her **blood pressure** [1] is 145/90mmHg.
- She is obese with a BMI of 32kg/m[2]. The **distribution of her obesity** [2] is central, involving the abdomen, trunk and neck. She has increased fat distribution over her upper back, causing a hump.
- Across her abdomen and thighs there are wide, purple **striae** [3].
- She has a rounded face with characteristic **'moon facies' and plethora** [4].
- Her upper limbs and lower limbs reveal many **ecchymoses** [5]; however, she denies any associated trauma.
- She has no **hirsutism or acne** [6] and she has no areas of **hyperpigmentation** [7].

- A **visual examination** [8] is unremarkable and of note she has no abnormalities of ocular movements, no diplopia, no papilloedema and no visual field defects.
- An upper and lower limb neurological examination reveals **proximal myopathy** [9]. She is unable to rise from a chair without using her arms for support. Otherwise, the neurological examination is unremarkable.
- On examination of her back, she has **point tenderness** [10] over the L1 vertebrae. No other point tenderness occurs on palpating.
- There is **no hip irritability or pain** [11] on testing hip movement.
- Examination of other organ systems is unremarkable.

1 Hypertension is a common comorbidity associated with Cushing's syndrome. The hypertension often improves once the Cushing's syndrome is treated.

2 Progressive central obesity is the most common feature of Cushing's syndrome. The distribution of adiposity typically involves the trunk, abdomen, face and neck. A dorsocervical fat pad is common and causes a buffalo hump.

3 Striae caused by Cushing's syndrome tend to appear as purple and wide due to increasingly thin and fragile skin over areas of progressively increasing obesity. The typical reddish-purple colour is because the colour of venous blood is no longer hidden by the thinning skin.

4 'Moon facies' is the classic rounded facial appearance in a patient with Cushing's syndrome; this is due to increased accumulation of adipose tissue in the cheeks. Plethora is thought to be a result of increased blood flow to superficial blood vessels.

5 The skin commonly becomes thin and fragile in Cushing's syndrome and results in ecchymoses not associated with trauma. A recent history of easy bruising may have been elicited by history taking with this patient.

6 Hirsutism and acne are signs of androgen excess, which is common in females with adrenal carcinomas. Women with ACTH-dependent Cushing's syndrome do not usually have signs of androgen excess or, if present, they tend to be mild.

7 Hyperpigmentation occurs due to increased ACTH secretion. Therefore it could be present in ACTH-dependent Cushing's syndrome but does not occur in ACTH-independent Cushing's syndrome. ACTH binds to melanocyte-stimulating hormone receptors resulting in pigmentation. The degree of hyperpigmentation is based on the duration and elevation of ACTH secretion. It is most common in ectopic ACTH-secreting tumours but can occur with pituitary ACTH-secreting tumours.

8 Optic nerve or chiasm compression by the tumour can result in visual field defects. The typical deficit of an enlarging pituitary adenoma is bitemporal hemianopia with central

visual field defect due to optic chiasm compression. Findings of raised intracranial pressure such as papilloedema are rare in pituitary adenomas as these are slow growing tumours. Diplopia and disconjugate eye movements are caused by single or multiple cranial nerve compressions by the tumour. The tumour can extend into the cavernous sinus and any or all of cranial nerves III, IV, V or VI can be affected.

9 Proximal muscle wasting and associated weakness is common in Cushing's syndrome and may present initially as difficulty rising from a chair without assistance. With more serious proximal myopathy it may present as being unable to mobilise up stairs. This muscle weakness and wasting is due to the catabolic effects of excess cortisol on skeletal muscle.

10 In the context of Cushing's syndrome and potential osteopenia or osteoporosis, point tenderness over a vertebral body may be suggestive of a compression fracture, even in the absence of a history of trauma, and needs further investigation.

11 Non-traumatic avascular necrosis of the femoral head can occur in patients with exogenous glucocorticoid use and can be a challenging diagnosis to make clinically. There should be a high index of suspicion for this diagnosis if a patient has persistent pain in the hip region in the context of chronic glucocorticoid use.

Investigations

- In the context of the patient's history and examination being **suspicious for Cushing's syndrome** [1] with no evidence of exogenous glucocorticoid use, the patient undergoes a **24-hour urinary cortisol collection and a late night salivary cortisol test** [2] which are both abnormally elevated. Both investigations are repeated and the results remain abnormal.
- With biochemical hypercortisolism shown on initial investigations, the patient then has further investigations to determine the cause of the hypercortisolism. She had a **plasma ACTH** [3] level which is elevated above the reference range.
- She then has a **high dose dexamethasone suppression test** [4] with a dexamethasone infusion

protocol. At 4 hours post the infusion, her plasma cortisol level is mildly suppressed at 25% of the reference range; the plasma cortisol level on testing the following morning has returned to baseline and is no longer suppressed.
- A **pituitary MRI brain** [5] is performed and a 7mm pituitary lesion is identified.
- The patient's fasting glucose is 4.2 and her **HbA1c is 5%. Fasting cholesterol levels** [6] reveal: LDL cholesterol 5, HDL cholesterol 0.8 and triglyceride level 3.
- The patient also has imaging of her lumbar spine **(X-ray and then CT)** [7] which do not show evidence of compression fractures.

1 The clinical diagnosis of Cushing's syndrome can be difficult as clinical presentation is highly variable and non-specific. Investigations to assess for Cushing's syndrome can also be unreliable, with various potential reasons for false positive and false negative results. Therefore, the decision to investigate further should be considered on the pre-test probability based on careful clinical assessment. Investigating

for Cushing's syndrome should be considered if a patient has multiple features of Cushing's syndrome, if they have a severe presentation such as severe osteoporosis or resistant hypertension, or in a young patient who presents with osteoporosis or hypertension, which would be unusual for the patient's age. Prior to investigating a patient with such a presentation, exogenous glucocorticoid use must be excluded as a potential cause. Pseudo-Cushing's syndrome should also be considered as this can result in false positive investigation results for the 1mg dexamethasone suppression test and 24-hour urinary free cortisol test. If a plasma cortisol at 11pm is high, this suggests Cushing's syndrome and may exclude pseudo-Cushing's syndrome. Differentiating pseudo-Cushing's syndrome from Cushing's syndrome can be very challenging and may require a specialist opinion.

2 Initial testing focuses on demonstrating biochemical hypercortisolism. Investigation options include 24-hour free urinary cortisol excretion, overnight 1mg dexamethasone suppression test and late-night salivary cortisol. Ideally to confirm biochemical hypercortisolism, two of these investigations should be performed and shown to be abnormal. 24-hour urinary free cortisol excretion, if elevated, is suggestive of Cushing's syndrome, and should ideally be confirmed with one or two additional measurements. It is possible to have false negative results so if there is a high degree of suspicion for Cushing's syndrome the test should be repeated. There can be difficulty obtaining 24-hour urine collections and instead, a 1mg overnight dexamethasone suppression test can be done. The patient takes 1mg of dexamethasone at 11pm and then the plasma cortisol level is measured at 8am the following morning. There should be normal suppression of the cortisol level in the absence of Cushing's syndrome. Late-night salivary cortisol levels can also be measured to show hypersecretion of cortisol. Hypercortisolism in Cushing's syndrome can be variable, so investigations of 24-hour urinary free cortisol and late-night salivary cortisol levels should be repeated to confirm abnormal results.

3 Once hypercortisolism is shown biochemically, the cause should then be determined. A plasma ACTH level is the first investigation to separate ACTH-independent Cushing's syndrome from ACTH-dependent Cushing's syndrome. A plasma ACTH level that is elevated above the reference range is suggestive of ACTH-dependent Cushing's syndrome, while a plasma ACTH that is low and below the reference range is suggestive of ACTH-independent Cushing's syndrome. A patient with a low plasma ACTH level would then undergo imaging of the adrenal glands to assess for presence of an adrenal mass. An equivocal plasma ACTH level is usually in keeping with ACTH-dependent Cushing's syndrome.

4 In this patient with testing suggestive of ACTH-dependent Cushing's syndrome, the next set of investigations aims to determine the source of ACTH secretion. The most common cause of ACTH hypersecretion is a pituitary adenoma (Cushing's disease); other potential causes include ectopic ACTH secretion, and rarely, ectopic CRH secretion. The decision of which investigations to perform and their interpretation is typically guided by an endocrinologist. A high dose dexamethasone suppression test can help to differentiate between ectopic ACTH hypersecretion and pituitary ACTH hypersecretion by the negative feedback pathway discussed in the History section. ACTH secretion

by pituitary adenomas is only relatively resistant to negative feedback regulation by glucocorticoids, while ectopic ACTH secretion is completely resistant to this negative feedback regulation. High dose dexamethasone suppression tests can be performed in a variety of ways, including oral dexamethasone regimes and infusion dexamethasone regimes, and the choice of protocol is based on the centre and the endocrinologist involved. The patient in this case has undergone an infusion protocol: a 4mg infusion of dexamethasone with subsequent plasma cortisol testing hourly for 4 hours and then the following morning. A patient without Cushing's syndrome will have cortisol levels suppressed by at least 50% by 4 hours and which remain suppressed the next day. In Cushing's disease, such as in this patient, the cortisol may partially suppress, but rebounds the next day. In ectopic ACTH syndrome, there is no suppression of cortisol.

5 MRI is used to identify the presence of pituitary tumours. A tumour that is >6mm in diameter is suggestive of a causative Cushing's disease neoplasm. Up to 50% of confirmed Cushing's disease has no pituitary adenoma identified on MRI. In the case of a patient with ACTH-dependent Cushing's disease and no obvious causal tumour (a tumour that is >6mm in diameter), the patient should go on to have inferior petrosal sinus sampling to differentiate pituitary from an ectopic cause of ACTH-dependent Cushing's syndrome.

6 Diabetes mellitus and dyslipidaemia are common comorbidities associated with Cushing's syndrome. Patients with Cushing's syndrome are at increased cardiovascular risk and have higher rates of myocardial infarction, stroke and thromboembolism. Diabetes mellitus and dyslipidaemia should be identified and treated to reduce this risk.

7 Osteopenia and osteoporosis are common in Cushing's syndrome and there should be a low index of suspicion to investigate for potential fractures. There are no specific guidelines to recommend a DEXA scan at the time of diagnosis of Cushing's syndrome; however, this could be considered.

Management

- The diagnosis of Cushing's disease and the need for a neurosurgery opinion for **operative management** [1] is discussed with the patient.
- The patient is commenced on **perindopril 2mg daily for hypertension and atorvastatin 20mg daily for dyslipidaemia** [2] with a plan to up-titrate medications as required.
- Her vaccination schedule is reviewed and it is confirmed that she has previously received all age-appropriate vaccinations. She is given the influenza, herpes zoster and pneumococcal **vaccinations** [3].
- In discussion with the **patient, her general practitioner, endocrinologist and neurosurgeon** [4], the decision is made for a **transsphenoidal selective adenomectomy** [5] with the necessary medical peri-operative input.
- Potential **complications of the procedure** [6] are discussed with the patient and she is informed of the **postoperative monitoring** [7] required to assist in identifying these issues if they arise.
- **Postoperative glucocorticoid replacement** [8] is discussed.
- The patient is informed that there is a significant **recurrence rate** [9] of Cushing's disease and she may need **further medical or surgical treatment or radiotherapy** [10] after her initial surgery in order to achieve remission if the procedure is not successful or there is recurrence in the future.
- In the longer term, the patient is aware that a large focus of her management will be on her **cardiovascular health** [11].

[1] The aim for management in a patient with Cushing's syndrome is to treat the cause of hypercortisolism to achieve remission as well as manage hypercortisolism-associated comorbidities. This treatment aims to normalise cortisol levels and thus eliminate signs and symptoms of Cushing's syndrome, improve quality of life and improve mortality outcomes. Management of Cushing's disease requires neurosurgical opinion for resection of a causative pituitary adenoma.

[2] Hypercortisolism-associated comorbidities include hypertension, dyslipidaemia, obesity, diabetes, osteoporosis and psychiatric disorders. Many of these complications may persist post treatment despite normalisation of cortisol levels and therefore require ongoing monitoring and management.

[3] It is recommended that patients with Cushing's syndrome are up to date with the age-appropriate vaccinations as well as being immunised for herpes zoster if not immune, and pneumococcal vaccinations and yearly influenza vaccinations.

[4] A multidisciplinary team, including an endocrinologist, surgeon, radiologist, pathologist and the patient's GP, is an important aspect of managing a patient with Cushing's syndrome.

[5] Where feasible, resection of the causative lesion of Cushing's disease is the gold standard treatment. Transsphenoidal selective adenomectomy is the typical surgery performed if a clearly circumscribed microadenoma can be identified. If a microadenoma is not identified, subtotal resection of the anterior pituitary is performed.

[6] Operative complications include electrolyte disturbances, haemorrhage and meningitis. Patients with Cushing's syndrome have an increased risk of thromboembolism, especially during the peri-operative period. In conjunction with the treating neurosurgeon, when appropriate, patients who are not mobilising should be given prophylactic anticoagulation while in hospital.

[7] A combination of diabetes insipidus followed by the syndrome of inappropriate antidiuretic hormone secretion (SIADH) followed by diabetes insipidus can present in patients post pituitary surgery due to hypothalamus and posterior pituitary damage. Some patients will only have one of these phases, the most common being diabetes insipidus. The risk of sodium abnormalities increases with the size of the lesion being removed. Most cases resolve and are not permanent. Serum sodium monitoring and fluid balance assessment are performed for the first 5–14 days in the postoperative period to identify sodium abnormalities. Serum free thyroxine and prolactin testing should be performed within 1–3 weeks of surgery to assess for hypopituitarism. Hormonal deficits identified may be secondary to hypercortisolism and therefore transient and so require further follow-up to assess ongoing need for hormone replacement. Typically, a patient will have a repeat pituitary MRI scan 1–3 months post procedure to assess the appearance and provide a new baseline scan to assist in identifying future recurrence.

[8] The hypothalamus–pituitary–adrenal axis may take 6–12 months to recover post successful surgery for Cushing's disease. During this period, glucocorticoid replacement therapy is required. Patients must be educated on the importance of stress dosing for intercurrent illness and should be encouraged to wear a medical alert tag.

[9] Remission is defined as an undetectable morning plasma cortisol 3–7 days postoperatively. Persistently

detectable plasma cortisol levels indicate incomplete resection and likely recurrence. Remission rates for selectively resected microadenomas are 73–76%; remission rates for macroadenomas are approximately 43%. Other factors which influence remission rates include surgeon experience and the presence of dural invasion. Patients require ongoing long-term follow-up to identify recurrence.

10 There are various second-line therapies that can be used in the case of non-curative surgery or where surgery is not possible. Management options include repeat transsphenoidal surgery, radiotherapy, medical therapy and bilateral adrenalectomy.

11 Cardiovascular comorbidities, including obesity, hypertension, dyslipidaemia and diabetes, are common in Cushing's syndrome and are considered a primary cause of excess mortality in this patient group. These conditions tend to improve within weeks to a year of successful treatment; however, many of these comorbidities persist and require

intensive treatment and monitoring to reduce mortality risk. Patients should receive advice on quitting smoking, and alcohol consumption should not exceed 14 units of alcohol per week. Dietary recommendations include limiting salt to <6g/day and eating five servings of vegetables and two servings of fruit daily. Patients should be encouraged to engage in exercise – at least 2.5–5 hours of moderate-intensity activity or 75–150 minutes of vigorous intensity activity each week. Patients should aim for a BMI of <25kg/m^2 and a waist circumference of <94cm for males and <80cm for females. Antihypertensive management is as per the general population; with hypertension, however, mineralocorticoid blocking agents such as spironolactone may be more effective in this population with elevated serum cortisol levels and hypokalaemia. Lifestyle and medication therapy should be used to achieve a blood pressure target of <140/90mmHg, or lower if tolerated. Lipid targets are as follows: total cholesterol <4.0mmol/L, HDL cholesterol >1.0mmol/L, LDL cholesterol <2.0mmol/L, triglycerides <2.0mmol/L.

CASE 14: Hyperthyroidism

History

- A **29-year-old female** [1] presents with a 4-month history of a **constellation of symptoms** [2] including intermittent palpitations, sweating despite cold weather, increased frequency of bowel motions, restlessness and difficulty concentrating at work.
- She also reports three kilograms of **weight loss** [3] over a 6-month period despite a robust appetite and increasing oral intake.
- She has noticed **progressive bulging of her eyes** [4] and a swelling in the middle of her neck, but has not experienced any **neck pain or difficulty swallowing** [5].
- There has been no recent acute illness, including any **upper respiratory tract infection** [6].

- She has **not been pregnant previously** [7].
- She also reports some **irregularity in her menstrual periods** [8] for the past 3 months.
- She has no significant past medical history, but has a positive family history for thyroid disease in her mother and maternal grandmother. She has **no regular medications** [9] or allergies, and there has been no known exposure to any **significant iodine intake** [10] through radiocontrast agents or an iodine-rich diet.
- **Socially** [11], she works as a primary school teacher and consumes alcohol occasionally but does not smoke nor use **recreational drugs** [12].

[1] Thyrotoxicosis is a clinical state that results from excessive thyroid hormone levels, while hyperthyroidism specifically refers to thyrotoxicosis due to inappropriately elevated synthesis and secretion of thyroid hormone by the thyroid gland. The prevalence of thyrotoxicosis is 1–1.5%, with the incidence being highest between the ages of 20 and 50. Hyperthyroidism is approximately five times more common in females than males, and more common in smokers. The most common causes include Graves' disease, toxic multinodular goitre and toxic adenoma. Less common causes include thyroiditis, trophoblastic disease or germ cell tumours, exogenous hyperthyroidism, ectopic hyperthyroidism or TSH-producing pituitary adenomas.

[2] Thyroid hormone influences almost every organ system in the body, by increasing tissue thermogenesis and the basal metabolic rate. Hyperthyroidism can range from subclinical to overt, and may present with a range of symptoms including heat intolerance, increased sweating, palpitations, tremor, weakness, restlessness, anxiety, emotional lability and weight loss despite a normal or heightened appetite. Other possible symptoms include urinary frequency, frequency of bowel motions, erectile dysfunction in men, and menstrual dysfunction in women.

[3] A heightened appetite in combination with increased metabolism in hyperthyroidism can lead to the characteristic feature of weight loss despite increased oral intake, but it is also possible that the degree of excessive appetite stimulation may lead to weight gain.

[4] An ophthalmopathy in combination with other features of hyperthyroidism should raise suspicion of Graves' disease, an autoimmune thyroid disorder characterised by diffuse enlargement of the thyroid gland with hyperactivity due to TSH-receptor antibodies. Graves' ophthalmopathy occurs as a result of infiltration of periorbital connective tissues and extraocular muscles by inflammatory cells, leading to tissue swelling and fibrosis.

[5] A tender goitre with fevers, dysphagia and dysphonia is in keeping with the presentation of suppurative thyroiditis. Common aetiological organisms include *Staphylococcus aureus*, *Streptococcus pyogenes* and *Streptococcus pneumoniae*.

[6] A recent history of an upper respiratory tract infection in combination with symptoms of hyperthyroidism may indicate viral thyroiditis, in which case the patient may also report a painful goitre.

[7] There is an increased risk of autoimmune thyroid disease in the postpartum period, due to the immunological rebound after the partially immunosuppressed state of pregnancy. This is often a painless thyroiditis, occurring in individuals who may have a personal or family history of autoimmune or thyroid disease. Postpartum thyroiditis is associated with TPO-antibody positivity and expression of human leucocyte antigen haplotypes DR-3, DR-4 and DR-5.

[8] Women in a thyrotoxic state can experience various menstrual abnormalities, including amenorrhoea, oligomenorrhoea and menorrhagia, the last of which is the least common.

9 The onset of Graves' disease has been associated with initiation of several drugs, including lithium, interferon alfa and alemtuzumab.

10 Iodine-induced hyperthyroidism may occur after significant iodine intake in the presence of a multinodular goitre. The source of iodine may be dietary, radiographic contrast materials or drugs such as amiodarone.

11 Consider the social history of the patient, including occupational or dietary factors that may pose as a risk factor

for the development of thyrotoxicosis. Though it is rare, thyrotoxicosis factitia is a described cause of thyrotoxicosis, occurring due to exogenous thyroid hormone ingestion. One historical example of this is consumption of minced beef contaminated with bovine thyroid gland.

12 It is important to consider potential alternative causes for a presentation of anxiety and palpitations, including use of sympathomimetic drugs such as amphetamines or excessive caffeine intake.

Examination

- The patient is alert and oriented, but appears restless with an anxious affect. She is of **slim build** [1] and despite air conditioning in the clinic room, she is flushed and warm to touch.
- Her palms are **moist and mildly erythematous** [2], and she has a **fine tremor** [3].
- Her cardiac examination demonstrates **tachycardia with a regular pulse rate of 118bpm** [4], normal heart sounds with a non-displaced apex beat, and a normal blood pressure.
- On examination of her eyes, there is a **notable prominence of the eyelids** [5] with **visible sclera above the iris** [6], more prominent on the right.
- There is demonstrable **lid lag** [7] but her eye movements otherwise appear normal.
- On examination of her neck she is found to have a

midline swelling [8] that moves with swallowing of water, but not with tongue protrusion.
- The mass is **soft**, **smooth and diffusely enlarged** [9] with **no overlying scars** [10] or skin changes. It is non-tender on palpation and there is **no associated lymphadenopathy** [11], **tracheal deviation or retrosternal dullness** [12] on percussion.
- There is a **palpable thrill and a soft bruit** [13] on auscultation.
- On examination of her lower limbs there is **mild proximal muscle weakness** [14] and **bilateral lower limb pitting oedema** [15] with an erythematous appearance of the lower shins that is rough in texture on palpation.
- Examination of other organ systems is unremarkable, and she is **afebrile** [16].

1 On general inspection when assessing thyroid status, take note of body habitus, whether clothing is appropriate for the weather, behaviour and mental state.

2 Skin changes including palmar erythema and sweating can be seen in hyperthyroidism. Clubbing and swelling of the fingers is termed thyroid acropachy and is specific to Graves' disease.

3 Test for a peripheral tremor by asking the patient to place her arms straight out in front of her then place a piece of paper across the back of her hands and observe for any quivering of the sheet to indicate a fine tremor.

4 Hyperthyroidism leads to increased peripheral oxygen requirements and increased cardiac contractility, which can result in tachycardia, widened pulse pressure and systolic hypertension. Thyrotoxicosis can also lead to AF, diastolic dysfunction, dilated cardiomyopathy, pulmonary hypertension and congestive cardiac failure in severe cases.

5 The eye signs of hyperthyroidism relate to either sympathetic overactivity (lid lag and lid retraction) or autoimmune thyroid disease (chemosis, exophthalmos,

ophthalmoplegia). Clinically apparent ophthalmopathy can occur in up to one-third of patients with Graves' disease, with chemosis, conjunctivitis and proptosis. Exophthalmos is anterior displacement of the eye out of the orbit, and bilateral exophthalmos is associated with Graves' disease. Restriction of eye movements and diplopia may also be evident.

6 Observe for any stare in the resting position, or for sclera visible above the iris indicating the presence of lid retraction.

7 Test for lid lag by asking the patient to hold an initial upward gaze, then track your finger as you swiftly move it downwards.

8 A normal thyroid gland should not be visible. If a mass is observed during inspection of the neck, take note of the size and shape as well as overlying scars or skin changes, and then assess further by asking the patient to swallow some water and protrude their tongue. The thyroid gland and thyroglossal cysts will move with swallowing, while lymph nodes will not. Thyroglossal cysts will move upwards with tongue protrusion; however, the thyroid gland and lymph nodes will not.

9 The thyroid gland is diffusely enlarged in Graves' disease and the goitre is typically smooth, while it will be nodular in a multinodular goitre, and painful and tender in thyroiditis.

10 A patient with a scar suggests previous thyroidectomy and may be on thyroxine replacement. If such patient presents with thyrotoxicosis, this may indicate over-replacement and should prompt thyroxine dose reassessment.

11 Palpate for local lymphadenopathy during a thyroid exam, in particular assessing the supraclavicular nodes, the anterior cervical chain, the posterior cervical chain and submental nodes.

12 Assess tracheal position and percuss for retrosternal dullness after assessing the thyroid, as a large thyroid mass can result in tracheal deviation and may extend posterior to the manubrium.

13 A palpable thrill and audible bruit can occur in thyrotoxicosis associated with Graves' disease, and are due to increased vascularity.

14 The neurological examination in a patient with hyperthyroidism can feature proximal muscle weakness and brisk reflexes.

15 Graves' dermopathy can occur in a small percentage of individuals with Graves' disease. It is due to glycosaminoglycan accumulation and lymphoid infiltration, and often affects the pretibial region. Myxoedematous skin changes appear as erythematous infiltrative plaques on lower extremities, resembling orange peel in colour and texture.

16 In rare cases of severe hyperthyroidism, patients may present in a thyroid storm with tachycardia, fever, altered mental status, agitation, features of cardiac failure and impaired liver function. Another acute presentation of thyrotoxicosis is thyrotoxic periodic paralysis, where individuals present with acute muscle paralysis and severe hypokalaemia, often after oral carbohydrate intake, vigorous exercise or IV dextrose.

Investigations

- Thyroid function testing is performed with a **thyroid-stimulating hormone (TSH) level** [1] and a **free T4 level** [2].
- Her results reveal a markedly **elevated free T4 and free T3 level** [3], and a suppressed serum TSH level of <0.01mU/L. This is consistent with the clinical picture of thyrotoxicosis.
- To pursue a diagnosis of autoimmune thyroid disease, **thyroid antibodies** [4] including anti-thyroid peroxidase (anti-TPO) antibodies and thyrotrophin receptor antibodies (TRAbs) are requested.
- She is found to have moderately **elevated TPO antibodies** [5] and markedly **elevated TRAb levels** [6].
- A **radioisotope thyroid scan** [7] is not performed, given the clinical and biochemical findings are **highly suggestive of Graves' disease** [8].
- Further biochemical testing performed includes a **full blood examination (FBE)** [9], urea and electrolytes (U&E), and **liver function tests (LFTs)** [10].
- An **ECG reveals sinus tachycardia** [11] to a rate of 120bpm.
- **No further blood tests** [12] or imaging such as **ultrasound imaging** [13], X-ray, CT or MRI is undertaken.

1 Hyperthyroidism is diagnosed through history, physical examination and confirmatory blood testing, with the most sensitive and specific test to evaluate suspected hyperthyroidism being a serum TSH. The serum TSH level should be used for initial screening, with subsequent testing of T3 and T4 levels. Thyrotoxicosis is marked by suppressed TSH levels and elevated T3 and T4 levels, with the rise in T3 usually preceding the rise in T4.

2 Hyperthyroidism can be primary (due to disease of the thyroid gland) or central (due to pituitary or hypothalamic disease). It can be overt (suppressed TSH level with elevated T3 and T4) or subclinical (suppressed TSH level with normal T4 and normal or elevated T3), with the former being more likely to be associated with signs and symptoms. The free T4 level can aid differentiation between the two. Central hyperthyroidism is rare and is due to pituitary hypersecretion of TSH which can occur in the presence of a pituitary tumour.

3 Total triiodothyronine (T3) testing may be useful where the serum TSH is suppressed but the free T4 level is normal. Elevation of the T3 level only with a low TSH level has been termed T3-toxicosis and may signify early Graves' disease or the presence of an autonomous thyroid nodule.

4 Autoantibody testing in hyperthyroidism includes anti-TPO antibody and TRAb levels. They are associated with autoimmune thyroid disease, and therefore aid diagnostic work-up of the underlying aetiology of thyrotoxicosis. These autoantibodies are usually absent or found in only low titres in other causes of thyrotoxicosis such as toxic adenoma, either single or multiple (toxic multinodular goitre). The underlying mechanism here is nodule formation and development of autonomy over time, occurring due to somatic activating mutations of the genes that regulate thyroid hormone synthesis, rather than antibody driven.

5 Anti-TPO antibodies can be non-specifically raised in autoimmune thyroid disease, and this is found in approximately 85% of patients with Graves' disease. Anti-TPO antibodies are more likely to occur in patients with Hashimoto's thyroiditis, which may cause transient hyperthyroidism during the initial destructive phase.

6 TRAb positivity is more specific for Graves' disease, being found in 60–80% of affected individuals. TRAbs are the underlying mechanism for TSH receptor stimulation thyroid hormone overproduction in Graves' disease.

7 A radioactive iodine uptake scan can be performed if, after physical examination and other laboratory testing, the aetiology of thyrotoxicosis remains unclear. The degree and pattern of isotope uptake can indicate the type of thyroid disorder. In Graves' disease there is diffuse enlargement of the thyroid gland with homogeneous increased uptake throughout. If a toxic multinodular goitre is the underlying aetiology, the scan would demonstrate multiple areas of focal increased and suppressed uptake, with overall radioactive iodine uptake being mildly to moderately increased. A toxic adenoma would show focal uptake with suppressed uptake in the surrounding and contralateral thyroid tissue. In painless, postpartum, factitious or subacute thyroiditis there would be minimal radioactive iodine uptake. Thyrotoxicosis with normal or elevated radioiodine uptake may also be seen in a TSH-producing pituitary adenoma, trophoblastic disease, or resistance to thyroid hormone. Radioactive iodine uptake scans should be avoided during pregnancy, but Doppler ultrasound may be used to assess thyroidal blood flow if imaging is required for diagnostic clarification.

8 In this patient with a symmetrically enlarged thyroid, ophthalmopathy, and severe hyperthyroidism, there is sufficient evidence for the diagnosis of Graves' disease that there is no requirement for further investigations.

9 An FBE can be performed to assess for anaemia. A normochromic, normocytic anaemia can be seen in hyperthyroidism due to increased plasma volume exceeding the increase in red blood cell mass. Graves' disease may also be associated with other autoimmune haematologic conditions such as immune thrombocytopenia and pernicious anaemia.

10 Abnormal LFTs can occur with hyperthyroidism, in particular elevated serum alkaline phosphatase levels, and less commonly, a cholestatic picture of liver enzyme derangement.

11 An ECG is important to assess for AF as it occurs in 10–20% of patients with hyperthyroidism and the patient must be counselled on the risk of an arterial embolic event (e.g. stroke), and therefore the risk vs. benefit of anticoagulation. In patients with hyperthyroidism found to have AF, the rhythm converts to sinus rhythm spontaneously in 60% with treatment of hyperthyroidism.

12 Inflammatory markers such as erythrocyte sedimentation rate (ESR) and C-reactive protein (CRP) can be tested if subacute thyroiditis is suspected, as they are often elevated in this condition, as well as other infective or inflammatory states.

13 Thyroid ultrasound imaging is not routinely required in hyperthyroidism, as it does not reliably distinguish between the common underlying aetiologies, and it will frequently detect nodules that are unrelated to the hyperthyroidism. This can result in unnecessary investigations, increased healthcare burden and patient anxiety.

Management

- Hyperthyroidism can usually be managed in the outpatient setting, except in the case of a **thyroid storm** [1] or hypokalaemic periodic paralysis which may require inpatient management.
- Some cases may require **outpatient monitoring only** [2]. Management of thyrotoxicosis will vary depending on the underlying aetiology and severity, and also the patient's age, symptoms and comorbidities.
- Mainstays of treatment include **beta blocker therapy** [3], **antithyroid medications** [4], **radioiodine therapy** [5] and **thyroid surgery** [6].
- This patient is diagnosed with Graves' disease and commenced on **carbimazole** [7], a short course of beta blockade, and lubricating eye drops for her **mild ophthalmopathy** [8].
- A pathology form is given to her to have **repeat blood tests in 4 weeks** [9] for serum TSH, free T4 and free T3 levels.
- She is also referred to an **endocrinologist** [10] for ongoing management and carbimazole dose titration.

- She is provided with **written and verbal information**[11] on the signs and symptoms of hypothyroidism and hyperthyroidism, and the importance of follow-up.
- She is informed of the need for closer monitoring should there be medication changes or should she become **pregnant**[12].

- The diagnosis is clearly **documented**[13] in her medical record to aid assessment of treatment adequacy and the **development of complications**[14].

1 Patients can rarely present in a thyroid storm, with tachycardia, fever, altered mental status, agitation, and gastrointestinal symptoms of nausea, vomiting and abdominal pain. This is considered an endocrine emergency which can develop in patients with long-standing untreated hyperthyroidism, often precipitated by an acute event such as trauma, infection, surgery, an iodine load or childbirth. Therapeutic options include a beta blocker, a thionamide, glucocorticoids and iodine or Lugol's solution. ICU admission is often required for monitoring, and investigation for any precipitating factors should be undertaken once the patient is stabilised.

2 Subclinical hyperthyroidism is a state of suppressed TSH with normal free T4 and T3 levels, and patients are often asymptomatic. Mild subclinical hyperthyroidism may stabilise without intervention, but factors that may prompt treatment include underlying cardiovascular disease or symptoms of hyperthyroidism, especially in the elderly.

3 Beta blockers can be used in thyrotoxicosis for symptom relief of adrenergic symptoms such as tachycardia, anxiety and diaphoresis. Propranolol, a non-selective beta blocker given up to 3–4 times a day, is commonly used. In high doses, it also contributes to reduction of serum T3 levels by inhibiting the conversion of T4 to T3. Atenolol is a beta-1 selective longer-acting beta blocker which allows daily dosing. Reconsider the use of beta blockers, depending on disease severity, in patients with obstructive airways disease, Raynaud's phenomenon, bradycardia, heart block (second- or third-degree) or severe peripheral vascular disease.

4 Antithyroid medication options include carbimazole or propylthiouracil (PTU). These drugs decrease the production of thyroid hormone, and in high doses PTU also reduces peripheral conversion of T4 to T3. Antithyroid drugs are used first-line in Graves' disease if there are no contraindications; however, they are not considered first-line for autonomous nodules, as remission is unlikely and these drugs may be required indefinitely. Toxic adenomas and toxic nodular goitres should therefore be considered for radioactive iodine or surgical management. Carbimazole is more potent and longer-acting than PTU, but PTU can be used in the case of carbimazole allergy or thyroid storm, or in the first trimester of pregnancy. PTU is associated with a risk of hepatotoxicity, while carbimazole poses the risk of agranulocytosis and teratogenicity, leading to aplasia cutis and choanal or oesophageal atresia.

5 Radioiodine therapy (131-I) is administered as an oral capsule or liquid, and is absorbed by thyroid tissue. It induces tissue-specific inflammation that results in fibrosis and thyroid tissue destruction over weeks to months, and can lead to eventual hypothyroidism within 6–12 months. It is contraindicated if the patient is pregnant, breastfeeding, or intending to conceive.

6 Thyroidectomy is reserved for special circumstances, including in patients with a large goitre associated with thyroid ophthalmopathy with failure or anticipated inadequacy of antithyroid medications and radioiodine therapy. It is also considered in pregnant women who are not adherent or intolerant of antithyroid medications, and patients who are refractory to or unable to have radioactive iodine therapy. Surgery may also be required in patients who require urgent normalisation of thyroid function, such as patients who are pregnant or intending to conceive within 6 months, or patients with unstable cardiac conditions being aggravated by hyperthyroidism. Risks of surgery include hypoparathyroidism and recurrent laryngeal nerve palsy.

7 For Graves' disease, initial treatment dosing of thionamides depends on the severity of hyperthyroidism. Carbimazole can be started at a dose of 15–20mg for mild–moderate hyperthyroidism, or a dose of 30–40mg for severe hyperthyroidism. If effective, it can be used for 12–18 months before considering cessation of therapy with ongoing monitoring for sustained remission. Recurrence of Graves' disease is common within the first year after stopping antithyroid therapy. Consider radioactive iodine or surgery if antithyroid therapy is ineffective.

8 There are several treatment options for Graves' ophthalmopathy, depending on the severity. If mild, saline eye drops can be used as required and tight-fitting sunglasses utilised outdoors. For severe ophthalmopathy, high dose glucocorticoids are recommended, with consideration for orbital decompression surgery and ocular radiation therapy.

9 Serum TSH, free T4 and free T3 should be reassessed at 4–6 weeks to evaluate the effect of therapy. For patients commenced on antithyroid medications, if their serial thyroid function tests demonstrate a reduction in serum T3 and T4 at 4 weeks of follow-up, they may require a reduction in dosage of thionamides. Patients who reach a hypothyroid state quickly may need further 4-weekly assessment of their thyroid function. Some patients require repeat thyroid function testing without having commenced antithyroid therapy, if the suspected cause of thyrotoxicosis is thyroiditis. Thyroiditis characteristically has a triphasic course (of hyperthyroidism followed by hypothyroidism, then euthyroidism), in which case beta blockers may provide symptomatic benefit but no other treatment is typically required. Autoimmune thyroiditis may lead to sustained hypothyroidism requiring thyroxine replacement, while subacute viral thyroiditis is expected to fully recover.

10 The decision to refer to an endocrinologist depends on the experience of the clinician who makes the diagnosis and the severity of hyperthyroidism.

11 Patients must be adequately educated on the condition and the benefits and adverse effects of treatment. This will enable prompt medical attention if they fall into a state of undertreatment or overtreatment, or if there is worsening of their thyroid disease signifying treatment failure and the need to pursue the next line of therapy.

12 Thyroid function must be monitored throughout pregnancy and matched to trimester-specific reference ranges, targeting a euthyroid state. Gestational hyperthyroidism can occur in the first trimester due to increased thyroxine-binding globulin as a result of chorionic gonadotrophin stimulating the thyroid gland, and placental degradation of thyroid hormone. This can be more marked in women with high human chorionic gonadotrophin (hCG) levels, and usually resolves without intervention. Persistent hyperthyroidism may indicate a flare of Graves' disease in pregnancy, so TRAbs should be measured. Overt hyperthyroidism is associated with adverse outcomes in pregnancy including the risk of pregnancy loss, but subclinical hyperthyroidism can be a normal variant and is not known to result in adverse outcomes.

13 Individuals with Graves' disease are at increased risk of developing other autoimmune conditions such as coeliac disease, type 1 diabetes mellitus, Addison's disease, alopecia areata and myasthenia gravis. Graves' disease also has a familial tendency, and a known association with HLA-B8 and HLA-DR3. Monitor for these autoimmune conditions in the long-term follow-up of individuals at risk.

14 Long-term sequelae of chronic thyrotoxicosis include cardiac complications and osteoporosis due to accelerated bone loss. Thyroid hormone stimulates bone resorption and therefore can increase cortical bone porosity and reduce trabecular bone volume.

CASE 15: Hypothyroidism

History

- A **38-year-old female** [1] with a history of **type 1 diabetes mellitus (T1DM)** [2] presents with **3 months** [3] of a **collection of symptoms** [4] including progressive fatigue, constipation, feeling cold despite warm weather, and weight gain of 2kg despite a reduced appetite.
- She has observed some coarsening of her hair and skin, and slight **facial puffiness** [5].
- Upon further questioning she reports **normal menstrual periods** [6].
- She has no other past medical history apart from T1DM diagnosed at age 12, which has been stable and well controlled on a basal-bolus insulin regimen, with a recent glycated haemoglobin (HbA1c) of 6.0%, and no diabetic complications detected so far on regular screening.
- She has **not been pregnant** [7], and has had **no previous surgery or radiotherapy** [8], in particular no thyroid surgery or radiation to the head and neck region.
- Her family history is remarkable only for **Addison's disease** [9] in her maternal grandmother.
- Apart from insulin she is on **no other regular medications** [10], and has no known allergies. She works in an office job and is a non-smoker, with minimal alcohol intake.

[1] Hypothyroidism is a condition that occurs as a result of inadequate thyroid hormone, and it is 5–8 times more common in women than men, with an overall prevalence of 0.1–2%. The peak incidence occurs between 30 and 50 years of age.

[2] Patients with a history of an autoimmune disorder are at risk of developing other autoimmune conditions, in this instance autoimmune thyroid disease, and should therefore be screened yearly. Screening of the general population in the absence of symptoms is not recommended.

[3] Symptomatic onset of hypothyroidism usually develops insidiously over months to years.

[4] The features of hypothyroidism can be a product of slowing of metabolic processes, presenting as fatigue, cold intolerance, weight gain, cognitive dysfunction, constipation or growth failure. Children and infants can present with failure to thrive.

[5] Other features of hypothyroidism can result from an accumulation of connective tissue matrix substances, including dry skin, hoarseness and oedema. Less common symptoms of hypothyroidism include muscle weakness, myalgias, carpal tunnel syndrome, sleep apnoea, slowed speech, impaired cognition or slowed processing.

[6] A small percentage of women with hypothyroidism can experience menstrual abnormalities, with either oligomenorrhoea or amenorrhoea, or less commonly, hypermenorrhoea (menorrhagia). Men can experience decreased libido, erectile dysfunction and delayed ejaculation. These factors can result in reduced fertility.

[7] Major causes of hypothyroidism with onset in adulthood include autoimmune thyroiditis (Hashimoto's disease), prior radioiodine therapy, previous thyroidectomy, prior radiotherapy to the head and neck, postpartum thyroiditis, iodine deficiency and infiltrative disease. Central hypothyroidism is much less common than primary hypothyroidism and can occur as a result of pituitary disease (congenital, traumatic, drug-induced, tumour-related) or hypothalamic disease (congenital, inflammatory, infiltrative, iatrogenic due to surgery or radiotherapy).

[8] Pregnancy is a known precipitating factor for Hashimoto's thyroiditis, as it causes immunosuppression due to reduced function of T and B cells, with subsequent rebound in the postpartum period. Classical Hashimoto's disease eventually develops in one out of five women who experience postpartum thyroiditis.

[9] A familial predisposition to autoimmune disease can be seen in patients with autoimmune thyroiditis. There have been several susceptibility genes for Hashimoto's disease confirmed, including human leucocyte antigen (HLA) alleles such as DR3. Other familial conditions that can feature hypothyroidism include genetic mutations or defects resulting in type 1 autoimmune polyendocrinopathy, congenital hypothyroidism or congenital hypopituitarism.

[10] Hypothyroidism can occur as a result of drug therapy, either by inhibition of thyroid hormone synthesis, or by

drug-induced thyroiditis. Drugs that inhibit synthesis include thionamides, lithium, iodine (leading to transient thyroid dysfunction), amiodarone, or aminoglutethimide. Drug-induced thyroiditis can occur as a result of amiodarone, interferon alfa, interleukin-2, and tyrosine kinase inhibitors such as sunitinib and sorafenib. Immune checkpoint inhibitors, used increasingly in advanced neoplasias, are well associated with immune-related adverse events that affect the endocrine system. Two primary classes are the programmed cell death receptor 1 (PD-1) receptor checkpoint inhibitors (nivolumab and pembrolizumab) and cytotoxic T-lymphocyte-associated antigen 4 (CTLA-4) inhibitors (ipilimumab). Use of these agents has been found to result in primary hypothyroidism in 4–7%, and hypophysitis (leading to central hypothyroidism) in up to 3%. Primary hypothyroidism is more likely to occur with PD-1 receptor blockade, while hypophysitis is more common with CTLA-4 inhibition. Combination therapy with both PD-1 and CTLA-4 blockade is associated with an increased incidence of hypothyroidism (13%) and hypophysitis (6.4%).

Examination

- The patient is alert and demonstrates **intact mentation** [1].
- She has a height of 155cm and a weight of 65kg, with a BMI of 27kg/m², and is **dressed in winter attire** [2] despite a sunny day.
- On general inspection, she is noted to have **generalised non-pitting oedema** [3], primarily affecting both eyelids and bilateral feet.
- Her skin, hair and nails appear dry, and on palpation, her hands feel **cool to touch** [4].
- On examination of her neck she is noted to have a **midline swelling** [5] with no overlying scars or skin changes. It moves with swallowing of water, but not with tongue protrusion.
- The mass is **diffusely enlarged** [6] and symmetrically distributed, with a firm consistency and no tenderness on palpation [7].
- There is no palpable thrill, **no lymphadenopathy** [8], and the **trachea is midline** [9].
- There is no **retrosternal dullness** [10] on percussion, and no bruit on auscultation.
- A neurological examination demonstrates **hyporeflexia** [11] of the biceps jerk and knee jerk, and **no proximal myopathy** [12].
- Her heart sounds are normal and she is normotensive; however, she is found to be **bradycardic** [13] with a regular heart rate of 53bpm.
- Other observations including respiratory rate and oxygen saturations are within normal limits. Examination of other organ systems is unremarkable.

[1] Hypothyroidism can present variably as a spectrum from subclinical hypothyroidism to severe hypothyroidism manifesting as a myxoedema coma. Myxoedema coma is an endocrine emergency, the hallmarks of which are decreased mental status and hypothermia. It can also present with hypotension, bradycardia, hypoglycaemia and hypoventilation. It requires hospitalisation and intensive care for supportive management and administration of thyroxine.

[2] On general inspection when assessing thyroid status, take note of body habitus, whether clothing is appropriate for the weather, behaviour and mental state. Listen for any voice hoarseness or stridor, which can occur in the presence of a retrosternal goitre.

[3] Generalised non-pitting oedema, which can also affect the periorbital region, is a manifestation of hypothyroidism.

[4] As a result of slowed metabolism, hypothyroidism can lead to coolness of the skin and cold intolerance.

[5] A normal thyroid gland should not be visible. If a mass is observed during inspection of the neck, take note of the size and shape as well as overlying scars or skin changes, and then assess further by asking the patient to swallow some water and protrude their tongue. The thyroid gland and thyroglossal cysts will move with swallowing; however, lymph nodes will not. Thyroglossal cysts will move upwards with tongue protrusion, whereas the thyroid gland and lymph nodes will not. Goitre in the presence of hypothyroidism can be due to Hashimoto's thyroiditis, iodide deficiency, drug goitrogens (such as lithium, iodide, PTU or methimazole, amiodarone, interferon alfa, interleukin-2), or rarely, infiltrating disease (cancer, sarcoidosis).

[6] A thyroid gland can be diffusely enlarged, it can have a single enlarged node, or have multiple nodules. Diffuse enlargement is seen in Graves' disease, Hashimoto's thyroiditis and an endemic goitre. A single node can represent a cyst or tumour, or may be a dominant node of a multinodular goitre.

[7] A goitre that is firm in consistency is more suggestive of Hashimoto's thyroiditis, malignancy and other benign nodules. A soft goitre is seen in Graves' disease, and a tender goitre is suggestive of suppurative thyroiditis.

[8] Palpate for local lymphadenopathy after examining the thyroid, in particular assessing the central and anterior cervical chain. Local lymphadenopathy raises the likelihood of a malignant process.

9 Tracheal deviation can occur as a result of a large thyroid mass, so it is important to assess tracheal position after examining the thyroid gland and identifying the physical characteristics of any abnormalities found.

10 As part of the examination, percuss downwards from the sternal notch to identify any retrosternal dullness. This may indicate extension of a large thyroid mass posterior to the manubrium.

11 The neurological component of a thyroid exam prioritises testing of reflexes and power, as hyporeflexia and delayed relaxation can occur in hypothyroidism.

12 Proximal myopathy can occur in up to 80% of cases of hypothyroidism, and can be functionally limiting in severe

or untreated hypothyroidism. The underlying mechanism in hypothyroidism is reduced mitochondrial oxidative capacity and abnormal glycogenolysis with subsequent impaired muscle contractility and alteration in muscle fibres from fast to slow twitching fibres, as well as muscle deposition of glycosaminoglycans.

13 Hypothyroidism leads to increased peripheral vascular resistance, cardiac dysfunction, impaired contractility and decreased cardiac output. The cardiac examination of a patient with hypothyroidism can therefore feature bradycardia, diastolic hypertension, and distant heart sounds if a pericardial effusion is present.

Investigations

- **Thyroid function testing** [1] is performed with a TSH level and a free T4 level.
- The patient's results reveal an elevated TSH and a low free T4 level, confirming **primary hypothyroidism** [2].
- Given this and the clinical finding of a goitre, antibody testing is performed, specifically evaluating **thyroid peroxidase (TPO) antibody** [3] levels.
- Further biochemical testing performed include

a **cortisol level** [4], **FBE** [5], **U&Es** [6] and a **lipid profile** [7].
- A **thyroid ultrasound** [8] is performed due to the presence of a palpable goitre, demonstrating diffuse enlargement of the thyroid gland with a hypoechoic pattern and increased vascularity, consistent with **Hashimoto's thyroiditis** [9].
- No further imaging such as X-ray, CT or MRI is undertaken.

1 The diagnosis of hypothyroidism is made by taking a history and performing a physical examination, and then proceeding to blood tests as indicated to establish a diagnosis. Initial screening is performed by measuring the serum TSH level. If it is abnormal, assess thyroid function further with a peripheral hormone level (free T4). Request both TSH and free T4 upfront if there is a high degree of suspicion, if a goitre is found on examination or if there is known or suspected hypothalamic–pituitary disease.

2 Hypothyroidism can be primary (due to primary disease of the thyroid gland) or central (due to pituitary or hypothalamic disease). It can be overt (raised TSH level with decreased T4 level) or subclinical (raised TSH level with a normal T4 level), with the former being more likely to be associated with signs and symptoms. Treatment of subclinical hypothyroidism is recommended when the TSH level is above 10mU/L; however, in pregnant women there is a lower threshold to treat.

3 An autoimmune cause of primary hypothyroidism can be further assessed for by performing antithyroid antibody testing, in particular TPO antibodies. TPO antibodies are found in 10–15% of the general population, and both TPO and antithyroglobulin antibodies are positive in 95% of patients with autoimmune thyroiditis. However, antithyroglobulin antibodies are non-specific

and so are not routinely used for further assessment of hypothyroidism, but primarily used in the monitoring of thyroid cancer. TPO antibodies in the presence of subclinical hypothyroidism increases the likelihood of progression to overt hypothyroidism.

4 It is important to assess a cortisol level to exclude central adrenal insufficiency, as thyroxine replacement in the setting of this can precipitate an adrenal crisis.

5 An FBE can be performed to assess for anaemia. A normochromic, normocytic anaemia can be seen in hypothyroidism due to a decrease in red blood cell mass. A macrocytic anaemia may be seen due to pernicious anaemia, which can occur in a tenth of patients with autoimmune thyroiditis.

6 Hyponatraemia can occur in hypothyroidism due to the reduction in free water clearance. Individuals with hypothyroidism can also experience a reversible increase in serum creatinine levels.

7 Lipid clearance is decreased in hypothyroidism and can lead to hyperlipidaemia, in particular hypercholesterolaemia or less commonly, hypertriglyceridaemia.

8 Identifying hypothyroidism does not mandate thyroid imaging, and it is not part of the routine work-up of abnormal thyroid function unless there is a large goitre or nodular thyroid. Thyroid ultrasound can be performed to evaluate and characterise any clinical finding of structural thyroid abnormalities, e.g. palpable thyroid nodules. Ultrasound assessment is important due to the malignant potential of thyroid nodules, especially in hypothyroidism, given that the risk of malignancy in nodules rises with the degree of serum TSH elevation. Thyroid radionucleotide scanning does not have a role in the work-up of hypothyroidism.

9 Hashimoto's thyroiditis, or chronic lymphocytic thyroiditis, is a condition that commonly presents with painless, diffuse enlargement of the thyroid gland. It typically presents with hypothyroidism due to the underlying process being autoimmune destruction of the thyroid gland. The diagnosis can be made with testing of thyroid function tests and antibody testing. On ultrasound imaging Hashimoto's thyroiditis characteristically appears as focal or diffuse enlargement with coarse, heterogeneous and hypoechoic parenchymal changes.

Management

- Hypothyroidism can usually be managed in the outpatient setting, with the goals of therapy being to **ameliorate symptoms** [1], **normalise serum TSH level** [2] and reduce the size of any goitre, if present.
- The standard treatment of choice is oral synthetic thyroxine (T4, levothyroxine), prescribed as a once-daily dose, often in the **early morning** [3] on waking.
- Paired free T4 and TSH should be repeated 6–8 weeks after commencing treatment to **check the adequacy of replacement therapy** [4].

- Educate the patient on the need for ongoing monitoring, more frequently initially and then with **reduced frequency of testing** [5] once the TSH is within normal limits and remains stable.
- Provide written and verbal information on signs and symptoms of hypothyroidism and **hyperthyroidism** [6] to enable the patient to look out for signs of under- or overtreatment.
- Additionally, inform patients of the need for closer monitoring should there be **medication changes** [7] or in women, should they become **pregnant** [8].

1 Thyroid hormone replacement is indicated in patients with overt hypothyroidism, and subclinical hypothyroidism with a serum TSH level above 10mU/L.

2 The TSH level is a marker of thyroid status in primary hypothyroidism and is relied upon to adjust thyroid hormone replacement. The therapeutic target is a value within the normal reference range. In secondary (central) hypothyroidism, which is characterised by insufficient pituitary production of TSH, serum TSH is an unreliable indicator of thyroid status.

3 The absorption of levothyroxine can be affected by co-administration of food, so patients should be educated to take it on an empty stomach, at least 30 minutes and preferably 60 minutes before food or other medications.

4 The dose requirement of thyroxine replacement in a patient with hypothyroidism is dependent on body weight, TSH level and goal, the underlying cause of hypothyroidism, age and pregnancy. The full replacement dose is 1.6mcg/kg body weight, but the usual approach is to commence an initial dose of 50–100mcg/day with subsequent titration based on a thyroid function test (TFT) performed 6–8 weeks later.

5 Once a euthyroid state has been achieved, adult patients with hypothyroidism can undergo annual monitoring. A persistently elevated TSH level can occur in the setting of inadequate thyroxine dosing, poor adherence,

expired medications, thyroxine absorption reduced by co-administration with food or other medications, or malabsorption due to bowel disease.

6 Caution must be taken to avoid overtreatment and induce a thyrotoxic state in patients receiving thyroxine replacement. Iatrogenic thyrotoxicosis can lead to AF and osteoporosis, especially in older people and postmenopausal women.

7 It is important to monitor TSH when new medications are commenced, as some medications can alter the thyroxine requirement. This includes commencement or cessation of oestrogens and androgens, rifampicin, sertraline, or anti-epileptic drugs such as phenobarbital, phenytoin and carbamazepine.

8 Thyroxine requirements increase in pregnancy due to increased thyroxine-binding globulin as a result of chorionic gonadotrophin stimulating the thyroid gland, and placental degradation of thyroid hormone. Overt hypothyroidism during pregnancy is associated with increased risk of miscarriage, pre-eclampsia, placental abruption, preterm birth, low birth weight and reduced IQ in offspring. The significance of subclinical hypothyroidism during pregnancy is not yet fully established. Women with pre-existing hypothyroidism who may plan for pregnancy should be informed to discuss this with their treating clinician, to enable optimisation of their thyroxine dose targeting a

CASE 15: HYPOTHYROIDISM 81

serum TSH in the lower reference range. Upon confirmation of pregnancy, the thyroxine dose should then be increased by approximately 30%, with monitoring of serum TSH every 4–6 weeks until 20 weeks of gestation, then once in the third trimester. Thyroxine dosing should be adjusted to maintain serum TSH within the trimester-specific reference ranges, and the dose can be reduced to pre-pregnancy levels after delivery.

CASE 16: Osteoporosis

History

- A **53-year-old** [1] **female** [2] presents for review following a recent **wrist fracture** [3].
- She reports sustaining the fracture after falling from **tripping over a box on the floor** [4] in her living room.
- She denies any **previous fractures** [5].
- The patient reports experiencing occasional mild pain of fracture site, which improves with simple analgesia.
- She denies **pain elsewhere** [6].
- She has not noted any recent **change to her weight or height** [7].
- She does report episodes of **anxiety** [8] which she attributes to the stress related to her job as a senior corporate executive.

- She is otherwise well, and usually leads an **active life** [9] with her family.
- She went through **menopause** [10] at the **age of 48 years** [11].
- Her **past medical history** [12] includes asthma for which she uses **salbutamol** [13] as required.
- She does not take any **other medications** [14].
- She is a **smoker** [15] with a 20 pack year history.
- She is a social **drinker** [16].
- There is no **family history of fractures** [17].

[1] Older age (>50 years in women, >65 years in men) is a risk factor for osteoporosis, as there is an association of increasing age with a decrease in bone mineral density (BMD). Low bone mass and disruption of normal bone architecture characterises osteoporosis. Low bone mass is determined not only by the BMD, but also by other characteristics such as the rate of bone turnover, size and shape of bone and the microarchitecture of the bone.

[2] Female sex is another risk factor.

[3] Diagnosis of a fracture is the initial clinical feature of osteoporosis. Vertebral fractures are commonly seen – patients may or may not be symptomatic with these. Proximal femur, proximal humerus, pelvic and distal radial fractures are also seen. Fractures of the face and skull are unlikely to be indicative of osteoporosis.

[4] Minimal trauma fracture (i.e. from standing height) in patients should prompt further history taking and careful evaluation for osteoporosis. Minimal trauma fractures are a main cause of morbidity and mortality in patients, especially in older adults.

[5] Previous fracture with minimal trauma indicates a higher risk of new fractures.

[6] Absence of back pain does not exclude a vertebral fracture in patients with osteoporosis as they may occur slowly and insidiously. On the other hand, some patients with acute vertebral fractures may present with acute

back pain without any major preceding trauma (following bending, lifting or coughing). Pain may be described as sharp or nagging in nature, usually localised to a specific area of the vertebral column, and may be accompanied by muscle spasms. Acute pain can resolve in 4–6 weeks; however, in some patients a degree of pain may persist.

[7] Osteoporotic compression fractures can cause height loss. This process is gradual and can also occur due to disc space narrowing. Weight loss can increase the risk of fracture in women over the age of 50.

[8] Consider organic causes of symptoms of anxiety including hyperthyroidism, which is a risk factor for osteoporosis.

[9] Patients who are frail, use walking aids and have reduced functional mobility are prone to higher risk of fracture. Poor health and dementia are also considered as risk factors.

[10] Postmenopausal bone loss occurs due to oestrogen deficiency. The mechanism of normal bone remodelling is the resorption of bone matrix by osteoclasts followed by the synthesis of new bone matrix by osteoblasts. RANKL (receptor activator of nuclear factor kappa-B ligand) interacts with RANK receptors to facilitate osteoclastic formation. Osteoprotegerin is an inhibitory factor secreted by osteoblasts which inhibits excessive bone resorption by interfering with the RANKL-induced activation of RANK. In postmenopausal women, there is an overexpression of RANKL which surpasses the inhibitory effects of osteoprotegerin. This causes an imbalance in the bone remodelling, leading

to a lower quality of bone and lower bone density. This predisposes bone to fracture.

11 An earlier age of menopause is more likely to result in premature osteoporosis.

12 Several medical conditions are linked with an increased risk of fracture due to low BMD. Examples include chronic kidney disease, chronic liver disease, diabetes mellitus, coeliac disease, inflammatory bowel diseases, rheumatological/autoimmune conditions, malabsorption, chronic malnutrition, cystic fibrosis and as previously mentioned, hyperthyroidism.

13 Ask the patient about their control of asthma, particularly regarding any exacerbations which may have required management with steroids. Also ask about other medical conditions which may require long-term steroid medications such as rheumatoid arthritis, inflammatory bowel disease and many other immunologic and malignant disorders. Osteoporosis is a known adverse effect of chronic glucocorticoid therapy.

14 Check if the patient is on any other medications that can add to your risk assessment. For example, aromatase inhibitor treatment in women can lead to bone loss due to oestrogen deficiency, as it inhibits peripheral conversion of androgen to oestrogen. Other medications include androgen deprivation agents, anticonvulsants, proton pump inhibitors and selective serotonin reuptake inhibitors (SSRIs). Ask specifically about over-the-counter medications such as vitamins. Vitamin D deficiency increases risk of osteoporosis.

15 Smoking is associated with a rapid decline in bone mass in postmenopausal women.

16 Excessive alcohol use increases fracture risk. Enquire regarding any changes to the amount of alcohol consumed during weekends.

17 Family history, specifically parental history of hip fractures, is a risk factor unrelated to BMD in a patient.

Examination

- The patient has a **BMI of 26** [1].
- Her **vital signs** [2] are within normal range.
- She has a **Glasgow Coma Scale (GCS) score** [3] of 15.
- There are no **visual or hearing aids noted** [4].
- She has a normal **gait** [5].
- On general inspection the patient has mild **thoracic kyphosis** [6].
- **Lumbar lordosis** [7] is intact.
- There is no **cushingoid appearance** [8].
- There is a below-elbow plaster cast in place. **Hand examination** [9] is otherwise normal.

- There is no **tenderness of the spine** [10].
- The patient is able to demonstrate full passive and active **range of movement** [11] of the thoracic, cervical and lumbar spine.
- Both **hips** [12] are non-tender on palpation with normal range of movement.
- There is no **proximal muscle weakness** [13].
- An upper and lower limb **neurological examination** [14] is performed and does not reveal any impairment.

1 Low BMI can predispose to osteoporosis. There is an association of low BMI with an increased loss of BMD. Another contributing factor could potentially be small bone size. Recording the height of the patient during each visit can be helpful.

2 A tachycardia may point toward hyperthyroidism being an underlying cause. Also look for other signs such as a fine tremor of the hands, sweating, palmar warmth, presence of a goitre and pretibial myxoedema. Assess for orthostatic hypotension – this increases the risk of falls and insufficiency fractures in older patients.

3 Cognitive impairment, including dementia, is a risk factor for falls and fracture. Formal cognitive testing may be appropriate in older patients.

4 Sensory impairment predisposes to falls and thereby increases fracture risk in these patients.

5 Severe kyphosis may cause gait imbalance in some patients. Heel to toe walking and single limb stance might be more difficult. Also note any gait aids that the patient may be using – this can provide clues regarding their functional mobility status. An antalgic gait may be seen in patients with a hip fracture.

6 Kyphosis (dowager's hump) can be an indication of vertebral body compression fractures. In general, each compression fracture can result in approximately 1cm of loss in height. A buffalo hump, in patients with Cushing's disease, appears more as a fat deposition over the interscapular area rather than a curvature of the spine.

7 Patients may have subsequent loss of lumbar lordosis.

8 Look for evidence of long-term glucocorticoid therapy – moon-like facies, central obesity, bruising and excessive pigmentation. Consider your findings in combination with the clinical history.

9 Check for signs of coexisting medical conditions that can increase the risk of osteoporosis. In rheumatoid arthritis patients may have Z deformity, ulnar deviation, swan neck and boutonnière deformity.

10 Check for spinal tenderness, which may indicate a fracture. Commonly these occur in the mid-thoracic area and thoracolumbar junction.

11 In an acute fracture, movement would be limited by pain. Patients may restrict movement due to the fear of exacerbating the pain.

12 Hip fractures occur commonly in patients with osteoporosis. Tenderness may be elicited in the buttock, groin or thigh. Gait assessment would reveal an impaired ability to bear weight. Diminished range of movement, with restricted flexion and internal rotation, may be noted.

13 Weakness of muscles in the lower extremity, due to deconditioning or wasting, is an important clinical feature, especially in older patients, as this increases their falls risk and subsequent risk of fracture.

14 Assess for any neurological compromise that may occur secondary to undiagnosed vertebral fractures with bony fragments in spinal canal. Look for sensory deficits in a dermatomal distribution, upper motor neurone signs and focal weakness.

Investigations

- Based on a **clinical suspicion** [1] of osteoporosis further investigations are performed for confirmation.
- The patient undergoes a **DEXA (dual energy X-ray absorptiometry) scan** [2].
- The scan shows osteoporosis in the femoral neck with a **T score** [3] of –3.0.
- **Vertebral bone density** [4] shows a T score of +1.5.
- Her **Z score** [5] value is –1.5.
- A thoracic and lumbar spine X-ray is performed. This reveals a previous Grade 1 **compression fracture** [6] of T6.

- **Laboratory studies** [7] are performed including a **full blood count** [8], **biochemical studies** [9] (renal function, electrolytes, LFT), **calcium** [10], **magnesium** [11] and phosphate. These all return as normal.
- **Thyroid function tests** [12], **25-hydroxyvitamin D level** [13] and **alkaline phosphatase levels** [14] are also normal.
- **Bone turnover markers** [15] are not tested in this instance.

1 A diagnosis of osteoporosis may be made when there is a minimal-trauma fracture present. These should be fractures that occur either spontaneously or with a minor trauma, such as falling from a standing height. Essentially the mechanism of injury is not one that is normally expected to cause a fracture. A typical history and a common site of fracture such as the hip, spine, wrist or pelvis indicate osteoporosis. In contrast, fractures of skull, cervical spine, hand, feet and ankles work against the diagnosis. Stress fractures are also less likely to be due to osteoporosis.

2 This is the standard diagnostic test for identifying osteoporosis. It assesses BMD, measured as a T score or a Z score. A T score indicates the difference in standard deviation of the patient's BMD compared with a group of healthy young adults.

3 A T score less than –2.5 (below 2.5 standard deviations from the mean) is indicative of osteoporosis. A T score of –1.0 to –2.5 (1–2.5 standard deviations below the mean) is indicative of osteopenia. Normal BMD is a value above –1.0 (within 1 standard deviation of the mean). As this patient has a T score below 2.5 standard deviations of the mean, she is osteoporotic and is in the category of patients with the highest risk of fracture.

4 The discrepancy in the BMD at the two sites could be due to a previous fracture of the vertebral body, giving an artificially elevated vertebral BMD reading. Plain radiograph should be obtained.

5 The Z score is an age-adjusted measurement, with the value comparing the patient's bone mineral density to that of a population of similar age. A Z score below 2 standard deviations of the mean is an abnormal result. This indicates that osteoporosis may be caused by factors other than age alone, and should prompt further investigation for other causes (e.g. medication and coexisting medical conditions).

6 Osteoporotic compression fractures can occur gradually and patients may be completely asymptomatic with it. As in this case, healed or old fractures can be an incidental finding on X-ray imaging. Grading of compression fractures is determined radiographically by the percent height deformity. Imaging can also show wedge fractures of the spine. If a fracture is seen in a young patient, or seen as an isolated fracture of the cervical spine, an alternative diagnosis should be suspected. Exclude other causes of low bone mass, e.g. osteomalacia, metastatic disease and granulomatous disease.
Ensure that there are no neurological findings (refer to

Examination section); if abnormalities are present, urgent imaging with an MRI or CT should be performed with a view to surgical intervention.

7 In addition to assessing the BMD, blood tests can be performed to establish baseline levels and also look for evidence of secondary causes of osteoporosis.

8 Anaemia can be indicative of malabsorptive states or can be seen in sickle cell disease (can cause orthopaedic complications including osteonecrosis). Multiple myeloma should be considered as a differential diagnosis of patients with anaemia and reduced BMD, particularly in those aged over 60. Anaemia may also be seen in patients with alcohol abuse – correlate these with liver function test (LFT) results (usually elevated gamma-glutamyl transpeptidase (GGT)).

9 Renal function is used to assess for renal disease as a contributing factor for osteoporosis in this patient. Elevated creatinine may be seen in patients with multiple myeloma. If this is suspected in a patient, conduct serum and urine electrophoresis. LFTs can be used to check for chronic liver disease (as a cause of secondary osteoporosis) and excessive alcohol use.

10 Calcium level can be used to assess for other differential diagnoses of low BMD – hypercalcaemia can indicate malignancy or hyperparathyroidism (request parathyroid hormone levels in this case), whereas hypocalcaemia would be a contributing risk factor for osteoporosis. For patients with GI diseases (coeliac, inflammatory bowel disease), a 24-hour urinary calcium and creatinine measurement can be performed to assess for adequate calcium intake and absorption.

11 Low magnesium levels can impair calcium absorption and metabolism.

12 A low TSH level can indicate hyperthyroidism or subclinical hyperthyroidism.

13 Vitamin D deficiency increases fracture risk. In combination with anaemia and low urinary calcium excretion, this may indicate other medical conditions such as coeliac disease (tissue transglutaminase and anti-endomysial antibodies should be checked).

14 Serum alkaline phosphatase (ALP) is elevated in most patients with Paget's disease. ALP levels, alongside vitamin D and serum calcium levels, can be used to assess for osteomalacia (values depend on the cause of osteomalacia – in nutritional osteomalacia generally ALP is elevated with low vitamin D and calcium).

15 Bone turnover markers include markers of bone resorption (serum fasting collagen type 1 cross-linked C-telopeptide (CTX) and fasting spot urine N-terminal telopeptide to creatinine ratio (uNTx/Cr)) and markers of bone absorption (serum fasting type 1 procollagen (N-terminal) (P1NP)). These are generally not routinely performed in the general practice setting, but may be used in specialised settings to monitor progress of treatment.

Management

- Management in this patient includes both **lifestyle measures** [1] and **medical management** [2].
- Provide patients with advice to optimise their **diet** [3].
- Encourage participation in **regular exercise** [4].
- In this case, the patient's **smoking habits** [5] are discussed, where she expresses a wish to quit.
- The circumstances around her fall are revisited to **minimise the risk of further falls** [6].
- Assess the patient's **risk of fracture** [7].

- Commence on **bisphosphonate therapy** [8] if there are no **contraindications** [9].
- **Denosumab** [10] can be considered as an alternative.
- Other pharmacological options are **teriparatide** [11], **oestrogen therapy** [12] and **tibolone** [13].
- Monitor **tolerance of therapy** [14].
- **Vitamin D and calcium levels** [15] should be optimised.
- Patients should be linked in with an outpatient clinic for **ongoing follow-up** [16].

1 These steps are aimed at reducing bone loss in postmenopausal women.

2 Patients with a higher risk are likely to benefit more from pharmacological therapy. A secondary cause of osteoporosis should be excluded prior to commencing drug therapy. Medical management is appropriate in patients with a T score in the osteoporotic or osteopenic range.

3 Patients should be informed of the recommended daily intake of calcium (1300mg for patients aged >50) that is required in the management of osteoporosis – some patients may be able to reach this desirable target with diet alone, whilst others may require calcium supplementation. They should also optimise their calorie and vitamin D intake (approximately 600–800IU daily). Vitamin D levels are generally harder to maintain with dietary intake alone. In patients diagnosed with coeliac disease, a gluten-free diet can improve BMD.

4 It is recommended that patients with osteoporosis should engage in regular physical exercise – ideally 30 minutes per day, at least three times per week. Low impact aerobic exercises can be useful, with weight-bearing exercises recommended for patients with osteoporosis. However, patients should be encouraged to choose a form of exercise that they will enjoy, as this improves adherence to a regular exercise regimen.

5 Patients should be educated on the adverse effect of smoking on bone health. A motivational interviewing technique can be used to determine the patient's readiness for cessation of smoking.

6 Some general measures to reduce the risk of falls include minimising risks around the home, improving vision and hearing in those with impairment and providing gait aids as appropriate. A home visit by an occupational therapist can be helpful in establishing appropriate home modifications. Some patients may benefit from input from a physiotherapist (particularly following operative management of a fracture) or referral to falls clinic.

7 For patients with T score between –1 and –2.5, pharmacological therapy may be appropriate based on their clinical risk factors and fracture risk. A fracture risk assessment tool named FRAX is available to predict the 10-year probability of fracture in an untreated patient (hip or major osteoporotic fractures combined). Calculation requires the femoral BMD and information regarding the following clinical factors: advancing age, previous fracture, glucocorticoid therapy, parental history of hip fracture, low body weight, current cigarette smoking, excessive alcohol consumption, rheumatoid arthritis and secondary osteoporosis (inflammatory bowel disease, malabsorption, chronic liver disease, premature menopause and hypogonadism).

8 Bisphosphonates inhibit osteoclasts and thereby improve BMD and slow loss of bone. Suitable regimens include oral alendronate 75mg weekly, risedronate 35mg weekly, risedronate 150mg monthly or yearly zoledronic acid 5mg IV. Patients should be advised to take oral bisphosphonates on an empty stomach. They should avoid taking oral bisphosphonates within 2 hours of taking calcium, magnesium, iron and antacids as this can impair optimal absorption.

9 Alendronate and risedronate can exacerbate upper GI tract irritation and require weekly dosing, whilst zoledronic acid is only an annual dose with avoidance of GI side-effects. However, some patients may not be comfortable with the intravenous route of administration. All above options are contraindicated in severe renal disease. Patients with vitamin D deficiency, malabsorptive disorders or renal disease are at risk of hypocalcaemia if commenced on zoledronic acid. Therefore, these parameters should be measured prior to the first dose and then monitored throughout treatment.

10 Denosumab is another antiresorptive drug – it reduces the formation and differentiation of osteoclasts. It also acts by increasing apoptosis of osteoclasts. Inform the patient of the risk of spontaneous vertebral fractures if denosumab is withdrawn or dose delayed – emphasise the importance of adhering to the 6-monthly regimen (given as 60mg subcutaneously). If ceased, patient must be switched to a bisphosphonate to prevent rapid decline of BMD. Denosumab also can cause hypocalcaemia.

11 Teriparatide is a synthetic parathyroid hormone which increases bone formation, and is appropriate for use in postmenopausal women with a T score of less than –3 and two or more minimal trauma fractures with a fracture occurring following one year (minimum) of antiresorptive therapy. It can be administered as a daily subcutaneous dose for up to 24 months.

12 In younger postmenopausal women (typically below the age of 60), oestrogen therapy may be appropriate, especially if they have coexisting menopausal symptoms. There is risk of certain cancers with prolonged use – this risk is lower in women <60. Selective oestrogen receptor modulators (e.g. raloxifene) can be used. Raloxifene can increase the risk of venous thromboembolism. As it reduces the risk of breast cancer, this drug may be more appropriate for treatment of women with osteoporosis who are at high risk of breast cancer.

13 Tibolone is similar to oestrogen therapy in that it also has oestrogenic effects on bone.

14 A rare complication of bisphosphonate therapy is osteonecrosis of the jaw. Dental extractions, implants and periodontal disease increase this risk. Encourage patients to complete any necessary dental interventions prior to commencing therapy. They should maintain good oral hygiene and attend regular reviews with their dentist. For this patient, smoking would add to this risk (other factors increasing risk include diabetes, immune compromise, glucocorticoid therapy and diabetes). In general, the benefits of bisphosphonate therapy outweigh the risk of osteonecrosis. Antiresorptive agents can increase the risk of atypical femoral fractures – this can present as thigh or groin pain.

15 If dietary intake is insufficient, commence patients on calcium supplementation. Appropriate starting doses include calcium carbonate 1.25g (500mg elemental calcium) or 1.5g (600mg elemental calcium) daily or calcium citrate 2.38g (500mg elemental calcium) daily. Calcium citrate is better absorbed in patients who are also taking a proton pump inhibitor (calcium carbonate requires gastric acidity for absorption). For vitamin D optimisation, encourage measures to increase sunlight exposure as a first step. Consider commencing cholecalciferol 25–50mcg (1000–2000IU) daily in patients with limited sun exposure.

16 Progress should be monitored using BMD values, 2 years after commencement of treatment. In patients without a high risk of minimal-trauma fracture, consider ceasing bisphosphonate therapy after 5 years (if oral therapy) or 3 years (if IV therapy). Note that even after being ceased, bisphosphonates remain within the system – alendronate and zoledronic acid can persist for several years. In high risk patients, it can be continued up to 10 years (oral) or 6 years (IV). Patients' BMD should be measured approximately 2 years after ceasing treatment – treatment may need to be recommenced if they have a significant decrease in their BMD or experience a minimal trauma fracture. This should also prompt investigation of any new risk factors. Check patients' adherence to the therapy.

CASE 17: Paget's disease of bone

History

- A **65-year-old male** [1] is awaiting orthopaedic surgery for treatment of severe left knee osteoarthritis (OA).
- He has been referred for review following identification of **radiological abnormalities** [2] in the left tibia in keeping with Paget's disease of the bone.
- On further history from the patient, he reports **pain** [3] in the upper portion of his left shin for many years.
- He describes his shin pain as a **mild, aching pain which is present throughout the day and at rest and tends to be worse in the evening** [4].
- He reports symptomatic **osteoarthritis** [5] in his left knee for years which has become increasingly difficult to manage with analgesic agents over the last 12 months.
- He has never had a **fracture** [6] to his left lower limb.
- The patient denies any history of **hearing loss, significant headache, dizziness or vertigo** [7].
- He has no history of **significant back pain or lower limb sensation changes** [8].
- There is **no known family history** [9] of Paget's disease of the bone.
- The patient is overweight and has bilateral knee OA, but has no other known medical history. His current medications include regular paracetamol and occasional ibuprofen as required.

[1] Paget's disease of bone is a common focal disorder of bone metabolism. In this condition, there is an accelerated rate of bone metabolism resulting in overgrowth of bone at single sites (monostotic disease) or multiple sites (polyostotic disease), with subsequent impaired quality of the affected bony site. It is thought to be a disease of the osteoclast. Bony sites that are typically affected include the skull, spine, pelvis and long bones of the lower limbs. The condition generally occurs in patients >55 years and it is rare in patients <40 years old. Frequency of diagnosis increases with age and there is a slight male predominance.

[2] Paget's disease of bone is most commonly asymptomatic and may be identified when imaging is performed for an alternative reason.

[3] When Paget's disease of bone does present with symptoms, this is either pain due to the pagetic lesion or from secondary consequences of bony overgrowth and deformities. Secondary complications include OA, radiculopathy due to nerve compression syndromes, hearing loss, fracture and bony tumours.

[4] Pain associated with Paget's disease of bone is typically mild to moderate in severity and is described as deep and aching. The pain is often worse with weight bearing and patients often complain of worsening pain as the day goes by.

[5] Osteoarthritis can be associated with pagetic bony abnormalities, or in this case, may be idiopathic OA in the context of other OA risk factors. Osteoarthritis can occur in joints adjacent to the affected pagetic bones due to deformity of the bone involved in the joint or from abnormal forces transmitted to the joint from a bowed or shortened bone.

[6] Pagetic lesions cause weakened bone and, in long bones, can result in bowing deformities which can increase fracture risk caused by minimal trauma. Traumatic and pathological fractures are the most common complications of pagetic lesions in long bones, and are more common in the femur than the tibia. Paget's disease of bone causes increased risk of primary bone neoplasms, particularly osteosarcoma, which can present as a pathological fracture. Osteosarcoma more commonly presents with localised bony pain and swelling which does not respond to medical therapy. Transformation of pagetic bone to osteosarcoma is rare, with a lifetime risk of <1%. Giant cell tumours are benign primary bone neoplasms that present similarly to osteosarcomas; however, they tend to occur in the axial skeleton and can present as multiple neoplasms.

[7] The skull is a common site affected by Paget's disease of bone. Potential symptoms include hearing loss due to cochlear involvement, headache, dizziness and vertigo.

[8] Paget's disease of bone affecting the spine and pelvis can cause bone pain, spinal stenosis, nerve compression and compression fractures.

[9] There is family history of Paget's disease of the bone in 10–20% of cases. Familial forms tend to have an earlier onset and are more severe in clinical picture, with more skeletal involvement, deformity and fractures.

Examination

- The patient does not appear unwell and has **vital signs** [1] which are within the normal range.
- The patient has a slightly unstable gait as he avoids putting excess weight through his painful left lower limb. He does not use a gait aid.
- On assessment of the lower limbs, there is **increased warmth** [2] over the proximal anterior aspect of the left tibia where the patient experiences pain.
- There is no associated **fluctuant mass** [3].

- This area of tibia is also **increased in size and more irregular** [4] compared to the patient's right lower limb.
- The **skin is not red** [5].
- The left knee has **minimal restriction of range of movement** [6] on testing passive knee flexion and knee extension, and crepitations are present.
- On comparison of both legs, there is **no evidence of bowing** [7] of either femur or tibia.
- Examination of other body systems is unremarkable.

[1] A differential of a painful joint or painful area of bone is infection – a septic joint or osteomyelitis. Assessing a patient's vital signs, including their temperature, is part of this work-up.

[2] A pagetic bony area is typically warm to the touch. This is thought to be due to increased blood flow to an area with increased bone turnover.

[3] A fluctuant mass over a bone may be suggestive of a bony tumour, such as an osteosarcoma. Although rare, this is an important diagnosis to consider and requires targeted imaging with MRI. The diagnosis of osteosarcoma is made based on histopathological characteristics on a biopsy specimen.

[4] Bone that is increased in size and abnormal in shape is in keeping with skeletal deformity that is seen in Paget's disease of bone with abnormally increased bone turnover.

[5] The absence of skin erythema makes a diagnosis of cellulitis less likely.

[6] A septic or inflamed joint is exquisitely painful to move. Crepitations and some restriction of passive range of movement are seen with knee OA.

[7] Paget's disease of bone can cause bowing of lower limb long bones. Bowing may be seen on examination or may be better appreciated radiologically. Bowing of long bones can increase the risk of OA.

Investigations

- The patient has a **serum alkaline phosphatase (ALP)** [1] which is three times the upper limit of the reference range.
- The **remaining liver function tests** [2] are within the reference range.
- His **serum corrected calcium is 2.40mmol/L and serum phosphate is 0.85mmol/L** [3], both within the reference range.
- The patient's **renal function** [4] is within the reference range with a urea of 7.0mmol/L, a creatinine of 61μmol/L and an eGFR of >90ml/min/1.73m^2.

- He has a normal **vitamin D level** [5] of 60ng/ml.
- **Plain radiographs** [6] are taken of the left femur, left knee, left tibia and fibula and reveal a mixed lytic and sclerotic lesion in the proximal area of the anterior tibia with thickening of the associated cortical bone. There is also anterior curvature of the tibia noted. Radiological evidence of OA is identified at the left knee joint.
- The patient undergoes a **bone scintigraphy scan** [7] which identifies increased uptake in the skull and right pelvic bone as well as the left proximal tibia.

[1] The diagnosis of Paget's disease of bone is primarily radiological. However, the incidental finding of an elevated ALP, a marker of bone turnover, is a common initial finding that can then lead to diagnostic imaging to investigate for potential Paget's disease of bone. The ALP is frequently elevated in Paget's disease of bone; however, the degree of elevation is not always consistent with the degree of disease activity.

[2] ALP results must be interpreted cautiously as there is overlap with ALP from liver. If remaining LFTs are normal, an elevated ALP is more likely due to Paget's disease of bone. In the case of the remaining LFTs being abnormal, the ALP is difficult to interpret, and instead the bone turnover marker serum procollagen type 1 N propeptide (P1NP) can be measured. A serum P1NP will typically be elevated in Paget's disease of bone; however, its use is limited by expense.

3 The serum calcium and serum phosphate are typically normal in the setting of Paget's disease of bone. If these blood tests are abnormal, a secondary disorder should be considered. Of note, hypercalcaemia should raise the possibility of concurrent primary hyperparathyroidism which can commonly coexist with Paget's disease of bone.

4 Kidney function is important to assess as this impacts on treatment options. If the eGFR is <30–35ml/min/1.73m², zoledronic acid, the first-line treatment option for Paget's disease of bone, is contraindicated.

5 Vitamin D should be tested to assist with differential diagnosis as well as to guide therapy. Osteomalacia can present with bone pain and raised ALP. When treating Paget's disease, the patient should be vitamin D replete prior to zoledronic acid therapy to reduce the risk of post treatment hypocalcaemia.

6 Radiological findings of Paget's disease of bone are dependent upon the timing of the disease course. Early stage lesions are predominantly lytic lesions. With time, areas of sclerosis develop and mixed lytic and sclerotic lesions can be seen on radiographs. These mixed lesions have thickened trabecular bone expansion, cortical thickening and are associated with deformity. Later stage disease is more sclerotic in nature. Long bones, such as the femur and tibia, should be assessed for bowing on radiographs. This may correlate with clinical findings or be asymptomatic. Of note, bowing of long bones can be a risk factor for OA of an adjacent joint. Bony lesion radiographic features of Paget's disease of bone are characteristic; however, differential diagnoses of these lesions should be considered, such as metastatic malignancy.

7 Bone scintigraphy is useful in identifying the extent of disease, especially in the context of asymptomatic sites. Pagetic lesions have increased bone remodelling and increased blood flow which corresponds to enhanced radionuclide uptake on bone scintigraphy scanning. Bone scintigraphy can identify very early lesions that are not yet present on radiographs. When a patient has a response to treatment, the findings on bone scintigraphy scans may decrease or normalise.

Management

- In the setting of **symptomatic Paget's disease of bone** [1] and in a patient planned for **orthopaedic surgery** [2] at an active pagetic site, the patient is assessed for treatment with zoledronic acid infusion.
- His **blood tests** [3] are reviewed as above and he has **clearance from his dentist** [4] to proceed with the treatment.
- He goes on to have treatment with IV zoledronic acid 5mg as a single infusion and **no adverse effects** [5] are noted.
- He is encouraged to continue using regular paracetamol and to trial a short course of regular anti-inflammatory medications for **pain management** [6].

- He is reviewed by a **physiotherapist** [7] and is recommended to use a single point stick to improve his mobility while awaiting his surgery.
- The patient has a **repeat ALP level** [8] six weeks after the treatment and the ALP has reduced to the normal reference range.
- His left knee joint replacement surgery is scheduled. The patient is aware he will need **ongoing follow-up** [9] of his Paget's disease of bone and may need further imaging investigations in future if changes occur.

1 The aim of treating Paget's disease of bone is to improve pain and associated complications of bone remodelling at pagetic sites. By reducing the rate of bone remodelling, the goal is to improve deposition of normal lamellar bone, decrease bone vascularity and decrease rate of disease progression. Effective treatment improves bone histology, radiographic lytic lesions, bone scintigraphy uptake severity, pain and quality of life. Treatment is indicated in a symptomatic patient to improve symptoms of pain and reduce associated complications. Treatment is indicated in asymptomatic patients with one of the following added features: biochemically active disease (indicated by elevated ALP or bone turnover markers) with affected sites that may lead to complications; serum ALP 2–4 times the upper limit of normal reference; normal ALP but bone scintigraphy identifying pagetic involvement at a site where complications may occur; planned surgery at an active pagetic site; presence of hypercalcaemia in association with immobilisation.

2 Patients with Paget's disease of bone have increased risk of OA and in this context, may require joint replacement surgery as part of their management. Less commonly, surgical corrective osteotomy for long bone deformity, fracture fixation or tumour resection may need to be performed. Active pagetic sites have higher vascularity than normal bone and as such, there is an increase in peri-operative blood loss during surgery at these sites. Paget's disease of bone treatment, such as zoledronic acid, preoperatively reduces abnormal bone turnover and results in reducing this hypervascularity and associated bleeding risk.

3 Zoledronic acid is a highly potent bisphosphonate agent and is the treatment of choice for management of Paget's disease of bone. It is the most effective available agent for Paget's treatment and most patients will achieve remission after a single dose. Prior to treatment, patients require assessment for appropriateness of receiving the medication. Blood tests including calcium, vitamin D and renal function should be performed. Patients should have a normal corrected calcium and be vitamin D replete prior to receiving zoledronic acid, to reduce the risk of hypocalcaemia. Renal function should be assessed, as zoledronic acid is contraindicated if the creatinine clearance is <30–35ml/min.

4 Osteonecrosis of the jaw (ONJ), the presence of non-healing exposed bone in the maxillofacial region, is a rare but serious complication associated with zoledronic acid. Poor dentition can increase the risk of this complication, making it important that a patient is reviewed by a dentist prior to commencing the medication. The risk of ONJ is much higher in the oncology patient population group, as these patients receive high doses of causative medications at frequent intervals. In comparison, the risk of ONJ in patients with Paget's disease of bone having bisphosphonate treatment is very low.

5 Zoledronic acid is infused over 15–20 minutes. A flu-like illness is seen in approximately 25% of patients and this is the most common adverse effect. Uveitis and other inflammatory changes in the eye occur in 1% of patients and require urgent ophthalmology review and commencement of topical steroids.

6 Zoledronic acid usually improves pain dramatically. Adjunctive analgesics should be used for management of both pain related to Paget's disease of bone and, in this patient, pain related to OA.

7 Physiotherapy assessment is useful to assess and aim to improve a patient's mobility that may be affected by pain as well as structural changes from Paget's disease of bone. Mobility aids and physical therapy may be useful management aids to improve functional status.

8 ALP or other baseline disease activity markers such as P1NP are tested at 6–12 weeks post zoledronic acid infusion to assess response to treatment. The reduction in ALP or other activity markers reflects the decrease in bone turnover. Maximal remission is seen in patients who have bone turnover markers reduced below the midpoint of the reference range. Most patients will only require a single dose of IV zoledronic acid to achieve remission.

9 Retreatment with bisphosphonates may be indicated if there is evidence of increased or recurrent abnormal bone turnover which is suggested by increasing serum ALP, radiographic progression of disease or recurrent pain. The decision to re-treat based on symptoms or based on laboratory and radiological progression alone is variable in practice. Retreatment is typically done with IV zoledronic acid.

CASE 18: Primary hyperparathyroidism

History

- A **52-year-old female** [1] is reviewed following a routine blood test as part of a wellness check-up that identifies **hypercalcaemia, with an elevated parathyroid hormone (PTH)** [2] level on additional testing.
- The patient has no **family history** [3] of conditions related to abnormal calcium or PTH levels.
- On further questioning, the patient has **no symptoms** [4] of **hypercalcaemia or hyperparathyroidism** [5].

- She denies fatigue, weakness, low mood, poor appetite or difficulties with her thinking.
- The patient has no medical or surgical history, particularly that of **nephrolithiasis** [6] or renal colic.
- She has no previous **fractures** [7].
- She does not take regular **medications** [8].
- She is a non-smoker and drinks occasional alcohol. She works as a primary school teacher and **exercises** [9] regularly.

[1] PTH, secreted by the parathyroid glands, is vital in regulating serum ionised calcium within a narrow range. PTH secretion occurs as a rapid response to parathyroid gland calcium-sensing receptors detecting a serum ionised calcium level lower than the target range. PTH acts directly to increase the serum ionised calcium level by increasing calcium resorption from the bone to the blood and by reducing renal clearance of calcium. PTH also indirectly increases the serum calcium level through its effect on the kidneys to increase active vitamin D synthesis, which increases efficiency of intestinal calcium absorption. Through the calcium-sensing receptors, increasing serum calcium levels have a negative feedback mechanism on PTH secretion. Primary hyperparathyroidism is a condition of abnormal regulation of PTH secretion by calcium. It can be diagnosed at any age but is most common in adults between 50 and 65 years of age. Women are twice as commonly affected as men. Other forms of hyperparathyroidism are secondary and tertiary hyperparathyroidism, which will not be the focus of this Case. Secondary hyperparathyroidism is an increased PTH level in response to hypocalcaemia in an attempt to restore calcium homeostasis. Causes include low calcium intake and vitamin D deficiency. In the context of chronic kidney disease (CKD), secondary hyperparathyroidism occurs due to a low concentration of 1,25-dihydroxyvitamin D. Tertiary hyperparathyroidism occurs typically in the setting of CKD and is a result of prolonged hypocalcaemia causing parathyroid gland hyperplasia. In this setting, there is autonomous oversecretion of PTH causing hypercalcaemia.

[2] More than 90% of cases of hypercalcaemia are caused by malignancy and primary hyperparathyroidism. Non-parathyroid causes of hypercalcaemia include hypercalcaemia of malignancy, granulomatous disease such as sarcoidosis, hypervitaminosis D and milk-alkali syndrome.

The hypercalcaemia caused by these conditions will result in a suppressed PTH through the above described calcium homeostasis mechanism. Primary hyperparathyroidism is suggested by hypercalcaemia with an associated elevated PTH level, or an inappropriately normal range PTH level. Primary hyperparathyroidism, in 80–85% of cases, is caused by a single abnormal gland with most often, a single adenoma. These adenomas are usually benign. Two adenomas are present in 2–5% of patients with primary hyperparathyroidism. Multiple gland hyperplasia is the cause in 6% of cases. Parathyroid carcinomas are rare and are the cause of primary hyperparathyroidism in 1–2% of cases.

[3] Familial forms of primary hyperparathyroidism are rare but are important to assess for. Multiple endocrine neoplasia (MEN) type 1 syndrome is the most common cause of familial primary hyperparathyroidism. MEN-1 is an autosomal dominant condition caused by inactivating mutations of the *MEN1* tumour-suppressor gene with resulting predisposition for tumours of the parathyroid glands, anterior pituitary gland and pancreas, along with other non-endocrine tumours. MEN-1 syndrome most commonly presents as multiple parathyroid tumours causing primary hyperparathyroidism. Other familial causes of primary hyperparathyroidism include familial isolated hyperparathyroidism, familial hyperparathyroidism-jaw tumour syndrome, MEN-2A syndrome and familial hypocalciuric hypercalcaemia.

[4] Primary hyperparathyroidism is most commonly diagnosed following an incidental finding of hypercalcaemia in an asymptomatic patient. It can be difficult to differentiate between asymptomatic primary hyperparathyroidism and symptomatic primary hyperparathyroidism in the case of patients with non-specific symptoms such as fatigue, weakness, mild depression and anorexia, that may

be overlooked without specific questioning. With time, approximately 30% of patients with initially diagnosed asymptomatic primary hyperparathyroidism may develop clinical manifestations of the condition. The classical manifestations of primary hyperparathyroidism of 'bones', 'stones', abdominal 'moans' and psychic 'groans' are uncommon in developed countries.

5 There is an overlap in some of the symptoms caused by hypercalcaemia with those attributed to hyperparathyroidism. Classical manifestations of hyperparathyroidism include bone disease, nephrolithiasis, proximal renal tubular acidosis, gout, neuromuscular symptoms of weakness and fatigue and neuropsychiatric symptoms such as lethargy, depressed mood, psychosis and cognitive dysfunction. Hypercalcaemia symptoms include anorexia, nausea, vomiting, bowel hypomotility and constipation; musculoskeletal symptoms of weakness, bone pain and osteoporosis; renal symptoms of polyuria, nephrolithiasis, nephrocalcinosis, distal renal tubular acidosis, nephrogenic diabetes insipidus and renal insufficiency; neurological presentations including decreased concentration, confusion, fatigue and coma; and cardiovascular complications such as QT interval shortening and bradycardia. A rare atypical presentation of primary hyperparathyroidism is a parathyroid crisis, which is characterised by symptoms of severe hypercalcaemia. There is a 1–2% risk in untreated patients with primary hyperparathyroidism to progress to this state. It is unclear why it occurs; however, it may occur in the context of severe intercurrent illness or significant volume depletion.

6 Nephrolithiasis is the most common complication of primary hyperparathyroidism. While 15–20% of patients with hyperparathyroidism have nephrolithiasis, 5% of patients with nephrolithiasis are found to have hyperparathyroidism. Nephrolithiasis occurs in the context of prolonged PTH excess. Most stones are made of calcium oxalate. Other contributing factors for stone formation include dietary risk factors (low calcium intake, high animal protein intake, low fluid intake), hypercalciuria, hyperoxaluria and hypocitraturia. Nephrocalcinosis, the deposition of calcium in the kidneys, can also occur from hyperparathyroidism, but is less common than nephrolithiasis.

7 Bone disease in the context of hyperparathyroidism is related to prolonged PTH excess. Classically, primary hyperparathyroidism bone disease is osteitis fibrosa cystica, where the bone becomes soft and deformed and cysts may develop. Patients present with bone pain. This is now very rare, and if it occurs, will typically occur in patients with very severe disease, such as with the very high levels of PTH caused by a parathyroid carcinoma. More commonly, primary hyperparathyroidism bone disease causes decreased BMD resulting in increased fracture risk. The reduction in BMD tends to occur at cortical sites (for example the hip and the forearm) compared with trabecular sites (for example the spine).

8 Lithium and thiazide diuretic use can be associated with primary hyperparathyroidism and their use should be questioned in a patient such as this. Thiazide diuretics reduce calcium excretion and can cause a mild hypercalcaemia. Their use can unmask underlying primary hyperparathyroidism. If hypercalcaemia persists following cessation of a thiazide diuretic, this is more suggestive of primary hyperparathyroidism than the medication effect. Lithium can induce a defect in calcium-PTH regulation and can cause an increase in serum total and ionised calcium and an increase in PTH levels.

9 Parathyroidectomy is a curative treatment for primary hyperparathyroidism and so history taking in a patient such as this should be assessed for anaesthetics risk if an operative procedure is required.

Examination

- On **examination** [1] the patient does not appear unwell and has observation signs which are within the normal range, including a blood pressure of **120/80mmHg** [2] and a heart rate of 70bpm.
- She is **euvolaemic** [3] on fluid assessment with moist mucous membranes, warm peripheries, normal skin turgor, a JVP of 3cm when lying at 45 degrees, lungs clear to auscultation and no peripheral oedema.
- She is **oriented** [4] to time and place and able to do simple and complex maths calculations rapidly.
- She has a **euthymic affect** [5].
- A **neck examination** [6] is unremarkable, with no palpable neck mass.
- An assessment of upper limb and lower limb **muscle strength** [7] is normal.
- Examination of the patient's **eyes** [8] with a slit-lamp examination does not show band keratopathy.
- Examination of other body systems is unremarkable.

1 Examination of a patient with primary hyperparathyroidism is usually unremarkable. There are no specific examination findings for primary hyperparathyroidism; however, hydration status is important to assess in the context of hypercalcaemia.

2 Hypertension is a common finding in patients with primary hyperparathyroidism. The causal association of primary hyperparathyroidism and HTN is unclear and of note, it does not improve with cure of primary hyperparathyroidism.

3 Patients with significant hypercalcaemia may be hypovolaemic on assessment. This is important to assess accurately to determine if IV fluid treatment is required.

4 Neurocognitive symptoms, ranging from lethargy and confusion to stupor and coma, are important to assess for and may be secondary to increased serum PTH and/or calcium. Lethargy is common and non-specific for primary hyperparathyroidism. Confusion, stupor and coma are associated with more severe primary hyperparathyroidism.

5 Mild depression can be identified in patients with primary hyperparathyroidism and this has been seen to be improved in some studies post treatment of hyperparathyroidism, but not in all. Neuropsychiatric symptoms are not listed as a criterion for surgical treatment of primary hyperparathyroidism.

6 Examination of the neck in the context of primary hyperparathyroidism is typically unremarkable. Parathyroid adenomas are rarely palpable. If a neck mass is detected during a neck examination, it is more likely to be a thyroid nodule or a parathyroid carcinoma.

7 In the context of earlier diagnosis of primary hyperparathyroidism, profound muscle weakness is not typically present. Weakness and muscle wasting may also be a finding associated with malignancy.

8 Band keratopathy is a very rare finding in hypercalcaemia. It is a horizontal band across the cornea that is exposed between the eyelids, which may be seen on slit-lamp examination. It is caused by subepithelial calcium phosphate deposits in the cornea.

Investigations

- The patient has blood pathology tests taken with the following results:
  - **corrected calcium** [1] 2.95mmol/L (normal range 2.10–2.60mmol/L)
  - **PTH** [2] 18.5pmol/L (normal range 1.0–7.0pmol/L)
  - **vitamin D** [3] 70mmol/L
  - **phosphate** [4] 0.78mmol/L (normal range 0.75–1.50mmol/L)
  - **Kidney function** [5] tests show urea 8mmol/L (normal range 3.0–9.2mmol/L), creatinine 90µmol/L (normal range 60–110µmol/L) and eGFR >90ml/min/1.73m^2.
- A **24-hour urinary calcium** [6] is in the normal reference range.
- The patient has an **abdominal X-ray and renal tract ultrasound** [7] which are both normal.
- A **DEXA scan** [8] is performed and reported with the following T scores: lumbar spine −1.5, hip −2.5, distal third of radius −2.8.

1 Serum calcium should be tested and then repeated to confirm an abnormal result. A corrected calcium level should be determined based on serum albumin levels. An ionised calcium level can also be tested to confirm the presence of hypercalcaemia. Normocalcaemic hyperparathyroidism is a known variant of primary hyperparathyroidism. This is mostly an indolent condition but may progress to hypercalcaemic primary hyperparathyroidism. To make a diagnosis of normocalcaemic hyperparathyroidism, secondary causes of hyperparathyroidism need to be ruled out and the serum corrected calcium and ionised calcium levels must be within normal ranges.

2 Serum PTH is elevated in most patients with primary hyperparathyroidism. Parathyroid cancer and secondary hyperparathyroidism associated with chronic kidney disease tend to cause much higher levels of serum PTH. About 10–20% of patients with primary hyperparathyroidism have serum PTH levels in the normal range; in the presence of hypercalcaemia, normal range PTH levels are considered inappropriately high.

3 Vitamin D needs to be measured in all patients with suspected primary hyperparathyroidism. Primary hyperparathyroidism disease activity appears to be higher when the patient is vitamin D insufficient (<20ng/ml) or deficient (<10ng/ml). Secondary hyperparathyroidism from vitamin D deficiency may be challenging to differentiate from primary hyperparathyroidism with coexisting vitamin D deficiency. Primary hyperparathyroidism may not be recognised until the vitamin D level is replete and hypercalcaemia develops.

4 In patients with mild primary hyperparathyroidism, serum phosphate level is typically in the lower half of the normal range. With more severe primary hyperparathyroidism, the phosphate levels become lower. This reduction in serum phosphate is due to increased phosphate excretion by the kidneys, with PTH inhibiting proximal tubular reabsorption of phosphate.

5 Primary hyperparathyroidism can cause renal impairment and is a criterion for operative management. Renal function is important to assess as the differentials of secondary and tertiary hyperparathyroidism are commonly related to CKD.

6 A 24-hour urinary calcium is helpful to assess the risk of renal complications in asymptomatic primary hyperparathyroidism. A urinary calcium excretion of >400mg per day is associated with higher risk of long-term renal complications and is a criterion for operative management of primary hyperparathyroidism. Low daily calcium excretion may suggest a possible diagnosis of familial hypocalciuric hypercalcaemia (FHH). FHH is an autosomal dominant disorder and, in most cases, is a result of an inactivating mutation in the calcium-sensing receptor in the parathyroid gland and kidneys. FHH typically causes mild hypercalcaemia, normal serum PTH levels and low urinary calcium excretion. Urinary calcium levels assist in differentiating FHH from primary hyperparathyroidism with minimally elevated or inappropriately normal PTH levels.

7 Baseline abdominal imaging may be performed to assess for asymptomatic nephrolithiasis and presence of nephrocalcinosis.

8 Primary hyperparathyroidism is an important secondary cause of osteoporosis. DEXA imaging should be performed at diagnosis of primary hyperparathyroidism to assess BMD. The distal radius, a site which is rich in cortical bone, is the most sensitive DEXA marker for early detection of bone loss in patients with primary hyperparathyroidism. The distal radius often has the lowest BMD in primary hyperparathyroidism compared with other sites scanned. The spine is the least sensitive site as it instead has a high proportion of trabecular bone which is less affected in primary hyperparathyroidism. This patient's investigation results are in keeping with osteoporosis secondary to primary hyperparathyroidism.

Management

- The patient's treating physician reviews the above investigations and discusses the importance of being reviewed for **surgical** [1] management even though the patient is **asymptomatic** [2].
- The patient is given information regarding the management options of **decreased bone mineral density** [3] in the context of primary hyperparathyroidism.
- She is also advised on **preventive strategies** [4] to reduce the risk of disease progression while awaiting surgical review.
- The patient is agreeable to consideration of surgery and is an appropriate **operative candidate** [5].
- **Localisation studies** [6] are performed to guide surgical decision-making.
- A neck ultrasound scan is performed and detects a homogenously hypoechoic nodule with

internal vascularity peripherally located near the left hemithyroid and is favoured to represent a parathyroid nodule. A nuclear medicine parathyroid scan with technetium-99m sestamibi is also performed and shows increased uptake in the left-sided parathyroid gland. The patient is referred to and seen by an endocrine surgeon for consideration of parathyroidectomy. Given localisation of a single parathyroid gland being the likely cause for her primary hyperparathyroidism, a **minimally invasive parathyroidectomy** [7] approach is discussed.

- The patient is informed that **follow-up** [8] after the procedure will involve blood tests to monitor her calcium and PTH levels as well as follow-up with both the endocrinology and the endocrinology surgical teams.

1 The definitive treatment for primary hyper-parathyroidism is removal of the parathyroid gland or glands causing the increase in PTH levels. In most cases, the causative issue is a parathyroid adenoma, and excision of the gland and the adenoma will result in a biochemical cure of the patient's primary hyperparathyroidism. Parathyroidectomy results in a decrease in kidney stone risk and improvement in BMD. There is limited and conflicting evidence to suggest that parathyroidectomy improves non-specific neuropsychiatric symptoms associated with primary hyperparathyroidism and therefore these symptoms alone are not indication for surgery.

2 Operative treatment is indicated for any patients with symptomatic primary hyperparathyroidism, such as nephrolithiasis, fractures and symptomatic hypercalcaemia.

Indications for operative management in asymptomatic patients relates to predicting which patients will have progressive disease and may therefore develop end-organ effects of primary hyperparathyroidism. Although most asymptomatic patients do not have progressive disease, approximately one-third of patients will progress. Current recommended indications for operative management include any one of the following: patient with serum calcium levels more than 0.25mmol/L above the upper limit of normal, age <50 years old and renal and skeletal indications. Renal indications are: a creatinine clearance <60cc/min; 24-hour urine for calcium >400mg/d and increased stone risk by biochemical stone risk analysis; presence of nephrolithiasis or nephrocalcinosis by X-ray, ultrasound or CT. Skeletal indications are: a BMD reduction with a T score of <–2.5 at lumbar spine, total hip, femoral neck, or distal third of radius; vertebral fracture by X-ray, CT or MRI. Patients who have a diagnosis of primary hyperparathyroidism and are not symptomatic and do not meet any of the criteria for operative management, require ongoing monitoring to identify progressive disease such as worsening hypercalcaemia, renal impairment or bone loss which would warrant reconsideration of operative management. Typical monitoring would be yearly serum calcium and creatinine and bone density testing every 1–2 years. There is no recommendation for repeat abdominal imaging to screen for nephrocalcinosis or asymptomatic nephrolithiasis.

3 Patients with decreased BMD in the context of primary hyperparathyroidism will have improvements in their BMD post parathyroidectomy. Along with this, the fracture risk is also improved. An alternative treatment option for decreased BMD is bisphosphonate agents. Longer-term benefit of these agents for BMD and fracture risk is lacking. Given the paucity of evidence, surgical management remains the treatment of choice rather than bisphosphonates.

4 Patients who are not having surgery or who are awaiting surgery for primary hyperparathyroidism should avoid potential precipitators of worsening hypercalcaemia. Patients should avoid thiazide diuretics and lithium carbonate therapy. They should be encouraged to maintain adequate hydration to minimise the risk of nephrolithiasis. Vitamin D levels should be at least 50–75mmol/L as deficiency stimulates PTH secretion and bone resorption. There are no trials to suggest repletion strategies; however, this should be done cautiously as increased vitamin D levels in this setting can worsen hypercalcaemia and hypercalciuria.

5 Patients who are poor surgical candidates may be managed with medical therapy. For a symptomatic patient or a patient who has severe hypercalcaemia, cinacalcet is used. Cinacalcet is a calcimimetic which activates the calcium-sensing receptor in the parathyroid gland, resulting in inhibition of PTH secretion. In patients with hypercalcaemia and low BMD, a combination of a bisphosphonate agent and cinacalcet may be used; however, there are only small observation studies that support this combination. If the patient's calcium level and BMD levels are appropriate, no pharmacological treatment is required.

6 In a patient with biochemically confirmed primary hyperparathyroidism and who is recommended for operative management, localisation studies are useful in identifying a patient who could have a minimally invasive operative approach. Imaging studies should not be used to make the diagnosis of primary hyperparathyroidism due to high false positive rates. The choice of imaging modalities varies from centre to centre. Ultrasound is highly sensitive to localise a parathyroid adenoma, but requires expertise for the most reliable results. Sensitivity of ultrasound is reduced in the setting of concurrent thyroid pathology. A nuclear medicine parathyroid scan with technetium-99m sestamibi is useful and highly sensitive in detecting and localising hyperfunctioning, enlarged parathyroid glands or tissue, including in ectopic locations. Sestamibi scanning can be negative in cases of parathyroid hyperplasia, multiple parathyroid adenomas or coexisting thyroid disease. In a patient who meets the operative criteria but fails to localise on the imaging studies, a bilateral neck exploration procedure is conducted.

7 The standard approach for parathyroidectomy involves a bilateral neck exploration and adenoma removal based on visual and weight-based estimates of the parathyroid gland size. With improved imaging modalities, minimally invasive parathyroidectomy is now the procedure of choice. There are similar cure rates from both procedures at 90–95% and although complication rates are low for both procedures, the minimally invasive approach has even lower complication rates. Potential complications include recurrent laryngeal nerve injury causing vocal cord paralysis, symptomatic hypocalcaemia and persistent hyperparathyroidism. Intra-operative PTH levels guide how successful the procedure is with an expectation of the PTH level dropping by more than half if the procedure is successful. If the PTH level does not decrease, further exploration for another source of the hyperparathyroidism is warranted.

8 Calcium and vitamin D supplementation is typically commenced postoperatively until stable results are obtained. Histopathology samples from the procedure are important to review and confirm a benign adenoma rather than a rare carcinoma. If persistently elevated PTH levels are identified at postoperative follow-up appointments, the patient may require further work-up for another source of hyperparathyroidism, such as another adenoma.

CASE 19: Type 1 diabetes mellitus

History

- A **10-year-old** [1] **female** [2] is brought to the ED with **abdominal pain and vomiting** [3] .
- On further history taking, there is a 4-week history of **polyuria** [4] and **polydipsia** [5] .
- The parents report they have noticed the patient to have experienced some **weight loss** [6] over this period of time.
- There is associated **lethargy** [7] .
- She has been **well** [8] prior to these 4 weeks.
- On further **systems review** [9] , there is no recent history of cough, cold, fever, sweats, rigors, diarrhoea, constipation, dysuria or headache.

- There is no known **past history of diabetes** [10] .
- The patient does not have any **regular medications** [11] .
- **Family history** [12] includes pernicious anaemia in her mother and hypothyroidism in her uncle.
- There is no **history of T1DM** [13] within the immediate family.
- The **developmental history** [14] is largely unremarkable.

[1] There is a bimodal distribution of childhood onset type 1 diabetes mellitus (T1DM): a peak at 4–6 years old and another at 10–14 years of age (early puberty).

[2] No particular gender difference in the overall incidence of childhood T1DM has been noted. However, in certain populations, it occurs more frequently in males.

[3] In some patients, the initial presentation of T1DM can be the acute complication of diabetic ketoacidosis (DKA), where they may present with symptoms of acidosis and dehydration such as abdominal pain, nausea and vomiting. In normal regulation of glucose homeostasis, insulin reduces gluconeogenesis and glyogenolysis. Insulin inhibits glucagon secretion and allows glucose uptake by adipose tissues and skeletal muscles. In DKA, insulin deficiency results in an inability to utilise glucose in adipose tissues and skeletal muscles. There is a subsequent stimulation of glucagon and other counter-regulatory hormones which oppose the action of insulin. The increased secretion of glucagon, catecholamines, growth hormone and cortisol leads to an increase in glucose via gluconeogenesis and glycogenolysis. Increased lipolysis from peripheral fat stores in the absence of insulin leads to ketone production. Ketones act as an alternative source of energy in the setting of reduced glucose availability. This results in hyperglycaemia and anion gap metabolic acidosis.

[4] As glucose concentration increases there is increased urinary glucose excretion. Glycosuria then causes osmotic diuresis, leading to polyuria and hypovolaemia. In children, polyuria can present as bed-wetting or nocturia. In children wearing nappies, ask the parents about an increase in the

number of wet nappies or unusually 'heavy' wet nappies. Other causes of polyuria for consideration in patients may include diabetes insipidus (related to lack of ineffective antidiuretic hormone) and other electrolyte abnormalities such as hypercalcaemia.

[5] Polydipsia occurs as a result of hyperglycaemia and hypovolaemia leading to an increase in serum osmolality. This causes an increased sensation of thirst.

[6] Weight loss occurs due to hypovolaemia and increased catabolism. In patients with T1DM, deficiency of insulin prevents the absorption of glucose and thereby impairs use in skeletal muscles. Therefore, the breakdown of fat and muscle increases. Other differentials for weight loss would include malignancy, chronic infection, hyperthyroidism and malnutrition (less common in this scenario).

[7] Patients with undiagnosed T1DM can present with vague symptoms such as lethargy. Classic symptoms such as polyuria and polydipsia may not be the initial complaints, and require a systematic approach to a careful history.

[8] Subclinical beta-cell destruction can exist for a period of time of months to years as inflammation of beta cells (insulitis). The patient can be euglycaemic and asymptomatic during this period of time. A substantial number of beta cells must be lost prior to symptomatic hyperglycaemia occurring.

[9] DKA can be precipitated by infection. It is important to complete a thorough systems review to check for any localising symptoms which may suggest an infection.

[10] Approximately 20% of patients presenting with DKA do not have a previous diagnosis of T1DM.

11 In patients with known diabetes, it is important to clarify their adherence to insulin administration and accuracy of dosing of insulin. A precipitant for DKA can be variable adherence or non-adherence to insulin. In certain instances, it may be precipitated due to errors in dose calculation of insulin.

12 Family history of autoimmunity can suggest a predisposition to autoimmune disease. Adolescents and children with T1DM are at a higher risk of developing other autoimmune diseases, such as coeliac disease and autoimmune thyroiditis.

13 The risk of T1DM is increased in close relatives of a patient with T1DM (siblings and offspring), with a markedly increased risk (50%) in identical twins. Type 1 diabetes occurs as a result of the destruction of the insulin-producing beta cells in the islets of Langerhans in the pancreas, causing an insulin deficiency; it can be further classified as type 1A and type 1B diabetes mellitus. Type 1A occurs due to the destruction of the beta cells through an autoimmune process. It occurs in genetically susceptible individuals. There are multiple genes that are reported to influence the risk of type 1A diabetes in individuals. Patients can have the autoantibodies glutamic acid decarboxylase; insulin; and a tyrosine-phosphatase-like molecule, islet autoantigen-2 (IA-2). Patients with type 1B or idiopathic diabetes mellitus do not have any evidence of autoimmunity or another known cause for beta-cell destruction.

14 Certain perinatal and pregnancy-related factors are associated with a slight increase in risk of type 1 diabetes, including pre-eclampsia, jaundice and neonatal respiratory distress.

Examination

- On general inspection, the patient is **lean** [1] and appears tired and lethargic.
- She is alert but confused with a **GCS** [2] of 14 (E4 V4 M6).
- Her vital signs reveal a blood pressure of 117/70mmHg with **a postural drop of 20/10mmHg and tachycardia** [3].
- Respiratory rate is 32 with **deep respiration** [4] noted. She is afebrile with normal SpO_2 levels.
- There is **reduced skin turgor and dry mucous membranes** [5].
- There is no palpable **goitre** [6].
- On palpation, the abdomen is soft with minimal generalised tenderness. There is no **rigidity, guarding or rebound tenderness** [7].

1 Note the patient's body habitus and assess for any evidence of recent weight loss. In T1DM, weight loss can indicate uncontrolled glycosuria. On the other hand, an increased BMI (overweight or obese) in a patient with T1DM should prompt a conversation regarding lowering caloric intake and inducing weight loss, given the increased risk of comorbidities associated with excess adipose tissue.

2 Altered conscious state can result from diabetic ketoacidosis. Comatose states occur secondary to the acidosis, dehydration or plasma hyperosmolality. Patients are at risk of DKA-related cerebral injury. The Glasgow Coma Scale (GCS) or other assessment can be used for objective measurement of neurological status. This assessment should be repeated at regular intervals to monitor improvement until conscious state has normalised.

3 In this context, tachycardia and postural hypotension suggest volume depletion.

4 Observe for evidence of Kussmaul's breathing. This can be present in patients with DKA as a result of the acidosis created by the increased metabolism of fat. This leads to excess production of acetyl-coenzyme A, which is then converted into ketone bodies in the liver. The tachypnoea is as a result of the respiratory system compensating for the metabolic acidosis by increasing the respiratory rate to blow off CO_2. This may fully or partially compensate for the acidosis. In DKA, there may also be distinctive ketotic-smelling breath.

5 A thorough fluid status assessment is vital as the osmotic diuresis caused by elevated glucose levels in the urine can lead to massive fluid loss. Assess the degree of dehydration. An accurate assessment allows guidance of management with IV fluid for volume repletion. However, in children, clinical signs alone (skin turgor, dryness of mucous membranes) can lead to an underestimation of the degree of dehydration. Therefore, a general target of fluid replacement assuming a 5–10% fluid deficit can be used.

6 Rarely, young patients with T1DM may be hyperthyroid, with a prevalence of approximately 1%.

7 As the patient is presenting with abdominal pain and vomiting, the examination should also aim to exclude other causes, including acute surgical conditions.

Investigations

- Given the suggestion of DKA on history taking and presentation, a panel of **further investigations** [1] are requested.
- **Random plasma glucose** [2] is 22mmol/L.
- Results are as follows:

Na [3]	132mmol/L
K [4]	5.7mmol/L
Urea [5]	10.0mmol/L
Creatinine [6]	125μmol/L
pH [7]	7.15
Bicarbonate [8]	9mmol/L
Glucose [9]	23mmol/L

- **Lactate** [10] is normal.
- A **full blood examination** [11] is also performed, showing the following results:

Hb	13.4g/dl
WCC [12]	23 x 10⁹/L
Plt	380 x 10⁹/L

- Urine dipstick reveals a result of **ketones +++** [13], glucose +++.
- Red blood cells, **white blood cells and nitrates** [14] are not detected.
- **Blood cultures and urine cultures** [15] are obtained.
- An **ECG** [16] is performed which shows a sinus tachycardia with no other acute changes.

[1] Early recognition of DKA based on history and clinical examination is vital; however, further tests are required to confirm the diagnosis, guide management and assess progress.

[2] Plasma glucose is elevated in DKA. An initial fingerprick test can be performed for a fast result; however, a formal plasma glucose measurement should be performed. Blood glucose of >11mmol/L confirms hyperglycaemia. Fasting glucose can be done at a later stage, particularly if there is no previous documented diagnosis of diabetes. An HbA1c level can be performed to assess the degree of hyperglycaemia in the preceding 3 months.

[3] Low or borderline sodium levels can be seen in patients with DKA. This is due to the high plasma glucose level.

[4] Potassium elevation is due to the acidosis that is present in DKA. Potassium is shifted from the intracellular space to the extracellular space.

[5] In DKA, urea may be normal or elevated secondary to dehydration.

[6] Elevated creatinine may be seen in severe cases due to prerenal failure.

[7] The acid–base status can be used to categorise the severity of the DKA:

Mild	pH 7.2 to <7.3	bicarbonate 10 to <15mEq/L
Moderate	pH 7.1 to <7.2	bicarbonate 5–9mEq/L
Severe	pH <7.1	bicarbonate <5mEq/L

A pH of <7.3 indicates an acidosis. The cause of the acidosis may be metabolic or respiratory. Metabolic acidosis can be classified as having an increased anion gap or normal anion gap. Causes of metabolic acidosis with an increased anion gap (generally due to increased acid production or ingestion) include ketotic acidosis (diabetes, alcohol ingestion), lactic acidosis (increased lactate production due to infection, hypoxia, circulatory insufficiency and shock), uraemia (secondary to renal failure) or toxins/drugs (methanol, salicylate, ethylene glycol, etc.). Metabolic acidosis with normal anion gap can result from diarrhoea (loss of HCO_3^-), renal tubular acidosis, Addison's disease (absorption of H^+ ions) or certain drugs (e.g. acetozolamide).

[8] A low bicarbonate with a low pH indicates a metabolic acidosis, consistent with DKA.

[9] High plasma glucose level, in combination with the findings of a metabolic acidosis with urinary ketones, confirms the diagnosis of DKA.

[10] Blood lactate can be measured to assess the amount of lactic acid, which could also be contributing to the acidosis. In patients with sepsis, shock or severe dehydration, lactic acidosis is more likely to occur.

[11] A full blood examination can allow the detection of raised inflammatory markers suggestive of infection. This is important as infection can be a precipitant for DKA. It may also reveal an underlying anaemia which may be contributing to generalised weakness and lethargy.

[12] An elevated white cell count can suggest an underlying infection. However, the WCC of a patient with DKA may be elevated without a significant associated infection. A complete septic screen may be required as in some instances infection is difficult to rule out.

[13] Presence of ketones in the urine is because of the excretion of ketones due to deranged metabolism of glucose and the production of ketone bodies including acetone, acetoacetate and beta-hydroxybutyrate (BOHB). BOHB is the predominant ketone body present in DKA (concentrations ≥3mmol/L are consistent with DKA). The urine dipstick method detects acetoacetate. Therefore, whilst the presence

of urine ketones supports DKA, it should not be used to assess the severity of ketonaemia, as this test cannot measure the blood BOHB.

14 The absence of pyuria and nitrates rules out a differential diagnosis of a urinary tract infection in a patient presenting with abdominal pain.

15 Where it is unclear what the precipitant of the episode of DKA is, investigations can be performed to rule out a source of infection. This may not be necessary if there is a clear cause (such as non-adherence to insulin injections). If the patient presents with respiratory symptoms, sputum cultures may also be sent off. If respiratory pathology is suspected, a CXR as an initial imaging study may also be warranted.

16 An electrocardiogram should be requested in patients with diabetes presenting with DKA, particularly in the older age group as myocardial infarction can precipitate DKA. These patients may not necessarily present with chest pain (silent myocardial infarction). However this is unlikely in this case due to the young age of the patient. In this situation, it is important to check for any ECG changes consistent with electrolyte disturbances such as hyperkalaemia (peaked T waves) which may require urgent attention.

Management

Immediate

Patients can be treated in various **clinical environments** [1] including the **emergency department** [2], **inpatient ward** [3] or in **specialised settings** [4]. Use **IV isotonic saline** [5] (0.9% sodium chloride NaCl) as a bolus initially. Administer **additional boluses** [6] as required. **Maintenance IV fluid** [7] should be administered.

Short-term

Following initial fluid bolus administration, **IV insulin infusion** [8] should be commenced. IV insulin can be commenced as an infusion of **0.1 unit/kg/hour** [9]. **IV dextrose** [10] should be administered to prevent hypoglycaemia whilst the insulin infusion continues. IV insulin should continue until **ketoacidosis** [11] has resolved. **Potassium** [12] levels should be measured and replacement commenced when appropriate.

Electrolyte levels [13] should be closely monitored during therapy. Monitor the **calculated anion gap** [14] as treatment continues. When appropriate, the patient can be commenced on their **usual regimen of insulin** [15].

Long-term

Monitoring of **glycated haemoglobin (HbA1c) levels** [16] and **glucose** [17] is required in the long-term management of patients with T1DM. For newly diagnosed T1DM patients, a **basal-bolus regimen of insulin** [18] should be commenced. The insulin regimen should be adjusted as appropriate during **follow-up reviews** [19]. It is important to prevent DKA given its associated **mortality and complications** [20]. A **multidisciplinary team approach** [21] can be used to provide the patient, carer and family with information regarding early diagnosis of diabetes and ongoing management.

1 It is important to determine the most appropriate clinical unit and setting for the management of a patient with DKA. Patients should be managed in an environment which can facilitate frequent monitoring of clinical symptoms, vital signs, fluid status and blood test outcomes. The severity of the patient's DKA can guide the most appropriate place for ongoing management.

2 Patients with known T1DM with only mild DKA, who may show significant improvement with IV fluids and insulin therapy, may be managed in the ED with outpatient follow-up. The appropriateness of this would depend on whether the patient has a sick day management strategy in place, access to monitoring of glucose and ketone at home and has specialised diabetes team follow-up organised.

3 For patients with mild to moderate DKA, IV insulin infusions and IV therapy can be provided in a regular inpatient setting, provided that the unit is capable of close monitoring of the patient.

4 Patients with severe DKA may require treatment in an ICU setting. This is especially appropriate for patients who are at risk of developing cerebral injury. This can include patients with severe acidosis, severe electrolyte disturbances, altered consciousness or very young patients. The clinical management policies and guidelines of some healthcare services mandate that a patient be admitted to the ICU if they require IV insulin.

5 Administering an initial IV fluid bolus aims at restoring the circulating volume and allowing the clearance of glucose and ketones from the bloodstream.

6 The aim of the fluid boluses is to achieve haemodynamic stability. Although rare, hypovolaemic shock can occur in DKA and requires prompt management.

7 Once initial volume expansion has been achieved, the remaining fluid deficit (based on the estimated percentage of fluid loss) must be corrected with a slower infusion of IV therapy. The rate, amount of IV fluid and composition should be adjusted based upon close monitoring of laboratory results and the patient's fluid balance. Increasing fluid volume also allows lowering of serum glucose concentration by dilution. Further, the rehydration with IV fluids increases renal perfusion, stimulating removal of excess ketone bodies.

8 Administration of insulin permits the uptake of circulating glucose, allowing normal metabolism to be stimulated. Insulin reduces hepatic glucose output and ketogenesis. Insulin stimulates the metabolism of ketoacid anions. This results in gradual resolution of ketosis and lowering of serum glucose.

9 This is a recommended rate of insulin infusion; slower rates (e.g. 0.05units/hour/kg) can also be used. The insulin can be administered as a mix with normal saline through an infusion pump. There are hospital- or health service-specific guidelines which can be used for the monitoring and adjustment of insulin infusions.

10 In most cases of DKA, the hyperglycaemia resolves with IV fluid and IV insulin therapy prior to the resolution of ketoacidosis. This means that the blood glucose may normalise whilst a residual ketoacidosis is present. Continuous insulin is required for complete resolution of the ketoacidosis. Therefore IV dextrose can be given to maintain serum glucose concentration at a safe level (e.g. 5.5–8.3mmol/L). Blood glucose levels should be closely monitored and the dextrose infusion adjusted accordingly in response.

11 If metabolic acidosis continues despite IV insulin therapy, consider the possibility of other causes of acidosis. This may include infection or sepsis.

12 Insulin stimulates transfer of potassium into the intracellular space in exchange for hydrogen ions. This causes a decline in serum potassium levels as the ketoacidosis is gradually resolved. If the potassium level was in the normal range at presentation, generally potassium replacement can be commenced at the time of commencement of the insulin infusion. If, as in this case, the patient was hyperkalaemic on presentation, serum potassium level can be repeated during the course of treatment and potassium replacement commenced when potassium normalises. It is important to ensure that renal function is preserved prior to commencing potassium. Potassium replacement should be delayed in the case of renal failure. If the patient is hypokalaemic on presentation, then potassium replacement should be commenced promptly, monitored frequently and replaced as required. Monitor serum potassium concentrations every 2–4 hours during initial therapy.

13 As the hyperglycaemia is corrected, the serum sodium concentration should gradually increase. In many cases, the serum sodium is mildly low or borderline at presentation; this can be due to the osmotic effect of hyperglycaemia. A corrected sodium can be calculated for a more accurate measure, taking into account the degree of hyperglycaemia. Serum phosphate should be intermittently monitored and replaced, as hypophosphataemia can occur during DKA treatment.

14 A normal anion gap with a venous pH of >7.3 indicates that the ketoacidosis has resolved. It is important to note that ketonuria can persist despite resolution of DKA. Insulin infusion can be discontinued when the ketoacidosis has resolved, serum glucose is <11.1mmol/L and the patient is tolerating oral intake.

15 The transition to subcutaneous insulin should ideally be done prior to a meal. Continue the IV insulin infusion for 15–30 minutes following the injection of rapid-acting insulin, prior to discontinuing the infusion.

16 HbA1c levels should be monitored every 3–6 months to assess long-term glucose control. The target HbA1c is variable, specific to the patient. This is due to a need to balance the risk of micro- and macrovascular complications with the risk of hypoglycaemia. In general, most adults should have a HbA1c target of <7.0.

17 For patients with established T1DM, it is important to ensure that the patients and/or carers are proficient in self-monitoring of blood glucose and insulin administration. Some patients may benefit from continuous glucose monitoring, particularly those with frequent or severe hypoglycaemic episodes and/or hypoglycaemic unawareness.

18 There are a variety of ways in which an insulin regimen can be created. Essentially the regimen consists of a basal insulin (long- or intermediate-acting, administered once or twice daily), with bolus doses of a rapid- or short-acting insulin (mealtime boluses). Choice of insulin regimen depends on multiple factors including patient preference (consider the impact of multiple daily injections), lifestyle and cost. Advise the patient on administration technique – referral to a diabetic educator can be made to optimise patient education. Advise patients to alternate injection sites. A continuous subcutaneous infusion of insulin (insulin pump) may be more appropriate for some patients.

19 All recorded glucose reading data should be reviewed during clinic visits (glucose meters, continuous glucose monitors and glucose pumps). Observe for glycaemic trends such as postprandial hyperglycaemia and fasting hyperglycaemia. Identify potential to reduce hypoglycaemic episodes whilst maintaining glycaemic targets.

20 Cerebral injury accounts for the majority of deaths related to DKA. Other complications of DKA include cognitive impairment, venous thrombosis and, rarely, cardiac arrhythmias (secondary to electrolyte disturbances) and acute kidney injury.

21 Higher rates of involvement of patients and their families with a diabetes care team should be encouraged through regular phone calls and clinic visits. Patients' confidence in self-management, including sick day management, should be optimised. Dietitian input is helpful in providing patients with nutrition education, as it can be challenging to match insulin requirement to carbohydrate consumed. Psychological strategies may also be helpful for patients who experience significant stress associated with a new diagnosis of this chronic condition or due to self-care responsibilities.

CASE 20: Type 2 diabetes mellitus

History

- A **58-year-old male** [1] presents with a **five-week history** [2] of increased thirst, urinary frequency, fatigue and two kilograms of weight loss.
- He has been passing urine 8–10 times during the day, **without any associated dysuria or lower urinary tract symptoms** [3].
- On further questioning, he reports mild exertional central chest pain for several months that resolves with rest and sounds typical for **angina** [4]; however, it has not yet been investigated.
- He denies any **visual changes** [5] or **recurrent infections** [6]. He has a past medical history of **obesity** [7], schizophrenia and hypertension.

- His medications are **olanzapine** [8] and amlodipine, both of which he has been on for several years, and he has **no other regular medications** [9] and no allergies.
- He is of **Caucasian background** [10], and has a **positive family history** [11] of T2DM in his mother and maternal grandfather.
- He lives alone and works a **desk job** [12] in a call centre.
- He **smokes five cigarettes a day** [13] and does not consume alcohol.

[1] Type 2 diabetes mellitus (T2DM) is a progressive condition characterised by hyperglycaemia, insulin resistance and relative impairment in insulin secretion. T2DM makes up the majority of cases of diabetes, and usually develops in adults over the age of 45 years. The prevalence of T2DM has increased significantly with the rising rates of obesity and physical inactivity.

[2] Many individuals with T2DM are asymptomatic, and may only be diagnosed on routine screening. Symptoms of T2DM include polyuria, polydipsia and weight loss, which occur as a result of osmotic diuresis. Fatigue, poor wound healing, recurrent infections and blurry vision can also be reported as presenting symptoms.

[3] Some of the symptoms of T2DM are non-specific and it is important to consider and exclude potential differential diagnoses. Symptoms may represent coexisting conditions; e.g. urinary frequency may be a manifestation of T2DM, but infection of the urinary tract may coexist, given that glycosuria and hyperglycaemia increase the risk of infection.

[4] Complications of T2DM are broadly divided into microvascular and macrovascular. Macrovascular complications include CAD, stroke and peripheral vascular disease. Due to the commonly asymptomatic nature of T2DM, diagnosis may only occur after presentation with an acute myocardial infarction or stroke, or a non-healing infection. This patient has reported symptoms concerning for both T2DM and CAD, both of which should be promptly investigated and treated. The macrovascular complication of peripheral arterial disease can present with a range of clinical symptoms from

mild, moderate or severe claudication to ischaemic rest pain, and in the latter stages, ulceration or gangrene.

[5] Microvascular complications include retinopathy, neuropathy and nephropathy. Diabetic retinopathy is often asymptomatic until advanced stages, where potential symptoms include blurred vision, distortion, floaters and progressive visual acuity loss. Diabetic neuropathy can manifest variably as a distal symmetric polyneuropathy, autonomic neuropathy, focal mononeuropathies, polyradiculopathies or mononeuritis multiplex. Distal symmetric polyneuropathy is the most common form, where distal sensation loss may be reported or results in distal limb injury manifesting as ulcers and infection. Autonomic neuropathy affects multiple organs and can manifest as dizziness due to postural hypotension, nausea or vomiting due to gastroparesis, diarrhoea or constipation due to an enteropathy, and erectile dysfunction.

[6] The link between infection and diabetes is well established, with the underlying pathophysiology being hyperglycaemia causing an impaired immune response, contributed to by factors such as altered lipid metabolism and neuropathy. For any wound or ulceration, take a detailed history about the origin and current symptoms, to aid differentiation of whether the underlying process is vascular or neuropathic disease, or a combination of both.

[7] T2DM forms part of the collection of conditions referred to as the metabolic syndrome, accompanied by abdominal obesity, hypertension, dyslipidaemia (specifically high LDL cholesterol concentrations, and low serum HDL cholesterol).

Another condition associated with metabolic syndrome is polycystic ovarian syndrome, which features insulin resistance and therefore an increased risk of T2DM.

8 Atypical antipsychotic agents, in particular olanzapine and clozapine, are associated with weight gain, hypertriglyceridaemia and the development of T2DM. An individual's cardiovascular risk profile must be considered when prescribing these agents, and screening for metabolic syndrome should be performed when these drugs are used long-term. Alternative antipsychotic drugs that are safer from a metabolic perspective include aripiprazole or ziprasidone.

9 Drug-induced hyperglycaemia can occur through various mechanisms including impaired glucose tolerance, reduced insulin secretion, increased hepatic glucose production and increased insulin resistance. Drugs implicated include glucocorticoids, the oral contraceptive pill, beta blockers, thiazide diuretics, nicotinic acid, calcineurin inhibitors, atypical antipsychotic agents, protease inhibitors, statins and gonadotrophin-releasing hormone agonists.

10 The risk of developing diabetes has been found to be higher in individuals of Asian, Hispanic, and African-American ethnic background, compared to those of Caucasian background.

11 There is a genetic risk associated with the development of T2DM, with 40% of affected individuals having at least one parent with the disease.

12 Social factors also play a role in the development of T2DM. A sedentary lifestyle promotes weight gain and increases the risk of T2DM, even independently of weight gain. A dietary history is informative as the consumption of sugar-sweetened beverages, red meat and processed meat heightens the risk of diabetes and is a modifiable risk factor.

13 Cigarette smoking increases the risk of T2DM, with each cumulative pack year correlating to a higher risk. Potential mechanisms include impaired insulin sensitivity, increased abdominal fat distribution and higher blood glucose levels after smoking.

Examination

- He is **alert and oriented** [1] , and is measured to have a **body mass index** [2] of 32kg/m² (height 178 cm, weight 101 kg).
- There is a central distribution of adiposity, with a **waist circumference** [3] of 130cm, and **neck circumference** [4] of 41cm.
- He has a blood pressure of 150/95mmHg without a **postural drop** [5] , a heart rate of 85bpm, and he is afebrile with normal oxygen saturations and respiratory rate.
- There are no features of **Cushing's syndrome or acromegaly** [6] .
- His cardiovascular examination demonstrates normal heart sounds with no murmur, and his apex beat is undisplaced. There are no signs of **congestive cardiac failure** [7] , and he is clinically euvolaemic.
- There is no **acanthosis nigricans** [8] , and the abdomen is soft and non-tender with no **signs of chronic liver disease** [9] .
- A **neurological examination** [10] demonstrates normal power and tone throughout the upper and lower limb and intact reflexes in the upper limbs, but there are reduced ankle reflexes and reduced sensation to light touch and vibratory sensation below the ankles.
- On **monofilament testing** [11] there is one point on the left fifth metatarsal head which is insensate, but there is normal sensation reported at five other points tested across both feet.
- **Peripheral vascular examination** [12] identifies no carotid bruits, a capillary refill time of 2 seconds distally in the fingers and toes, and palpable femoral, popliteal, tibialis posterior and dorsalis pedis pulses bilaterally.
- He has **worn and poorly fitted shoes** [13] with poor foot hygiene and **evidence of tinea pedis** [14] bilaterally, but no ulceration or cellulitic changes.
- His visual acuity is 6/6 bilaterally with corrective lenses, and **fundoscopy** [15] is performed demonstrating clear fundi with no evidence of retinopathy.

1 T2DM can rarely present as hyperosmolar hyperglycaemic state (HHS) or even less commonly, diabetic ketoacidosis (DKA). HHS is marked by severe hyperglycaemia, severe dehydration and obtundation, without ketoacidosis. DKA is very rarely the presentation of T2DM, but can occur in children or in the setting of severe concurrent illness. These illnesses often result in altered conscious state and marked biochemical abnormalities, and require inpatient management and monitoring.

2 Obesity heightens the risk of developing T2DM, and independently increases cardiovascular risk. In individuals with obesity, consider secondary causes and also complications, including T2DM, obstructive sleep apnoea, malignancy, CAD, venous thromboembolism, venous insufficiency, infection, fatty liver disease and osteoarthritis. Potential secondary causes of obesity include hypothyroidism, Cushing's syndrome, polycystic ovarian syndrome and medication-related weight gain. Identifying and treating secondary causes may improve or reverse the associated T2DM.

3 Waist circumference is a better estimate of visceral fat than BMI, and is therefore deemed a more accurate predictor of cardiovascular risk and metabolic syndrome. An increase in risk is suggested by a waist circumference ≥102cm in males, and ≥88cm in females.

4 Neck circumference is another indicator of overweight and obesity, as well as a predictor for obstructive sleep apnoea, with the upper limit of normal being 35.5cm in males and 32cm in females.

5 This patient is hypertensive, which contributes to his profile of metabolic syndrome. The need to measure a lying and standing blood pressure in T2DM relates to the complication of autonomic neuropathy, which can result in postural hypotension.

6 Both acromegaly and Cushing's syndrome can lead to weight gain, hypertension and T2DM. Assessing for other clinical features of these syndromes will guide the need for further investigations. Individuals with Cushing's syndrome can develop moon facies, thin skin and bruising, a dorsocervical fat pad ('buffalo hump') and abdominal striae. A targeted exam for acromegaly includes assessing for coarsened facial features, frontal bossing, a protruding lower jaw, enlarged hands and feet, goitre, skin tags, bitemporal hemianopia and organomegaly.

7 Cardiovascular complications can occur in T2DM due to CAD and the development of ischaemic cardiomyopathy. Assess for clinical evidence of cardiac failure, including a displaced apex beat due to cardiomegaly, cardiac murmurs due to valvular lesions, crackles on auscultation of lung fields due to pulmonary oedema, and pitting lower limb oedema.

8 Acanthosis nigricans is a cutaneous sign related to insulin resistance, appearing as thickened brown velvety-textured patches of skin, most commonly in the axillae, groin and back of neck. It can also occur as a hereditary or malignant process, the latter of which is associated with GI tumours.

9 T2DM is associated with liver disease, ranging from asymptomatic deranged LFTs to NAFLD, liver cirrhosis, hepatocellular carcinoma and acute liver failure. Given this association, an abdominal examination assessing for hepatomegaly, stigmata of chronic liver disease and signs of decompensation is of value in a diabetes examination.

10 Diabetic neuropathy is a complication of T2DM that can result in variable neurological signs. In a neurological examination focus especially on power, reflexes and sensation, including vibration sensation (with a 128Hz fork)

and proprioception. A distal symmetric polyneuropathy will result in a glove–stocking distribution of sensory loss and reflex loss, with progression leading to motor weakness in advanced stages. The neurological deficits may alternatively be in keeping with a focal mononeuropathy, polyradiculopathy or a mononeuritis multiplex, in which case differential diagnoses for the underlying aetiology should also be considered and excluded.

11 Monofilament testing is used to gauge protective foot sensation and therefore risk of ulceration. A 10g monofilament is used, meaning that the buckling force is 10g when pressure is applied to the patient's skin. It should be tested on the plantar aspect of the first, third and fifth toe metatarsal head, with pressure applied until the filament bends. If it is not sensed by the patient, the site is considered insensate.

12 Peripheral arterial disease is a major macrovascular complication of T2DM and a vascular examination is a necessary part of the diabetes examination. This includes evaluating for pallor, coolness, hair loss and thin skin, timing capillary reperfusion and palpating for pulses in the dorsalis pedis, posterior tibialis and popliteal arteries. Auscultation for bruits to indicate arterial stenosis can be performed over the carotid arteries, the aorta (above the umbilicus) and the renal arteries (above the umbilicus lateral to the midline bilaterally). Bedside ankle brachial index (ABI) can be performed if there is clinical evidence of peripheral vascular disease. The ABI is the ratio of systolic blood pressure in the brachial artery to that in the posterior tibial artery after resting in a supine position, which is considered abnormal when it is below 0.90.

13 A foot assessment in an individual with T2DM involves a neurological and vascular examination, in addition to examining the patient's footwear. In doing so, note the pattern of wear on the soles, check that the sizing is correct, and note defects or materials that could lead to foot injury.

14 Describe and document foot wounds or ulcerations to enable accurate monitoring. Assess for secondary infection over any wounds, and consider the possibility of infection of underlying bone. Fungal infections such as tinea pedis should be treated promptly to avoid progression or superimposed bacterial cellulitis.

15 Fundoscopic examination should be performed for anyone newly diagnosed with T2DM. The pupil should be dilated with mydriatic drops, such as tropicamide or atropine, before the exam. Diabetic retinopathy is classified as non-proliferative or proliferative, the latter of which is characterised by neovascularisation. The earliest sign of diabetic retinopathy is microaneurysms which appear as small, red dots in the superficial retinal layers, occurring due to capillary wall outpouching. With progression, fundoscopy will also reveal dot and blot haemorrhages, flame-shaped haemorrhages, cotton-wool spots, retinal oedema and hard exudates. Increasing retinal ischaemia can lead to venous beading and venous loops, which predicts progression to proliferative diabetic retinopathy.

Investigations

- A random blood glucose level (BGL) tested in the clinic room is **15.5mmol/L** [1] and a urine dipstick demonstrates **glucose ++** [2] and **protein ++** [3] with no leucocytes or nitrites.
- The urine sample is sent for a spot **albumin-to-creatinine ratio** [4], which returns elevated and confirms the presence of microalbuminuria.
- Formal pathology testing is performed to assess his **HbA1c** [5], **lipid profile** [6], **urea, electrolytes, creatinine (UEC)** [7], and **LFT** [8].
- To work up the reported **exertional chest pain** [9], an ECG, chest X-ray and a full blood examination is requested in addition to the aforementioned blood tests. He is also referred for a cardiac stress test, to assess for evidence of reversible ischaemia that would warrant an angiogram.
- Given his distal predominant sensory neuropathy, other causes of **peripheral neuropathy** [10] are considered, and further blood tests are performed followed by nerve conduction studies.
- No **other blood tests** [11] or **imaging** [12] are undertaken.

[1] The diagnostic criteria for diagnosis of T2DM include one of:
- a random plasma glucose ≥11.1mmol/L
- a fasting plasma glucose ≥7.0mmol/L
- 2-hour plasma glucose after 75g oral glucose tolerance test ≥11.1mmol/L
- HbA1c >48mmol/mol (6.5%).

[2] Use of a urine dipstick is a non-invasive bedside test that can be performed to assess for the presence of urinary glucose, ketones, protein, blood, nitrites and leucocytes. Glycosuria occurs when there is hyperglycaemia above the 'renal threshold', as seen in T2DM. Glycosuria can also occur in the absence of diabetes as a result of drugs or rare conditions such as renal glycosuria. Limitations of this test include that it is qualitative only, and its error-prone nature given the impact of urine concentration, timing of the test and timing of interpretation.

[3] Proteinuria on dipstick has multiple potential causes, including recent strenuous exercise, acute illness, pregnancy, infection, congestive cardiac failure and proteinuric kidney disease. Persistent proteinuria confirmed on two or more consecutive positive dipsticks over 2 weeks warrants further quantification with a urine albumin–creatinine ratio (ACR) or protein–creatinine ratio. ACR has higher sensitivity than protein–creatinine ratio for low concentrations of protein, and albumin is the main protein excreted in most proteinuric renal disease.

[4] Screening for microalbuminuria should be performed yearly in T2DM, as it is a risk factor for macrovascular disease and for further renal impairment. The ACR or protein–creatinine ratio in a spot urine sample estimates albumin or protein excretion, respectively, in milligrams daily. Spot urine samples should be collected in the early morning as the sample will be more concentrated. More accurate quantification can be performed with a timed urine specimen collection, but a spot urine sample generally suffices. Microalbuminuria is defined differently depending on gender, with the range for men being 2.5–25mg/mmol, and for women 3.5–35mg/mmol. Macroalbuminuria is defined as >25mg/mmol in men and >35 mg/mmol in women.

[5] HbA1c testing provides an average of glycaemic control over the 3 months preceding testing. An HbA1c between 5.7 and 6.4% (39–46mmol/mol) is indicative of an increased risk of developing T2DM, and is termed impaired glucose tolerance. An HbA1c above 6.5% is considered diagnostic for T2DM. It is important to consider if there are any factors that may lead to a false reading, including haemolysis or conditions of increased cell turnover (falsely low HbA1c) or conditions of decreased cell turnover (falsely elevated HbA1c).

[6] Lipid abnormalities are common in T2DM, in particular high total cholesterol, triglycerides and LDL cholesterol, and low HDL cholesterol.

[7] Assessment of renal function is relevant in T2DM to detect the presence of renal impairment secondary to diabetic nephropathy, and enable renal dose adjustment of drugs used in diabetic management.

[8] T2DM is associated with the development of non-alcoholic fatty liver disease, with the underlying pathological process being insulin resistance. Identifying LFT derangement enables further investigation and treatment of contributing factors, and initiation of routine monitoring for the development of cirrhosis.

[9] Chest pain in an individual with T2DM warrants early investigation, given the associated elevated cardiovascular risk. This can be worked up with an ECG looking for any ischaemic changes, a chest X-ray to assess for features of cardiac failure, and subsequent to these first-line investigations, a cardiac stress test and consideration of revascularisation procedures.

[10] Diabetes is the most common cause of peripheral neuropathy, but alternative contributing factors must be identified and treated if possible, including nutritional deficiencies, toxins, drugs, alcohol, hypothyroidism, infections, vasculitic processes, infiltrative diseases, hereditary disorders, paraproteinaemia-related neuropathies, paraneoplastic conditions and demyelination. Screening tests, based on

history and exam findings, may include a vitamin B12 level, thyroid function tests, erythrocyte sedimentation rate, vasculitic screen and a serum protein electrophoresis. Nerve conduction studies may identify a pattern that is more indicative of a particular aetiology.

11 Measurement of BGLs and an HbA1c are usually adequate for the diagnosis of T2DM, but occasionally antibody testing is performed if there is question about the diagnosis and the presence of an underlying autoimmune process. Atypical phenotypic characteristics may lead a clinician to consider antibody testing; antibody-positive diabetes is associated with lower BMI, better blood pressure control and better lipid status compared to those without antibodies. Latent autoimmune diabetes of adults (LADA) is a slow-onset T1DM that is seen in middle-aged adults. It can be misdiagnosed as T2DM, and differentiated by testing for antibodies against the 65-kd isoform of glutamic acid decarboxylase (GAD65). This is an enzyme in pancreatic beta cells, which is elevated in T1DM but not T2DM. These patients may respond to insulin secretagogues for a brief period but will require early transition to insulin therapy. Diagnostic clarification allows early treatment with the most appropriate therapy and therefore can delay disease progression.

12 There is no routine imaging required in the diagnosis or management of T2DM, unless complications develop that require further evaluation. For example, clinical or biochemical evidence of fatty liver disease may be worked up further with an abdominal ultrasound or Fibroscan. Peripheral vascular disease can be evaluated with a lower limb Doppler ultrasound, with CT arteriography as the next step if ultrasound imaging was inadequate or if planning for a revascularisation procedure. For diabetic retinopathy, fluorescein angiography can be used to evaluate retinal blood flow and optical coherence tomography scanning to measure retinal thickness.

Management

- The goals of diabetes management include tightening of glycaemic control according to an **individualised HbA1c target** [1] and **cardiovascular risk factor modification** [2].
- The patient is enrolled in several **education sessions** [3] with a dietitian and a diabetes nurse educator (DNE), and counselled on the benefits of weight loss through **increasing physical activity** [4] and **diet modification** [5].
- He is linked in with the **National Diabetes Services Scheme** [6] to provide access to support services and subsidised products for **self-monitoring of blood glucose** (SMBG) [7].
- Given his markedly **elevated HbA1c** [8], he is commenced on **metformin** [9] therapy, with a plan to reassess his HbA1c in **three months** [10].
- His usual antihypertensive drug amlodipine is ceased and he is commenced on an **ACE inhibitor** [11] for management of his hypertension and for the additional benefit of addressing proteinuria.
- He is referred to a **podiatrist** [12] and an **optometrist** [13] to commence a regular schedule of screening of diabetic complications.
- He continues to be monitored by the clinic and considered for **referral to specialists** [14] where required.
- His family members are made aware of the diagnosis and educated on risk factors and the need to consider **screening** [15] now that they have an affected first-degree relative.

1 In both type 1 and type 2 diabetes mellitus, achieving adequate glycaemic control is a priority as it reduces the risk of development and progression of diabetic complications. One measure of this is an HbA1c level of ≤7%, which is recommended for most patients based on large trials such as the Diabetes Control and Complications Trial (DCCT) and United Kingdom Prospective Diabetes Study (UKPDS), and reflected in national guidelines. The target HbA1c should be individualised depending on age, comorbidities, existing therapies and pregnancy. The HbA1c target in pregnancy or when planning pregnancy is ≤6.0% due to the adverse pregnancy outcomes associated with an HbA1c above this in pregnancy. A higher HbA1c target of ≤ 8.0% may be more appropriate in individuals with recurrent severe hypoglycaemia or hypoglycaemic awareness, where tight glycaemic control may outweigh the benefits. Symptomatic therapy only, with no specific HbA1c target, may be the goal when individuals with major comorbidities have a limited life expectancy.

2 Cardiovascular risk factor management includes addressing weight control, hypertension and hypercholesterolaemia, and considering the role of antiplatelet therapy.

3 The management of T2DM should involve an MDT including a dietitian and DNE to provide individualised instructions on nutrition, physical activity, metabolic control, BGL monitoring and management, and complication prevention. Structured education should be provided to individuals diagnosed with T2DM and their carers where relevant, providing information and advice in a culturally sensitive manner that considers preferences and lifestyle.

4 Lifestyle modification is the first line of management for T2DM, with the goal of weight loss and improving glycaemia. This includes improving physical activity, dietary modification and cessation of smoking or alcohol consumption. Adults with diabetes are encouraged to perform at least 30–60 minutes of moderate-intensity aerobic activity most days a week, achieving at least 150 minutes per week over at least three days. Regular exercise in T2DM reduces insulin resistance and improves glycaemic control.

5 Medical nutrition therapy is the process by which nutritional therapy and counselling is provided to people with diabetes, to provide a nutritional prescription suited to lifestyle, personal factors and medical issues. It takes into consideration weight management, nutritional content, timing and consistency of carbohydrate intake, and physical activity. Dietary modification to achieve negative caloric balance can aid weight loss and improve glycaemic control and hypertension. Recommended dietary composition will vary between individuals, with potential approaches including a low carbohydrate diet, a low fat diet, or a pattern such as the Mediterranean diet, which has been demonstrated to reduce the incidence of diabetes independent of weight loss.

6 Diabetes UK is a charity that assists individuals with diabetes understand and manage their diabetes, and access services, support and subsidised diabetes products. Similar health schemes to support individuals living with diabetes may be available in other countries.

7 All individuals with T2DM should engage in SMBG, and the frequency and timing should be individualised. Generally, the BGL targets are 6–8mmol/L fasting and preprandial, and 6–10mmol/L two hours postprandial.

8 People with newly diagnosed T2DM can be offered a trial of lifestyle modification, but with markedly elevated BGLs or HbA1c, pharmacotherapy may be necessary upfront.

9 Metformin therapy is the preferred initial agent for the pharmacologic management of T2DM as long as there are no contraindications. Metformin is a biguanide, which acts to decrease hepatic gluconeogenesis, decrease intestinal absorption of glucose, and improve insulin sensitivity by increasing peripheral glucose uptake and utilisation. It rarely causes hypoglycaemia and facilitates modest weight loss. Adverse effects include GI symptoms and risk of lactic acidosis. It should be avoided in individuals who are acutely unwell, used in caution in people with an eGFR of 30–45ml/min/1.73m^2, and is contraindicated with an eGFR <30ml/min/1.73m^2.

10 An individual's HbA1c level should be checked at 3–6-monthly intervals until the HbA1c is stable on a particular therapy, then checked at 6-monthly intervals. If glycaemia is not improved within 3 months, a second agent can be commenced in addition to the first, as guided by patient characteristics including age and comorbidities. Other groups of oral hypoglycaemic agents include sulphonylureas (insulin secretagogues), dipeptidyl peptidase IV (DPP-4) inhibitors (prolong incretin hormone action), sodium glucose transporter 2 (SGLT-2) inhibitors (increase urinary glucose excretion), thiazolidinediones (insulin sensitisers) and glucagon-like peptide-1 (GLP-1) agonists (stimulate glucose-dependent insulin release), the last of which is also available as an injectable agent. If initial combination therapy does not achieve target HbA1c, more intensive therapy may be required with further agents including insulin. National and local guidelines should be consulted to inform the choice of agents for escalation of therapy, and thresholds to do so.

11 ACE inhibitors have been shown to have a reno-protective effect in people with microalbuminuria, independent of the blood pressure lowering effect. Commencement of an ACEi in this patient would aid in treating hypertension, and also help to prevent or delay progression from microalbuminuria to overt nephropathy.

12 Foot care is important in T2DM given the risk of ulceration, infection and amputations, especially if there is established diabetic neuropathy. Educate patients on the importance of daily self-checks and regular foot care; referral to a podiatrist should be made for annual review at a minimum. A painful neuropathy can be treated with amitriptyline, venlafaxine, duloxetine or pregabalin. These options are preferred, while opioid use is not recommended.

13 All individuals with T2DM should have an eye assessment at diagnosis, and then regularly at least every two years, to screen for changes of diabetic retinopathy. Routine screening is crucial as it can progress quickly and there are available therapies to delay deterioration and improve symptoms. Pharmacologic therapy includes intravitreal triamcinolone or bevacizumab, and with progression laser photocoagulation is used for areas of non-proliferative diabetic retinopathy, while pan-retinal photocoagulation (sparing the macula) is used for proliferative diabetic retinopathy.

14 Involvement of specialty units may be indicated when complications develop, with commonly involved specialties including Endocrinology, Nephrology (for advancing diabetic nephropathy), Cardiology (for management of ischaemic heart disease), Infectious Diseases (for advice on recurrent infections) and Vascular Surgery (when peripheral vascular disease requires revascularisation or non-healing ulcers require amputation). With progressive obesity and rising insulin requirements, suitable patients may be referred for consideration of bariatric surgery, which can result in significant weight loss and remission of diabetes.

15 In addition to treating T2DM in affected individuals, it is important to identify individuals at risk who may benefit from preventive measures. Individuals at risk include those with a sedentary lifestyle, HTN, hypercholesterolaemia, cardiovascular disease, polycystic ovarian syndrome, obesity, a high risk ethnicity, or a family history of diabetes mellitus in a first-degree relative.

CASE 21: Acute pancreatitis

History

- A **41-year-old female** [1] presents to the ED with a 6-hour history of **immense abdominal pain that has progressively worsened** [2].
- The pain is localised **above the umbilicus with radiation to the back** [3].
- She also complains of **multiple episodes of nausea, vomiting, sweating** [4] **and dyspnoea** [5].
- She denies **haematemesis** [6], reflux or **recent changes in bowel habits** [7].
- **No recent loss of weight** [8] is noted.

- Prior to her presentation, **she consumed multiple glasses of wine** [9] at a party.
- The other **partygoers are well** [10] and not complaining of any symptoms.
- Her medical history is positive for **cholelithiasis** [11], but she is otherwise well.
- She is **not sexually active, and her last menstrual period was 5 days ago** [12].
- She has **no obstetric or gynaecological history and her last Pap smear was negative** [13].

[1] The risk of acute pancreatitis progressively increases with age. Cases under 20 years of age are uncommon. There is equal gender distribution, with gallstones and alcohol the main contributors to acute pancreatitis. The third most common cause is idiopathic. There is also a risk of iatrogenic pancreatitis post endoscopic retrograde cholangiopancreatography (ERCP). Metabolic disorders such as hypercalcaemia and hypertriglyceridaemia have also been implicated.

[2] The pathophysiology of acute pancreatitis depends on its aetiology. In biliary obstruction such as gallstones or cancer, outflow obstruction causes the accumulation of bile salts and disrupts pancreatic ductal activity. Alcohol triggers increased pancreatic enzyme activity and can disrupt pancreatic cell membranes. In both cases, the build-up of pancreatic enzymes leads to autodigestion and cell death. This process is exacerbated by activation of the inflammatory cascade with the translocation of neutrophils into the pancreatic tissue. Proteolysis and interstitial oedema occur, resulting in the characteristic severe abdominal pain.

[3] Visceral pain is poorly localised and refers to the corresponding embryonic origin. In acute pancreatitis, this is felt in the upper abdominal regions as the pancreas is derived from the foregut region. Furthermore, as the pancreas is considered a secondary retroperitoneal organ, any inflammation within that compartment can cause pain to be felt in the back.

[4] In acute pancreatitis, the underlying mechanisms involved in these non-specific symptoms are complex and encompass psychological states, the central nervous and autonomic nervous system, gastric dysrhythmias and the endocrine system.

[5] In cases of severe acute pancreatitis, the pancreatic inflammatory process may extend and affect multiple organs, resulting in a condition known as severe inflammatory response syndrome (SIRS). SIRS is characterised by two or more of the following criteria:
- Hypo-/hyperthermia
- Tachycardia (heart rate >100/min)
- Tachypnoea (>20 breaths/min)
- White blood cell count <4 x 10^9/L, >12 x 10^9/L or at least 10% bands.

Dyspnoea is an early indicator of SIRS and may be related to the increased metabolic stress from inflammation and cellular hypoperfusion resulting in anaerobic metabolism.

[6] Haematemesis is not a common symptom of acute pancreatitis, although patients experiencing severe vomiting or dry retching are at risk of Mallory–Weiss tears in the oesophageal mucosa. In most cases, haematemesis indicates non-pancreatic pathology such as gastritis, peptic ulcer disease or vascular malformations such as varices.

[7] Changes in bowel habit with abdominal pain often lead clinicians to consider non-pancreatic diseases such as bowel obstruction, inflammatory bowel disease, coeliac disease or GI infections.

[8] Patients with unplanned loss of weight in the preceding months must always be evaluated for malignancy. Head of pancreas tumour must be ruled out, as in patients with concurrent weight loss and pancreatitis.

[9] Alcohol is one of the leading causes of pancreatitis, with the risk of disease increasing as more alcohol is consumed. The pathophysiology remains uncertain; however, the two main by-products of ethanol metabolism, fatty acid ethyl ester (FAEE) and acetaldehyde, have been shown to

predispose the pancreas to acute pancreatitis. Pancreatic acinar cells, the main cells responsible for digestive enzyme production, are dependent on calcium-mediated pathways to function and secrete their zymogens. FAEE causes a sustained increase in intracellular calcium within these acinar cells, leading to inappropriate activation.

10 Infectious causes of abdominal pain, such as gastroenteritis, have similar symptoms. Always enquire about recent travel history, vaccination status, consumption of foods and beverages and whether contact with other sick individuals has occurred.

11 One of the main causes of acute pancreatitis is gallstones which can get lodged and stuck in the ampulla of Vater (also known as the hepatopancreatic ampulla). This tract is formed by the union of the pancreatic duct and the common bile duct. Obstruction can cause impaired pancreatic drainage, leading to pancreatitis and autodigestion.

12 Pregnancy and ectopic must be ruled out in all females of childbearing age that present with sudden onset abdominal pain.

13 A variety of gynaecological conditions, including endometriosis, ruptured ovarian cysts, pelvic inflammatory disease, uterine fibroids, ovarian torsion and gynaecological cancers, can present with severe abdominal pain and mimic pancreatitis.

Examination

- The patient is **overweight** [1] and **lying on her side on the bed with her legs flexed in the foetal position** [2].
- General examination reveals she **is distressed and tachypnoeic (RR 24/min)** [3].
- Other vital signs include a **regular heart rate (HR) of 120bpm, BP: 115/80mmHg, SpO$_2$: 99% and temperature of 38.1°C** [4].
- Peripheral examination is unremarkable with no **hepatic flap** [5].

- Facial examination reveals no abnormalities such as conjunctival pallor or central cyanosis.
- The patient's **abdomen is distended and significantly tender** [6].
- Organs are unable to be palpated due to **guarding; however, there is no rigidity** [7].
- **Reduced bowel sounds** [8] are noted.
- No **peristalsis, pulsations or ecchymosis** [9] is noted on the patient's flanks or abdomen. A digital rectal exam was not performed.

1 Excess fat can accumulate in intra-abdominal areas and surround viscera. In acute pancreatitis, inflammation can also affect peri-pancreatic adipose tissue. Compounding this finding, numerous studies have shown that excess adipose tissue generates more pro-inflammatory cytokines, such as leptin and less anti-inflammatory adiponectin. The net result is an inflammatory milieu which can exacerbate pancreatitis. Obesity also increases numerous risk factors which can precipitate pancreatitis, including gallstones and hypertriglyceridaemia.

2 The foetal position helps relieve abdominal pain by physiologically relaxing abdominal muscles. Psychologically it is an instinctive reaction to immense stress, pain or trauma.

3 During episodes of pain, the sympathetic nervous system becomes highly activated. This can influence breath flow, frequency and volume of breaths. Tachypnoea in acute pancreatitis is also an early indicator of multi-organ failure. It is a compensatory mechanism for hypoxia due to ventilation perfusion mismatch associated with circulatory shock. Acute pancreatitis is also associated with a number of respiratory complications such as pleural effusion (transdiaphragmatic lymphatic blockage or pancreaticopleural fistulae secondary to leak and disruption of the pancreatic duct or pseudocyst caused by an episode of acute pancreatitis), atelectasis (diaphragmatic impairment from inflammation) and acute respiratory distress syndrome, ARDS (considered a poor prognostic sign). ARDS is diagnosed when there is:
- acute onset <1 week
- respiratory failure not secondary to heart failure or volume overload
- widespread bilateral radiographic infiltrates
- decreased PaO$_2$/FiO$_2$ ratio.

The pathophysiology of pancreatitis-induced ARDS is not well known but could be due to a combination of inflammatory mediators, increased leucocyte activation and agglutination, neutrophil migration and complement-mediated injury.

4 Increased frequency of observations is necessary to monitor for SIRS which is characterised by hypo-/hyperthermia, tachycardia, tachypnoea and elevated leucocyte count. SIRS can also increase the risk of concurrent infection. It is a component of numerous pancreatitis severity scores to guide management.

5 Asterixis is a sign of hepatic or metabolic encephalopathy. It is never seen in pancreatitis and its presence may indicate a non-pancreatic cause of abdominal pain such as acute hepatitis and hepatic failure.

6 Abdominal distension and tenderness are common signs in pancreatitis. In acute pancreatitis, inappropriate activation of pancreatic enzymes produces severe abdominal pain. Neuronal tissue in the pancreas becomes inflamed, causing visceral pain. As the inflammation extends and irritates the peritoneum, this causes somatic pain. Pressing down on inflamed tissues during examination can further exacerbate this pain.

[7] Abdominal guarding is a characteristic finding of an acute abdomen. Abdominal tensing reduces the amount of pressure placed upon inflamed organs. Rigidity indicates peritonitis, which is a known complication of acute pancreatitis.

[8] Reduced or tinkling bowel sounds can indicate ischaemic bowel or a bowel obstruction which are important differentials to consider in patients presenting with severe abdominal pain.

[9] The classic flank discolouration (Grey Turner sign) or umbilical bruising (Cullen sign) is rarely seen unless retroperitoneal haemorrhage with tracking along tissue planes occurs. The presence of these signs may indicate multi-organ failure.

Investigations

Pathology

- After a thorough **history and examination, further investigations were ordered** [1].
- FBE revealed **elevated white blood count** [2].
- **LFTs** [3] were normal, although **serum lipase** [4] and **C-reactive protein** [5] were elevated.
- Retrospective **cholesterol and triglycerides and CMP** [6] were also ordered, which were normal.
- **Beta-hCG** [7] was also negative.

Imaging

- **CT abdominal scan** [8] demonstrated **obscure pancreatic margins with diffuse parenchymal enlargement, pockets of hypodense regions, retroperitoneal fat stranding** [9].
- A CT severity index **(CTSI) score** [10] of 4 was given.

[1] Acute pancreatitis is diagnosed when clinical features such as abdominal pain and vomiting correlate with elevations of pancreatic enzymes. In cases where clinical and biochemical markers are inconclusive, imaging may be used to confirm diagnosis. These investigations can also determine pancreatitis severity, guide therapy and identify precipitants. The Ranson criteria or Glasgow score can assist in determining the severity of pancreatitis and whether ICU admission is warranted. Scoring systems such as the APACHE-II are also used to predict prognosis.

[2] In acute pancreatitis, the release of inflammatory signals from acinar cells mediates the recruitment and activation of circulating inflammatory cells such as neutrophils. Elevated white blood counts are also correlated with poorer outcomes.

[3] In biliary pancreatitis, ALP, GGT and direct bilirubin are generally higher. However, normal LFTs should not preclude acute pancreatitis as these enzymes may not be elevated in autoimmune or idiopathic pancreatitis.

[4] Lipase is a catalyst produced by the pancreas that hydrolyses fat and aids in its absorption into the body. When pancreatic cells are injured, lipase levels increase in the blood. Acute pancreatitis should be considered when lipase concentrations are 2–3 times the upper limit of normal. Note that the magnitude of elevation does not predict disease severity. Lipase is the preferred biochemical test over amylase

due to its improved sensitivity and longer diagnostic window, as it can remain elevated for up to 2 weeks. Other conditions that can cause elevated lipase include cholecystitis, pancreatic cancer, intestinal ischaemia and renal failure.

[5] CRP is a non-specific marker of acute inflammation; a rise >90 from admission or absolute value of >190 at 48 hours of disease onset is the best single predictor of pancreatitis severity.

[6] Identifying the main triggers for acute pancreatitis can help prevent recurrence. Metabolic disorders such as hypertriglyceridaemia and hypercalcaemia increase the risk of pancreatitis. In patients with a history of pancreatic cancer, CA 19-9 should also be considered in acute pancreatitis as it is a surrogate marker for malignancy relapse.

[7] A negative beta-hCG indicates that ectopic pregnancy is unlikely to be the main cause of the patient's pain.

[8] The role of abdominal CT scans in acute pancreatitis is to confirm diagnosis, assess severity, determine possible causes and identify possible complications such as ischaemic and necrotic areas of the pancreas. However, CT scans done <12 hours of symptom onset may demonstrate normal findings. MRI is a good alternative to CT as it offers superior characterisation of pancreatic and peripancreatic collections and necrotised debris. However, costs and availability prevent

its widespread use. Abdominal ultrasound is rarely used as it poorly visualises the pancreas due to its retroperitoneal location.

9 As the pancreas becomes inflamed, the organ enlarges due to an influx of immune cells. Peripancreatic inflammation can also occur, causing hazy or reticular stranding of the surrounding fat. Hypodense regions may indicate multiple fluid collections due to a build-up of oedema.

10 The Balthazar CT severity index (CTSI) is used to stratify the severity of acute pancreatitis and predict mortality. Scores of 0–3, 4–6 and 7–10 indicate mild, moderate and severe acute pancreatitis, respectively.

Findings	Points
Normal	0
Pancreatic enlargement	1
Peripancreatic inflammation	2
Single acute peripancreatic fluid collection	3
>2 acute peripancreatic fluid collections	4

Pancreatic necrosis	
None	0
<30%	2
30–50%	4
>50%	6

Severity is an important indicator of mortality and facilitates management decisions about the need for ICU admission and nutritional support. The Atlanta classification is commonly used:

- Mild acute
  - no organ failure or local or systemic complications
- Moderate acute
  - transient organ failure of <48 hours
  - local complications (peripancreatic fluid collection, pancreatic necrosis) or systemic complications (exacerbation of pre-existing disease)
- Severe acute
  - persistent organ failure of >48 hours
  - high mortality rate of 20–30%.

Management

Immediate

The patient was made **nil by mouth** [1]. Intravenous access was gained and **fluid replacement therapy** [2] initiated. **Fentanyl** [3] was also prescribed. If SIRS was suspected, **supplemental oxygen** [4] would be necessary and **ICU admission** [5] warranted. **Prophylactic antibiotics** [6] were not recommended.

Short-term

As the patient was under bowel rest, a **dietetics** [7] referral was made to determine whether parenteral nutrition was needed. Because CT scans identified the presence of gallstones in gall bladder and pancreatic duct, an **ERCP** [8] was performed. Once the patient was stable, a **cholecystectomy** [9] was also recommended. If **pancreatic necrosis** [10] is suspected, surgical drainage may be necessary.

Long-term

It is important to monitor for **complications** [11] of acute pancreatitis. Identifying the **causative factor** [12] will also prevent future relapses.

1 During digestion, the pancreas is stimulated to secrete enzymes. Therefore, to prevent the exacerbation of pancreatitis, strict bowel rest is required. Most patients will eventually recover from mild pancreatitis.

2 Fluid resuscitation is the cornerstone therapy in acute pancreatitis. The rationale behind fluid replacement stems from the need to resolve hypovolaemia that occurs from reduced oral intake, vomiting and extravasation of fluid from the intravascular space as capillaries become leaky from pro-inflammatory mediators. Ensuring adequate intravascular volume prevents severe acute pancreatitis and necrosis. The ideal choice of fluids is yet to be determined. Crystalloids such as normal saline and Ringer's lactate are distributed in both the plasma and the interstitial compartments, and large volumes are therefore required for circulatory restoration. This can lead to pulmonary oedema. Colloids such as hydroxyethyl starch or gelatins are theoretically superior to crystalloids as they are retained in the intravascular space due to their larger molecular size, resulting in better haemodynamic support. They also assist in osmosis of fluid from interstitium to the vascular compartment. However, colloids can cause intravascular volume overload, hyperoncotic renal impairment, coagulopathy and anaphylactic reaction. Protocols differ between hospitals, although crystalloids are more commonly used due to their lower costs.

Rates of fluid resuscitation is another controversial topic, with multiple studies demonstrating that aggressive hydration can increase morbidity and mortality even though the intravascular compartment is restored more quickly, leading to more effective end-organ tissue perfusion and reversing pancreatic ischaemia. Those in favour of non-aggressive hydration suggest that pancreatic necrosis is already non-reversible by the time diagnosis has been made and intervention begun, and aggressive fluid therapy will only lead to respiratory failure and increased intra-abdominal pressure. Bolus doses with vasopressor support have also been investigated, with recommendations mimicking those for septic shock.

3 Pain management is complex and critical to preventing shock in patients with acute pancreatitis. Therapies range from simple analgesia in very mild cases to the potent opioids and surgery in severe cases. Previously, opioids were rarely used as they were thought to cause the sphincter of Oddi to spasm, leading to increased pancreatic enzyme and bile activity and movement. However, this has since been dispelled and opioids are routinely prescribed. Intravenous morphine provides good analgesia, although this should be avoided in patients with renal impairment as it is renally excreted. Poor glomerular filtration can cause the accumulation of toxic metabolites, leading to CNS depression. Instead fentanyl is a viable short-term alternative as it is broken down by the liver and its metabolites are inactive. However, like morphine, high doses can also lead to central nervous system (CNS) depression. Therefore, pain management must be carefully monitored, and dosages titrated according to the patient's physiological status.

4 In SIRS, supplemental oxygen should be provided to maintain arterial oxygen saturation. This can be provided via a nasal cannula or Hudson mask, depending on the optimal flow rate. In certain situations, ventilator support may be necessary. Failure to maintain or increase oxygenation is correlated with a poorer prognosis in acute pancreatitis.

5 In severe acute pancreatitis, patients are at risk of developing SIRs. A large proportion of patients require continuous care and therefore ICU admission is necessary. These departments can provide special equipment and therapeutic interventions such as mechanical ventilation, renal replacement therapy and invasive monitoring.

6 Opinion on the use of prophylactic antibiotics remains divided, as it has not been shown to reduce mortality. Therefore, it is not routinely recommended in mild or moderate pancreatitis. However, patients with severe acute pancreatitis are at risk of developing other infections such as urinary tract infections and hospital-acquired pneumonia. In these cases, antibiotic use is recommended. The choice of antibiotics depends on individual hospital protocol although broad-spectrum cover is prescribed initially, pending cultures and sensitivity. If no source of infection is found, or investigations are negative, antibiotics should be ceased. If patients develop pancreatic necrosis and consequently sepsis, antibiotics in conjunction with drainage and surgical debridement are necessary.

7 Patients with mild–moderate pancreatitis do not require nutritional support. Oral feeding can be restarted approximately a week after their admission, as early feeding can result in pain or reactivation of pancreatitis. Around 20%

of patients relapse when refeeding begins. Diet should be reintroduced slowly and gradually, beginning with clear fluids for the first 24 hours. If tolerated, this can transition to soft, low fat diets and eventually a regular diet. Enzyme supplements are also recommended due to pancreatic exocrine insufficiency which occurs as a result of pancreatitis. This eventually resolves as the pancreas recovers. For patients with severe acute pancreatitis, nutritional support is recommended. Route of administration is clinician dependent, although enteral feeding is cheaper, more physiological and has fewer adverse effects relative to parenteral delivery. A combination may be recommended if caloric requirements cannot be met through a single approach. Nutritional supplements can be delivered via nasojejunal tubes or intravenously.

8 ERCP should be performed within 72 hours of presentation if abdominal CT suggests gallstones are the main cause of pancreatitis. Gastroenterologists may also decide to perform a biliary endoscopic sphincterotomy which ligates the sphincter muscle of the common bile duct using a specialised knife. This enlarges the opening of the bile duct, allowing gallstones to be removed from the duct into the bowel. This procedure also assists with pancreatic enzyme drainage that may have been blocked by the gallstone. In some cases of chronic pancreatitis, stents may be placed if strictures or narrowed parts of the duct are noted.

9 Prior to discharge, all patients with gallstone-induced pancreatitis should undergo cholecystectomy to prevent a relapse.

10 Pancreatic infection is the major risk factor in necrotising pancreatitis. Abdominal CT may reveal retroperitoneal gas locules or circumscribed fluid attenuations. Radiological guided or surgical drainage of the infected sites will prevent sepsis and guide antibiotic therapy. Open necrosectomy may be performed to debride infected or ischaemic areas. Minimally invasive techniques have also been developed. Further studies are necessary to evaluate the efficacy of different techniques.

11 The most common complication of acute pancreatitis is an abscess, especially after surgical intervention. Percutaneous drainage is widely applied. Accumulation of pancreatic secretions due to damaged pancreatic ducts may also form pseudocysts (also known as pancreatic ascites). These are monitored and managed conservatively, especially if they are not growing. Pancreatic haemorrhage is a life-threatening complication of pancreatitis. This is a result of weakened arterial walls that encounter proteolytic enzymes. Angiography and embolisation is the gold standard diagnostic and therapeutic technique.

12 Apart from cholecystectomy in biliary pancreatitis, patients should be educated to reduce smoking and consumption of alcohol, limit fatty food consumption, exercise regularly but not reduce weight drastically. There should be regular health check-ups to monitor electrolyte and mineral levels.

CASE 22: Cholelithiasis, choledocholithiasis and cholecystitis

History

- A **45-year-old obese Caucasian female** [1] presents to her family practitioner complaining of a **dull pain in the right upper abdomen** [2], which occasionally radiates up her right shoulder.
- She describes this pain as **episodic and occurring after large fatty meals** [3].
- The pain remains unrelieved with **antacids or positional changes** [4] but eventually subsides within 30 minutes of onset.

- She also experiences **nausea, dyspepsia and bloating** [5].
- However, she denies vomiting, **recent loss of weight** [6], changes in bowel habit or uncontrollable **fever and shaking** [7].
- Her past medical history is significant for **dyslipidaemia** [8], hypertension and **type 2 diabetes mellitus** [9].
- She does not eat **healthily** [10] and lives a **sedentary life with minimal exercise** [10].

[1] The majority of gallstones are formed in the gall bladder when there is:
- biliary supersaturation with cholesterol
- accelerated transition from liquid bile to solid form, and
- gall bladder hypomotility retaining this abnormal bile.

Multiple risk factors contribute to this process. Obesity is an important risk factor for cholesterol gallstones as it increases the activity of beta-hydroxy-beta-methylglutaryl (HMG) coenzyme A, leading to increased biliary cholesterol. Pregnancy and being female also increases the risk of gallstones, as oestrogen increases the hepatic secretion of biliary cholesterol, which, in turn, leads to an increase in cholesterol saturation of bile. Chronic haemolysis can also contribute to gallstone formation. Genetic studies also demonstrate that the prevalence of cholelithiasis varies widely, from <5% in Asian and African populations to 30% in the European and Northern American population. A classic mnemonic to remember the risk factors for cholelithiasis are fat (BMI >30), forty (age ≥40), female, fertile (current pregnancy) and fair.

[2] Most patients with cholelithiasis are asymptomatic. Symptoms tend to arise when gallstones impact within the cystic duct, causing ductal spasming and increased motility and stretching of the gall bladder. The presence of gallstones within the common bile duct is known as choledocholithiasis. Since visceral pain is poorly localised, symptomatic gallstones are felt along the overlapping somatic afferent nerve. In this case, pain is felt in the right upper abdominal quadrant with the occasional radiation to the shoulder blade (known as Boas' sign). Pain that radiates to the arm warrants investigation for possible cardiac disease, especially in patients at high risk of acute coronary syndrome.

[3] The gall bladder plays a critical role in digestion and promoting absorption of lipids. It stores and concentrates bile produced by the liver. When the body detects fatty meals, the duodenum releases cholecystokinin which promotes gall bladder contraction of bile into the small intestine to assist with fat digestion. Bile is rich in bile salts and micelles which allow emulsification and hydrolysis of triglycerides in gastric contents, allowing intestinal absorption and eventually re-esterification and incorporation as cholesterol for later use. Gall bladder contraction, however, can also expel stones from the gall bladder into the cystic or common bile duct. Small stones may pass by themselves; however, large stones may obstruct these ducts, causing spasm, irritation and severe pain. Bile stasis is predisposed to bacterial infection, leading to cholecystitis which is a medical and surgical emergency.

[4] Epigastric pain relieved with antacids or sitting upright suggests gastro-oesophageal reflux disease (GORD) or peptic ulcer disease.

[5] These are common symptoms associated with biliary colic. Fatty meals require a longer time for digestion, which is exacerbated by impaired gall bladder function.

[6] All patients who report unplanned loss of weight must be investigated for a malignancy. In the case of epigastric or right upper quadrant (RUQ) pain, gastric, gall bladder and hepatic carcinomas must be ruled out.

[7] The presence of fever with RUQ pain may suggest cholecystitis. 90% of acute cholecystitis episodes are caused by gallstones which block the cystic duct. Blockage of bile leads to thickening and an enlarged tense gall bladder. If left untreated, the gall bladder can become extremely distended

and inflamed. If bile becomes infected, then an empyema may form and lead to sepsis. Chronic inflammatory changes can also lead to adhesions forming between the gall bladder and the duodenum. This can lead to fistulas. Rarely, the gall bladder can become gangrenous, increasing the risk of rupture and peritonitis. Surgical removal of the gall bladder is the recommended therapeutic option in combination with antibiotics.

8 Most gallstones are composed of cholesterol with black pigment stones and brown stones making up the minority. Black pigment stones (calcium bilirubinate) are associated with haemolytic diseases such as thalassaemia. Brown pigment stones tend to occur with recurrent biliary tree

infections. Metabolic abnormalities such as dyslipidaemia are associated with gallstone disease.

9 There is a strong association between insulin resistance and gallstone formation. Gall bladder motility is reduced in patients with T2DM although the molecular mechanism is unknown.

10 A western diet, high in fat, refined carbohydrates and low in fibre, is a potent risk factor for cholelithiasis. Furthermore, the metabolic syndrome, a cluster of conditions such as hypertension, obesity, reduced insulin sensitivity and elevated cholesterol, is strongly associated with gallstone disease.

Examination

- On examination, the patient's **vital signs are stable and she is afebrile** [1].
- She is **overweight** [2] with stretch marks over her abdomen.
- She appears calm and alert with nil respiratory distress. There is no marked cachexia or **visible jaundice** [3].
- Peripheral examination is unremarkable. Cardiac and **respiratory exams** [4] are also insignificant.

- **No masses, pulsations or peristalsis are visible** [5].
- There is some mild tenderness on deep palpation in the RUQ of her abdomen, especially when she is asked to **breathe in** [6].
- There is no **iliac fossa tenderness** [7].
- No **organomegaly** [8] is noted.
- Rebound tenderness is not apparent and **bowel sounds** [9] are present and normal.

1 Patients with simple cholelithiasis or choledocholithiasis will not have abnormal vitals. In contrast, cholecystitis or cholangitis may demonstrate fevers and tachycardia or in extreme cases, tachypnoea and hypotension if sepsis occurs.

2 Obesity is associated with gallstone disease and its pathogenesis involves increased hepatic *de novo* cholesterol synthesis and hepatobiliary cholesterol efflux. Obesity also causes gall bladder hypomotility and bile stasis, which promotes gallstone formation.

3 Obstruction of the bile duct by a gallstone can prevent the excretion of bilirubin into the bowels, causing accumulation of conjugated bilirubin and therefore jaundice. Elevated levels of bilirubin are excreted renally, resulting in darker urine. Patients may also pass clay-coloured stools due to the absence of stercobilin in faeces, a breakdown product of bilirubin in the intestine.

4 RUQ pain can also be caused by irritation of the pleural layer in the right lower lung zone. This can be caused by pleurisy, pleural effusions and pneumonia. Patients should be screened for respiratory illnesses to prevent misdiagnosis.

5 Check for the presence of hernias, tumours or aneurysms, which can often present with symptoms of nausea and abdominal discomfort, to rule out differential diagnoses.

6 Murphy's sign has a high sensitivity but poor specificity for acute cholecystitis. During inspiration, abdominal organs are pushed inferiorly as the diaphragm moves downwards. If the gall bladder is tender due to distension and inflammation, the patient will stop inspiration as it meets the clinician's fingers.

7 In patients with right iliac fossa tenderness, acute appendicitis must be ruled out.

8 In patients with a painless palpable gall bladder accompanied by jaundice, gallstones are unlikely to be the main cause of disease and instead gall bladder malignancy or pancreatic cancer must be investigated. This is known as Courvoisier's sign.

9 If bowel sounds are absent consider an intestinal obstruction, especially in elderly patients. Gallstone ileus is also an important differential, especially in patients with chronic cholecystitis that develop adhesions and fistulas.

Investigations

- Baseline **blood tests** [1] were taken which reveal normal FBE, CRP and UEC.
- **LFTs** [2] are deranged with an elevated **GGT and ALP** [3].
- **Total bilirubin** [4], **AST and ALT** [5] are not elevated.
- An **abdominal ultrasound** [6] was ordered and the report noted **multiple shadows, gall bladder wall thickening and multiple gallstones**.

- A **CT abdomen** [7] was considered, but later abandoned due to unnecessary radiation exposure to the patient.
- Instead, an **MRCP** [8] or **endoscopic ultrasound** [9] would be organised as it was a safer alternative.

[1] An elevated white cell count is suspicious of concurrent biliary infection such as acute cholecystitis or cholangitis. Simple cholelithiasis or choledocholithiasis should not elevate acute inflammatory markers. A raised WCC with an elevated CRP in this patient is suspicious for an acute infection such as cholecystitis or cholangitis. UEC are generally taken to assess renal function and determine whether there are metabolic abnormalities. It can also be used to guide therapy, as certain medications may be contraindicated in patients with poor eGFR.

[2] LFTs may reveal elevated direct bilirubin, AST, ALT, ALP and GGT. LFTs are often used as a screening tool to determine whether there is any hepatobiliary involvement in any patient with abdominal pain. They are also used to gauge the extent of liver injury, distinguish between different types of liver disorders and monitor response to therapy. The parameters are reflective of cellular integrity (ALT, AST), the biliary tract (GGT, ALP) and functionality (albumin).

[3] ALP is an enzyme found in several tissues including the liver and bone. Elevations indicate damage to cells lining the biliary duct. However, it should not be used in isolation to determine the presence of liver disease as it is not specific. GGT, an enzyme found predominantly in biliary epithelial cells and hepatocytes, should then be used to confirm whether elevated ALP is due to hepatic injury. If both GGT and ALP are elevated, it is highly suggestive of biliary tract obstruction and is known as a cholestatic picture.

[4] Total bilirubin includes both conjugated and unconjugated bilirubin. Haemoglobin breaks down to form unconjugated bilirubin. The liver metabolises unconjugated bilirubin and allows it to be water soluble before excreting it renally and faecally. Elevations in unconjugated bilirubin indicates pre-hepatic disease such as haemolysis. Elevations in conjugated bilirubin may indicate intrahepatic or posthepatic disease such as viral hepatitis or obstructive gallstones. Increased bilirubin may manifest clinically in jaundice as it is deposited in mucous membranes, sclera and skin.

[5] Aspartate aminotransferase (AST) and alanine aminotransferase (ALT) are transaminases found intracellularly in hepatocytes. Damage to these cells causes these enzymes to leak into the vascular system. ALT is more specific than AST for liver injury, as AST is also present in skeletal and cardiac muscle and the kidneys. Isolated elevations in AST and ALT tend to indicate intrahepatic disease, with different ratios and absolute counts indicating possible precipitants of liver injury. In cholelithiasis, there may be a minor increase in AST and ALT but not to the same extent as ALP and GGT.

[6] Abdominal ultrasound is the primary imaging modality given that it is safe, accessible, non-invasive and quick. It has a specificity and sensitivity of up to 95% and can identify stones as small as 2mm in diameter. In addition to anatomical information, ultrasound detects intramural gas and pericholecystic fluid collection suggestive of active gall bladder inflammation. It can also highlight bile duct dilation which may indicate an obstructed stone plus gall bladder wall thickening for chronic disease. Classic findings on abdominal ultrasound include stones of varying sizes or shadowing caused by the reflection of ultrasound waves, gall bladder wall thickening (in cholecystitis), pericholecystic fluid during acute gall bladder inflammation and distension. Gall bladder sludge, a precursor to stone formation, may also be detected.

[7] Although CT abdomens are not as reliable at detecting cholelithiasis as ultrasound, they are superior in demonstrating dilated biliary ducts and assessing complications of gallstones, such as perforations and abscesses. They are also useful for ruling out other causes of epigastric pain. X-rays are rarely ordered as cholesterol gallstones are not radio-opaque. However, pigmented and mixed stones composed of calcium may show up in X-rays if large enough.

[8] Magnetic resonance cholangiopancreatography (MRCP) should be used if choledocholithiasis is suspected from abdominal ultrasound reports. MRCP is a novel non-invasive technique that uses an MRI scan to evaluate the hepatobiliary system. It can detect parenchymal abnormalities as well as assess for inflammation, fluid collections and underlying infections. It provides valuable anatomical information and can assess for bile duct dilations. Patients with metal implants are contraindicated from using this technique because it uses magnets. Patients with pacemakers are also required to determine if they are MRI-compatible. Fasting prior to this

investigation is required to reduce gastroduodenal secretions, bowel peristalsis and related motion artefact, and to promote distension of the gall bladder.

9 In endoscopic ultrasonography (EUS), a tiny ultrasound device embedded within an endoscope is guided through the oesophagus and into the small intestine. When adjacent to the gall bladder, it can transmit ultrasound images which are more accurate than standard abdominal ultrasound. This is not a first-line test and is generally only used when staging hepatobiliary and pancreatic cancers.

Management

Immediate

The patient was given **paracetamol and ibuprofen** [1] with good effect. An **anti-emetic** [2] was also administered for nausea along with an **anti-spasmodic** [3] for her abdominal cramping. Because she was at high risk of cholecystitis, **prophylactic antibiotics** [4] were administered. She was also made nil by mouth. As the MRCP noted choledocholithiasis, an **ERCP** [5] was organised for the next day.

Short-term

To prevent further cholelithiasis, **ursodeoxycholic acid** [6] was also prescribed. Because the patient was responding well to antibiotics, she would be placed on an elective list for a **cholecystectomy** [7]. She was educated on the warning signs of cholecystitis and told to present to the ED if they were to occur. If she was septic, a **cholecystostomy tube** [8] would be inserted until she was medically fit for surgery. After her cholecystectomy, she would be monitored carefully for **complications** [9].

Long-term

The patient was also advised to make several lifestyle modifications such as **dietary changes** [10] and increasing her level of exercise. Given her cardiac risk factors, she was also prescribed a statin to reduce her cholesterol.

1 Simple analgesia should relieve biliary colic. If pain continues to be uncontrolled, a step-up approach according to the World Health Organization (WHO) pain ladder should be considered. Patients tend to respond well to oral opioids such as oxycodone. Intravenous opioids such as morphine or fentanyl can also be considered in patients unresponsive to oral analgesia. If further relief is required, consult an acute pain specialist.

2 Anti-emetics such as metoclopramide or ondansetron can provide temporary relief for nausea and vomiting. Metoclopramide binds to and antagonises the D_2 (dopamine) receptors in the chemoreceptor trigger zone of the CNS. This prevents nausea and vomiting associated with biliary colic. Ondansetron is a highly specific serotonin 5-HT_3 receptor antagonist that binds peripherally along the vagus nerve and centrally in the chemoreceptor trigger zone, preventing nausea and vomiting.

3 Antispasmodics such as hyoscine butylbromide can relieve abdominal cramping, spasming and distension. Hyoscine is an anticholinergic drug with high affinity for GI smooth muscle muscarinic receptors. It exerts a smooth-muscle relaxing/spasmolytic effect and therefore is effective in targeting biliary spasms.

4 Surgical antibiotic prophylaxis is only required if patients are elderly, immunocompromised or at risk of a perforated viscus. Empiric coverage targeting predominantly Gram-negative enteric organisms is recommended. Ampicillin and ceftriaxone or gentamicin combinations are commonly used, depending on the patient's allergies. Expert advice should be sought in the pre- and postoperative stage. Patients with multiple comorbidities and at risk of postoperative sepsis should be referred and monitored in an ICU.

5 ERCP is the preferred diagnostic and therapeutic intervention in high risk patients. A flexible endoscope is passed through the stomach and into the small intestine via the oesophageal tract. A thin catheter is then passed through the scope and into the ampulla of Vater. A radio-opaque contrast agent is injected through the catheter into the bile ducts and images are taken to detect any abnormalities such as obstructed ducts. Small surgical instruments can be attached to the end of the scope. A sphincterotomy of the sphincter of Oddi can be performed to allow stones to spill out into the intestine on their own. A grasping catheter can also be run through the endoscope to trap and pull embedded gallstones in the duct but not the gall bladder.

6 Ursodeoxycholic acid (USDA) is a bile acid that markedly reduces biliary cholesterol saturation by inhibiting its absorption in the intestine. However, gallstones tend to recur on cessation of this bile acid. To reduce saturation of biliary sludge, USDA must be taken for 6–12 months. Although some stones do dissolve, most patients end up requiring cholecystectomy a few years down the track. Therefore, this therapy has limited use and is only warranted for patients not eligible for surgery.

7 Cholecystectomy is the definitive therapy for symptomatic cholelithiasis or choledocholithiasis. This can be performed laparoscopically, which is minimally invasive and therefore at less risk of infection and a shorter hospital stay. Open cholecystectomy is reserved for high risk patients and those where the gall bladder is severely inflamed and hard to resect.

8 A cholecystostomy tube can be percutaneously inserted by interventional radiologists using ultrasound guidance to drain infected bile and allow for resolution of symptoms. This bridging therapy reduces gall bladder inflammation and risk of adhesions prior to cholecystectomy.

9 Post cholecystectomy complications include haematoma in the gall bladder bed, infection, bile leak, inadvertent bowel or bile duct injury and retained stone in the bile duct. Further surgery may be needed to repair the bile duct or to join the bile duct to the bowel by anastomosis.

10 Patients are advised to reduce their dietary fat intake. Bile is essential for the breakdown of fats; however, during the postoperative period, it is less concentrated due to the absent gall bladder. Patients may experience watery, loose and frequent bowel motions post cholecystectomy. This will eventually resolve within a few weeks.

CASE 23: Coeliac disease

History

- A **52-year old** [1] **Caucasian woman** [2] with a **20-year history** [3] of **anaemia** [4] and **chronic fatigue** [5] is referred to a digestive health clinic for further investigation and management.
- She has experienced multiple episodes of **diarrhoea** [6] , **abdominal bloating and discomfort** [7] , in particular after **consuming bread and pasta** [8] .
- She has also recently developed **lactose intolerance** [9] .
- Recent blood tests have also revealed **vitamin D and calcium deficiency** [10] .
- Her past medical history includes **type 1 diabetes mellitus, hyperthyroidism** [11] **and chronic itchy rashes on her knees and elbows** [12] .
- **Family history** [13] is significant for coeliac disease.

[1] Coeliac disease is most commonly diagnosed between the 4th and 6th decades of life; however, symptoms can manifest at any age from infancy to the elderly. There is an increasing frequency of paediatric patients, which may be partially explained by improvements in diagnosis and awareness of this disease.

[2] Like most autoimmune diseases, coeliac disease is more common in women than men. Numerous theories attribute this disparity to sex hormones and chromosomes. Globally, people of Caucasian, Jewish, north Indian and Middle Eastern descent have a higher frequency of coeliac disease. It is rarely diagnosed in the African, East Asian and Hispanic populations.

[3] Due to non-specific and variable symptoms and signs, coeliac disease is often incorrectly diagnosed or undiagnosed. Other diseases that have similar presentations include food intolerances, inflammatory bowel disease (IBD) and irritable bowel syndrome (IBS). No single test is available to diagnose coeliac disease. Instead diagnosis is dependent on a thorough history, examination and investigations.

[4] Chronic anaemia is a consequence of malabsorption of nutrients. Small bowel inflammation results in mucosal disruption, limiting the body's ability to absorb nutrients, especially iron, minerals and vitamins. Frequent bouts of inflammation eventually lead to villous atrophy, which exacerbates nutritional deficiencies.

[5] Chronic fatigue is another common complaint due to malabsorption of nutrients. In the paediatric population, failure to thrive and grow is also observed.

[6] The diarrhoea in coeliac disease has a secretory and osmotic component. Prolamin antigens in wheat (gliadin), rye (secalin), barley (hordein) and other grains activate both the innate and adaptive immune systems. Immune cells, such as dendritic cells and macrophages, stimulate intestinal

intra-epithelial lymphocytes, augmenting the secretion of inflammatory mediators and cytokines. This can augment gut motility, leading to secretory diarrhoea. Lymphocytes also secrete reactive oxygen species, which damage intestinal epithelial cells. Immature epithelial cells replace these damaged cells; however, they lack brush border enzymes and poorly absorb nutrients and water. These solutes in the bowel lumen are osmotically active and therefore also contribute to the diarrhoea observed in coeliac disease.

[7] Abdominal bloating involves the following interrelated components:
- a subjective sensation of fullness
- objective abdominal distension
- volume of intra-abdominal contents, and
- muscular activity of the abdominal wall.

This heterogeneous symptom is not well understood in coeliac disease, although it is often relieved with restriction of gluten.

[8] Coeliac disease is caused by an immune reaction to prolamin antigens such as gliadin, secalin, hordein and glutenin which are found in wheat, rye, barley and other related grains. As patients with coeliac disease are unable to digest these peptides, symptoms arise after the consumption of these foods.

[9] Lactase is a brush border enzyme produced by cells in the small bowel. As villous atrophy occurs, enterocytes are unable to produce adequate amounts of this enzyme, leading to lactose intolerance. Care must be taken to also differentiate between coeliac disease and other commonly associated conditions such as fructose/sucrose/sorbitol intolerance and exocrine pancreatic insufficiency. The latter conditions often exhibit similar symptoms.

[10] Dietary vitamin D is absorbed in the intestine and its absorption is dependent upon the presence of fat in the lumen, which triggers the release of bile acids and lipase. In

turn, bile acids initiate the emulsification of lipids, pancreatic lipase hydrolyses the triglycerides into monoglycerides and free fatty acids, and bile acids support the formation of lipid-containing micelles, which diffuse into enterocytes. Calcium is also absorbed in the proximal part of the small intestine; however, its transport is dependent on vitamin D. In patients with coeliac disease, villous atrophy limits the effective absorption of both vitamin D and calcium. This can significantly increase the risk of osteopenia or osteoporosis, especially in postmenopausal women.

11 There is a genetic association between coeliac disease and other autoimmune diseases such as thyroid disorders and diabetes mellitus. Mechanisms that underlie the coexistence of these diseases can be partially explained by the over-expression of HLA-DQ2 and DQ8 haplotypes in patients.

12 Dermatitis herpetiformis is a chronic pruritic skin condition associated with HLA-DQ2 and HLA-DQ8. These papulovesicular rashes erupt on extensor surfaces of the body and are often exacerbated after the ingestion of gluten. Patients who continually scratch these rashes increase the risk of secondary skin infections caused by skin flora. Crust formations and excoriations can also occur. Biopsy of these vesicles reveals immunofluorescent IgA deposits.

13 A positive family history for coeliac disease is the strongest risk factor for its development. Several genes have been implicated in its development, notably HLA-DQ2 and HLA-DQ8. These two variants have been found in >95% of patients with coeliac disease. These genes code for receptors that bind to gliadin proteins more tightly, increasing the risk of T-cell activation and autoimmunity. The frequency of these genes varies widely, with the highest prevalence in western Europe.

Examination

- The patient has a **small body habitus** [1], appears calm, alert and in no respiratory distress.
- She is **haemodynamically stable and afebrile** [2].
- Over the extensor surfaces of her arms and legs are **darkened patches of skin with excoriations** [3].
- **Peripheral examination is non-specific** [4] with **brittle nails** [5], **conjunctival pallor and multiple oral aphthous ulcers** [6] noted in the inner cheeks.
- Abdominal examination is also unremarkable apart from some **central tenderness** [7].
- **Bowel sounds are highly active** [8]. Digital rectal examination was declined.

1 UK guidelines recommend an average daily intake of 2000 calories (8700kJ), although this varies between individuals depending on age, height, metabolism, weight, exercise activity and other factors. Villous atrophy in coeliac disease can lead to malabsorption and therefore malnutrition. This increases the risk of anaemia, weight loss, osteoporosis and infertility. In children, short stature and failure to thrive are common presenting complaints in untreated coeliac disease.

2 Vital signs in coeliac disease generally do not fall outside normal ranges. However, a rare but life-threatening complication known as a coeliac crisis can cause derangements in heart rate, respiratory rate and blood pressure. In this syndrome, profuse diarrhoea can cause severe hypoproteinaemia, metabolic and electrolyte disturbances, acidosis, dehydration and neurological dysfunction. Hospitalisation is required with careful correction of electrolytes and rehydration, along with systemic glucocorticoid therapy to reduce immune reactivity.

3 Dermatitis herpetiformis is exacerbated after the consumption of gluten. Continual scratching of these pruritic rashes can form crusts, excoriations and skin discolouration.

4 Because there are no pathognomonic signs or symptoms of coeliac disease, a large number of people are incorrectly diagnosed or undiagnosed.

5 Nail changes are commonly seen in patients suffering from malabsorption. Consider zinc, calcium or protein deficiency in patients with leuconychia (multiple white spots), koilonychia (spoon shape), horizontal ridging (vertical ridging occurs normally with ageing) and weak splitting nails.

6 The pathophysiology of recurrent oral aphthous ulcers in coeliac disease is unknown but is most likely related to haematinic deficiency. Likewise, anaemia results in the shunting of blood away from the skin and other peripheral tissues, and redistributing flow to vital organs. This manifests as pallor, with its presence in the conjunctiva suggesting haemoglobin <90g/L.

7 Inflammation in the small bowel in coeliac disease leads to a viscera-somatic response with pain and tenderness felt centrally due to its midgut embryonic origin.

8 Highly active bowel sounds, known as borborygmi, result from increased peristalsis as a consequence of gluten consumption.

Investigations

Pathology

- **FBE** [1] demonstrates a low Hb, mean corpuscular volume (MCV) and mean corpuscular haemoglobin concentration (MCHC).
- **Iron studies** [2] also reveal elevated transferrin and total iron-binding capacity (TIBC) with low transferrin saturation and ferritin concentration.
- Serum CMP studies displayed **hypocalcaemia** [3].
- Serology for **anti-endomysial (EMA)** [4], **anti-transglutaminase (tTG) antibodies** [5] and **total serum IgA were elevated**.
- **IgG antibodies** [6] were not performed.
- Serum **vitamin B12** [7] was reduced.
- **TFT** [8] revealed an elevated TSH and low T4.
- The patient's immediate family was recommended to undergo **gene testing** [9].

Imaging

- An **abdominal X-ray and CT** [10] was considered to rule out other pathology.

Endoscopy

- Due to the positive IgA results, an **oesophagogastroduodenoscopy (OGD)** [11] was ordered.
- **Intraluminal examination** [12] revealed scalloping of the small bowel folds, a 'cracked-mud' mosaic mucosal pattern and submucosa blood vessel prominence.
- Biopsies taken in **5 different locations** [13] noted **intra-epithelial lymphocytes, villous atrophy and crypt hyperplasia** [14].

[1] Malabsorption of nutrients can result in anaemia, which is defined as a Hb <130g/L in adult males and <120g/L in adult females. Haemoglobin has a quaternary structure, with each subunit containing a haem group with an iron atom centre. Iron allows for oxygen binding and therefore each haemoglobin molecule is able to carry four oxygen molecules. During the initial stages of malabsorption, the body is able to depend on its iron stores (known as ferritin) for haemoglobin production. However, as this becomes depleted, haemoglobin formation is limited, impacting on the level of normal functioning red blood cells. Iron deficiency causes a microcytic, hypochromic anaemia, and vitamin B12/folate deficiency leads to a macrocytic, megaloblastic anaemia.

[2] When iron is transported around the body, it is bound to a glycoprotein known as transferrin. However, villous atrophy leads to poor absorption of iron and therefore low transferrin saturation. The body increases transferrin production as a compensatory mechanism, causing an increased transferrin expression. This results in a corresponding increase in TIBC and low transferrin saturation.

[3] Coeliac disease is often associated with hypocalcaemia due to malabsorption.

[4] Serological studies are the first-line investigations; however, seronegative findings do not rule out coeliac disease. Patients must be consuming gluten-rich foods as blood tests may normalise on gluten-free diets. Both anti-EMA and anti-tTG antibodies have similar sensitivities and specificities for coeliac disease. Anti-EMA is more labour intensive and costly with a greater specificity but lower

sensitivity to anti-tTG. Endomysium is a connective tissue layer that surrounds smooth muscle fibres. Antibodies to EMA are produced in response to gluten-induced intestinal inflammation.

[5] Tissue transglutaminase enzymes are found in the endomysium that form epitopes when they react with gliadin. These epitopes are thought to be antigenic and cause gut inflammation.

[6] Total serum IgA should be performed in parallel as approximately 5% of patients with coeliac disease are deficient in IgA and this therefore renders anti-tTG IgA tests unreliable. In these cases, IgG-tTG is performed instead.

[7] Vitamin B12 deficiency is common in patients with coeliac disease due to poor dietary absorption. This vitamin is absorbed in the terminal ileum and this segment can be affected by coeliac disease. Its concentration generally normalises after commencement of a gluten-free diet and with supplementation.

[8] There is evidence to suggest that patients with coeliac disease are predisposed to developing other autoimmune diseases such as hypothyroidism. The coexistence of coeliac disease and autoimmune thyroid disease is thought to be due to over-representation of HLA-DQ2 and DQ8 haplotypes. Outside the HLA region, both diseases are associated with the gene encoding cytotoxic T-lymphocyte-associated antigen-4 (CTLA-4), a candidate gene for conferring susceptibility to thyroid autoimmunity. Therefore, patients with coeliac disease should concurrently be screened for thyroid disorders. Mild elevation in TSH and low T4 levels indicate hypothyroidism, whilst low levels of TSH and high T4 indicate hyperthyroidism.

9 OGD remains the gold standard diagnostic test. If serological studies are positive, then an OGD is highly recommended to confirm diagnosis. If serological studies are negative but clinical suspicion remains high, OGD should still be performed. This day procedure involves visualisation of the oesophagus, stomach and duodenum under light sedation using a flexible telescopic camera known as a gastroscope. Patients with coeliac disease often have a normal-appearing small intestine on macroscopic evaluation. Biopsies are taken from multiple sites for further histopathological analysis.

10 Radiological imaging is generally not required unless to rule out other differential diagnoses. Nevertheless, clinicians should be aware of certain characteristic findings. Small bowel follow-throughs may show fewer jejunal folds, an increased number of ileal folds, small bowel dilation, wall thickening and intussusception. Extraintestinal abnormalities include mesenteric lymphadenopathy, vascular changes and splenic atrophy.

11 There is a strong genetic link in coeliac disease, meaning all immediate family should be screened following the diagnosis of one family member. Genetic testing with the HLA DQ2/DQ8 test can be helpful in certain circumstances. Given that >99% of patients with coeliac disease carry one or other of these markers, a negative test effectively excludes coeliac disease.

12 Patients are advised to remain on a gluten-rich diet prior to endoscopy. Macroscopic examination, although not diagnostic, can demonstrate scalloping of duodenal mucosal folds, a mosaic pattern on the mucosa leading to a 'cracked-mud' appearance and blood vessel prominence due to increased inflammation.

13 Biopsies must be taken from multiple locations as not all areas of the intestinal tract are affected equally. This reduces the risk of false negatives.

14 The Marsh classification is commonly used to grade the severity of coeliac disease. Grading the immunological reaction to gliadin is difficult and therefore intra-epithelial lymphocytes act as a surrogate marker. Crypt hyperplasia precedes villous atrophy and involves elongation of the length of the crypts of Lieberkühn. Elongation is caused by the expansion of the lamina propria due to inflammatory cell influx, proliferation of stromal cells and tissue remodelling. Villous atrophy is generally pathognomonic for coeliac disease with the height three times its width.

Marsh stage	Characteristics		
	Villous atrophy	Crypt hyperplasia	Intra-epithelial lymphocytes per 100 enterocytes
0	Normal	Normal	<30
1	Normal	Normal	>30
2	Normal	Increased	>30
3a	Mild	Increased	>30
3b	Moderate	Increased	>30
3c	Severe	Increased	>30

Management

Immediate

The patient was advised to immediately **cease consumption of gluten** [1]. Electrolyte and vitamin **supplementation** [2] was initiated.

Short-term

A referral to a **dietitian** [3] specialising in coeliac disease was made. If symptoms persist, **steroids** [4] may be considered.

Long-term

Follow-up and continuum of care with a **primary care physician is recommended** [5]. **DEXA scans** [6] for patients at risk of osteopenia and osteoporosis should also be considered. Failure to respond to gluten-free diet necessitates referral to a **digestive health subspecialist** [7]. The patient would also be monitored for **gastrointestinal T-cell lymphoma** [8].

1 As no medications are available, ceasing gluten consumption is the mainstay therapy. This prevents intestinal inflammation, allowing the GI tract to heal and, eventually, resolution of symptoms. Failure to comply can cause a relapse in disease. Withdrawal of gluten is also used as a diagnostic test. In patients who continue to have symptoms despite a gluten-free diet, a careful dietary history should be taken. Symptoms may in fact be due to other diseases such as small intestinal bacterial overgrowth, lactose/fructose/sucrose/ sorbitol intolerance, pancreatic insufficiency and microscopic colitis.

2 Villous atrophy prevents optimal absorption of nutrients, minerals and vitamins. Patients may be required to take dietary supplements, infusions or injections to treat nutritional deficits. Calcium and vitamin D supplements are recommended in most patients to reduce the risk of osteoporosis.

3 Dietitians can educate and assist patients in choosing gluten-free products. Numerous countries have differing guidelines on what are acceptable levels of gluten in 'gluten-free' products. Dietary counselling is also essential as gluten-free diets may be low in fibre, vitamin and nutrients and high in simple carbohydrates and fats. In addition to gluten withdrawal, some people need to follow a low-FODMAP diet or avoid consumption of commercial gluten-free products that contain preservatives and additives which may trigger GI tract symptoms.

4 Immunosuppressants are generally used on an off-label basis if villous atrophy continues to occur despite gluten withdrawal. Steroids are often the first-line pharmacotherapy used. Other immunosuppressive medications prescribed include azathioprine and ciclosporin. These medications are rarely used as their side-effects often outweigh their benefits.

5 Coeliac disease is rarely life-threatening and is managed with diet modifications. Follow-up with primary care physicians is recommended to monitor for nutritional deficits. Regular blood tests for vitamins, electrolytes and minerals is recommended to optimise the patient's health.

6 Patients with coeliac disease are at risk of osteoporosis due to low vitamin D and calcium levels. At-risk patients (postmenopausal women) should be considered for a DEXA scan to determine bone mineral density.

7 A small subset of patients may have refractory disease which can generally be attributed to poor diet adherence. However, other differentials such as small intestinal bacterial overgrowth, microscopic colitis or other dietary intolerances should be considered. Referral to a coeliac specialist may be necessary for further investigations and management.

8 Enteropathy-associated T-cell lymphoma is a rare complication of coeliac disease in which T-cell lymphomas develop in areas of the small intestine with active inflammation. Its aetiology is not well understood. When this malignancy is detected, surgery is to prevent spread and reduce the risk of bowel obstruction and perforation. Adjuvant chemotherapy is also required to limit its spread.

CASE 24: Decompensated liver cirrhosis

History

- A 65-year-old man is brought in by ambulance to the ED after his partner found him **vomiting frank blood** [1] in their lounge.
- Paramedics report **multiple syringes** [2] and a **strong smell of alcohol** [3] upon entering their house.
- Collateral history from the partner reports that the patient has become **increasingly confused** [4] over the past two weeks.
- His skin has become increasingly **yellow** [5] and his partner reports he has been getting **more swollen in the abdomen** [6].
- His partner has also noticed that he has **not**

been eating [7] as much food lately and has been developing bruises [8] on his arms spontaneously.
- Over the past few months, she also reports that he has been suffering from **erectile dysfunction** [9].
- She has also noted that he has been leaving **very offensive stools** [10] and dark red **streaks of blood** [11] in the toilet bowl.
- His past medical history is positive for **hepatitis C** [12] and **alcoholic liver disease** [13].
- She reports that the patient consumes on average a bottle of spirits per day. However, this has increased to two in the past month ever since he was fired from his job. Both of them are **IV drug users** [14].

[1] Haematemesis is a medical emergency and originates from the upper gastrointestinal tract. Causes include oesophageal varices, Mallory–Weiss tears, gastritis, peptic ulcer disease and vomiting ingested blood from ear/nose/throat haemorrhage. It is imperative that bleeding is controlled to prevent hypovolaemic shock.

[2] Multiple syringes can indicate the patient may be an active IV drug user.

[3] Overconsumption of alcohol can irritate stomach lining and cause gastritis. The area postrema, a structure in the medulla oblongata controlling vomiting, is activated triggering nausea and eventually vomiting as the body attempts to rid itself of this toxin. In the above stem, multiple bouts of vomiting can cause a tear within the mucosal layers of the oesophagus and therefore bleeding. Long-term consumption of alcohol can also cause cirrhosis, which is discussed further below.

[4] Increasing confusion in a patient with cirrhosis indicates the presence of hepatic encephalopathy. Other symptoms include changes in mood, personality and movement. In healthy individuals, the liver metabolises nitrogen compounds produced by intestinal bacteria. In patients with cirrhosis, this process is impaired due to a reduced number of hepatocytes, causing accumulation of nitrogenous products in the systemic circulation. Certain compounds such as ammonia can cross the blood–brain barrier where it is metabolised by astrocytes into glutamine. Glutamine exerts osmotic pressure, leading to an increase in cerebral oedema and therefore confusion. Furthermore, ammonia

is a neurotoxin and can influence other neural pathways with an imbalance between excitatory and inhibitory neurotransmission. There is direct interaction of ammonia with the GABA-A-benzodiazepine receptor complex, leading to increased sedative effects. Hyperammonaemia also exerts oxidative stress and increases neuroinflammation.

[5] The presence of jaundice indicates an elevated bilirubin >3mg/dl. In cirrhosis, hepatocyte death reduces the ability to metabolise and excrete bilirubin, leading to systemic accumulation. Furthermore, portal hypertension can cause splenomegaly, increasing haemolysis and production of bilirubin.

[6] The pathogenesis of ascites in patients with advanced cirrhosis is extremely complex and is caused by portal hypertension. As the liver becomes increasingly scarred, there is structural distortion of the intrahepatic vasculature, reducing contractility of the hepatic vascular bed. This is further exacerbated by a reduced vasodilatory response and increased production of vasoconstrictors, eventually leading to an increase in portal venous pressure. Portal hypertension causes backflow into the splanchnic circulation and the resulting stasis of vasodilatory compounds such as nitric oxide in this system. Consequently, splanchnic vasodilation occurs with resultant systemic hypoperfusion. This typically affects renal function, leading to activation of the renin–angiotensin–aldosterone system (RAAS). In response to a decrease in vascular pressure, renin is secreted from the renal juxtaglomerular apparatus. It in turn will convert angiotensinogen to angiotensin I which is further converted to angiotensin II in the lungs. Angiotensin II

causes the release of aldosterone from the zona glomerulosa of the adrenal cortex, and secretion of vasopressin from the posterior pituitary, leading to fluid acquisition and retention intravascularly. In patients with advanced cirrhosis, hypoalbuminaemia lowers oncotic pressure and therefore allows fluid to extravasate. Together with an increased hydrostatic pressure from retained blood volume, this overwhelms the capacity of the lymphatic and peritoneal surface to reabsorb this fluid, causing accumulation in potential spaces such as the peritoneal cavity.

7 Abdominal distension from ascites may reduce a patient's level of appetite.

8 The liver is responsible for the production of numerous proteins including clotting factors I, II (prothrombin), III, IV, V, VI, VII, IX, X, XI, XII and fibrinogen and prothrombin. Furthermore, the liver also synthesises thrombopoietin, a hormone that regulates platelet production in the bone marrow. Therefore, damage to the liver from cirrhosis can impair coagulation, leading to spontaneous bruising and bleeding.

9 Patients with advanced liver disease often have low serum testosterone which manifests clinically as erectile dysfunction, decreased libido and testicular atrophy. In alcoholic liver disease, ethanol also has a direct toxic effect on testicles. In liver cirrhosis, pituitary production of luteinising hormone is suppressed. This is thought to be a consequence of elevated inflammatory cytokines, such as IL-1, IL-6, and tumour necrosis factor alpha that artificially downregulate gonadotrophin-releasing hormone.

10 Melaena is black tarry stool that is extremely offensive due to the enzymatic digestion of haemoglobin by intestinal bacteria. The most common cause of melaena is peptic ulcer disease. Chronic alcohol consumption increases the risk of peptic ulcer development and when combined with

coagulopathy arising from advanced liver disease, can result in increased bleeding.

11 Haematochezia may be secondary to fissures, haemorrhoids or in the case of patients with decompensated liver cirrhosis, anorectal varices. Venous resistance in the portal venous system is increased in portal hypertension. When this pressure is greater than the systemic venous pressures, blood is shunted through portosystemic anastomosis. Such collateral routes include varicosities in the rectum, oesophagus and para-umbilical regions. Oesophageal and anorectal varices are prone to bleeding and must be treated as a medical emergency.

12 Around 30% of patients with untreated hepatitis C will develop cirrhosis. Globally, viral hepatitis is the leading cause of liver cirrhosis. An increasing number of patients with non-alcoholic fatty liver disease are also developing cirrhosis.

13 Alcoholic liver disease is the second most common cause of liver cirrhosis globally and the leading cause in western countries. Alcohol is a toxin that causes liver-related damage through steatosis, hepatitis and eventually cirrhosis. The metabolism of alcohol into acetaldehyde, then aldehyde dehydrogenase into acetic acid and finally CO_2 and water, generates NADH (nicotinamide adenine dinucleoside (NAD) + hydrogen (H)) which induces fatty acid synthesis and hepatic accumulation. Excessive accumulation of fat can also induce steatohepatitis. Alcohol, through its metabolism, also generates free radicals which can induce hepatocyte death. This signals the immune system to activate inflammatory pathways. Prolonged inflammatory responses lead to further hepatocyte death. Consequently, hepatic stellate cells deposit collagen at sites of injury which replace normal parenchyma. Eventually this culminates in liver cirrhosis.

14 Sharing needles increases the risk of viral hepatitis, as the hepatitis B and C viruses are bloodborne.

Examination

- On examination, the patient is **confused, not oriented to time or place** [1] , and unsteady on his feet; he has some **weakness in eye movements** [2] .
- He is **febrile, tachypnoeic and tachycardic** [3] and normotensive.
- Peripheral examination reveals **palmar erythema** [4] and a positive **hepatic flap** [5] .
- His **nails** [6] are pale and **contractures** [7] are noted on some of his left metacarpals.
- Facial examination reveals **scleral jaundice** [8] , a strong smell of alcohol on his breath and **swollen parotid glands** [9] .

- Examination of his neck and chest reveals **multiple spider naevi** [10] .
- **Gynaecomastia** [11] is also present along with patchy chest hair growth.
- His abdomen is **extremely distended** [12] with **superficial veins present and dilated** [13] .
- Palpation of the RUQ is difficult; however, the **liver is hard with a nodular liver edge** [14] .
- **Splenomegaly** [15] is also present. There is no other organomegaly.
- Percussion note is resonant and bowel sounds are muffled. **Shifting dullness** [16] is also elicited.

1 Confusion is a common sign of decompensated liver disease. This can be attributed to hepatic encephalopathy. In cases of alcoholism, patients may be deficient in vitamin B1, which can cause neurological impairments such as Wernicke–Korsakoff syndrome.

2 Wernicke's encephalopathy triad comprises ophthalmoplegia, confusion and ataxia. Classic triad is present only in 10–20% of patients.

3 The occurrence of fever, tachypnoea or tachycardia in the setting of decompensated liver disease may indicate concurrent infection due to impaired immunity, accumulated endotoxins as the liver is unable to clear it from the body or in the case of active bleeding, hypovolaemic shock.

4 In liver cirrhosis, there is impaired hepatic metabolism of oestradiol. This causes elevated serum oestradiol levels which increases vascularity of the thenar and hypothenar surfaces of the hand.

5 Hepatic flap (asterixis) consists of infrequent involuntary flexion–extension movements of the hand which is a result of neurotoxins such as ammonia impairing the diencephalic motor centres of the brain. Hepatic flap is not pathognomonic for decompensated liver disease and may occur in uraemia, hypoxia and hypercapnia.

6 Muehrcke's nails (pale transverse bands extending all the way across the nail) are cutaneous manifestations of liver disease. Muehrcke's nails are specific for hypoalbuminaemia.

7 Dupuytren's contractures are associated with alcoholic liver disease. Its exact pathogenesis is unclear; however, one theory suggests alcohol-induced damage to palmar fatty tissues, provoking a fibrotic response.

8 Scleral jaundice is a misnomer as bilirubin stains the conjunctival membranes overlying the sclera and not the sclera itself.

9 Sialadenosis is a chronic, asymptomatic, bilateral enlargement of the parotid glands that may be secondary to malnutrition, liver disease and alcoholism.

10 Spider naevi are vascular lesions characterised by a central red spot with reddish extensions that radiate outwards like a spider's web. They are generally found in the distribution of the SVC such as the face, neck, arms and chest. They arise secondary to failure of the sphincteric muscles surrounding the arteriole, causing it to be permanently vasodilated. Elevated oestrogen levels, as seen in patients with advanced liver disease, are thought to be responsible for its development.

11 Oestrogen levels are frequently elevated in men with cirrhosis due to impaired hepatic metabolism. Furthermore, chronic liver disease causes a disproportionate increase in sex-hormone binding globulin which has a stronger affinity to bind free testosterone than oestradiol. This causes an imbalance in free oestrogen-to-androgen ratio. Clinically, this causes gynaecomastia and the development of a female body habitus.

12 Ascites tends to accumulate in the peritoneal space. Large amounts can progressively distend the abdomen and be painful, limiting activities of daily life.

13 Caput medusae is the name given to the appearance of dilated superficial epigastric veins that radiate from the umbilicus across the abdomen. It is caused by portal hypertension.

14 In most patients with no hepatic diseases, the liver should not be palpable. Firmness and irregularity of the liver edge is often caused by cirrhosis, as scar tissue is much firmer than normal parenchyma. Nodular edges may also be suspicious of neoplasms as it becomes infiltrated with cancerous cells. Percussion can be used to map the size of the liver which is on average 7–10cm. Patients with moderate liver disease may have hepatomegaly. In advanced liver disease and cirrhosis, the liver size reduces as normal parenchyma is replaced with fibrotic tissue.

15 Splenomegaly occurs in advanced liver disease due to venous congestion of blood in the spleen from portal hypertension. The release of inflammatory mediators may also activate splenic lymphoproliferation of immune cells.

16 Shifting dullness indicates the presence of fluid in the peritoneal cavity. However, false positives can arise in patients with faecal loading and in obese individuals. Furthermore, this test is only accurate when there is >500ml of fluid present.

Investigations

Pathology

- **FBE** [1] reveals a normocytic anaemia and thrombocytopenia and **UECs** [2] demonstrate elevated urea, creatinine and reduced eGFR.
- **LFTs** [3] are globally deranged with an elevated AST, ALT, bilirubin, ALP and GGT.
- **Hypoalbuminaemia** [4] is confirmed along with a **prolonged INR** [5].
- **Serum ammonia** [6] and **alpha-fetoprotein (AFP)** [7] is elevated.
- **Hepatitis serology** [8] is positive for hepatitis C but there are no other derangements on the liver screen panel.

Imaging

- **Abdominal ultrasound** [9] reveals excessive fluid in the abdomen along with a large nodular liver.
- **CT abdomen** [10] was used to assess for malignancy.
- A **gastroscopy** [11] also reveals multiple varices along the patient's oesophageal tract.
- As the patient was coagulopathic, a **liver biopsy** [12] was contraindicated.

- **Peritoneocentesis** [13] were sent off for microscopy and culture.
- **Wedge pressures** [14] were also considered once the patient was stable.
- On discharge, he would require 6-monthly **FibroScans** [15] to monitor the extent of his cirrhosis.

[1] Anaemia may be secondary to GI haemorrhages and iron deficiency. Furthermore, thrombocytopenia occurs due to hypersplenism which is a consequence of portal hypertension.

[2] Reduced eGFR and elevated creatinine may be due to hepatorenal syndrome, a complication of portal hypertension. Splanchnic dilation reduces kidney perfusion, leading to kidney injury.

[3] LFTs are generally deranged in patients with cirrhosis with moderately elevated AST and ALT. However, normal aminotransferases do not preclude cirrhosis as levels of these enzymes are dependent on functioning hepatocytes that are damaged. In patients with alcohol cirrhosis, GGT will also be elevated. With decompensation, bilirubin tends to drastically rise, causing jaundice. LFTs provide important information for grading the severity of liver disease. Scoring systems such as the Child–Pugh score or MELD score provide prognostic information and can influence management of cirrhosis.

[4] In cirrhotic patients, hypoalbuminaemia occurs due to impaired hepatic synthesis, increased albumin catabolism and increased vascular leakage.

[5] The coagulation proteins factors II, VII, IX and X are synthesised within hepatocytes. Cirrhosis impairs this production leading to increased prothrombin time.

[6] Patients with cirrhosis with hepatic encephalopathy tend to have elevated ammonia levels. In patients with cirrhosis, the liver is unable to fully metabolise nitrogenous compounds produced by intestinal bacteria, leading to its accumulation in the systemic circulation.

[7] Alpha-fetoprotein is a biomarker for hepatocellular carcinoma (HCC). Other causes of elevations include testicular cancer and germ cell tumours. It is not routinely used as a diagnostic or monitoring test but as an adjunct to imaging.

[8] Hepatitis serology should be done in all patients with suspected liver disease to determine their infection and immunisation status. Serology commonly tests for HAV, HBV and HCV (hepatitis A, B and C virus, respectively). In patients with known chronic infections and on antiviral therapy, viral loads should be attained to determine efficacy of treatments.

[9] Abdominal ultrasound is the first-line imaging technique due to its ease of access, safety profile, non-invasiveness and low cost. Patients with cirrhosis will typically have hypoechoic nodules in liver parenchyma which may represent regenerative regions or small hepatomas. In some individuals the liver may also be atrophied. Fatty changes may also be observed. Patients with additional portal hypertension will also have a dilated portal vein (>1.5cm) and a reduced blood flow velocity on Doppler. Portosystemic collateral veins may also be visualised along with splenomegaly and ascites.

[10] CT is not generally used during early cirrhosis as it is less sensitive than ultrasound. In established disease, however, it can be used to determine the extent of cirrhosis and screen for malignancy. Characteristic findings include surface and parenchymal nodularity due to regeneration or malignancy, portal vein enlargement – if portal hypertension is present – and lobar atrophy.

[11] Gastroscopy is both a diagnostic and therapeutic technique for the assessment of oesophageal varices which are common complications of portal hypertension from cirrhosis. Gastric varices may also be observed although they are less prevalent.

[12] A liver biopsy is rarely performed unless clinicians are unable to determine a cause for the patient's liver disease. It is considered the gold diagnostic standard; however, it is invasive. Liver biopsies may also be used to determine the severity of cirrhosis, although imaging techniques such as transient elastography (FibroScan) are preferred.

[13] Peritoneal taps are only conducted in patients with ascites. A needle is introduced into the abdomen under ultrasound guidance to drain fluid for diagnostic and therapeutic purposes. Fluid analysis may reveal an infection if leucocytes and bacteria are elevated, or malignancy if dysplastic cells are detected.

[14] Portal hypertension can be determined through the introduction of a catheter into a hepatic vein, occluding it and measuring the pressure of proximal static blood. This indirectly measures the hepatic sinusoidal pressure which generally reflects the portal vein pressure. This is known as the wedged hepatic venous pressure. The normal pressure in the portal vein in 5–10mmHg. When compared with the free

hepatic venous pressure, the difference calculated is known as the hepatic venous pressure gradient. A gradient ≥5mmHg is diagnostic for portal hypertension. Gradients >10mmHg are clinically significant and >12mmHg has an extreme risk for variceal bleeding.

15 Transient elastography (FibroScan) is a cheap, safe and non-invasive technique used to monitor and measure the degree of liver fibrosis. Using an ultrasound transducer probe, vibrations are transmitted through the liver tissue. This creates a shear wave that travels through the liver tissue. The probe then utilises ultrasound to follow the propagation of the shear wave and to measure its velocity (which is directly related to tissue stiffness and correlates with fibrosis). Limitations include its inaccuracy in patients with ascites, obesity and concurrent hepatitis and the fact that it is operator-dependent. Nevertheless, it is extensively used to monitor progression of fibrosis in patients with cirrhosis.

Management

Immediate

After insertion of **two large-bore cannulas** [1], **intravenous antibiotics** [2] but not **proton pump inhibitors** [3] were prescribed. A **strict fluid balance chart and gentle albumin infusion** [4] was administered. To reduce the rate of active bleeding, splanchnic blood flow and portal hypertension were reduced with an **octreotide** [5] infusion. An emergency endoscopy was also organised to confirm the presence of varices which would require **endoscopic banding** [6].

Short-term

After the patient was stabilised, **paracentesis** [7] was conducted to drain large volumes of his ascitic fluid. He was also prescribed **diuretics** [8] to reduce sodium renal retention. **Lactulose** [9] was initiated with consideration of **rifaximin** [10] if encephalopathy persisted. Replacement **thiamine and vitamin B12 injections** [11] were also administered.

Long-term

The patient was advised to avoid **hepatotoxins, cease alcohol intake** [12] and begin IV drug rehabilitation. He was also encouraged to consume a **high protein, low salt, high caloric** [13] diet. A **transjugular intrahepatic portosystemic shunt (TIPS)** [14] would also be available if his portal hypertension worsened. In order to be eligible for **liver transplantation** [15], the patient was advised to cease alcohol consumption and begin **antiviral medications** [16] for his hepatitis C. He was also advised to regularly visit his GP and gastroenterologist for **monitoring and screening of HCC** [17] and **hepatorenal syndrome** [18].

1 In patients presenting with haematemesis, two large-bore cannulas are crucial to facilitate rapid fluid transfusion in cases of hypovolaemic shock.

2 IV antibiotics are recommended for patients with haematemesis and cirrhosis to reduce the risk of infection. Ceftriaxone IV is most commonly used although ciprofloxacin IV can also be administered in patients allergic to beta-lactams. Once patients are haemodynamically stable, switching to oral prophylaxis is recommended. Duration of prophylaxis is uncertain although the shortest possible duration (3 days) is recommended. Consider ceasing antibiotics once bleeding has resolved and octreotide has been stopped.

3 The use of high dose proton pump inhibitors (PPIs) remains controversial and they should not be routinely prescribed unless the patient is suspected to have active gastric ulcer bleeding. PPI use has been associated with an increased risk of spontaneous bacterial peritonitis, *C. difficile* infection and increased overall mortality.

4 Fluid balance charts with urinary indwelling catheter insertion should be mandatory to assess the patient's fluid status, especially if they are actively haemorrhaging or there is sequestration of fluids in the extravascular space due to low albumin. Albumin is the most abundant circulatory protein and maintains intravascular volume and colloid osmotic pressure. As patients with cirrhosis suffer from hypoalbuminaemia, albumin infusions are necessary to maintain adequate perfusion. This reduces the risk of renal impairment and mortality due to shock.

5 In cirrhosis, intrahepatic resistance and splanchnic blood flow are increased, causing the development of portal hypertension. Octreotide is a somatostatin analogue that increases vasoconstriction of the splanchnic arterial bed, reduces portal venous pressure and reduces splanchnic blood flow. Octreotide also inhibits the release of glucagon, which is a splanchnic vasodilator. Its effect on portal pressure is transient and therefore it is used as an infusion. An alternative is terlipressin, a vasopressin analogue that is as commonly used in the UK.

6 In patients with active bleeding, gastroscopy will allow visualisation of bleeding varices. Banding helps to control active bleeding, although sclerotherapy may also be employed in difficult cases. If bleeding remains uncontrolled, a temporary balloon tamponade may be inflated which applies traction to the oesophageal tract. This is only a temporary measure, as oesophageal necrosis may occur with prolonged inflation. A TIPS can then be performed to reduce portal hypertension.

7 Paracentesis is recommended in patients with large volume ascites, for symptomatic improvement. A large-bore needle with a long sheath is inserted under ultrasound guidance into the peritoneal cavity to allow drainage of the fluid. A sample is also sent off for microscopy, culture and sensitivity (MCS) to exclude spontaneous bacterial peritonitis (SBP). Albumin replacement therapy is recommended in patients undergoing paracentesis to prevent hypotension and prevent fluid shifts. Refractory ascites can be treated with repeat paracentesis or a percutaneous shunt between the hepatic and portal veins (TIPS). Patients suspected to have SBP should have their ascitic fluid drained and empirically treated with ceftriaxone IV until culture and sensitivities become available. Antibiotic prophylaxis (trimethoprim-sulfamethoxazole) may be considered in patients at high risk of SBP, such as those with Child–Pugh score >8.

8 Mild ascites can also be treated with adjunct medications such as spironolactone or amiloride, assuming their renal function and serum electrolyte functions are stable. Spironolactone and amiloride are aldosterone antagonists that prevent sodium retention, reducing fluid reabsorption in the distal tubules. Furosemide can be added for non-responders.

9 Lactulose therapy aims to reduce intestinal ammonia through multiple mechanisms. The metabolism of lactulose to lactic acid by intestinal microbiota results in acidification of the gut, favouring conversion of ammonia to non-absorbable ammonium, effectively reducing plasma ammonia levels and increasing its passage from tissues into the lumen. Gut acidification also inhibits ammoniagenic coliform bacterial growth in the colon. Its secondary laxative effect on the colon also facilitates increased bowel motions that aid in removal of nitrogenous compounds that contribute to hepatic encephalopathy.

10 Rifaximin is an antibiotic only used in persistent and recurrent hepatic encephalopathy. It reduces the level of intestinal ammonia-producing bacteria; however, long-term use can predispose individuals to resistance.

11 It is important to replace all vitamins such as thiamine and B12. This can be done once patients are haemodynamically stable through intramuscular injections (B12), intravenous route (thiamine) or oral supplementations. Supplementation will help optimise medical function and prevent further deterioration in overall health.

12 In patients with advanced cirrhosis, common hepatotoxins such as alcohol should be avoided. Medications such as paracetamol that require hepatic metabolism/clearance should also be substituted or dose reduced. This will prevent further strain and deterioration of remaining liver function. Vaccinations against hepatitis A and B should be encouraged if patients are not immune.

13 A high protein high caloric diet allows for maintenance of lean body mass and replacement of lost protein. Consider referral to a dietitian to optimise meal plans. Sodium restriction should also be encouraged to reduce fluid retention.

14 A TIPS procedure can be considered in patients with complicated portal hypertension and who are symptomatic with uncontrolled variceal bleeding or ascites. Under fluoroscopic guidance, a guidewire and sheath are inserted through the internal jugular vein in the neck and eventually into the hepatic vein. A needle is then pierced through the liver parenchyma into the portal vein to create a channel. An angioplasty balloon is inflated to maintain this tract and allows for a reduction in portal hypertension.

15 Liver transplantation remains the only cure for liver cirrhosis. The native liver is removed and replaced by a donor organ at specialised hospitals. Post-transplant immunosuppressive therapy will also be required to prevent organ rejection. Contraindications for liver transplantation include advanced HCC or liver metastases, uncontrolled viral hepatitis and active alcohol or substance abuse.

16 Antiviral medications for hepatitis C are highly recommended to prevent further deterioration of remaining liver function. Hepatitis genotyping is required to determine the most effective antiviral medication regimen. Chronic infections can now be cured in 95% of cases.

17 The risk of HCC is significantly increased in patients with cirrhosis and arises due to DNA alterations and mutations in cells that allow it to replicate uncontrollably. It is the most common complication of cirrhosis. Screening through blood tests and repeat ultrasound every 6 months is recommended. If detected, chemotherapy, percutaneous ablation, transarterial embolisation and/or surgical resection can be conducted. Liver transplantation should also be considered in patients with a single nodule.

18 Hepatorenal syndrome is a known complication of advanced liver disease with poor prognosis. Although its pathophysiology is not well understood, it is thought to be secondary to portal hypertension. The dilation of splanchnic vasculature reduces the circulatory volume and perfusion to the kidney. This activates the RAAS which causes vasoconstriction of renal vasculature. However, this effect is insufficient to counteract the mediators of vasodilation in the splanchnic circulation, leading to persistent renal hypoperfusion, aggravating kidney vasoconstriction and leading to eventual renal failure. Dialysis can prevent further deterioration of renal function; however, liver transplantation is the only definitive therapy.

CASE 25: GORD and oesophagitis

History

- A **60-year-old man** [1] presents to his GP with a 6-month history of **retrosternal burning chest pain** [2] that generally occurs **an hour after he consumes a large meal** [3].
- This is **exacerbated if he lies down** [4] and relieved slightly if he sits upright.
- Occasionally he feels extremely **nauseous** [5] and experiences some reflux which can cause him to **cough** [6].

- In the past few weeks, he has also been having **difficulty swallowing** [7] which can be uncomfortably **painful** [8] especially if food becomes stuck in his oesophagus.
- He denies recent **weight loss** [9] or changes in bowel habit and has not passed any **bloody stools** [10].
- He has a past medical history of chronic back pain which he treats with **diclofenac** [11].
- He drinks a **glass of wine with meals and smokes** [12] half a pack of cigarettes per day.

[1] Gastro-oesophageal reflux disease (GORD) affects up to 20% of the population and its prevalence is most likely higher due to the underreported nature of this disease. There is an increased incidence of GORD as age increases. There are no sex-related differences in prevalence although postmenopausal women are at higher risk of developing GORD because of the effects of oestrogen on gut motility. Hormone replacement therapy in perimenopausal woman has also been associated with GORD. Having first-degree relatives that suffer from GORD is also a risk factor.

[2] This is a cardinal symptom of GORD. The lower oesophageal sphincter (LOS) contains both smooth and skeletal muscles that contract and relax to allow food to pass from the oesophagus into the stomach. In individuals suffering from GORD, this sphincter may episodically relax, causing reflux of gastric contents into the oesophagus. As the stomach is highly acidic, patients will experience a burning sensation along the oesophagus which can cause sore throats and increased salivation as the body attempts to neutralise the gastric contents. Interestingly GORD can be divided into two further categories. One group typically experiences heartburn and reflux whilst the other tends to only experience chronic coughs.

[3] Eating large meals increases gastric distension, increasing pressure on the LOS and the risk of reflux. Patients are advised to eat smaller meals to reduce symptoms of GORD.

[4] Patients who sit upright after large meals are less likely to suffer from GORD due to the assistance of gravity in keeping gastric contents within the stomach.

[5] Repeated exposure of gastric contents to the oesophagus can cause reflux oesophagitis, waterbrash,

frequent coughing and burping. This can create nausea and in extreme cases, vomiting.

[6] The association of GORD with respiratory disorders such as bronchial asthma, laryngitis and nocturnal apnoea is well established. Aspiration of gastric contents into the airways can induce inflammation whilst activating the laryngopharyngeal reflex that induces coughing. This reflex helps to prevent exposure of the respiratory tract to gastric contents that may cause pneumonia.

[7] Chronic reflux can increase the risk of oesophageal stricture development, causing dysphagia and preventing normal peristaltic movement of food from the oesophagus into the stomach.

[8] Odynophagia is associated with severe oesophagitis, which is inflammation of the oesophagus. Patients with GORD are at an increased risk of reflux oesophagitis. Other causes of oesophagitis and their characteristics include:

- infectious: tends to occur in patients with immunodeficiency who are at risk of developing viral, fungal or bacterial infections; common pathogens include *Candida albicans*, cytomegalovirus and herpes simplex
- drug: related to medication use such as NSAIDs, antibiotics, potassium supplements, bisphosphonates and anticholinergics
- caustic: exposure to chemical fumes or swallowed toxins
- eosinophilic: autoimmune and associated with allergens and GORD.

[9] Weight loss coupled with chronic reflux, dysphagia, odynophagia and/or haematemesis are alarm symptoms which can indicate oesophageal metaplasia, otherwise

known as Barrett's oesophagus. In healthy individuals, the oesophageal mucosa is lined with stratified squamous epithelium. With repeated exposure to acid from GORD, this lining can abnormally change into simple columnar epithelium with interspersed column cells, the same cells present in the stomach. This premalignant change is associated with oesophageal adenocarcinoma.

10 Patients with GORD are often at risk of gastritis and peptic ulcer disease. This can cause melaena, especially in patients with actively bleeding ulcers.

11 Long-term NSAID and aspirin use is linked with several upper GI disorders such as gastritis, peptic ulcer disease

and GORD. The pathophysiology is most likely linked to its inhibition of cyclooxygenase (COX) enzymes which are crucial for gut protection. Other medications associated with GORD include anticholinergics, tetracycline antibiotics and vitamin supplements. Inappropriate bisphosphonate administration has also been associated with oesophagitis.

12 Behavioural factors such as alcohol consumption and smoking are risk factors for GORD. Alcohol can impair acid clearance in the stomach by reducing gut motility, increasing the risk of exposure of the distal oesophagus to gastric contents. Furthermore, alcohol stimulates gastrin secretion which increases acid production. Nicotine in cigarette smoke reduces LOS pressure and can exacerbate reflux.

Examination

- The patient is **obese** [1] but does not look systemically unwell and is **haemodynamically stable and afebrile** [2].
- Peripheral examination is unremarkable apart from some **nicotine staining** [3] on his fingers.
- Oral examination shows some **tooth enamel erosion, multiple mouth ulcers and halitosis** [4].
- His soft palate and **oropharynx are more erythematous** [5] than usual but there are no other significant findings.

- **Cardiac examination** [6] reveals no issues with dual heart sounds and no murmurs detected.
- Respiratory examination reveals a **hoarse voice** [7] and a **chronic dry and non-productive cough** [8]. His lung fields are clear, with good air entry and nil wheeze or stridor.
- GI exam is unremarkable although there is some epigastric tenderness on deep palpation. There is no organomegaly and normal **bowel sounds that radiate into the chest** [9].

1 Central obesity increases the pressure exerted between the abdomen and thorax, which can prevent optimal LOS functionality. This can also increase the likelihood of hiatal hernias, a protrusion of the stomach through the diaphragm into the thoracic cavity, which can exacerbate symptoms of reflux.

2 GORD is not a life-threatening illness. In cases of chronic reflux, acid may precipitate oesophagitis, increasing the risk of minor erosions to complete ulceration and/or dysplasia (as seen in Barrett's oesophagus). Alarm symptoms that may cause haemodynamic instability include anaemia, haematemesis, melaena and weight loss.

3 Patients who smoke are at risk of developing gastritis and GORD. Nicotine reduces LOS functionality and is also a gastric irritant.

4 Gastric contents are highly acidic, with a pH ranging from 2–6. When the acid encounters enamel, it can cause demineralisation, increasing the risk of erosions.

5 Refluxate can irritate the mucosa of the oropharynx, causing inflammation and hyperaemia of the highly vascular mucosa.

6 GORD can cause retrosternal chest pain. It is important to rule out cardiac red flags such as acute coronary syndrome (ACS), dissections, valvular heart disease and arrhythmias.

7 As reflux is highly acidic, it can irritate the larynx and vocal cords. This may cause local inflammation, resulting in a hoarse voice, frequent throat clearing and the sensation of a throat lump (globus sensation). This cluster of symptoms secondary to GORD is known as reflux laryngitis or laryngopharyngeal reflux.

8 GORD has been linked to chronic and nocturnal cough. Micro-aspiration of reflux contents means they enter the larynx, directly causing cough as a protective mechanism. Unless aspiration pneumonia occurs, patients with GORD are unlikely to have a productive cough.

9 These sounds may be transmitted due to a hiatal hernia.

Investigations

- The patient's **ECG and troponins** [1] are normal.
- **FBE, UEC and CMP** [2] are all within normal ranges.

- He was prescribed an 8-week **medication trial** [3] to see if his symptoms of GORD improve.

- If he continues to experience heartburn and GORD, he may require **endoscopic evaluation** [4].
- A **barium swallow** [5] would not provide as much information.

- If endoscopy reveals no mechanical or evidence of reflux oesophagitis, **ambulatory pH monitoring** [6] and/or **oesophageal manometry** [7] may be required.

[1] Troponins and ECG should always be done in patients presenting with chest pain, to rule out cardiac causes such as an ACS.

[2] Routine blood tests and biochemistry are generally normal in patients with GORD. Occasionally patients with bleeding from associated gastritis or peptic ulcer may have iron-deficiency anaemia, which warrants further investigation.

[3] A thorough history and examination is essential for a diagnosis of GORD. Patients are also trialled on therapeutic doses of PPIs. If symptoms of GORD improve then no further investigations are required.

[4] Endoscopy is only required:
- when a PPI trial fails to relieve symptoms of GORD, and an aetiological agent cannot be identified
- if patients experience alarm symptoms such as dysphagia, odynophagia, haematemesis, melaena, wheezing and weight loss
- prior to surgical intervention (discussed below)
- to monitor for complications of GORD.

Endoscopy should not be used as a first-line investigation due to its invasive nature. However, it can provide valuable macroscopic information, allowing visualisation of the oesophagus to the duodenum. Biopsies can also be taken to determine the aetiological agents, especially if fungal, viral or autoimmune causes are suspected. Histopathology will often demonstrate non-specific inflammatory changes such as lymphocytic and neutrophilic infiltration of the mucosal layer, oedema and metaplasia if patients are experiencing chronic reflux. Photographs and videos can also be taken during this investigation. This upper endoscopic technique is also used to grade severity of oesophagitis (Los Angeles classification) and to monitor complications of chronic reflux such as Barrett's oesophagus.

Grade (Los Angeles classification)	Characteristic
A	≥1 mucosal break <5mm in length
B	≥1 mucosal break <5mm in length but without continuity across mucosal folds
C	Mucosal breaks continuous between >2 mucosal folds, but involving <75% of the oesophageal circumference
D	Mucosal breaks involving >75% of the oesophageal circumference

[5] This technique involves ingestion of a contrast medium with concomitant X-rays to enhance visibility of the oesophageal tract. This allows for functional visualisation and can assist in diagnosing obstructive causes of dysphagia such as hiatus hernia, strictures and tumours as well as functional causes. Barium swallows are neither sensitive nor specific and therefore are not a good screening test for GORD.

[6] Oesophageal pH monitoring is considered the gold standard diagnostic technique as it provides objective information and is not subject to user bias. A small thin tube with a pH sensor tip is inserted through the nose and placed above the LOS. The end of the tube is attached to a portable recorder which monitors pH levels over 24–48 hours. The results are analysed and provide information regarding baseline pH status and the number of episodes of reflux.

[7] Oesophageal manometry is often combined with oesophageal pH monitoring and uses the same procedural technique. However, instead of pH it measures pressures along the oesophageal tract and can evaluate disorders of oesophageal motility.

Management

Short-term

The patient was advised to take an over-the-counter **antacid** [1] or **H$_2$ receptor antagonist** [2] for on-demand symptom relief as the **PPI** [3] would take a few days to take effect.

Long-term

Lifestyle modifications [4] were recommended to the patient to reduce symptoms of GORD. In the extreme case where pharmacological therapy was ineffective, **surgery** [5] may be required, especially if his hiatal hernia was a huge contributing factor. He was also recommended to visit his gastroenterologist yearly for consideration of **endoscopy** [6], especially if complications of GORD arose.

1 Antacids reduce stomach acidity and provide temporary relief from reflux. They come in tablet or liquid preparations and chemically neutralise gastric acid. Side-effects include diarrhoea (magnesium-based) and constipation (calcium or aluminium), and long-term use may cause kidney stones.

2 Histamine is released by enterochromaffin-like cells which stimulate H_2 receptors in gastric parietal cells to secret acid. H_2 receptor antagonists competitively bind and block this neuroendocrine signal and therefore reduce acid secretion. Like antacids, they provide only temporary relief and should be used in conjunction with a PPI during the acute period.

3 Proton pump inhibitors are considered the first-line treatment for patients with GORD and are used both diagnostically and therapeutically. Common PPIs include esomeprazole, pantoprazole and rabeprazole. All PPIs show equivalent efficacy and prescriptions are based on the prescriber preference. They are most effective in the post-prandial period and should be administered 30 minutes before meals. The proton pump in the parietal cell is directly responsible for secreting hydrogen ions into the gastric lumen. PPIs block this H^+/K^+ ATPase pump and therefore directly reduce acid secretion for up to 24 hours. Because PPIs have a short half-life, it takes about 2–3 days to reach steady state inhibition of acid secretion. Hence clinicians often prescribe a concurrent antacid or histamine antagonist during this interim period. The first course of treatment should take 1–2 months. If symptoms are adequately controlled, a step-down dose approach should be adopted. Clinicians should prescribe the lowest effective PPI dose, as it is associated with several side-effects and diseases and can interfere with the absorption of other medications (such as aspirin and clopidogrel). Common side-effects include nausea, diarrhoea, rash, abdominal cramping and rarely myopathies. Long-term PPI use has been associated with an increased risk of bone fractures, as PPIs reduce dietary calcium and magnesium absorption. Gastric acid is required for the breakdown of food and digestion of nutrients. Multiple studies have also linked chronic PPI use with *Clostridioides difficile* infections, spontaneous bacterial peritonitis, small intestinal bacterial overgrowth, interstitial nephritis, dementia and pneumonia. Therefore, the immunosuppressed and elderly should

be monitored accordingly to prevent any complications. Research is ongoing to determine the strength and causality of these relationships. If symptoms are not controlled after 2 months, check patient adherence and administration times. Patients who do not respond to high doses of PPIs should be referred to a gastroenterologist for further investigation.

4 Weight loss relieves abdominal pressure on the LOS and prevents reflux symptoms. Patients are encouraged to increase their level of physical activity whilst reducing their caloric intake. Eating healthily and decreasing intake of certain sugars will help sustain weight loss. Other lifestyle modifications such as smoking cessation, avoiding certain foods and beverages (chilli, caffeine, alcohol and acidic foods) may prevent triggering GORD. Other lifestyle modifications include elevation of the bed head and avoidance of meals 2 hours prior to sleep.

5 The Nissen fundoplication is the surgery of choice in patients with GORD, hiatal hernia and who have signs of microaspiration. The gastric fundus is wrapped and stitched around the LOS to reinforce its strength. The oesophageal hiatus is also repaired to prevent recurrence of hernia. When the stomach contracts, the newly strengthened LOS should hopefully be able to withstand the gastric pressures and prevent reflux of gastric contents into the oesophagus.

6 Patients presenting with alarm symptoms or untreated GORD are at risk of:
- oesophageal strictures: chronic reflux causes oesophagitis which is inflammation of the oesophagus. Prolonged mucosal oedema and inflammatory cell recruitment progressively leads to transmural inflammation. Fibrosis occurs, leading to the formation of oesophageal strictures. These are managed using stricture dilation or surgical excision of scar tissue.
- Barrett's oesophagus: chronic reflux leads to metaplastic changes in the oesophageal mucosa, increasing the risk of oesophageal adenocarcinoma. Barrett's oesophagus is monitored endoscopically, and biopsies taken can be categorised based on the level of dysplasia. High grade dysplasia and cancer will generally require resection and radiofrequency ablation. An oesophagectomy is indicated in extensive disease.

CASE 26: Hepatitis A, B and C

History

- A **45-year-old Vietnamese** [1] male is referred by his GP to the specialist hepatology clinic for persistently **deranged LFTs** [2].
- He reports he has been suffering from **chronic fatigue, myalgia and nausea** [3] since he was a young adult.
- Occasionally he notices that he passes **dark urine** [4], the whites of his **eyes turn yellow** [5] and his **skin becomes extremely itchy** [6]. These episodes occur when he is feeling run down.
- He travelled overseas to South Africa for work 2 months ago and engaged in **unprotected sexual intercourse** [7] with multiple partners. Overseas, he contracted gonorrhoea and chlamydia which were treated with antibiotics.
- A recent **HIV** [8] test was negative.
- He also suffered from bouts of diarrhoea and abdominal pain after **eating from a street vendor** [9] during his work trip.
- His past medical history is also significant for a left total knee replacement during his early 20s which required a **blood transfusion** [10].
- He denies any **IV drug use** [11] and does not consume **alcohol** [12].

[1] About 350 million people have hepatitis B globally, with highest prevalence in China, south-east Asia and throughout the African continent. Similarly, hepatitis C – with a global prevalence of approximately 150 million – is endemic to central and east Asia, North Africa and the Middle East. Both vertical and horizontal transmission are possible for both strains of the virus. The true incidence of viral hepatitis is likely to be higher, as most patients are asymptomatic. Disease prevalence is also higher in the prison population and in those who share needles.

[2] Many viral illnesses can cause liver function enzyme derangements during the acute phase of infection. When the hepatitis B virus (HBV) or hepatitis C virus (HCV) infects a hepatocyte, its viral DNA (or RNA in HCV) is incorporated into the host genome. As the immune system detects the viruses, it induces hepatocyte apoptosis to reduce its rate of replication. This causes the release of intracellular enzymes such as AST and ALT which can be measured in the patient's serum.
Viral hepatitis typically has marked elevations in AST and ALT with minimal to no elevation in ALP or GGT.

[3] Acute viral hepatitis typically follows four predictable phases:
- Incubation period: patients are generally asymptomatic in the immediate days after infection.
- Prodromal phase: non-specific, flu-like and constitutional symptoms such as anorexia, malaise, nausea and vomiting, myalgia and occasionally urticaria.
- Icteric phase: after 2 weeks, jaundice develops with darkening of urine. Patients may also develop abdominal discomfort.

- Recovery phase: between 2 and 4 weeks, jaundice slowly fades, with resolution of prodromal symptoms.
In some patients, acute infection can cause fulminant hepatic failure which requires intensive care admission and support.

[4] In acute hepatitis, hepatic metabolism and excretion of bilirubin is impaired due to cellular damage and necrosis. Bilirubin transport to the hepatocytes may also be mechanically obstructed by hepatocellular oedema secondary to acute inflammation. In long-standing viral hepatitis, cirrhosis may develop and cause a degree of obstructive jaundice. This causes an accumulation of unconjugated and conjugated bilirubin in the blood. When excreted by the kidney, this clinically manifests as dark amber-coloured urine.

[5] The presence of jaundice indicates an elevated bilirubin >3mg/dl. Bilirubin can be deposited in the conjunctival membrane of the eye, giving the appearance of yellow eyes.

[6] Intrahepatic disorders such as cholestasis of pregnancy, viral hepatitis and primary biliary cirrhosis can impair hepatic bile flow to the duodenum. Consequently, the accumulation of bile salts and bilirubin in a patient's plasma and tissues can cause pruritus.

[7] Several strains of viral hepatitis can cause hepatic injury, with hepatitis A, B and C the most well-known. The hepatitis B virus (HBV) is highly infectious and can be spread through sexual contact, sharing of needles, improperly screened blood transfusions and mother-to-child transmission. Hepatitis B can also be spread between family members who share toothbrushes. Similarly, the hepatitis C virus (HCV) is primarily a bloodborne virus and is spread through blood to

blood contact. Intravenous drug use is the most common form of transmission in the developed world, along with blood transfusions that are not screened thoroughly and needlestick injuries from patients who are HCV positive. Sexual transmission is uncommon, although those who engage in practices involving high levels of trauma (anal sex) are at greater risk. Mother-to-child transmission is also uncommon.

8 Patients with HIV have an increased risk of contracting viral hepatitis due to their reduced immunity. People who engage in risky sexual practices should be screened for sexually transmitted infections.

9 Transmission of the HAV is faecal–oral. Patients are at high risk when they consume contaminated food or water from eateries with poor hygiene practices. Infection with

hepatitis A is self-limiting, with eventual resolution. Hepatitis A is not known to cause chronic liver disease. Patients who are immunocompromised are, however, at risk of acute liver failure.

10 Blood products were not routinely screened for the hepatitis virus until the early 1990s. HBV was only discovered in the late 1960s and HCV in the late 1980s. Therefore prior to this era patients may have unknowingly contracted viral hepatitis through blood transfusions.

11 The risk of viral hepatitis transmission is significantly increased in patients who share intravenous needles.

12 Long-term alcoholism is a risk factor for the development of chronic liver disease, as it is a hepatotoxin. Alcohol can also precipitate acute hepatitis.

Examination

- The patient is **oriented to time and place** [1].
- He is a **lean male** [2], **haemodynamically stable and afebrile** [3].
- Peripheral examination reveals **palmar erythema** [4] and some track marks in his cubital fossa but is otherwise unremarkable.
- **Hepatic flap** [5] is negative.
- Facial examination reveals **scleral jaundice** [6] but no other findings.

- Neck and chest examination demonstrates some **spider naevi** [7] and **gynaecomastia** [8].
- On inspection of his abdomen, there is **no visible distension** [9] or **engorged vasculature** [10].
- Some **right upper quadrant tenderness** [11] is noted on palpation and his **liver is enlarged** [12] on percussion.
- His **liver edge is smooth with no nodules** [13] felt.
- There is **no other organomegaly** [14] and bowel sounds are normal and present.

1 Hepatic encephalopathy can occur in patients with acute liver failure or advanced liver disease. The liver plays a crucial role in metabolising nitrogenous compounds produced by intestinal flora. As hepatic function is reduced, these compounds, such as ammonia, accumulate in the systemic circulation where they can cross the blood–brain barrier and affect neurological function. Sedation may occur as ammonia can interact with GABA inhibitory receptors. Ammonia is also neurotoxic, causing cerebral oedema and inflammation. Other symptoms include poor memory and inattention.

2 Patients with a large BMI may also have concurrent fatty liver disease. There is an increasing incidence of patients with normal BMIs being diagnosed with fatty liver disease.

3 Unless decompensation of liver disease occurs, patients tend to be haemodynamically stable and afebrile. During the acute phase of viral hepatitis infection, patients may develop fever and tachycardia.

4 The liver converts oestradiol into testosterone. In patients with impaired hepatic function secondary to liver disease, oestradiol may accumulate. This increases vascularity

of the palm, causing palmar erythema.

5 Positive hepatic flap is caused by impairment of the diencephalic motor centres of the brain that control static muscle positioning. This can be secondary to accumulation of neurotoxins such as ammonia in acute liver failure or decompensated chronic liver disease.

6 Bilirubin can accumulate in the conjunctival membrane overlying the sclera. This causes yellowing of the eyes, also known as icterus.

7 Patients with viral hepatitis are at risk of developing chronic liver disease. As oestradiol accumulates due to the liver's inability to convert it to testosterone, it can cause sphincteric muscle failure of arterioles along the SVC distribution. This causes spider naevi which are vascular lesions that have outward radiating branches like a spider's web.

8 Long-standing chronic liver disease can cause derangements in free testosterone and oestrogen. This results in men developing gynaecomastia due to enlargement of glandular tissue.

9 Patients with long-standing untreated viral hepatitis are at risk of developing cirrhosis and subsequently portal hypertension. As fibrosis builds up within the liver, there is an increase in tissue resistance leading to increased portal venous pressures. This can result in the development of ascites with fluid sequestering in the abdominal cavity.

10 Portal hypertension in cirrhosis occurs as there is increased venous resistance in the portal venous system due to the replacement of normal liver tissue with fibrosis. When this pressure exceeds the systemic venous pressures, blood is shunted through portosystemic anastomosis such as the paraumbilical and oesophageal veins. In the abdomen, this causes dilation of superficial veins known as caput medusae.

11 As the liver becomes inflamed, it becomes engorged from immune cells and vascular flow, causing the liver capsule to stretch. This in turn also causes the overlying nerves to stretch. Consequently, patients with liver disease may often describe a dull, throbbing pain in the right upper quadrant of the abdomen.

12 Hepatomegaly is a non-specific sign and is due to inflammation secondary to vascular swelling and increased immune cell infiltration. In certain infiltrative liver diseases, it can also be due to deposition of compounds such as iron in haemochromatosis. Percussion can be used to map the size of the liver which is on average 7–10cm. Patients with moderate liver disease may have hepatomegaly. This can be confirmed with abdominal ultrasound or CT. In advanced liver disease and cirrhosis, the liver size reduces as normal parenchyma is replaced with fibrotic tissue.

13 The liver should not be palpable in healthy adults or patients with mild liver disease. Firmness and irregularity of the liver edge is often caused by cirrhosis as scar tissue is much firmer than normal parenchyma. Nodular edges may also be suspicious for neoplasms as it becomes infiltrated with cancerous cells.

14 In chronic liver disease, portal hypertension may lead to splenomegaly which can be detected on palpation of the left upper quadrant of the abdomen. This is due to congestion of blood due to increased portal venous pressures, leading to pooling of blood within this organ. Other causes of splenomegaly include haematological malignancies, infiltrative diseases, metastases, infections (EBV, CMV) or immune-mediated (rheumatoid, sarcoidosis, endocarditis).

Investigations

Pathology

- The patient's **FBE** [1] reveals a normocytic anaemia and thrombocytopenia.
- **LFTs** [2] are globally deranged with an elevated AST, ALT, bilirubin but normal ALP and GGT.
- His **INR** [3] is prolonged, **AFP** [4] is elevated and **hepatitis serology** [5] positive for multiple strains.

Imaging

- **Abdominal ultrasound** [6] reveals hepatomegaly which is later confirmed by **CT abdomen** [7].
- A **liver biopsy** [8] was not required as the aetiology of his liver disease was most likely viral hepatitis.
- On discharge, he would require annual **FibroScans** [9] to monitor the extent of his cirrhosis.

1 Patients with chronic liver disease frequently have haematological abnormalities. In advanced disease, anaemia can indicate GI haemorrhage. Splenomegaly due to portal hypertension can also lead to secondary haemolysis. There is intrasplenic destruction of erythrocytes, megakaryocyte and leucocyte precursors, resulting in pancytopenia. Anaemia and thrombocytopenia are also common in patients receiving active antiviral therapy for HCV, as it suppresses the production of red blood cells in the bone marrow and induces apoptosis.

2 In acute viral hepatitis, there are marked elevations in AST and ALT (typically around 400–500IU/L). ALT tends to be higher than AST; however, the sensitivity and specificity of ALT:AST for viral hepatitis is low and should only be used to measure disease activity and response to therapy. Values increase early in the prodromal phase, peak before jaundice is maximal, and fall slowly during the recovery phase. Patients with jaundice will also have elevated serum bilirubin.

3 The liver is responsible for the production of coagulation proteins. Coagulation proteins such as factors II, VII, IX and X are synthesised within hepatocytes and these four factors are dependent on vitamin K. Chronic liver disease may impair this synthetic function, causing prolonged INR.

4 Alpha-fetoprotein is a biomarker for hepatocellular carcinoma (HCC), testicular cancer and germ cell tumours. Elevated levels can also indicate acute liver disease without malignancy. It is not routinely used as a diagnostic or monitoring test but as an adjunct to imaging.

5 Diagnosis of viral hepatitis is confirmed by the presence of specific antigens, serum antibodies and viral load.
Hepatitis A
- Single-stranded RNA packaged in a protein shell. A positive IgG antibody test indicates the person had an HAV infection in the past or has been vaccinated. A positive IgM antibody indicates acute infection.

Hepatitis B

- Partially double-stranded DNA virus consisting of an outer lipid envelope and an inner core. The outer lipid layer contains proteins that assist in embedding and entry into hepatocytes. The inner core contains the virion which allows for replication within the host cell.
  - HBsAg: this surface antigen on the outer lipid envelope is the earliest indicator of acute infection and tends to peak 4–10 weeks after exposure. A positive result means the patient is potentially infectious. Patients who clear HBV will eventually have a negative HBsAg. Persistently detectable HBsAg beyond 6 months indicates chronic infection.
  - anti-HBs: the specific antibody to HBsAg. Its appearance months after onset of symptoms indicates clinical recovery and subsequent immunity to HBV. These antibodies also appear in patients who have been vaccinated against HBV.
  - anti-HBc: the specific antibody to the core antigen of the HBV. The presence of IgM identifies an early acute infection. In the absence of HBsAg and anti-HBs, interpretation is unclear and can indicate a resolved infection, false positive, low level chronic infection or resolving acute infection. IgG with no IgM may be present in chronic and resolved infections. If in doubt, further DNA testing can be considered.

Hepatitis C

- Small enveloped, single-stranded RNA virus which is divided into 6 main genotypes and multiple sub-types.
  - the most common test detects antibodies to HCV which are detectable approximately 6–8 weeks after infection. Patients with suppressed immune systems may take up to 6 months to create enough antibodies to be detectable. Interpretation of results should be made carefully, as once seroconverted, it will always remain positive. Positive HCV antibody tests can indicate the patient is either a chronic carrier (most common), has been infected but has resolved infection, or is recently infected. This test should then be followed up with HCV RNA test to determine whether the virus is present and the viral load. The negative predictive value of HCV antibody test result is very high. However, to account for the 6-month window period, people who engage in risky behaviours should be retested every year.

6 Abdominal ultrasound is often used to assess the degree of hepatomegaly and remains the first-line imaging modality as it is safe, cheap, non-invasive and readily available. It can also be used to assess for structural abnormalities and screen for cirrhosis and malignancy. Portal hypertension can also be diagnosed if patients have a dilated portal vein (>1.5cm) with a reduced blood flow on Doppler.

7 CT can be used to determine the size of the liver; common findings include extension of the inferior lobe of the liver into the pole of the right kidney. Nodules and scarring can also be assessed, although CT is not as sensitive compared to ultrasound for early cirrhosis.

8 Liver biopsy is not routinely done as it is invasive. In addition, only a small sample of liver is taken which can lead to incorrect diagnosis or disease staging due to sampling errors. It is only conducted if clinicians are unable to determine the definitive cause for the patient's liver disease. Liver biopsies may also be used to determine the severity of cirrhosis, although imaging techniques such as transient elastography (FibroScan) are preferred. Histopathology of liver biopsies infected with viral hepatitis tend to be non-specific, with:

- patchy cell dropout
- acidophilic hepatocellular necrosis
- mononuclear inflammatory infiltrate
- histologic evidence of regeneration
- preservation of the reticulin framework.

9 FibroScan is a relatively new non-invasive technique that assesses the stiffness of the liver via transient elastography. The patient lies supine and an ultrasound probe is placed over the RUQ of the abdomen. The probe generates a vibration wave and the device measures the velocity and time taken for the wave to travel through the liver (known as the shear wave). As cirrhotic tissue is harder than normal liver due to scarring, the degree of fibrosis can be inferred from the liver stiffness. Accurate readings are hard to obtain in patients who are obese or have ascites, due to technical limitations. Overall FibroScan is a quick and easy technique with no side-effects and an instantaneous result.

Management

Short-term

The patient was immediately started on an **antiviral therapy** [1]. He was advised to avoid **hepatotoxins** [2] such as alcohol and counselled on the dangers of IV drug use. A referral to a **dietitian** [3] was also made, to optimise his nutritional intake.

Long-term

He was also advised to regularly visit his GP and gastroenterologist for **hepatocellular carcinoma (HCC) surveillance** [4]. His family and friends who received HBV screening and tested negative were advised to be **vaccinated** [5]. In case of decompensation, he was also placed on the **liver transplant list** [6].

1 Hepatitis A is generally self-limiting and does not require antiviral therapy. Vaccination or previous exposure to HAV provides lifelong immunity.

For acute hepatitis B infections, treatment is generally supportive, and most adults clear the infection spontaneously. Patients who develop acute liver failure or are immunocompromised may be eligible for hepatitis B immunoglobulin-VF, a protein derived from donors that contains antibodies, after exposure. For patients who have chronic HBV infection, there are two classes of drugs used to suppress viral replication. The optimal timing and choice of treatment is extremely complex and relies on the patient's age, sex, viral load, ALT and degree of liver fibrosis.

Family	Examples	Advantages	Disadvantages
Interferon	Pegylated interferon alfa-2a	No viral resistance	Weekly subcutaneous injections, poor response in patients with HBV genotypes C or D or normal ALT Side-effects: influenza-like symptoms, anorexia, mood disturbance, thyroid dysfunction, bone marrow suppression
Nucleoside analogue	Tenofovir, entecavir	Oral dosing, well-tolerated	Risk of viral resistance if poor patient compliance, disease flare if therapy abruptly stopped Side-effects: renal impairment, osteoporosis (tenofovir)

Historically, pegylated interferon and ribavirin has been widely used as the mainstay therapy for chronic HCV infections, with varying levels of success due to lower cure rates and adverse side-effects. Ribavirin is associated with haemolytic anaemia and peg-interferon can cause bone marrow suppression.

Treatment for chronic HCV has changed dramatically with direct antiviral combination therapy and there remains a very limited role for pegylated interferon and ribavirin. These new regimens are extremely effective with a cure rate of at least 90%; they are well tolerated, have minimal side-effects and demonstrate effective responses within 3 months. Before therapy begins, it is important to identify HCV genotype as this will dictate the choice of medications. Commonly used medications are listed below:

Class	Examples
Protease inhibitor	Paritaprevir
Nucleotide polymerase inhibitor	Sofosbuvir
Non-nucleotide polymerase inhibitor	Dasabuvir
NS5A inhibitor	Ledipasvir, ombitasvir, elbasvir, pibrentasvir
NS3/4A inhibitor	Grazoprevir, glecaprevir

These are generally prescribed by specialists in the UK due to their costs. HCV RNA should be measured at baseline, at the end of treatment, and 12 weeks after the end of treatment to check for sustained virological response. Checking HCV RNA after 4 weeks of treatment may also be useful to check and reinforce adherence. No modifications to planned doses or duration of therapy should be made if HCV RNA is detected during the treatment course.

2 In patients with chronic liver disease, common hepatotoxins such as alcohol should be avoided. Medications such as paracetamol that require hepatic metabolism/clearance should also be substituted or dose reduced. This will prevent further insult to and deterioration of the remaining liver function.

3 A high protein, high caloric diet allows for maintenance of lean body mass and replacement of lost protein. Consider referral to a dietitian to optimise meal plans. Sodium restriction should also be encouraged in patients with chronic liver disease and ascites, to prevent fluid retention.

4 Chronic HBV and HCV is one of the leading causes of cirrhosis. HCC is the leading complication of cirrhosis. Regular ultrasound surveillance and repeat blood tests are recommended.

5 Vaccination against HBV is highly recommended for patients who are non-immune to HBV. It routinely forms part of the paediatric immunisation schedule. Vaccinations are given in three doses over six months. Testing for protective response is recommended, with a positive anti-HBsAg titre indicating successful vaccination. People with occupations that are at risk of exposure to blood and body fluids should also be vaccinated. Unlike HBV, there are no vaccines for HCV. Primary prevention aims to reduce risk of exposure, especially in high risk populations. These include free needle exchanges, safe disposal of sharps, promotion of condom use and comprehensive testing of donated blood for HBV and HCV.

6 Liver transplantation remains the only curative option for patients with hepatic cirrhosis. Patients with HCV are generally required to demonstrate virological clearance prior to transplantation. Post-transplant immunosuppressive therapy will also be required to prevent organ rejection. Contraindications for transplantation include advanced HCC, uncontrolled viral hepatitis and active alcohol/substance abuse.

CASE 27: Inflammatory bowel disease

History

- A **27-year-old Caucasian male** [1] has been referred to a gastroenterologist by his GP.
- He has been experiencing **abdominal cramping** [2] for the past month which has been unrelieved with antispasmodics and simple analgesia.
- This has been associated with **perianal discomfort** [3] and **loose stools** [4] **with occasional episodes of mucous and bloody diarrhoea** [5].
- He reports the feeling of **incomplete bowel evacuation and an increase in daily bowel motions** [6].
- Over the past month, he has also noticed **joint pain** [7], **some eye discomfort** [8] **and a skin nodule on his shin** [9].

- Although he is sleeping well, he feels more **fatigued and reports an unplanned 2kg weight loss** [10] over the past month.
- He has no past medical or surgical history and was previously fit and healthy and had a well-balanced diet. He does not take any **medications** [11], denies any recent **overseas travel or consumption of spoiled food or water** [12].
- His **grandfather** [13] also experiences similar symptoms and was diagnosed with **irritable bowel syndrome** [14].

1 The highest incidence of inflammatory bowel disease (IBD) occurs in cooler climates and in western areas such as Europe, Scandinavia and North America. Genetic studies have revealed Caucasians are at a higher risk of IBD than south Asians, east Asians and the African population. There are two peaks of onset; 15–40 years and 60–80 years of age.

2 The two main types of IBD, Crohn's disease (CD) and ulcerative colitis (UC), share similar symptoms. Abdominal cramping is a common complaint and is predominantly localised in the lower abdominal region. Visceral hypersensitivity in IBD is thought to be due to the upregulation of neurotrophin growth factor in response to enhanced production of inflammatory mediators in the colon wall.

3 Perianal discomfort tends to occur more with CD than UC and is a marker of severe disease. Transmural inflammation can cause fissures, swelling and ulceration, leading to an increased risk of fistulising disease. These can communicate with the bladder or vagina, causing significant pain, abscesses, discharge and restriction of sexual activity. Antibiotics are used to treat resulting perianal infections, along with surgical incision and drainage of abscesses and seton insertion to aid fistula healing.

4 The pathogenesis of IBD-associated diarrhoea is multifactorial and is an outcome of mucosal damage caused by persistent inflammation resulting in dysregulated intestinal ion transport, impaired epithelial barrier function and increased accessibility of the pathogens to the intestinal mucosa. Altered expression and/or function of epithelial ion transporters and channels is the principle cause of

electrolyte retention and water accumulation in the intestinal lumen, leading to diarrhoea in IBD. Aberrant barrier function further contributes to diarrhoea. Mucosal penetration of enteric pathogens promotes dysbiosis and exacerbates the underlying immune system, further perpetuating IBD-associated tissue damage and diarrhoea. Colonic inflammation also causes reduced GI transit time, limiting contact time of faecal material with colonic mucosa, reducing the rate of absorption of water and electrolytes.

5 Bloody and mucous diarrhoea tends to occur in UC where superficial ulcers along the colonic tract may bleed. Persistent bleeding can cause anaemia if left untreated.

6 Gut smooth muscles generate three types of contractions in the intestinal tract; rhythmic phasic contractions (RPCs), giant migrating contractions (GMCs) and retrograde giant contractions (RGCs). RPCs occur postprandially and in the interdigestive phase, mixing ingested meals and taking place in the stomach, small intestine and colon. GMCs propagate in the anal direction extremely quickly and over large distances spontaneously in the small intestine and colon. RGCs on the other hand originate in the mid small intestine and propagate in the oral direction. In IBD, the increased frequency of GMCs and suppression of RPCs produces frequent mass movements with distal propulsion of luminal contents. As the rectum senses increased matter, afferent signals are stimulated, generating the urge to defecate as well as causing relaxation of the internal anal sphincter. Strong GMCs can result in faecal incontinence and the number of unformed motions corresponds with colitis severity.

7 There are two main forms of IBD-associated arthritis: peripheral arthritis and axial arthritis. Peripheral arthritis can be oligoarticular or polyarticular, affecting limb joints including the elbows, wrists, knees, and ankles. This arthritis is non-deforming and non-erosive. Axial arthritis affects the sacroiliac and lumbar spine. Unlike peripheral arthritis, axial arthritis may cause permanent damage if the bones of the vertebral column fuse together—thereby creating decreased range of motion in the back. Other musculoskeletal manifestations of IBD include enthesitis (tendon insertion site inflammation), dactylitis (digit swelling) and arthralgia (joint pain without inflammation). IBD-associated arthritis is seronegative with negative rheumatoid factor. Up to 20% of patients with IBD will eventually develop a form of enteropathic arthritis. The link between intestinal and joint inflammation in IBD is not fully understood but genetics plays a role, with HLA-B27 strongly associated with both diseases.

8 Ocular complications of IBD tend to occur more frequently in CD than UC and include episcleritis, scleritis and uveitis. Episcleritis is the most common complication, where inflammation affects the highly vascular connective tissue between the sclera and conjunctiva. Scleritis affects the sclera of the eye, is associated with significant visual morbidity and has a bluish purple hue on examination. Finally, uveitis, grouped into anterior (iris), intermediate (vitreous) and posterior (retina) is an established complication and associated with HLA-B27. A common complaint of uveitis is light sensitivity, blurred vision and headache, and a characteristic ciliary flush is often seen on ophthalmic examination.

9 Skin manifestations of IBD affect up to one-third of patients with IBD and can be classified as specific, reactive and secondary to malnutrition. Specific skin manifestations share similar histopathology and include non-caseating granulomas and dermal infiltrates with multinucleated giant cells, lymphocytes, plasma cells and eosinophils. Reactive manifestations do not share the same histopathological findings of intestinal IBD. The most common lesions are erythema nodosum and pyoderma gangrenosum. Skin manifestations secondary to malnutrition result from malabsorption of vitamins and trace elements. These include stomatitis-glossitis-angular cheilitis (vitamin B12 and iron), scurvy (vitamin C), seborrhoeic dermatitis (vitamin E), bleeding, bruising and petechiae (vitamin K), hypopigmentation and nail abnormalities (amino acids, protein) and delayed wound healing (zinc).

10 Fatigue and weight loss can be a result of malnutrition and anaemia. Anaemia is the most common extraintestinal complication due to bleeding and malabsorption of iron and other vitamins and nutrients. Weight loss can also occur due to inadequate caloric intake, as patients with IBD may experience postprandial nausea and pain.

11 Pseudomembranous colitis must be suspected in all patients presenting with offensive diarrhoea with a recent history of antibiotic use. *Clostridioides difficile* normally resides in the intestinal tract. Antibiotics can disrupt normal healthy gut bacteria, leading to *C. difficile* overgrowth.

12 People who have recently travelled overseas to developing countries may experience viral or bacterial gastroenteritis. Enterotoxic *Escherichia coli* is the most common cause of infective diarrhoea, along with *Campylobacter*, *Salmonella*, and *Shigella*. Protozoal parasites such as Giardia, *Entamoeba histolytica*, and *Cryptosporidium* are infrequent causes of gastroenteritis but should be suspected if diarrhoea persists for more than a few weeks.

13 The risk of IBD is significantly higher among first-degree relatives, with up to 20% of patients with CD having a positive family history. This genetic component is well-recognised, and several genes such as *NOD2* are associated with CD.

14 Many patients with IBD are misdiagnosed with irritable bowel syndrome (IBS). This occurs because diarrhoea, abdominal cramping and pain are common to both illnesses and the specific symptoms for IBD – such as bloody stool and weight loss or fever – are absent in mild IBD. IBS remains a diagnosis of exclusion.

Examination

- The patient is **haemodynamically stable but has a fever of 37.6°C** [1].
- He has a low **BMI** [2] and appears **pale** [3], but no palmar or conjunctival pallor is noted.
- Oral examination reveals **multiple oral ulcers** [4] on his bottom lip.
- Limb examination identifies some **red nodules on his shin** [5].
- There is also some **wrist tenderness but no joint deformity** [6].
- His cardiac and respiratory exam is unremarkable. Abdominal examination notes some **tenderness** [7] on palpation in the central and right abdominal quadrants but is otherwise **soft with nil guarding or rigidity** [8].
- **Bowel sounds** [9] are highly active.
- Rectal examination reveals **multiple anal tags** [10] and increased **erythema and discharge** [11] near the anus.
- **PR exam is painful** [12] but no **bleeding or abnormal masses** [13] are felt in the rectal canal.

1 Patients with a clinical disease flare-up may have a low grade fever in mild to moderate colitis. A high grade fever only occurs in patients with severe colitis, a superimposed infection or toxic megacolon. Most patients are haemodynamically stable unless shock occurs. This may be due to sepsis or hypovolaemia from significant fluid losses.

2 Reduced caloric intake and increased nutritional requirements during active inflammation increase the risk of malnutrition and weight loss in patients.

3 Anaemia is a decrease in circulating haemoglobin in the body. Therefore, less oxygenated blood is visible through superficial layers of the skin such as the palm, oral mucosa and conjunctiva. Pallor is not a specific sign for IBD and is present in vasoconstrictive states such as sepsis or exposure to cold environments.

4 Oral manifestations of IBD tend to occur more in CD than UC (as it can affect the whole GI tract). Specific oral lesions include indurated mucosal tags, fissured swollen buccal mucosa and mucogingivitis. Secondary lesions such as recurrent aphthous ulcers, stomatitis, glossitis, cheilitis or perioral dermatitis may occur with deficiencies of B vitamin complex, albumin, iron, folate, zinc and/or other trace elements.

5 The most common reactive IBD-associated dermatological condition, erythema nodosum, is characterised by raised, tender, red subcutaneous nodules up to 5 cm in diameter on the anterior portion of the lower extremities. It is often associated with systemic symptoms of fevers and arthralgias and tends to erupt with disease flare-ups. The second most common cutaneous disease is pyoderma gangrenosum, which can occur all over the body but typically affects the leg and peristomal sites. Lesions often begin as pustules that rapidly ulcerate and form crater-like holes overlying pus-filled fistulous tracts.

6 Arthropathy is often seen in patients with long-standing IBD. The pathophysiology is not completely understood although current theories propose aberrant migration of intestinal immune cells from inflamed mucosa to the joint in genetically predisposed individuals. These macrophages may expose bacterial antigens that activate CD4+ T cells, causing the development of arthritis.

7 Abdominal tenderness is a common complaint in patients with IBD. Patients with CD may have abdominal tenderness in all regions, depending on the section of the intestinal tract affected. Those with UC are tender in the central and left lower abdominal region, as it affects the rectum upwards and tends to be confined to the colon.

8 Patients will not have guarding unless peritonitis occurs. This tends to occur more frequently in UC than CD as toxic megacolon predisposes to intestinal perforation and translocation of intestinal bacteria into the peritoneum. Toxic megacolon is characterised by non-obstructive colonic dilation and systemic toxicity and should be considered in patients with significant abdominal distension, acute or chronic diarrhoea and abdominal pain. CT abdominal findings tend to identify a dilated colon >6cm, multiple air-fluid levels and deep mucosal ulcerations between large pseudo-polypoid projections extending into the colonic lumen.

9 Hyperactive bowel sounds are non-specific and can be heard in early obstruction or any condition which increases gut motility, such as gastroenteritis. Hypoactive bowel sounds indicate diminished bowel motility and may be due to peritonitis, ileus or late bowel obstruction. Absent bowel sounds after 5 minutes generally indicates very late intestinal obstruction, which necessitates immediate intervention.

10 Anal tags are noted in one-third of all patients with CD. They are raised painless fleshy growths that occur secondary to lymphatic obstruction from intestinal inflammation. They are generally not excised.

11 Erythema and discharge near the anus can indicate the presence of an abscess or fistula. An acute swelling, induration and fluctuation may be noted and gentle pressure on any visible tract may elicit purulent discharge. Antibiotics and surgery may be necessary to prevent perianal sepsis.

12 Perianal disease is a recognised complication of IBD and incorporates multiple conditions such as abscesses, fistulas, skin tags and fissures. Anal fissures in IBD are either due to direct ulceration from the disease process itself or secondary to increased internal sphincter pressure from increased bowel motions. Fissures are painful but are relieved with topical analgesics.

13 UC is associated with an increased risk of colon cancer. This must be ruled out in all patients with a palpable mass on PR examination.

Investigations

- The patient's pathology investigations reveal a **mild microcytic anaemia** [1] and an **elevated CRP and ESR** [2].
- **Low ferritin and transferrin saturation** [3] and **vitamin B12** [4] are also noted.
- **Stool culture polymerase chain reaction (PCR)** [5] is negative for *E. coli* and *C. difficile*; however, **faecal calprotectin** [6] is extremely elevated.

- Abdominal X-ray showed **no significant pathology** [7]; however, **CT abdomen enterography** [8] reveals some bowel wall thickening and increased attenuation of mesenteric fat.

- A decision was made to book a **colonoscopy** [9] the following week where **biopsies** [10] would be taken and sent off for histological analysis.

1 A full blood examination may show anaemia secondary to a chronic disease process or elemental/nutrient deficiency. A low MCV and MCHC is suggestive of iron deficiency, while a high MCV indicates likely B12/folate deficiency.

2 C-reactive protein (CRP) is an acute phase protein produced by hepatocytes in response to circulating pro-inflammatory cytokines. Although CRP is elevated in IBD, higher values are typically seen in CD, due to its transmural inflammation, than in UC where inflammation is confined to the mucosa. ESR indirectly measures the rate at which red blood cells (RBCs) migrate through the plasma. When inflammation is present, factors such as fibrinogen cause RBCs to clump and settle quicker. This protein peaks later and more slowly relative to CRP but is useful as a measure of long-term inflammation. Both CRP and ESR are useful for confirming IBD, although normal values do not exclude the presence of inflammation.

3 Iron studies are valuable to determine the presence of iron deficiency. A low ferritin with low saturation indicates iron deficiency. Note that ferritin may also be elevated in active IBD flare-up, as it is an acute inflammatory protein.

4 Vitamin B12 is absorbed in the small bowel. In CD, active inflammation can contribute to malabsorption, especially in children. In patients with a low normal serum B12 level, further testing for serum homocysteine or methylmalonic acid can be used to confirm the diagnosis.

5 Stool culture is only used to rule out infective causes of diarrhoea. This test should not be routine unless patients have recently returned from overseas and there is persistent diarrhoea for longer than 1 week.

6 In the presence of inflammation, neutrophils are chemoattracted to the site of injury and engage in respiratory burst to degranulate and release antimicrobial enzymes. During this process, a protein known as calprotectin is also released. Therefore, its utility is to distinguish between IBD and non-inflammatory diseases such as IBS. This biomarker is simple, reliable and non-invasive and provides a quantitative measure of intestinal neutrophil activity. Faecal calprotectin is not disease-specific for IBD and should only be used to supplement endoscopy or serve as a screening test. False positives may occur with recent consumption of alcohol or concurrent NSAID use. Research into the use of faecal calprotectin to monitor response to treatment and predict clinical disease flare-ups remains ongoing.

7 Abdominal X-ray is generally the first-line modality used in patients with generalised abdominal pain as it is quick and cheap. Complications of IBD such as colonic dilation (suggesting toxic megacolon), perforation, obstruction or ileus may be visible. Barium enemas are rarely used unless other radiographic techniques such as CT scans are not available, as they can only be used in mild disease and may precipitate toxic megacolon. Ultrasound is rarely used unless biliary diseases are also suspected.

8 CT enterography (CTE) is a modified abdominopelvic CT examination which involves consumption of oral contrast along with IV contrast to enhance and maximise detection of small bowel pathology. In younger patients, abdominal MRI is recommended over CT to reduce radiation exposure. Mural enhancement and bowel wall thickening (due to oedema and engorgement of vasa recta) are commonly identified in CTE. In UC, these tend to occur in the rectum upwards, whilst in CD they tend to occur in the small bowel. Strictures may also be observed in patients with long-standing CD and in some cases, fistulas can be visualised as linear, enhancing tracts with or without communication with adjacent structures.

9 Endoscopy remains the gold standard diagnostic technique. It allows macroscopic visualisation of the GI tract and can assess disease severity, monitor response to medications and screen for dysplasia and other complications. Colonoscopy should be considered in all patients suspected to have IBD, although it is contraindicated if there is severe disease or toxic megacolon. CD under endoscopic evaluation reveals classic skip lesions, with areas of normal mucosa interspersed with inflamed regions. UC has continuous inflammation, and is generally localised in the colon distal to the splenic flexure. Proctitis may also be visible.

10 Histopathological analysis of biopsies can also distinguish between CD and UC. Specimens should be obtained from multiple locations including normal and diseased mucosa. Features of chronic inflammation include architectural disruption, increased inflammatory cell infiltrate into the lamina propria and plasmacytosis. The presence of non-caseating granulomas in the lamina propria suggests CD, although its presence is not pathognomonic.

Management

Short-term

The patient was diagnosed with active Crohn's disease and was screened for **several infections** [1]. He was given several **inactivated vaccinations** [2]. Subsequently, he was commenced on high dose **steroids** [3] and carefully monitored for response. As his disease was refractory to corticosteroid induction, he was prescribed another **immunomodulator** [4]. A **one-off serum thiopurine methyltransferase (TPMT) polymorphism test and weekly blood tests** [5] were required during the first month of therapy and every fortnight after that. He was also advised to seek **dietary counselling** [6] to correct any nutritional deficits. **Bone protection** [7] through pharmacological and non-pharmacological means was also recommended.

Long-term

After 3 months of immunotherapy, his private gastroenterologist repeated a colonoscopy and noted fistulising disease. He was switched to **infliximab** [8] infusions every 2 months. He was also referred to a **colorectal surgeon** [9] to optimise fistula healing. **Antibiotics** [10] were prescribed in preparation for surgery. He was also required to undergo endoscopic **surveillance** [11] for colorectal cancer for the rest of his life. He was alo warned that diseased segments that do not respond to pharmacological therapy and are severely scarred may require **surgery** [12]. A referral to a **psychologist** [13] was also made to optimise his mental health.

[1] Patients who are about to receive immunomodulatory medications must be screened for previous immunisation status or natural immunity to vaccine-preventable diseases such as diphtheria, tetanus, polio, pertussis, hepatitis B and varicella zoster. Evidence of immunity can also be elicited through immunological testing for specific antibodies. As immunomodulatory medications reduce the activity of the immune system, reactivation of latent infections can have serious health implications. Patients need to have a chest X-ray and interferon gamma release assays to rule out latent pulmonary TB.

[2] Live vaccinations (measles, mumps, rubella (MMR), varicella zoster, Bacillus Calmette–Guérin (BCG), rotavirus, oral typhoid, oral poliomyelitis) should be avoided in patients who have commenced immunomodulatory therapy, due to the risk of disease development. Instead all live vaccinations should be given 1 month prior to starting immunomodulatory therapy. Inactivated vaccinations can be given at any time.

[3] High dose steroids such as prednisolone are used to manage active IBD. Once a clinical response is achieved, prednisolone should be slowly weaned, as high dose corticosteroids can suppress adrenal function. Patients with severe colitis may require hydrocortisone or methylprednisolone intravenously and should be monitored as an inpatient in hospital. Long-term use should be avoided due to increased risk of osteoporosis and Cushing's syndrome. In patients who remain on high dose prednisolone (20mg equivalent) for more than a month, chemoprophylaxis against *Pneumocystis jirovecii* should be considered. In UC, if colitis is limited to the rectum, oral administration and enemas of

5-aminosalicylates (mesalazine) may also assist in inducing disease remission and symptom resolution.

[4] In patients with IBD who do not tolerate steroids, or whose disease is refractory to initial therapy, stronger immunomodulators such as azathioprine, mercaptopurine or methotrexate can be used.

Medication	Mechanism of action	Side-effects
Azathioprine	Purine synthesis inhibitor leading to reduced DNA and RNA production in white blood cells	*Common*: nausea, skin sensitivity/rashes, liver enzyme derangement *Rare*: hepatitis, anaemia, neutropenia, pancreatitis, increased risk of infections and cancer
Mercaptopurine	Interferes with white blood cell RNA and DNA synthesis	
Methotrexate	Folate antagonist leading to reduced T- and B-cell regulation and synthesis	*Common*: flu-like symptoms, mouth sores *Rare*: neutropenia, hepatitis, pulmonary fibrosis

[5] The enzyme TPMT is needed to metabolise immunomodulator medications such as azathioprine and mercaptopurine. Patients lacking this enzyme are at risk of increased drug-induced bone marrow suppression.

FBE, UEC and LFT should be performed regularly as immunomodulators can cause liver enzyme derangements, anaemia and leucopenia, which increase the risk of infections and cancer.

6 During an IBD flare-up, weight loss is common due to decreased appetite and increased nutritional requirement. A high energy protein diet rich in vitamins and minerals is recommended, along with increased fluid intake to offset fluid losses from diarrhoea. A low residue diet can also reduce stool output. Oral nutritional supplementation is also recommended. In cases of severe IBD, enteral feeding may be necessary. During disease remission, patients should also avoid specific foods that can trigger abdominal pain. Nutritional deficits such as iron-deficiency anaemia are common in IBD and therefore patients are encouraged to consume iron-rich foods daily or seek vitamin supplementation. Incorporation of omega-3 fatty acids is also recommended due to their anti-inflammatory effect. Adequate serum vitamin D levels are also essential for bone health. There is insufficient evidence to recommend pre- and probiotics and further research is needed to determine their effectiveness. Fermentable oligo-, di-, mono-saccharides and polyols (FODMAP) diets may also benefit patients with concurrent IBS and IBD.

7 Patients with IBD are at an increased risk of osteoporosis due to poor nutritional intake and as a side-effect of their medications. Corticosteroids reduce calcium absorption in the gut, stimulate osteoclast activity and increase urinary calcium excretion. Active inflammation also disrupts bone metabolism, with disease gut mucosa unable to adequately absorb nutrients, notably vitamin D. Patients should be counselled to avoid alcohol and smoking, partake in weight-bearing exercise and consider calcium and vitamin D supplementation. An endocrinologist may assist in optimising osteoporosis therapy.

8 Patients who do not respond to the above therapy after 3 months may require a specific immune inhibitor such as infliximab or adalimumab (anti-TNF) or vedolizumab (anti-integrin antibody). These medications require specialist monitoring.

9 Colorectal surgeons can assist in patients with fistulising disease. Perianal abscesses accompany fistulas and require incision and drainage. Seton placement also encourages drainage without closure of the fistula tract, limits recurrent abscess formation and increases the effectiveness of pharmacological therapy. The duration of seton placement is not clear and is practitioner-dependent. After resolution of perianal infection and start of IBD remission, surgeons may conduct a fistulotomy, where overlying tissue surrounding the tract is divided and the base curetted to allow the wound to naturally close through secondary healing. Alternatively, glue containing fibrinogen and thrombin may be injected to fill the tract to induce clot formation and seal the fistula.

10 Antibiotics should be considered in patients with active perianal fistulas to prevent sepsis. Metronidazole or ciprofloxacin are commonly used as they target anaerobes and Gram-negative enteric bacteria, respectively. However, long-term use is associated with an increased risk of *C. difficile* infection, especially in patients on immunosuppressive therapy.

11 Patients with long-standing IBD are at an increased risk of colonic dysplasia and cancer. The regularity of routine colonoscopies depends on the patient's extent of colitis, family history, age of onset and whether structures are present. Most guidelines recommend screening to commence no later than 8 years after symptom onset, with repeat colonoscopy every 2–3 years.

12 Surgery is indicated in patients with IBD when pharmacological therapy is ineffective at controlling symptoms or mechanical complications arise (strictures, obstructions, bleeding, fistulas or perforation). Strictures can be treated through strictureplasty, although multiple disease segments may require a resection. In CD ileocaecal resections may be necessary, as the terminal ileum is often severely diseased. In UC a colectomy of the affected segment is generally curative; however, patients will require education and ongoing care to manage a stoma.

13 All patients with chronic diseases are well-recognised to be at risk for psychological issues such as anxiety and depression. In IBD, psychological morbidity has a poor prognostic factor, reducing independent activity and quality of life. Young patients with IBD may be disadvantaged, especially if their disease impairs day-to-day activity.

CASE 28: Non-alcoholic fatty liver disease

History

- A **56-year-old morbidly obese** [1] **male** [2] is referred to a hepatologist following multiple blood tests showing **liver enzyme derangements** [3].
- He is otherwise **asymptomatic except for lethargy** [4].
- His past medical history is significant for **hypertension, hypercholesterolaemia and type 2 diabetes mellitus** [5].
- He has poor medication compliance but has been prescribed multiple medications. He also remembers receiving some **vaccinations** [6] to protect his liver a few years ago.

- **Family history** [7] is significant for metabolic syndrome but no **genetic disorders** [8].
- A nutritional history reveals **poor dietary choices** [9], with fast food consumed daily.
- There is a lack of fresh fruit and vegetables in his diet and he consumes large quantities of **soft drink** [10] daily.
- He does not drink **alcohol** [11], smoke or use any **intravenous drugs** [12].
- He rarely engages in **physical activity** [13] and has a **sedentary lifestyle** [14].

[1] The peak prevalence of non-alcoholic fatty liver disease (NAFLD) in men and women is noted to be between 50 and 60 years of age, with a general trend of increasing prevalence with age. Indeed, 25% of the general population in the western world suffers from NAFLD. The prevalence is increased in T2DM (70%) and morbid obesity (90%). Once thought to be a disease of the developed world, NAFLD and in its most severe form, non-alcoholic steatohepatitis (NASH), has become increasingly common in developing countries that are industrialising. This has been attributed to the adoption of a calorie-dense westernised diet.

[2] Gender differences exist, with premenopausal women at a reduced risk of NAFLD compared with men. After menopause, there is a comparable prevalence of NAFLD in men and women, leading many researchers to postulate the protective effect of oestrogen.

[3] It is estimated that one in four individuals has NAFLD, with many unaware due to the asymptomatic nature of this disease. NAFLD and NASH are the most common cause of chronic liver enzyme derangements. ALT is in the hepatocellular cytosol; AST is mostly within the mitochondria and GGT within the cell membranes of the biliary tract. AST, ALT and GGT are most commonly elevated in NAFLD/NASH. In the absence of any causative agents such as hepatotoxins, viruses or genetic disorders that affect the liver, further investigation and referral to a hepatologist are warranted.

[4] Most patients with NAFLD are asymptomatic. NAFLD is often an incidental finding in patients who are being reviewed for other metabolic diseases such as diabetes mellitus, hypertension and hyperlipidaemia. NAFLD exists as a spectrum, with its most severe form being NASH. Until its

conversion to NASH or cirrhosis, fatigue is the most common complaint. Very rarely do patients have specific symptoms such as the stigmata of liver disease (palmar erythema, hepatic flap, spider naevi) or symptoms of decompensation (jaundice, ascites, oedema, GI bleeding and encephalopathy). Fatigue may also be related to obstructive sleep apnoea, which is extremely common in obese patients.

[5] The metabolic syndrome is a cluster of diseases that increases the risk of cardiovascular disease, stroke and diabetes mellitus. Patients must have at least three of the five following medical conditions: central obesity, hypertension, impaired glucose tolerance, elevated triglycerides and low levels of high density lipoprotein (HDL). NAFLD is considered the hepatic manifestation of the metabolic syndrome. Insulin resistance promotes adipose tissue lipolysis, allowing free fatty acids to deposit in the liver, leading to steatosis.

[6] Apart from NAFLD/NASH, other common causes of chronic liver disease include alcoholism and viral hepatitis (HBV and HCV). Hepatitis B is a vaccine-preventable disease.

[7] Family history plays an important role for the development of NAFLD/NASH, with robust evidence demonstrating strong heritability for this disease and its associated comorbidities such as T2DM. Although its inheritance pattern is unknown, several genes as well as environmental factors are implicated in its pathogenesis.

[8] Genetic diseases such as haemochromatosis and alpha-1 antitrypsin deficiency can also cause hepatic injury.

[9] Poor dietary intake is one of the main perpetrators in the pathogenesis of NAFLD/NASH. Common foods in the western diet (processed sugars and fat, refined grains, soft drinks

and confectionery) can cause rapidly increased postprandial plasma glucose and insulin levels. This leads to increased *de novo* lipogenesis, one of the main contributors to hepatic steatosis. The western diet is also low in fibre. Diets high in fruits and vegetables are protective against NAFLD/NASH due to their high fibre content, phytochemicals and antioxidants. Fibre helps to normalise and maintain blood glucose fluctuations, while phytochemicals and antioxidants are anti-inflammatory compounds that prevent the conversion of simple steatosis to steatohepatitis. The type of fat consumed also influences fatty acid synthesis and insulin sensitivity. Multiple studies have shown that an increased intake of trans fats leads not only to poorer cardiac health but increased lipid peroxidation in the liver.

10 Numerous animal models of NAFLD and NASH have shown the importance of fructose in the pathogenesis of this disease. Fructose has been demonstrated to:
- promote *de novo* lipogenesis in the liver, resulting in hepatic steatosis
- induce oxidative stress, which is a necessary step to initiate hepatic inflammation
- impair normal hepatic fatty acid oxidation
- alter intestinal microbiota, with growing evidence to support the role of microflora in the pathogenesis of NAFLD.

The mechanisms through which fructose and NAFLD are linked are complex but its association is well-established.

11 Alcohol remains one of the leading causes of chronic liver disease in the developed world. Its mechanism of injury is complex and multifactorial. Like NAFLD, chronic alcohol consumption can also cause hepatic steatosis and chronic liver injury. When ethanol is enzymatically broken down, it forms acetaldehyde which is a direct hepatotoxin. It is toxic to mitochondria in the hepatocyte, causing oxidative stress and promoting cell death. The metabolism of alcohol also induces the production of NADH, a cofactor that promotes steatosis by stimulating the synthesis of fatty acids and opposing their oxidation.

12 Several strains of viral hepatitis can also cause chronic liver disease (HBV and HCV). HBV is highly infectious and can be spread through sexual contact, sharing of needles, improperly screened blood transfusions and mother-to-child transmission. Similarly, the hepatitis C virus (HCV) is primarily a bloodborne virus and spread through blood to blood contact. Intravenous drug use is the most common form of transmission in the developed world. It is important to screen for these infections when taking a history.

13 Prior to the advent of the modern world, humans expended significant energy gathering food to meet their nutritional intake. This has meant our physiology is well adapted to storing excess nutrients for times of famine. However, in modern times minimal physical activity is required to obtain our caloric load. Physical inactivity has been associated with reduced insulin sensitivity, increased visceral and peripheral fat deposition, and an increase in free fatty acid uptake by the liver. This predisposes to hepatic steatosis and the development of NAFLD/NASH.

14 Sedentary time is defined as lengthy periods of inactivity and minimal movement, such as in television watching, sleeping or sitting. Sitting for prolonged periods reduces cumulative energy expenditure produced by muscle contractions during movement and impairs the exercise/muscle contraction-stimulated uptake of glucose from the circulation and lipoprotein lipase activity, thus hampering fat handling. This can compound the detrimental effects caused by a lack of exercise, as mentioned above, leading to an increased risk of NAFLD/NASH.

Examination

- The patient is **morbidly obese and weighs 230kg** [1].
- He is calm, alert and **oriented to time and place** [2] but is slightly **tachypnoeic** [3].
- Apart from some mild **hypertension** [4], he is haemodynamically stable and afebrile.
- Peripheral examination reveals **palmar erythema** [5] and some **darkened patches** of **skin in his axilla** [6] but is otherwise unremarkable.
- **Hepatic flap** [7] and **scleral jaundice** [8] are not observed.

- Chest examination reveals **gynaecomastia** [9] and **spider naevi** [10] along with an increased work of breathing. Cardiac and respiratory sounds are normal.
- He has significant abdominal girth and no **caput medusae** [11] are visible.
- Deep abdominal palpation elicits minor **right upper quadrant tenderness and hepatomegaly** [12] with a smooth **liver edge** [13].
- There is no other **organomegaly** [14] and bowel sounds are present and normal.

1 Although obesity is objectively defined using BMI, several studies note the importance of fat distribution in the development of the metabolic syndrome. Notably, truncal or central obesity has been strongly implicated in the development of other cardiovascular and metabolic diseases. An estimated 90% of morbidly obese patients have NAFLD.

2 When patients with NASH cirrhosis decompensate, they can present with complications of portal hypertension, such as varices and ascites. Hepatic encephalopathy is also a hallmark feature, caused by the accumulation of nitrogenous compounds in the brain secondary to impaired hepatic clearance. This causes confusion and impaired memory and concentration.

3 Obese individuals tend to have a rapid, shallow breathing pattern, predominantly due to mechanical factors. There is a reduction in respiratory compliance due to increased weight on the thoracic cage and abdomen, associated with the accumulation of fat. Severe obesity can lead to obesity-hypoventilation syndrome and sleep apnoea overlap with decreased responsiveness to oxygen and CO_2, accompanied by alterations in respiratory muscle function.

4 Hypertension is a component of the metabolic syndrome.

5 Palmar erythema is associated with chronic liver diseases such as NAFLD/NASH. As the damaged liver is unable to metabolise oestradiol, this accumulates in the blood, causing increased vascularisation of surface hand capillaries.

6 Acanthosis nigricans is a dermatological condition characterised by hyperpigmentation and hyperkeratosis of skin, particularly in skin fold regions such as the groin, back of the neck and axilla. It is related to insulin resistance, with increased circulating insulin activating receptors responsible for keratinocyte and dermal fibroblast proliferation. The prevalence of NAFLD in patients with T2DM is approximately 70%.

7 Hepatic flap can be indicative of hepatic

encephalopathy. The damaged liver is unable to break down toxic ammonia into urea for excretion, causing it to accumulate in the brain. It is believed this affects the diencephalic motor centres of the brain which maintain the full extension of elbow and wrist.

8 Elevated bilirubin can manifest clinically as scleral jaundice. In NASH, hepatocyte death reduces the liver's ability to metabolise and excrete bilirubin, leading to an accumulation of unconjugated bilirubin in the blood.

9 The accumulation of oestradiol in male patients with cirrhosis causes the development of female body characteristics. There is proliferation of glandular tissue in the breast, causing gynaecomastia.

10 Elevated oestrogen levels, as seen in patients with advanced liver disease, are thought to be responsible for these vascular lesions. They are characterised by a central red spot with reddish extensions like a spider's web. Its pathogenesis is not well understood but stems from failure of the sphincteric muscle around the arteriole. Spider naevi are also found on pregnant women.

11 Caput medusae tend to only occur in decompensated liver disease. Portal hypertension causes the dilation of superficial epigastric veins that radiate from the umbilicus across the abdomen.

12 Abdominal examination is generally unremarkable. Some patients may complain of RUQ tenderness due to hepatomegaly, which can cause stretching of the capsule enclosing the liver parenchyma.

13 Patients with NAFLD/NASH tend to have smooth enlarged livers due to the accumulation of fat within the parenchyma. It is extremely unusual for the liver edge to be hard or nodular unless there was cirrhosis or an underlying malignancy.

14 Other features of hepatic decompensation include ascites, oedema and splenomegaly which can cause abdominal distension.

Investigations

Pathology

- The patient's FBE and biochemistry are normal. His **liver function tests** [1] demonstrate an elevated ALT, AST and GGT but no changes in ALP.
- His **albumin and bilirubin** [2] are not elevated.
- **Fasting cholesterol and lipids** [3] are elevated and **fasting blood sugar is deranged** [4].
- **Hepatitis screen, iron studies and antinuclear antibodies (ANA)** [5] are normal.

Imaging

- As NAFLD was clinically suspected, a **liver ultrasound** [6] was ordered to confirm the clinician's diagnosis.
- A follow-up **CT scan or MRI** [7] or **liver biopsy** [8] would be considered if the ultrasound findings were not definitive.
- **Transient elastography** [9] could be used to measure the degree of liver fibrosis.

1 There are no specific blood tests to diagnose NAFLD/NASH. As patients are asymptomatic, this disease is often incidentally diagnosed during health screens. LFTs are typically deranged, with a mild elevation in ALT and AST and an ALT/AST ratio of approximately 1 to 1.5, depending on the level of fibrosis. Occasionally there is minor elevation in GGT, especially if cholestasis is involved.

2 When NASH progresses to advanced liver disease and cirrhosis, complications such as portal hypertension and synthetic dysfunction can occur. This leads to hypoalbuminaemia as the liver is one of the main producers, and hyperbilirubinaemia due to reduced ability to metabolise and excrete this by-product. Thrombocytopenia and a prolonged INR may also be observed.

3 Dyslipidaemia is a common finding in NAFLD/NASH.

4 Fasting blood glucose tends to be deranged, as insulin resistance is a key component of NAFLD/NASH.

5 Patients with abnormal LFTs should also be investigated for other aetiological agents. These include alcohol excess, viral hepatitis, autoimmune liver disease, haemochromatosis, coeliac disease and Wilson's disease.

6 Ultrasound should be the first-line investigation for suspected NAFLD as it provides extensive information regarding fatty infiltration and size, and can screen for suspicious nodules. It is cheap, easily accessible, safe and effective in diagnosing established steatosis. However, it is unreliable with mild steatosis and therefore a negative result on ultrasound does not rule out NAFLD. Findings include diffuse hyperechoic liver with an increased echotexture relative to the renal cortex or spleen due to increased fatty infiltration. There may also be poor delineation of the intrahepatic architecture.

7 Non-contrast CT or MRI abdomen is not commonly used unless ultrasonography is unavailable or there is diagnostic uncertainty. Common findings include diffuse, low density hepatic parenchyma. Hepatomegaly may also be detected. MRI has been shown to most accurately detect lower levels of steatosis than those detected by US and CT.

8 Liver biopsy is not frequently used to diagnose NAFLD although it is considered the gold standard diagnostic technique. The histological spectrum of NAFLD ranges from simple steatosis through steatohepatitis to fibrosis and cirrhosis. It also allows for the staging of disease and can provide prognostic information, therefore influencing management. Characteristic findings on histopathology include:

- macro- and microvesicular steatosis resulting from the accumulation of triglycerides within hepatocytes
- hepatocyte ballooning with lobular inflammation and necrosis
- periportal fibrosis in NASH.

9 Transient elastography (FibroScan) is a relatively new and non-invasive method for assessing liver fibrosis. It uses ultrasound-based technology to measure the velocity and time for a vibration to travel through the liver. As cirrhotic tissue is harder than normal liver due to scarring, the degree of fibrosis can be inferred from the liver stiffness. Although it is not used as a diagnostic investigation, it is useful as an adjunct to assess for cirrhosis and monitor for disease progression.

Management

Lifestyle

The patient was advised to **reduce his caloric intake** [1] and seek advice from a **dietitian** [2] for a modified diet **high in omega-3 fats** [3] which are **minimally processed**, and **low in high fructose corn syrup** [4] . He was also encouraged to engage in **physical exercise** [5] and counselled to **abstain from alcohol** [6] . **Coffee consumption** [7] was encouraged due to its protective role in liver disease.

Medication

There are **no specific medications for NAFLD/NASH** [8] and instead **vitamin E** [9] was recommended to the patient. **Associated comorbidities** [10] such as diabetes mellitus, hypercholesterolaemia and hypertension were also treated accordingly.

Surgical

Failing lifestyle modifications, the patient would be recommended to undergo **bariatric surgery** [11] . He would also be **monitored regularly** [12] due to the increased risk of complications. If he developed liver cirrhosis, he would be placed on the waiting list for **liver transplantation** [13] .

1 The goal of NAFLD therapy is to prevent further disease progression to cirrhosis, reverse steatosis and fibrosis and improve other components of the metabolic syndrome. The first-line option involves dietary changes. Weight loss tends to occur when there is a negative caloric balance, which can be achieved through a reduction in energy intake and an increase in energy expenditure. Patients are counselled to reduce their high glycaemic index carbohydrates whilst increasing their protein and fibre intake. This has been shown to improve satiety. Interestingly, research has shown that snacking, a common feature in the westernised world, independently contributes to hepatic steatosis. There is a global consensus that gradual weight reduction achieved through dietary restriction leads to improved inflammatory markers, liver enzymes, hepatic inflammation and fibrosis in obese patients with chronic liver disease. It is important to note, however, that adherence to lifestyle interventions is poor, with many patients eventually regaining their lost weight.

2 Dietitians play an important role in optimising the patient's health. Treatment of NAFLD/NASH involves an MDT and dietitians play the most important role. They can provide nutritional guidance, develop diets to optimise weight loss and educate patients on how to maintain long-term weight loss.

3 Research has shown that diets high in omega-unsaturated fatty acids improve insulin sensitivity, reduce hepatic steatosis and inflammation. Omega-3 is an inhibitor of hepatic lipogenesis and improves dyslipidaemia. It can also activate peroxisome proliferator-activated receptor alpha, which in turn stimulates fatty acid oxidation.

4 Dietitians also recommend a reduction in processed and high fructose products. Advanced glycation end products are formed during the digestion of processed foods and have been linked to the development of metabolic disorders. Such foods have also been positively associated with insulin resistance and a reduction in the protective hormone adiponectin.

5 Increasing physical activity with exercise assists in weight loss by increasing energy expenditure. Research has also shown that exercise may aid in the reduction of hepatic steatosis, prevent progression to cirrhosis, and improve both metabolic and cardiovascular health. Physical activity is a cheap and easy intervention with therapeutic and preventive value. Exercise regimens should be tailored based on patients' preferences and likelihood of continuation in the long term. The beneficial effects of exercise on NAFLD are multifactorial:
- improved appetite control by enhancing satiety signalling
- reduction in circulating free fatty acids due to increases in the uptake and utilisation by the liver and skeletal muscle, leading to subsequently reduced hepatic fat accumulation
- improved hepatic and muscle insulin resistance through a reduction in hepatic fat content and an increase in muscle glucose transporter expression and muscle glycogen synthase activity.

6 As part of minimising ongoing liver damage, patients diagnosed with NAFLD are counselled to avoid hepatotoxins such as alcohol.

7 Coffee drinking has been linked to a reduced risk of decompensation in advanced liver disease and the development of hepatocellular carcinoma (HCC). Although research is still in its infancy, the hepatoprotective effects of coffee may be linked to caffeine and the multiple polyphenols from the coffee bean itself. Chlorogenic acid, a coffee polyphenol, has been shown to inhibit hepatic stellate cells *in vitro*, the main cell responsible for fibrosis.

8 There are no pharmacological agents that directly target NAFLD/NASH and no therapies can reverse histological fibrosis.

9 High dose vitamin E is an antioxidant that has been shown to have some benefit in reducing inflammation in NAFLD/NASH. Furthermore, vitamin E has been shown to break down lipids and exert anti-atherogenic activities.

10 Although there are no direct therapies for NAFLD, other components of the metabolic syndrome should be targeted. Insulin resistance can be treated with sensitisers such as metformin. In addition, metformin has been shown to cause weight loss but has no effect on NAFLD/NASH histology. On the other hand, there are some improvements in histological scores and liver enzymes in patients treated with thiazolidinediones. Their benefits, however, are offset by their multiple side-effects and therefore they are not routinely used. Hypertension should be controlled with antihypertensives to prevent cardiovascular mortality, and dyslipidaemia with statins to reduce the risk of coronary artery disease.

11 Bariatric surgery is highly recommended in morbidly obese individuals who have failed an adequate exercise and diet programme and suffer from an obesity-related comorbid condition. Multiple procedures are involved, the most common being gastric banding or sleeve gastrectomy, which reduces the capacity of the stomach. This physically limits caloric intake and helps to supplement weight loss. Bariatric surgery has been shown to drastically improve weight loss and address concurrent hypertension, diabetes and hypertriglyceridaemia. For patients with NAFLD/NASH there is significant improvement in steatohepatitis and fibrosis.

12 Patients who develop NASH have an increased risk of HCC development, which is further compounded if it transitions to cirrhosis.

13 Liver transplantation remains the only cure for patients that develop cirrhosis. However, this is limited by shortages in donor livers. There are multiple contraindications for liver transplantation including advanced HCC, uncontrolled viral hepatitis and active alcohol or substance abuse.

CASE 29:   Oesophageal achalasia

History

- A **66-year-old Caucasian male** [1] has been admitted under the respiratory team for treatment of **aspiration pneumonia** [2].
- The gastroenterology team has been providing consultation following reports that he has been suffering from increasing **dysphagia** [3] over the past year.
- He recounts **no previous history** [4] of swallowing difficulties.
- However, he now has issues swallowing **both solids and liquids** [5].
- Sometimes **food gets stuck in his oesophagus** [6] and he has occasional episodes of **regurgitation** [7].

- He also suffers from **nocturnal reflux** [8] and can wake up with immense coughing fits.
- Other symptoms include **heartburn** [9] and some **mild unplanned weight loss** [10] over the past 6 months.
- He denies any **haematemesis, coffee ground vomit** [11], changes in bowel habit or melaena.
- He reports his **grandfather** [12] also suffered from a similar disease that affected his swallowing.
- He is otherwise healthy with no past medical history, has not travelled to **South America** [13] and is not aware of any **genetic disorders** [14].

[1] There is equal frequency of achalasia in men and women, with the mean age of diagnosis between 50 and 60 years of age. No ethnic differences have been noted in developed nations.

[2] Respiratory complications are a common cause of hospitalisations for patients with achalasia, especially in the young and the elderly. This is due to aspiration of food and liquids that occurs due to impaired peristalsis. Chemical pneumonitis may also occur if gastric contents contain acid.

[3] Oesophageal peristalsis and relaxation of the lower oesophageal sphincter (LOS) are coordinated by a network of myenteric neurons of the enteric nervous system. Its activity is modulated by the vagus nerve from the CNS. The neurons that control motility and peristalsis are in a plexus between the circular and longitudinal smooth muscle layers of the oesophagus. Inhibitory neurons in this complex use nitrous oxide and vasoactive intestinal peptide as neurotransmitters and lead to muscle relaxation. Excitatory neurons, meanwhile, use acetylcholine as a neurotransmitter and enable muscles to contract. In achalasia, these inhibitory neurons are damaged or absent, leading to impaired swallowing.

[4] The aetiology of idiopathic (primary) achalasia involves inflammatory-mediated destruction of Auerbach plexus, inhibitory neurons that control oesophageal peristalsis and relaxation of the LOS. No single trigger has been identified and instead multiple factors, including viruses, autoimmunity and neurodegeneration, most likely contribute to its aetiology.

[5] In the initial stages of oesophageal achalasia, patients describe having difficulty swallowing solids. Individuals often develop positional strategies to increase intrathoracic pressure to overcome the increased lower oesophageal sphincter pressure, allowing the transmission of food from the oesophagus to their stomach. Such manoeuvres include raising their arms, standing up straight during mealtimes and arching their neck backwards. As the disease progresses and more myenteric neurons are destroyed, the ability of the oesophagus to push liquids is also impaired.

[6] As peristalsis is impaired, food can get stuck along the oesophageal tract, leading to this sensation. This may also cause retrosternal chest pain.

[7] Retention of food and liquids in the oesophagus occurs when the tract becomes dilated. Patients are at risk of regurgitation when in a supine position, as there is no assistance of gravity.

[8] Patients often regurgitate undigested food or saliva in their sleep. This can cause patients to wake up coughing and choking from their aspirate.

[9] Heartburn is a common complaint and is commonly reported in patients with achalasia. The mechanism for chest pain is unclear and is most likely multifactorial. This includes secondary or tertiary oesophageal contractions, oesophageal distension by retained food, and oesophageal irritation by retained medications and food, and by bacterial or fungal overgrowth. Oesophagitis may also contribute to chest pain. Interestingly, younger patients tend to experience chest pain

more frequently. As patients get older, their chest pain tends to resolve, suggesting increasing neurodegeneration leads to reduced sensitivity to oesophageal pain.

10 As patients are unable to consume enough calories, mild weight loss is common. A thorough history and investigation should also rule out other sinister causes of dysphagia, such as thyroid disorders or oesophageal malignancy. Cancer is an important cause of secondary achalasia and induces symptoms through three main mechanisms:
- direct mechanical obstruction of the distal oesophagus
- infiltration of the LOS by neoplastic cells can disrupt the myenteric neurons and cause reduced peristalsis and increased tone
- paraneoplastic syndrome, where tumours express a neuronal antigen which the host's immunity targets, causing reactions in parts of the enteric nervous system; this is commonly observed in small cell lung cancer.

11 Patients with haematemesis are unlikely to have idiopathic achalasia. They should instead be investigated for peptic ulcer disease and oesophageal or gastric cancer.

12 There is a weak association between family history and risk of developing oesophageal achalasia. Multiple case series note familial achalasia is horizontally transmitted due to consanguineous relationship, suggesting an autosomal recessive inheritance. Further genetic research is necessary to elicit this relationship.

13 The parasite *Trypanosoma cruzi* is endemic to regions of Central and South America and Mexico and can result in Chagas' disease. Individuals develop a chronic oesophageal infection which can manifest as achalasia many years after initial infection. Antibodies directed at targets within the myenteric plexus have been demonstrated in patients with Chagas' disease and achalasia.

14 Triple-A syndrome is a genetic disorder characterised by alacrima (difficulty producing tears), adrenocorticotrophic hormone-resistant adrenal insufficiency and achalasia. Pathological studies have demonstrated absence of ganglion cells in the oesophagus as well as atrophy resulting in achalasia.

Examination

- The patient is **haemodynamically stable and afebrile** [1] and receiving **IV fluids and antibiotics** [2]. He is alert and oriented, with no respiratory distress.
- He looks slightly **underweight** [3] for his height but is not cachectic. Peripheral examination is unremarkable, and his pulse is strong and regular.
- Oral inspection reveals some **mouth ulcers** [4] and **candidiasis** [5].
- There are **no neck swellings or protrusions** [6] noted and his trachea is midline.
- **Chest examination** [7] is normal with dual heart sounds and no detectable murmurs.
- Respiratory auscultation notes some **minor right lower basal crepitations** [8]. His abdomen is soft and non-tender with no masses noted on palpation.

1 Patients with achalasia and no resultant complications usually do not have any clinical signs. However, patients with aspiration pneumonitis or pneumonia may be febrile, tachycardic and tachypnoeic.

2 Aspiration pneumonia is a common complication of achalasia due to recurrent regurgitation of food and aspiration into the lungs. IV fluids assist in maintaining hydration and replacing lost electrolytes. Antibiotics help to target bacteria that are causing the respiratory infection.

3 Physical examination of patients with achalasia is usually remarkable for weight loss due to reduced caloric intake. Patients may have smaller body habitus, sunken cheeks and peripheral muscle wastage, depending on the extent of weight loss.

4 Oral ulcers are common in patients with achalasia and are a result of nutritional deficiencies such as vitamin B complex.

5 Oral candidiasis is a common finding in patients with advanced achalasia. This opportunistic infection is caused by overgrowth of *Candida* spp. Stasis of food and saliva can lead to oesophagitis, a reduction in local immunity and eventually fungal overgrowth.

6 Neck swellings, if large enough, can physically impair swallowing and breathing in some patients. This may be secondary to thyroid disorders such as a goitre, malignancy, enlarged lymph nodes or a pharyngeal pouch. It is important to conduct a thorough examination to rule out these differentials.

7 Cardiac examination is done to rule out other causes of chest pain including valvular heart disease, structural heart disease or arrhythmias.

8 The right middle and lower lung lobes are the most common sites where aspiration pneumonia occurs, as the right bronchus is larger and has a more vertical orientation. These areas of consolidation can lead to crepitations during auscultation and percussion dullness.

Investigations

- FBE shows a **microcytic hypochromic anaemia** [1] with his iron studies also noting an increased transferrin level.
- **CRP and ferritin are elevated** [2].
- The patient's **biochemistry panel** [3] is normal; however, his **nutritional screen** [4] demonstrates multiple vitamin deficiencies.
- **Oesophageal manometry** [5] would also be conducted over the following days to confirm achalasia.

- A **timed barium swallow** [6] was also ordered to confirm this diagnosis.
- As he had suffered recent weight loss, he was also booked in for a **gastroscopy** [7] to exclude an oesophageal malignancy.
- If a suspected lesion was detected, a **biopsy** [8] would be taken and a **CT neck, chest and abdomen** [9] would be ordered to assess for infiltration and metastases.

1 Patients with long-term achalasia will have a reduced caloric intake. Iron deficiency is commonly detected, resulting in a microcytic hypochromic anaemia.

2 These are markers of inflammation and will be elevated during the acute phase of inflammation/infection – in this case, aspiration pneumonia. In contrast, in absence of concurrent inflammation/infection, a typical iron-deficiency picture shows low ferritin and transferrin saturation levels.

3 Achalasia does not have a direct effect on kidney or liver function tests.

4 As there is a reduction in intake, many patients will experience nutritional deficits such as vitamin B complex, folate, iron, vitamin C and essential elements such as zinc.

5 Oesophageal manometry is considered the gold standard diagnostic investigation as it is highly sensitive. A catheter with pressure sensors is introduced into the oesophageal tract to measure the varying pressures. Data collected can be used to create a topographic map and allow classification of the types of achalasia according to the pattern of oesophageal peristalsis (see table below):

Type	Characteristics	Integrated relaxation pressure (IRP)	Response to therapy
Normal	Normotensive, propulsive peristalsis	≤15mmHg	n/a
1	No evidence of oesophageal pressurisation, pan-oesophageal pressure generation <20%, peristalsis absent	>15mmHg	good
2	Pan-oesophageal pressurisation ≥20%, peristalsis absent	>15mmHg	very good
3	Peristalsis absent, >2 spastic contractions	>15mmHg	poor

6 Barium swallow will show the characteristic 'bird beak' appearance at the gastro-oesophageal junction with a dilated oesophageal tract. A timed barium swallow can also assess the degree of peristalsis, with poor emptying into the stomach indicative of severe disease. Radiology is not necessarily diagnostic as it is less sensitive than manometry. However, this investigation remains important to rule out other causes of obstruction, pharyngeal pouches or structural abnormalities and to estimate the diameter of the oesophagus. An additional role for barium swallow is to provide objective assessment of oesophageal emptying after therapy.

7 The primary goal of endoscopy is to exclude anatomical lesions and malignancies as the cause of achalasia. Any mechanical obstruction can mimic the features of achalasia on manometry with impaired LOS relaxation and abnormal peristalsis or spastic contractions. During the early stages of achalasia, endoscopy is less sensitive than manometry. Advanced disease, however, will often show a dilated oesophagus with retained food and increased resistance at the gastro-oesophageal junction. A classic pop may be felt when the endoscope passes into the stomach. Endoscopic ultrasonography with biopsies can also be considered to rule out cancer or other infiltrative diseases. Endoscopy can also assess for GORD post achalasia therapy.

8 A biopsy of suspected malignancy may show metaplasia. Biopsies are not routinely taken if no lesions are observed. However, histopathological analysis of oesophageal achalasia specifically demonstrates significant infiltration of cytotoxic lymphocytes, evidence of complement activation within myenteric ganglia and ganglionitis. In advanced disease there may be an absence of myenteric ganglion cells.

9 In older patients with profound weight loss, CT is a useful subsequent investigation to exclude gastro-oesophageal infiltration by invading malignancy. Asymmetrical thickening on CT may suggest pseudo achalasia.

Management

- During his inpatient stay, the patient would be referred to a **speech pathologist** [1] for education on several lifestyle modifications along with dietitian input to **optimise nutrition** [2].
- After discharge, he would be eligible for an outpatient **pneumatic dilation** [3] to treat his achalasia.
- If this failed, a surgical **myotomy** [4] would be considered.
- While he is on the waiting list, **pharmacological agents** [5] could be trialled.

- Patients who fail both surgical and conventional medical therapies would require **botulinum toxin injections** [6] to relieve oesophageal sphincter tone.
- A **gastrostomy** [7] or **oesophagectomy** [8] would be the last option if his achalasia continues to progress.
- Regardless of the treatment chosen, the patient would be regularly **monitored** [9] for the rest of his life.
- He would also require ongoing **oesophageal cancer** [10] surveillance.

1 Patients with achalasia will need to be educated on the importance of eating slowly and chewing their food very well to prevent stasis and regurgitation of food in the oesophageal tract. Drinking water during meals and positional changes such as upright sitting during eating will also assist in transition of food. Patients are also advised to avoid eating before bedtime, to reduce the risk of regurgitation and aspiration.

2 Even in mild–moderate achalasia, nutrition is generally affected, but if dietary modifications are followed, loss of weight and malnutrition can be easily prevented. Along with adequate chewing, dysphagia diets should be highly individualised, including modification of food texture or fluid viscosity. Food may be chopped, minced or puréed, and fluids may be thickened and fortified with extra minerals and vitamins. This should be done in conjunction with a speech pathologist.

3 Pneumatic dilation is considered the first-line therapy for oesophageal achalasia. After a prolonged fast (to prevent accumulation of food and liquids in the oesophageal tract), a preliminary endoscopy is performed to assess the anatomy of the gastro-oesophageal junction and the cardia, and to screen for any lesions. Subsequently, a plastic pneumatic cylindrical balloon mounted on an endoscope is introduced into the oesophageal tract until it reaches the LOS. Using a guide wire, the balloon is inserted until its waist is within the sphincter. The balloon is then slowly inflated to forcefully stretch the sphincter, held in place for a minute and then deflated. This disrupts the oesophageal sphincter muscle fibres, assisting in the transition of food and liquids. The

smallest balloon is generally used and subsequent dilations with larger balloons over the next few weeks are only necessary if symptoms are not relieved or there are no improvements on objective measurements from manometry. The patient is observed for the next 5–6 hours to assess for complications, such as perforation. Other complications include haematomas and chronic retrosternal chest pain. Some patients may also experience GORD due to the stretched LOS.

Pneumatic dilation provides excellent symptomatic relief in up to 90% of patients; however, one-third will eventually have a relapse within 5–10 years. Long-term remission can be achieved by repeat dilation. Contraindications for pneumatic dilation include poor cardiopulmonary status or other comorbid illnesses that would prevent surgery should an oesophageal perforation occur.

4 A Heller myotomy involves a lengthwise transection along the oesophagus, starting from the LOS and extending into the stomach. The inner mucosal layer is preserved, as only the muscular layers are causing compression. This procedure can be done laparoscopically, using an open thoracoscopic technique or through a per-oral endoscopic approach.

Due to the disruption of the LOS, reflux is a common side-effect. Therefore, upper GIT surgeons tend to offer a concurrent fundoplication. Both pneumatic dilation and a myotomy have comparative success rates; however, a myotomy is generally better tolerated in younger patients. Success is also determined by how straight the patient's oesophagus is, as tortuosities in the distal part result in more difficult myotomies. Patients with type 3 achalasia respond better to myotomy than medical or dilation therapy. Recurrent symptoms after Heller myotomy can be safely treated with pneumodilation or, if such conservative treatment fails, by repeat laparoscopic Heller myotomy.

5 All pharmacological agents aim to lower the resting pressure of the LOS; however, they are generally the least effective mode of therapy. Commonly prescribed medications include calcium channel blockers (nifedipine) or nitrates (isosorbide dinitrate). Nifedipine taken sublingually an hour before meals inhibits LOS contraction by blocking cellular calcium uptake and lowers resting oesophageal resting pressure. Nitrates similarly relax the LOS through dephosphorylation of the myosin light chain. Nitrates have been shown to be more effective than calcium channel blockers but are less tolerated. This is attributed to their multiple side-effects including headaches, hypotension and tachyphylaxis. Patients may also develop tolerance to nitrates with long-term use. Therefore they are generally only prescribed on an as-needed basis pending definitive surgical therapy.

6 The current pathophysiological theory surrounding achalasia revolves around loss of myenteric inhibitory neurons, resulting in unopposed excitation of the LOS. Botulinum toxin (Botox) is a potent inhibitor of acetylcholine release and has been widely used in diseases with similar mechanisms, such as sphincter of Oddi dysfunction and gastroparesis. Therefore, injection of this neurotoxin into the LOS can attenuate increased tone and allow it to relax. Endoscopic injections of botulinum toxin are reserved for patients who are poor responders to conventional medical and surgical therapies. Injections are very effective although symptomatic relief is only temporary, with repeat injections every 6 months highly recommended. Common side-effects include episodic reflux and, very rarely, neuromuscular blockade. As Botox causes surrounding inflammation,

multiple and repeat injections can increase the risk of fibrosis which can interfere with the success of subsequent surgery if this is required.

7 In some patients, oral intake is often not adequate even in the absence of significant swallowing difficulties. If a patient is unable to eat or drink or the risk of pulmonary aspiration is high, enteral feeding should be provided. This can be done through a nasal feeding tube or through the insertion of a percutaneous gastrostomy tube. Both options are effective, with gastrostomy tubes generally more comfortable for patients. Long-term complications include tube obstruction and wound infection.

8 In patients with late and end-stage achalasia, oesophageal resection might be necessary to improve quality of life. The risk of needing oesophagectomy is higher if the oesophagus is already markedly dilated >4cm after the first invasive intervention.

9 Most patients receive immediate symptomatic relief with a return to near-normal swallowing and improved quality of life. Patients must be reminded to swallow only when sitting upright to prevent aspiration of gastric contents. Many patients eventually relapse and will require intermittent top-up procedures. Patients should be monitored annually with either a timed barium swallow or oesophageal manometry.

10 Accumulation of food and saliva can occur with suboptimal therapy. This can result in bacterial growth and chemical irritation due to decomposition, resulting in oesophagitis. This significantly increases the risk of dysplasia, and eventually malignant transformation of oesophageal epithelial cells. Because dysphagia is also a common symptom for oesophageal carcinoma, its diagnosis is often delayed as it is frequently attributed to exacerbation or recurrence of achalasia. Therefore, an endoscopic surveillance programme should be initiated for early detection of cancer.

CASE 30: Peptic ulcer disease

History

- A **55-year-old** [1] **refugee** [2] presents to his GP complaining of long-standing **epigastric pain** [3] that **occurs after meals** [4].
- The pain is typically dull and gnawing in nature and is **relieved with antacids** [5].
- Sometimes at **night, he is also woken up by the same pain** [6].
- Associated symptoms include **reflux, nausea and halitosis** [7].
- Recently, he has been feeling more bloated than usual and his **bowel motions have become increasingly offensive and darker** [8]. He denies vomiting or **haematemesis** [9] and has not had any recent weight loss.
- Apart from regular **ibuprofen** [10] for back pain, he takes no other regular **medications** [11].
- He is otherwise fit and healthy and is not under any recent **stress** [12].
- Other family members have similar episodes of **abdominal discomfort** [13].

1 Peptic ulcer disease (PUD) incorporates gastric and duodenal ulcers. The incidence of PUD increases with age, with gastric ulcers peaking in the 5th to 7th decades and duodenal ulcers in the 4th to 5th decades. There are no gender differences in prevalence. In the developed world, the incidence of *Helicobacter pylori*-induced peptic ulcers has been slowly decreasing due to improvements in hygiene and therapy. NSAID-induced ulcers, however, have been increasing due to their widespread use.

2 The bacterium *Helicobacter pylori* is the major cause of peptic ulcer disease. *H. pylori* infection is more prevalent in developing nations or populations with a lower socioeconomic status. Density of living, lack of sanitation and low hygiene levels all contribute to an increased risk of infection. Transmission generally occurs between cohabiting family members and, given the bacteria live in the gastric mucosa, ingestion through gastro–oral, oral–oral or faecal–oral routes are the most likely. Interestingly, half the world's population is infected with *H. pylori* yet only 5% develop ulcers.
The pathophysiology of *H. pylori* is not well understood but involves a combination of genetic, environmental and immunological factors. In gastric ulcers, *H. pylori* infection with concurrent inflammation degrades gastric mucin, causing epithelial cell death by disrupting tight junctions between cells throughout the stomach. In duodenal ulcers, *H. pylori* impairs somatostatin secretion and consequently increases gastrin release, leading to gastric acid hypersecretion.

3 The stomach and first part of the duodenum is embryologically derived from the foregut. The visceral afferent nerves from this section are non-specific and overlap with somatic afferent nerves. Therefore, the visceral pain distribution follows the distribution of the somatic afferent nerves, and in the case of peptic ulcers, between the T5–T9 dermatomes. Other causes of epigastric pain that should be considered include GORD, malignancy, abdominal aortic aneurysm, pancreatitis, functional dyspepsia, cardiac disease and pleurisy. A thorough history and examination will help distinguish between these diseases.

4 Although not well understood, the timing of epigastric pain may help distinguish the location of the ulcer. Post-prandial pain is associated with gastric ulcers, as gastric acid production is increased as food enters the stomach. This causes further inflammation and corrosion of the wound.

5 *H. pylori* can induce hyperchlorhydria, which exacerbates mucosal inflammation. Antacids provide rapid symptomatic relief as they neutralise stomach acids. H_2 histamine antagonists also provide temporary relief, as they inhibit gastric parietal cells from secreting acid.

6 Nocturnal or fasting pain is associated with duodenal ulcers. The pyloric sphincter is open during the fasting state, allowing a small amount of stomach acid to flow through to the duodenum. During digestion, this valve is closed to enhance chyme formation and therefore prevents stomach acid from reaching the duodenum.

7 Dyspepsia, nausea and halitosis are common non-specific symptoms of PUD. Other symptoms include weight loss and abdominal bloating.

8 Melaena is black tarry stool that results from degradation of blood in the GI tract. It is extremely offensive due to the enzymatic digestion of haemoglobin by enzymes and intestinal bacteria. The most common cause of melaena is PUD, although tumours must also be ruled out. Actively bleeding ulcers are at risk of perforation, characterised by sudden-onset intense abdominal pain, and are a medical emergency.

9 Haematemesis indicates an upper GI bleed. This can occur in severe PUD where there is erosion of the gastric mucosa into an underlying artery. Duodenal ulcers can erode the gastroduodenal artery, while gastric ulcers can affect branches of the left gastric artery. Patients with persistent haematemesis are at risk of hypovolaemic shock. Therefore, a risk assessment tool (Rockall score) should be used to identify high risk patients at risk of deterioration.

Variable	Score			
	0	1	2	3
Age (years)	<60	60–79	>80	–
Shock	Nil	HR >100, BP normal	HR >100, systolic BP <100mmHg	
Comorbidity	Nil	–	Cardiac disease, GI tract cancer, other major comorbidities	Renal/liver failure, disseminated malignancy
Diagnosis	Mallory–Weiss tear	All other diagnoses	Malignancy of upper GI tract	–
Recent haemorrhage signs on endoscopy	Nil	–	Blood in the upper GI tract, adherent blood clot, visible or spurting vessel	–

10 Chronic NSAID use is the second leading cause of PUD. NSAIDs induce stomach mucosa damage through the systemic inhibition of the enzyme cyclooxygenase (COX). COX is responsible for prostaglandin synthesis, which plays a protective role for the gut mucosa by stimulating gastric mucus production. Therefore, blocking COX exposes the underlying stomach mucosa to increased acid-induced ulceration. The loss of mucosal integrity is followed by tissue reaction amplified by luminal content such as acid, pepsin, food and *H. pylori*. Locally, NSAIDs also decrease mucosal blood flow and bicarbonate secretion, which may delay ulcer healing.

11 Apart from NSAIDs, other medications which can cause PUD include aspirin and selective COX-2 inhibitors such as celecoxib. Patients taking anticoagulants are also at risk of GI bleeds. Alcohol can also irritate the gastric lining and cause minor bleeds.

12 There is no clinical evidence to suggest a causal link between stress and the development of peptic ulcers. Interestingly there has been a surge in *H. pylori*-negative, NSAIDs-negative and aspirin-negative PUD. Further research is necessary to determine why this occurs.

13 *H. pylori* is contagious and can be passed on by saliva, faecal–oral and poor hygiene practices. It is common in communities that live in crowded conditions and share living areas, such as families.

Examination

- The patient appears calm and oriented and is **haemodynamically stable and afebrile** [1].
- No obvious **weight loss or cachexia** [2] is noted.
- Peripheral examination is unremarkable apart from **nicotine-stained fingers** [3].
- **Cardiac and respiratory examination** [4] reveals no abnormalities.
- Abdominal examination is non-specific, with no scarring or **visible peristalsis** [5].
- Palpation reveals **epigastric tenderness** [6] but no **guarding or rigidity** [7] or **pulsatile masses** [8].
- There is no **organomegaly** [9] and bowel sounds are present with no **succussion splash** [10].
- **Rectal examination** [11] is also unremarkable.

1 Patients with uncomplicated PUD do not have haemodynamic compromise. However, if ulceration and perforation occur, shock may develop. In these cases, tachycardia, tachypnoea and hypotension may occur. Presence of fever may also indicate bacterial or chemical peritonitis due to leakage of bowel contents. Both are medical emergencies and require urgent intervention.

2 Intra-abdominal malignancies such as stomach cancer can present as epigastric pain. This must be ruled out, especially if unplanned weight loss is noted.

3 Tobacco is a risk factor for peptic ulcer development, as it alters gastroduodenal mucosal protective mechanisms. It can inhibit mucosal cell renewal and induce cell death whilst reducing gastric immunity. This increases the risk of *H. pylori* infection.

4 PUD usually does not manifest clinical signs in other organ systems unless hypovolaemic shock occurs. Such patients may have tachypnoea, tachycardia and in severe cases of bleeding, hypotension.

5 Visible peristalsis may indicate intestinal obstruction, especially if patients have concurrent nausea, vomiting and inability to pass bowel motions or gas.

6 Most patients with PUD have epigastric pain that can occasionally radiate to either the left or right upper quadrants. Radiation to the back is uncommon unless pancreatic involvement occurs.

7 Guarding can indicate a perforated peptic ulcer. If stomach contents irritate the peritoneum, peritonitis can occur, leading to abdominal rigidity.

8 Patients with tender pulsatile masses must always be investigated for an abdominal aneurysm. An enlarged abdominal aorta may present initially as abdominal pain and is at risk of rupture.

9 PUD does not present with organomegaly. If a mass is detected in the epigastric region, consider vascular, hepatic or splenic causes of abdominal pain. These include abdominal aneurysms, hepatitis or splenomegaly secondary to infection.

10 A succussion splash is an auscultative sign elicited by rocking abdominal movements. Retained gastric material more than three hours after a meal will generate a sloshing sound and suggests the presence of obstructed gas or fluid. Although non-specific, it may indicate gastric outlet obstruction such as pyloric stenosis, which is an important differential of epigastric pain.

11 In anaemic patients, a digital rectal exam can determine the presence of melaena. This may indicate an actively bleeding ulcer.

Investigations

- **FBE** [1] is unremarkable with metabolic panels, **LFTs and UECS** [2] all within normal ranges.
- The GP advises that a **urea breath test** [3] or **stool antigen test** [4] will be required.

- If the diagnosis is still unclear, then an **oesophagogastroduodenoscopy** [5] may be warranted instead of **radiological imaging** [6].
- A **biopsy** [7] could also be taken for further analysis.

1 A low haemoglobin may be present if the patient has evidence of GI bleeding or is clinically anaemic. This test is not diagnostic but can determine whether intensive investigations and therapy are necessary.

2 Liver and kidney function tests should be normal in patients with PUD. They are used as baseline tests to guide treatment. LFT derangements may indicate altered hepatic function of clotting factors, which can increase the risk of gastric bleeding. Elevated urea with a normal eGFR may indicate GI haemorrhage.

3 Patients <55 years of age from low risk areas do not require endoscopic evaluation. Instead a C^{13} urea breath test is preferred as it is less invasive but still accurate. *H. pylori* secretes urease, an enzyme that breaks down urea into carbon dioxide and ammonia, to create alkaline environments that assist in its survival. The breath test exploits this reaction by measuring the levels of isotope C^{13}, which is not naturally occurring in gastric mucosa. After consumption of enriched C^{13} tablets or drinks, breath samples are taken. If post dose levels are elevated, this implies the presence of urease-excreting *H. pylori* in the stomach. To minimise false negatives, antibiotic, PPI and bismuth therapy should be withheld for at least a few weeks prior to testing.

4 Stool antigen tests are cheaper and require less specialised equipment for analysis compared to urea breath tests; however, they are not as accurate. As with the urea breath test, antibiotics, PPI and bismuth therapy should be withheld to minimise false negatives. Serology for IgG specific to *H. pylori* is rarely used as it is less sensitive and specific and cannot distinguish between active and past infections.

5 OGD is considered the gold standard diagnostic test and is recommended in patients >55 years of age, especially those with concurrent weight loss. Endoscopy allows the direct visualisation of ulcers and can determine location and severity. If no ulcers are visualised, an alternative diagnosis of epigastric pain should be considered, such as malignancy. Biopsies of ulcers and lesions may also be taken to confirm diagnosis. Macroscopically, ulcers are oval with a smooth base, flat straight borders and are well-demarcated from surrounding tissue. The presence of elevated mass lesions, irregular borders and abnormal adjacent mucosal folds may suggest malignant changes. Endoscopy is also therapeutic and can be used to manage minor active bleeding.

6 Barium X-rays are rarely conducted as they can miss small ulcers and are not as accurate. This test involves swallowing a liquid suspension of barium sulfate prior to a series of X-rays that can map regions of the GI tract. The barium is radio-opaque and enhances the borders of the GI tract.

7 When a biopsy is taken, two diagnostic modalities, usually histology and urease test, are required to optimise yield. Microscopically, the surface is covered with inflammatory debris. An abundance of polymorphonuclear leucocytes are present in the underlying layers. *H. pylori*

may also be visualised as spiral-shaped bacterium, although specialised stains (Giemsa and Genta) may be necessary to enhance detection. Chronic infection may also demonstrate mucosal atrophy. When biopsy samples are submerged into a urea medium and a pH indicator, *H. pylori* produces urease that hydrolyses urea to ammonia, changing the colour of the solution. Sensitivity and specificity for this test is high; however, the process to obtain samples is expensive and invasive relative to breath or stool tests.

Management

Immediate

If perforation is suspected, **timely endoscopic treatment or surgery** [1] is necessary to prevent further complications. **Fluid resuscitation** [2] may be necessary if patients develop hypovolaemic shock. Correcting any **anticoagulation** [3] therapy should be on a case-by-case basis.

Short-term

The patient was advised to **cease oral ibuprofen** [4] for his back pain. A strict **antibiotic regimen** [5] was prescribed to eradicate *H. pylori* infection with an

addition of a **proton pump inhibitor** [6] to promote ulcer healing. **Bismuth** [7] may also be used as an adjunct. A **repeat breath test** [8] should be conducted one month after completion of antibiotics.

Long-term

Prostaglandin analogues [9] were considered if the patient's ulcer was refractory to natural healing. **Long-term PPI use** [10] should be avoided due to numerous side-effects. Patients with chronic *H. pylori* infections but no active ulcers should also be monitored for **gastric cancers** [11].

1 Scoring systems such as the Glasgow–Blatchford score can assist clinicians in determining whether patients will require an endoscopic intervention and transfusion. Scores >6 require urgent inpatient intervention. Endoscopy with cautery or adrenaline injections is most commonly employed for ulcers showing active bleeding. Surgery or angiographic embolisation should be reserved for cases of uncontrollable bleeding.

Component	Score
Urea (mmol/L)	
6.5–8.0	2
8.0–10.0	3
10.0–25	4
>25	6
Hb (g/L for males)	
120–129	1
110–119	3
<100	6
Hb (g/L for females)	
100–119	1
<100	6

Systolic blood pressure (mmHg)	
100–109	1
90–99	2
<90	3
Other	
Pulse >100/m	1
Melaena	1
Syncope	2
Liver disease of any sort	2
Cardiac failure of any sort	2

2 Recognition of early symptoms of shock, such as tachypnoea, cool clammy skin, tachycardia, agitation, hypotension, chest pain and confusion, will prevent patient deterioration. If hypovolaemic shock from actively bleeding ulcers is suspected, fluid resuscitation is necessary to prevent end-organ damage. Maintaining a systolic blood pressure >90mmHg with crystalloids or colloids ensures adequate perfusion. Blood transfusions should be considered in patients with a Hb <70g/L. Intravenous PPIs can also suppress bleeding and assist in platelet aggregation and prevent clot lysis.

3 The decision to cease antiplatelet or antithrombotic therapy must be conducted on a case-by-case basis. This should be discussed with the haematology team. Patients on warfarin can be temporarily treated with vitamin K, fresh frozen plasma, prothrombin complex concentrates or recombinant factor VIIa. Warfarin should be restarted once haemostasis is achieved, with low molecular weight heparin as a bridging therapy until the target INR is reached.

4 NSAID use should be ceased immediately, to promote ulcer healing. A selective COX-2 inhibitor such as celecoxib may be considered to reduce the risk of ulceration. However, it is contraindicated in patients with a history of cardiovascular events. Alternative analgesics should be considered if required.

5 Antibiotics are the first step in PUD, as they eliminate the underlying *H. pylori* infection. The choice of eradication regimen is made based on knowledge of locally determined antimicrobial resistance rates. The typical 'triple therapy' involving two antibiotics and a PPI is the recommended first-line therapy. Clarithromycin 500mg bd plus amoxicillin 1g bd and esomeprazole 20mg bd for 7 days is extremely successful in clearing 90% of infections. Patients with penicillin hypersensitivity should substitute amoxicillin with metronidazole 400mg bd.
Treatment failure occurs predominantly due to pre-treatment poor patient adherence and clarithromycin resistance. Susceptibility testing is strongly recommended after one treatment is unsuccessful. For rescue treatments, expert guidance from gastroenterologists and infectious diseases physicians should be sought.

6 PPIs should be prescribed with antibiotics as they irreversibly bind to gastric H^+K^+ ATPase pumps in the stomach and inhibit basal and stimulated acid secretion. This creates an alkaline environment that minimises mucosal irritation and promotes ulcer healing. Choice of PPIs is clinician-dependent and numerous clinical trials have shown no differences in efficacy between the different subtypes.

7 Bismuth subcitrate is used in quadruple therapy as it is bactericidal. Bismuth is incorporated into the bacterial membrane and inhibits iron uptake by *H. pylori*, limiting its growth. This is known as the oligodynamic effect and applies to other metals such as copper, silver and zinc.

8 The outcome of eradication therapy should be considered in all patients as it provides patient and clinician reassurance and can guide management if symptoms persist. This should be conducted a month after completion of antibiotic therapy, and PPIs and bismuth withheld for at least 1–2 weeks to minimise false negatives. Urea breath tests are recommended over antibody levels for *H. pylori* as serology is unreliable due to long and variable times for levels to fall. Endoscopy is usually not required unless complications persist such as continual bleeding.

9 Prostaglandin analogues such as misoprostol can be considered, especially in cases of NSAID-induced PUD. However, these should not be prescribed in pregnant women as they can cause uterine contractions and miscarriages.

10 PPIs remain one of the most overprescribed medications. Common side-effects such as headache, diarrhoea and abdominal bloating are well-tolerated. However, their long-term use is associated with serious adverse events, notably GI infection (including *C. difficile*), pneumonia and interstitial nephritis. Gastric acid inhibition by PPIs also can affect the uptake of certain vitamins, minerals and medications leading to iron deficiency and hypomagnesaemia. A step-down approach should be considered as ulcers heal and infection is cleared.

11 *H. pylori* infection can cause chronic gastritis. Long-term inflammation leads to gastric mucosal atrophy with dysplasia, increasing the risk of gastric cancers and mucosa-associated lymphoid tissue (MALT) lymphoma.

CASE 31: Acute myeloid leukaemia

History

- A **45-year-old** [1] male who is **previously well** [2] presents with **fatigue** [3], **gum bleeding** [4] and **a non-blanching rash** [5].
- He has also had recent **pharyngeal pain** [6] associated with **swelling in the cervical** [7] area. This was not associated with rhinorrhoea, myalgias, coryzal symptoms or cough.

- Aside from recent paracetamol use for the sore throat he does not take any **medications** [8].
- There is no personal history of **malignancy** [9], **bone marrow or blood disorders** [10].
- He **works as a plumber** [11] and has a wife and young family.
- The patient has two **siblings** [12].

[1] Acute myeloid leukaemia (AML) can affect people of all ages although is more common in the older adult. It accounts for 80% of adult acute leukaemias. Acute lymphoblastic leukaemia is more common in children (incidence highest between age 3 and 7 years) but can occur uncommonly in adults.

[2] AML can occur secondary to pre-existing haematological conditions including myeloproliferative diseases, primary myelofibrosis and myelodysplasia. However, many patients will have no known risk factors, or may have evidence of an underlying undiagnosed pre-existing haematological condition. Other possible predisposing factors include previous chemotherapy (especially alkylating agents), exposure to ionising radiation and chemical exposure.

[3] Fatigue is a common presenting symptom. This is usually multifactorial:
- due to anaemia
- may be due to infection, and
- the burden of the increased cell turnover of malignancy requiring significant energy availability.
In hindsight fatigue may have been present for weeks to months prior to the diagnosis. Other common symptoms include joint pain and bone pain due to marrow infiltration. Some patients are diagnosed incidentally on routine blood tests.

[4] Mucosal bleeding is common due to thrombocytopenia. In some patients it may be the main presenting complaint or reason to undergo a blood test. Certain subtypes of acute leukaemia can predispose to disseminated intravascular coagulation (DIC), resulting in bleeding.

[5] A petechial rash suggests the presence of thrombocytopenia. Ask about easy bruising. Check whether there are wet purpura or petechiae in the mouth.

[6] The patient may have a bacterial pharyngeal infection due to neutropenia occurring in acute leukaemia. This aetiology of infection is similar to bacterial throat infection in healthy individuals.

[7] Cervical lymphadenopathy due to infiltration of the nodes with leukaemia is uncommon but does occur. The patient is likely to have lymphadenopathy due to the bacterial throat infection. Ask about dental pain or recent dental procedures or infections.

[8] Drug causes must be considered in regard to neutropenia. Common agents include chemotherapy, anti-epileptics and immunosuppressants such as azathioprine. Ask the patient whether there has been any previous treatment for any autoimmune, arthritic or rheumatological disorders.

[9] Previous treatment for cancer is a risk factor for leukaemia, especially the use of alkylating chemotherapy agents. The risk of second malignancy is a concern after treatment for malignancies in younger age groups, such as testicular cancer and Hodgkin lymphoma.

[10] Leukaemia can occur from underlying bone marrow disorders including myelodysplasia and myeloproliferative neoplasms. This is called 'transformed' or 'secondary' leukaemia and generally confers a poorer prognosis.

[11] It is important to be aware of the patient's social situation in the context of a very serious and life-threatening diagnosis. Support should be offered to the family. The patient is unlikely to be able to work for weeks to months and many will never return to work after a leukaemia diagnosis, due to the high morbidity and mortality rates of the condition. In those returning to work, infection risk needs to be considered.

[12] Clinicians treating acute leukaemia will be considering management options from diagnosis. There is a likelihood

of this patient being recommended to receive an allogeneic bone marrow transplant (allograft) at some stage in the future. The preferred donor for an allograft is a matched sibling, therefore there is usually an attempt to obtain HLA typing from the patient and all siblings soon after diagnosis. This process is performed even if an allograft is not immediately likely, as it can take weeks to months to find a matched donor.

Examination

- The patient appears to be **pale** [1] and has a **low grade fever** [2].
- Respiratory rate, blood pressure and **heart rate** [3] are within normal limits.
- There are occasional **purpura** [4] on the forearms and a **petechial rash** [5] is noted.
- The **gums** [6] are not hypertrophied. Examination of the throat reveals erythematous tonsils.
- There is anterior **cervical lymphadenopathy** [7] of <1cm bilaterally.
- Examination of the oral cavity demonstrates white plaques consistent with **oral candidiasis** [8].
- **Fundoscopy** [9] is normal.

[1] Pallor is common due to the associated anaemia. In young patients or in early disease this may be the only noticeable feature on examination.

[2] Fever may be due to the leukaemia itself causing release of cytokines. If this is the cause, it will usually resolve after commencing chemotherapy. However, fever is also a sign of infection and should be treated as such until proven otherwise.

[3] Anaemia can cause tachycardia due to increased cardiorespiratory demand; however, younger patients are often able to compensate. In those presenting with coagulopathy or severe thrombocytopenia, tachycardia may be a sign of occult haemorrhage. Tachycardia may also be present due to infection. Ensure an ECG is performed.

[4] Purpura is concerning for thrombocytopenia or may even be a sign of life-threatening DIC. Easy bruising may have been noted for weeks prior to the diagnosis.

[5] Low platelets are a common presenting feature of acute leukaemia, and when the level is below 20–30 x 10^9/L a petechial rash may be seen. Examine the lower limb, particularly around the ankles, forearms and abdomen. Examine the mouth for wet purpura and oral petechiae.

[6] Blasts can infiltrate into all tissues of the body, including the gums, causing the tissue to swell. Other common sites include the liver, spleen and central nervous system. Examine the skin for nodular abnormalities or papular discolouration which could indicate the presence of leukaemia cutis (skin involvement).

[7] Mild lymphadenopathy is likely due to concomitant bacterial infection. Lymphadenopathy due to the disease at diagnosis is rare in AML and is more likely in lymphoid malignancies, e.g. acute lymphoblastic leukaemia (ALL).

[8] Immunosuppression can result in thrush due to overgrowth of candida within the oral cavity.

[9] Fundal haemorrhages can occur due to thrombocytopenia and coagulopathy. All patients should have screening tests and any patients with visual symptoms should be reviewed by an experienced ophthalmologist. The more common findings include macular haemorrhage and cotton-wool spots. In some cases, leukaemia can directly infiltrate the structures of the eye, including the optic nerves.

Investigations

- FBE demonstrates **anaemia** [1], **thrombocytopenia** [2] and **neutropenia** [3], but an **elevated total WCC** [4] of 72.
- Blood film demonstrates the presence of **blasts** [5].
- There are no **Auer rods** [6] seen.
- **Liver function tests** [7] and **UEC** [8] are normal; however, the **uric acid** [9] and **LDH levels** [10] are elevated.
- Coagulation studies demonstrate the presence of **disseminated intravascular coagulation** [11], with low fibrinogen, elevated INR and aPTT and a high D-dimer.
- **Chest X-ray** [12] is normal.
- Bone marrow aspiration and trephine demonstrated a **hypercellular marrow** [13] infiltrated with immature blasts of **>30%** [14], consistent with acute myeloid leukaemia.

- **Cytogenetics** [15] demonstrates a balanced translocation between **chromosome 15 and 17** [16], found in a subset of AML called **acute promyelocytic leukaemia** [17].

- **Cerebrospinal fluid examination** [18] is negative for abnormal cells.

---

1 Normochromic normocytic anaemia occurs due to reduced production of red cells in the marrow. The erythrocyte precursor cells are 'crowded' out by the presence of abnormal leukaemic blasts in the marrow. Anaemia also occurs due to the dysfunctional bone marrow forming abnormal red cells which have reduced survival in the circulation.

2 Thrombocytopenia is due to the reduced production in the bone marrow. This, combined with coagulation defects, leads to significant bleeding risk in this patient.

3 The normal neutrophil count varies with age and race. Those of African heritage (including American and Afro-Caribbean) often have lower neutrophil counts than Caucasian individuals. As with the red cells and platelets, the production of neutrophils is also halted due to suppression by production of blasts in the marrow.

4 Elevated total white cells with neutropenia suggests the presence of abnormal cells (such as immature blasts) making up the differential. Acute infections can raise the white cells in the blood but this should not be associated with anaemia or thrombocytopenia. Acute leukaemia can present with decreased, normal, slightly increased or markedly increased total WCC. Markedly elevated white cells raises the risk of hyperviscosity and leucostasis, a condition which can result in organ infiltration and rapid fatality.

5 Blast cells are immature white blood cells which are present in the bone marrow in small numbers. The presence of blast cells in the peripheral blood is always associated with an underlying pathology in the bone marrow. In many cases the type of leukaemia can be determined initially by the morphology of the peripheral blast cells under the microscope by an experienced haematologist.

6 Auer rods contained within the blast cells are diagnostic of AML. They are cytoplasmic inclusions formed from azurophilic granules due to the defect in production, formation and aggregation in leukaemic blasts. They are not always seen or may be missed in the small sample size that is the blood film, so a lack of presence does not prohibit the diagnosis of AML. When Auer rods are seen in cells in groups forming the appearance of 'bundles of sticks' these are termed faggot cells.

7 Abnormal renal or liver function may reflect infiltration of the organ. Assessment of renal and hepatic function must be undertaken prior to starting therapy. If there is dysfunction of either organ the chemotherapy dosage will need to be

adjusted. A 24-hour urine collection for creatinine clearance is routine even in those with normal serum creatinine.

8 Abnormal renal function may occur in tumour lysis syndrome (TLS). TLS is a well-recognised complication of the rapid cell turnover of acute leukaemias. It can occur spontaneously in high tumour burden conditions, or in response to cytotoxic chemotherapy. It is especially important to recognise elevations in the potassium occurring with TLS, which can affect the cardiac skeletal muscle and myocardium, causing life-threatening ventricular arrhythmia.

9 Uric acid is a by-product of increased cell production and turnover, as a product of purine nucleotides adenine and guanine which form the backbone of nucleic acids. Purines are metabolised via the enzyme xanthine oxidase to uric acid. Uric acid can crystallise and cause renal obstruction and dysfunction.

10 Elevation in lactate dehydrogenase (LDH) reflects the rapid apoptosis and turnover of leukaemic cells in acute leukaemia. An elevation of LDH in a patient presenting with one cytopenia (e.g. neutropenia) raises suspicion for an underlying malignancy. Markedly elevated LDH may reflect underlying tumour lysis.

11 Disseminated intravascular coagulation refers to activation of the entire coagulation process with intravascular clotting and fibrinolysis, resulting in consumption of all the coagulation factors, including platelets. This can result in severe bleeding and organ damage secondary to microvascular thrombosis. The presence of DIC can be due to infection or malignancy. However, in the context of acute leukaemia with coagulation deficit, acute promyelocytic leukaemia (APML) should be suspected.

12 Chest X-ray should be performed to rule out pneumonia, pleural effusion or, in rare cases, infiltration of the pulmonary vasculature with blasts (leucostasis). It may also demonstrate lytic lesions, or a mediastinal opacity caused by an enlarged thymus in T-cell ALL.

13 The bone marrow appears hypercellular due to the attempts of increased production of normal cells as well as the presence of abnormal cells.

14 A diagnosis of leukaemia generally requires a blast count of at least 20% in the bone marrow. Normal bone marrow contains <5% blasts. An exception to this is if a leukaemia-specific cytogenetic or molecular abnormality is found to be present.

15 Cytogenetic abnormalities are used to determine the type and prognosis of many leukaemias. These abnormalities are the major mechanisms for the failure of maturation and reduced apoptosis which leads to uncontrolled proliferation of immature undifferentiated leukaemia cells that are called blasts.

16 The translocation between chromosomes 15 and 17 results in formation of the PML-RARα fusion gene. This arrests normal differentiation of the cells at the level of the promyelocyte. The presence of this translocation with clinical and biochemical features of acute leukaemia confirms the diagnosis of acute promyelocytic leukaemia.

17 Confirmation of the diagnosis of APML is important prior to starting induction therapy. This subset of leukaemia has an early mortality rate of 10%, due to haemorrhagic complications; however, the outcomes are highly favourable and complete remission is achieved in >90%. Treatment regimes are very different and often non-chemotherapeutic compared to other types of AML.

18 Acute leukaemia has a risk of infiltrating into the central nervous system. CSF is sampled by lumbar puncture and the fluid is sent for flow cytometry and cytology. Care must be taken to ensure platelet levels are adequate and coagulation studies are normal for this procedure and if not, a transfusion will need to be given beforehand. Patients who are at high risk of having CNS involvement are given 'intrathecal' chemotherapy directly into the spinal fluid during the lumbar puncture. Those with CNS involvement will need to have repeat lumbar punctures with intrathecal chemotherapy.

Management

Immediate

Commence **intravenous fluids** [1] and allopurinol to prevent tumour lysis. Administer **broad-spectrum antibiotics** [2]. Seek urgent advice from the haematology team and aim to transfer to a ward with **haematology or oncology trained nursing staff** [3]. Begin to correct the DIC by ordering **platelets** [4], **fresh frozen plasma** [5] and **cryoprecipitate** [6].

Short-term

The haematology team will assist with advising on further management for this patient in a specialised unit. In suspected APML, **all-trans retinoic acid** [7] should be given as soon as available. The patient should be closely monitored for signs of **differentiation syndrome** [8].
As well as broad-spectrum antibiotics, which can be modified once **microbial results** [9] are back, he will need to receive **bacterial** [10], **viral** [11] **and fungal prophylaxis** [12]. Insertion of a **central venous access device** [13] should be organised. He should be offered **fertility preservation** [14] prior to commencement of treatment. The patient will need to receive **intensive cytotoxic chemotherapy** [15] including **induction therapy** [16] to achieve remission, and post-remission **consolidation therapy** [17]. This is likely to include **CNS prophylaxis** [18]. Support with blood products including **irradiated** [19] red cell and platelet transfusions is routine. Offer **social work** [20] and **psychological support** [21].

Long-term

In this patient with APML, there is a strong likelihood of long-term remission. In **high risk patients** [22] with other types of AML, **allogeneic bone marrow transplantation** [23] may be recommended. There are many new agents under investigation, many of which are only available upon enrolment in a **clinical trial** [24].

1 IV fluids and a xanthine oxidase inhibitor are routinely commenced to protect against tumour lysis. High urine output minimises the risk of uric acid and phosphate deposition in the renal tubules. Diuretic therapy may be required in those with underlying cardiac or renal dysfunction who cannot tolerate large volumes of fluid.

2 Infection in a neutropenic patient can become rapidly life-threatening and should be recognised and treated promptly with broad-spectrum antibiotics. Fever may be the only sign of infection in a neutropenic patient, as without neutrophils pus will not be formed and the infection may not be able to be localised. It is typical to use a broad-spectrum penicillin such as piperacillin-tazobactam, which must be commenced immediately after cultures have been taken.

3 As well as assisting with prompt management of the patient, haematology trained nurses can provide valuable psychological support with this new diagnosis. Utilising experienced nursing staff is imperative to ensure the prioritisation of infusion of blood products, antimicrobials and medications. They will also have perspective on the appropriate and timely use of pharmacotherapy to minimise patient discomfort and side-effects such as nausea.

4 Platelet transfusions are derived from both apheresis donations (one donor) or multiple whole blood donations. Platelets are routinely leucodepleted (white cells removed) in the UK. However, not all platelets are irradiated (this is dependent on necessity). Antiplatelet medications are usually ceased during intensive chemotherapy due to bleeding risk and the likelihood of prolonged relative thrombocytopenia.

5 Fresh frozen plasma is separated from whole blood and frozen within 18 hours of collection. It contains all of the clotting and coagulation factors in whole blood. These coagulation factors are being consumed in DIC faster than they can be produced by the body, so need to be replaced with this blood product.

6 Cryoprecipitate is a blood product that can also be prepared from apheresis or pooled from multiple whole blood donations. It is made by thawing the fresh frozen plasma and collecting the precipitate. It contains factor VIII, factor XIII and von Willebrand factor, but it is mainly used to replace fibrinogen. It can be stored frozen for up to 12 months.

7 All-trans retinoic acid (ATRA) is a differentiating agent which can improve the life-threatening coagulopathy associated with the underlying leukaemia. It is able to induce terminal differentiation of the leukaemic cell lines, turning the malignant cells into functional haematopoietic cells.

8 The blast cells of APML are very sensitive to the differentiating effects of ATRA. This can result in differentiation syndrome – manifesting as respiratory distress, pulmonary infiltrates, pleural effusions and fluid gain. It appears to be related to cytokine release. This can rapidly become fatal, over just hours from the first signs. If there is evidence of differentiation syndrome, the intensive care unit (ICU) team should be notified and the patient needs to be monitored very closely.

9 Specific microbial causes of presumed neutropenic infection are often not found. Despite patient anxiety with regard to contact with infectious family members or general public, most infections arise from the patient's own commensal microbes. Gram-positive skin organisms (e.g. *Staphylococcus* and *Streptococcus*) are a concern in those with indwelling lines, and serious infection can occur even from organisms not usually thought to be pathogenic. Overwhelming sepsis can occur rapidly due to Gram-negative organisms, e.g. *Pseudomonas*, *Klebsiella*, *E. coli* and anaerobes.

10 Prophylaxis against infection is used in most leukaemia regimes. As well as profound neutropenia which can be measured for weeks, cytotoxic therapy causes hypogammaglobulinaemia and cellular dysfunction. Bacterial prophylaxis is not routinely used due to concerns relating to resistance.

11 It is routine to use viral prophylaxis against reactivation of herpes viruses such as herpes simplex (HSV), varicella zoster (VZV), Epstein–Barr virus (EBV) and cytomegalovirus (CMV). Most adults have been exposed to their viruses in childhood or young adulthood with latency resulting in lack of eradication from the host.

12 Fungal infection is a major cause of mortality in heavily immunosuppressed patients. There are two major subtypes:
- yeasts including *Candida* species
- moulds such as *Aspergillus* species.

Neutropenia is the major risk factor for fungal infection and fungal prophylaxis is very routine in those at risk. Diagnosis can be difficult, requiring invasive testing such as bronchoscopy. Fungal infection should be suspected in those with a persistent fever despite several days of broad-spectrum antibacterial treatment. Prophylaxis against *Pneumocystis jirovecii* pneumonia (PJP) is given in addition to antifungal prophylaxis.

13 A central venous access device (CVAD) is inserted in those requiring intensive IV therapy. It is usually inserted under local anaesthetic by a radiologist into a skin tunnel from the anterior chest into the SVC. It can be used to administer therapy, antibiotics, blood products and IV parenteral nutrition. It can also be used to take blood tests.

14 Fertility preservation must be discussed prior to commencing treatment and appropriate collection and storage should be offered. It should never be assumed that a patient (unless beyond menopause) is beyond childbearing age, physically or mentally. The majority of regimes used in acute leukaemia will affect sperm production and function. Sperm collection and storage is often available in big centres or can be arranged.

15 The use of intensive cytotoxic therapy is dependent on the age, general health and comorbidities of the patient. Dosage is usually reduced for patients over the age of 60 and alternative less toxic regimes used for elderly patients. Therapy is also dependent on the characteristics of the leukaemia, including genetic and molecular abnormalities, which can predict likelihood of long-term treatment success.

16 Induction therapy is an intense regime designed to induce remission, i.e. eliminate leukaemic cells from detection in the blood or bone marrow using conventional techniques. Some patients may receive two induction cycles. A proportion of patients will be refractory to induction therapy due to disease characteristics, and this portends a grave prognosis. Alternatives need to be used in those over 70 years or with comorbidities who will not tolerate the intensity of traditional induction therapy.

17 Consolidation therapy is required to maintain remission over a long period and eliminate the disease. Usually 3 or 4 consolidation treatments are given, unless an allograft is planned. The intensity of therapy needs to be balanced with the toxicity and complications of treatment.

18 Many types of leukaemia can seed in the CNS and proliferate in the brain and spinal cord, including cranial nerves. The therapy used to induce remission generally does not penetrate the CNS, so specific treatment is needed to protect against leukaemia in this area. Chemotherapy can be given into the nervous system via lumbar puncture and administration of the medication into the spinal fluid. The presence of CNS leukaemia can also be monitored by sampling of the fluid prior to administration.

19 Patients with acute leukaemia (and many other haematological disorders) need to receive irradiated blood products. Irradiation is a process which removes the donor T lymphocytes from the blood product. In very immunosuppressed patients, donor T lymphocytes can cause transfusion-associated graft-versus-host disease, a condition with very high mortality rates.

20 The diagnosis of acute leukaemia is almost always sudden and unexpected. Even in favourable risk patients there is always concern regarding treatment mortality and disease relapse. Many patients will have families and concerns about employment and finances. Leukaemia centres are often located in big cities, therefore travel may be a major concern for rural patients and their families. The vast majority of treatment will occur as an inpatient or require intensive and regular follow-up.

21 Psychological support is a key aspect of treatment of leukaemia. Patients are in hospital and physically unwell for weeks at a time. Many big centres will have psychology or psychiatry professionals integrated into the unit and be able to offer a relatively easy access to these services. Patient education and communication are important to assist with psychological assistance from the physician's perspective as the 'unknown' contributes to fear and anxiety.

22 Risk profiling at diagnosis is increasingly used to determine the treatment strategies in acute leukaemia. High risk patients include those with complex cytogenetic or molecular abnormalities, those who do not respond to initial therapy and secondary leukaemias.

23 Allogeneic bone marrow transplantation (allograft) is a risky procedure with high mortality rates. Decision to offer allograft must be made by an MDT of experienced transplantation clinicians. It is offered in select intermediate- and high-risk patients in first remission, or upon relapse in second remission. It is not performed in patients over 70 years or with major physical or psychological comorbidities. Despite improvement in immunosuppression and supportive care, transplant-related mortality occurs in around a third of patients.

24 Acute leukaemia attracts research funding due to the high mortality rates and propensity to affect children. Patients who fail to respond to conventional therapy, and fitter older patients who are unsuitable for intense regimes, may be offered further treatment though early phase clinical trials. This may include medications which are directly targeting a mutation present in their specific type of leukaemia. It is often uncertain with regard to whether the treatment will be effective due to lack of data and experience in the early phase trials.

CASE 32: Chronic lymphocytic leukaemia and non-Hodgkin lymphoma

History

- A **66-year-old male** [1] presents with **fatigue** [2], increasing **neck swelling** [3] and **weight loss** [4] which he has noted over the past **8 weeks** [5].
- He denies any **fevers** [6] but has experienced **night sweats** [7].
- Past medical history is significant for **chronic lymphocytic leukaemia (CLL)** [8] but he has **not received treatment** [9] for this.
- He has a history of chronic obstructive pulmonary disease with **recurrent pulmonary and sinus infections** [10].
- A history of **disseminated shingles** [11] requiring a hospital admission last year is also noted.
- He has a relative with a **white blood cell disorder** [12].

[1] The incidence of chronic lymphocytic leukaemia (CLL) increases with age and the median age of diagnosis is around 70 years. It does occur in much younger patients but this is uncommon. CLL is nearly twice as common in males. It is the most common leukaemia in the developed world, comprising up to 30% of adult leukaemias. As well as being a leukaemia, CLL is often classified as a type of non-Hodgkin lymphoma.

[2] Many patients with CLL and other indolent lymphoproliferative disorders are asymptomatic at presentation. Up to 80% of those with CLL will be diagnosed with leucocytosis seen on routine bloods. The initial presentation may also be due to incidentally discovered lymphadenopathy. Many patients will have a degree of fatigue which can be attributed to the condition itself, or to associated anaemia. Symptoms often correlate with the overall tumour burden.

[3] At least half of patients with CLL will have lymphadenopathy found on examination at diagnosis. Despite being termed a leukaemia, CLL is considered to be the same disease process as SLL, the indolent non-Hodgkin lymphoma called small lymphocytic lymphoma. They share identical pathologic features. The disease is called CLL when it is predominantly in the blood, and SLL when there is mostly nodal involvement. However, there is often considerable overlap, indicating it is a disease spectrum rather than distinct entities. It is important to reassure the patient that a chronic leukaemia has a very different natural history and prognosis to an acute leukaemia.

[4] Weight loss may be a sign of an active disease process. This is concerning in a patient with a history of a low grade or indolent lymphoma as it can indicate transformation to a high grade non-Hodgkin lymphoma requiring prompt treatment. In some patients this is the natural history of CLL.

[5] CLL is an indolent, chronic type of leukaemia and may be present for months to years without detection. Many patients will remain stable for years without treatment. A change in disease activity over weeks should be investigated for transformation to high grade disease.

[6] The presence of objective fever of >38.0°C can be a sign of infection as a cause for the symptoms. If fever is present, ask about associated symptoms such as cough, coryza, urinary frequency, dysuria, headache and diarrhoea. Fevers can also occur with haematological disease, mainly due to the burden of cytokine production.

[7] Night sweats can be a sign of transformation to high grade disease. This is specifically called Richter's transformation in patients with CLL and indicates that the indolent disease has become a high grade, progressive large cell lymphoma.

[8] A large subset of patients with early stage CLL often stay in that stage with low or mildly elevated lymphocytes for years. It is common for early stage CLL patients to have monitoring blood tests just once or twice per year. Many patients are discharged back to be monitored by their GP if they have been stable for many years without treatment. Patients who are only being observed may be lost to follow-up and present years later.

[9] A large proportion of patients with CLL will never have or need treatment for the condition and will have a normal life expectancy. Early or inappropriate treatment can result in unnecessary harm in stable patients. With increasing research into therapies in haematological malignancy, there may be benefit in waiting for clinical trials or newer therapies in appropriate patients. Although CLL is thought to be indolent, it is generally incurable and most therapies will not eliminate the condition altogether.

10 Early on in CLL there is an increase in common bacterial infections such as sinus and chest infections. This is due to a decrease in healthy immunoglobulin synthesis due to the monoclonal nature of the overproduction of one type of lymphocyte. Pneumococcal and seasonal influenza vaccines are recommended in all patients.

11 Presentation with unusual infections is due to low immunoglobulins (acquired hypogammaglobulinaemia). Shingles is a very common infection in immunosuppressed patients, especially in the elderly. However, it is unusual to have disseminated shingles in those with an intact and functioning immune system. These viral infections, as well as fungal infections, occur later on in the disease process.

12 There is likely to be a genetic component to CLL although the genes involved are currently largely unknown. It is very uncommon in Asian populations, even those who have immigrated to western countries. The risk of CLL in close relatives of those with the condition is up to sevenfold. Currently, screening for CLL in those with affected family members is not recommended due to the overall low risk of the condition in the general population and the indolent nature of the disease.

Examination

- The patient looks **well** [1] and not in distress.
- There is **firm, round, non-tender** [2] **cervical and inguinal lymphadenopathy** [3] found on examination.
- **Examination of the throat** [4] is unremarkable; however, there is evidence of **thrush** [5] on the tongue.
- The tip of the **spleen is palpable** [6] 5cm below the costal margin with no evidence of **hepatomegaly** [7]. There is mild non-specific abdominal tenderness.
- **Chest is clear** [8] to auscultation and **heart sounds are dual** [9] with no added sounds.
- The **skin across the T7 dermatome** [10] is faintly scarred, consistent with previous shingles.
- There are no other abnormalities of the **skin** [11].

1 The general appearance of the patient may assist with determining whether prompt inpatient investigations and treatment are required, or whether the patient can be investigated as an outpatient. The majority of CLL and non-Hodgkin lymphoma therapy is done as an outpatient. Other factors that may prompt inpatient admission for urgent treatment include bulk of disease, comorbidities and impending malignant obstruction on local structures (e.g. spinal cord, ureteric or biliary obstruction).

2 The lymphadenopathy of CLL/SLL is usually non-tender, involving multiple nodes which are not fixed or matted and not compressing surrounding structures. The nodes are usually discrete and mobile with palpation.

3 It is common to have multiple nodal groups involved; the most easily palpable being the cervical, supraclavicular and axillary and inguinal groups. Other lymph node areas to examine include the preauricular, postauricular, occipital, epitrochlear and popliteal groups.

4 Waldeyer's ring should be examined as this is an area of lymphoid tissue which can be potentially infiltrated by disease. This refers to the tonsils, nasopharynx and base of tongue. Tonsils may be asymmetrically enlarged and surrounding superficial nodes (cervical, preauricular) may be palpable.

5 Oral candidiasis or 'thrush' can occur in those who are immunosuppressed.

6 Around 25–50% of patients will have splenomegaly on examination; however, splenic infarction is a very uncommon presenting feature, likely due to the slow-growing nature of the splenomegaly. The spleen is usually non-tender with a smooth surface.

7 A minority of patients will have hepatomegaly on presentation. This is more likely to occur in those with splenomegaly.

8 Auscultate the chest to examine for signs of cardiac failure, or infection due to low immunoglobulins. Pleural effusions or, rarely, pericardial effusions can occur. This may be due to local obstruction, or due to pleural involvement with disease.

9 Auscultating the heart may reveal a pericardial friction rub which may indicate presence of pericardial effusion.

10 The rash of shingles generally starts as a crop of papules, usually post the onset of pain. Over several days it erupts to become blistering over the dermatome. The rash then crusts over. Most patients will have minimal cosmetic abnormality once it has healed over several weeks, but some may be left with scarring.

11 The skin is a common site for extranodal lymphoma or leukaemia. Carefully examine for any suspicious areas. Ask the patient if they have noted any tenderness or erythema. Look for any rashes which could indicate infection.

Investigations

- FBE shows a mild **normochromic normocytic anaemia** [1] with elevated **lymphocyte count** [2] and **normal platelet count** [3].
- Blood film shows **small, mature lymphocytes** [4] and **smear cells** [5].
- The **red cells** [6] appear normal. UEC is normal.
- **LDH** [7] is elevated; however, **haptoglobin and bilirubin** [8] are within normal limits.
- **Direct Coombs test** [9] is negative.
- **Peripheral flow cytometry** [10] reveals a **clonal population** [11] almost entirely consisting of **B cells** [12].

- Immunoglobulin testing reveals a markedly **reduced serum IgG** [13].
- CT of the neck, chest, abdomen and pelvis shows **widespread lymphadenopathy** [14] including a 5cm abdominal lymph node mass.
- **CT-guided biopsy** [15] of the abdominal area demonstrates **poorly differentiated large cells with high metabolic activity** [16].
- **Bone marrow biopsy** [17] shows a diffuse infiltration of small, mature lymphocytes.
- **CSF examination** [18] is negative for malignant cells.

[1] In advanced disease, the increased numbers of small lymphocytes crowd the normal bone marrow and affect production of blood cells. This results in a lack of production of red cells, white cells such as neutrophils, or platelets. The anaemia will likely be normochromic and normocytic because the cells which are being produced are drastically reduced in number but of normal phenotype. Alternatively, anaemia can occur due to the increased destruction of autoimmune haemolytic anaemia in CLL, rather than reduced production.

[2] The elevated lymphocyte indicates an increase in bone marrow output of lymphocytes. This can occur in response to infection, but in someone of this age group in the absence of infection a lymphoproliferative condition should be suspected. Infections such as EBV, pertussis and *C. difficile* are associated with lymphocytosis but levels will return to normal within weeks. In CLL, lymphocyte counts can be elevated over 300 x 10^9/L (normal is 4–11 x 10^9/L) and may be up to 99% of the white cells in the blood. Even at these high levels the lymphocytosis does not usually cause complications of leucostasis in the microcirculatory system.

[3] Thrombocytopenia can occur in advanced disease with marrow infiltration. Immune thrombocytopenia occurs in a minority of patients and is likely to improve with treatment of the disease.

[4] The malignant and abnormal cells of this chronic leukaemia have evolved further from the stem cell origin than the immature 'blast cells' of acute leukaemia and therefore are termed 'mature' cells. The level of maturation of the malignant cell can be identified by:
- the appearance on the blood film
- the clinical presentation of the disease, and
- the specific surface markers that are expressed by the cell.

[5] Smear cells are commonly reported on the blood film in patients with CLL. The 'smear' is induced by the production

of the blood film and is not actually a form that is present in the blood. CLL cells are fragile and burst, causing an artefact. Smear cells are also seen in EBV infection.

[6] Concomitant autoimmune haemolytic anaemia is strongly associated with CLL. The blood film will have evidence of spherocytes and possibly red cell fragments.

[7] LDH is a marker of cell turnover and in uncomplicated CLL is usually normal. Elevation of LDH in a patient with enlarging lymph nodes, increasing lymphocytosis or increasing 'B symptoms' is concerning for transformation to large cell, progressive disease. Consider testing for elevations in the beta-2 microglobulin in addition to LDH.

[8] LDH, haptoglobin and bilirubin are markers of haemolysis, along with reticulocytes and the direct Coombs test. A normal haptoglobin suggests haemolysis is less likely, despite the elevated LDH.

[9] The direct Coombs test will be positive in up to a third of patients with CLL. This may be due to overt autoimmune haemolytic anaemia, or may be a non-specific marker of the immune system activation associated with the disorder. The positive predictive value of a patient with a positive direct Coombs test developing haemolytic anaemia is low.

[10] Flow cytometry is a key diagnostic test in haematological malignancy. It involves using labels to sort the cells by the signal expressed. These signals are used to identify the cell of origin. For example, B-cell malignancies will express markers such as CD19 and CD20, while T cells will express CD3 and CD4.

[11] A clonal population refers to a large group of identical cells which have been identified to have formed from one cell. This has resulted in a mutation from one stem cell which has divided and passed on the mutation to all daughter cells. The malignant immunoglobulin population will be seen to express a single light chain rather than a wide variety.

12 CLL is almost always a disease of the mature B lymphocytes, with <5% being due to T lymphocytes.

13 Hypogammaglobulinaemia occurs due to clonal immunoglobulin synthesis leading to a reduced spectrum of synthesis of different immunoglobulins. Usually the measured IgG, IgM and IgA will all be low. This predisposes patients to recurrent bacterial infections.

14 A CT scan is a useful test for demonstrating the presence of abnormal lymph nodes throughout the body. Individual enlarged nodes can easily be measured and compared to prior scans using this imaging modality. There may also be some appreciation of the abnormal structure of affected nodes. CT can be useful to determine the most easily accessed nodes for arrangement of a biopsy.

15 CT-guided biopsy is used to access the deep abdominal nodes for core biopsy. There are many structures in the abdomen which need to be avoided by the biopsy needle, such as bowel and the large vessels. Abnormally enlarged nodes can be visualised and targeted. This is usually performed under local anaesthetic.

16 The biopsy is confirmation of transformation to high grade lymphoma; this patient has progressed to a Richter's transformation. This patient has evidence of both the underlying CLL and the new high grade lymphoma. In CLL, histology of a lymph node will show well-differentiated small uniform lymphocytes, which is not the case here. It is likely the patient now has the most common form of high grade lymphoma called diffuse large B cell lymphoma (DLBCL).

DLBCL can occur sporadically or secondary to an underlying low grade lymphoma. The pathologist will perform immunohistochemistry stains for B cell markers to confirm this diagnosis.

17 Bone marrow biopsy in CLL is used to confirm the diagnosis and facilitate additional tests such as cytogenetics. The procedure can be performed as a day procedure in the clinic or in a hospital ward. The patient is often given sedation or light anaesthesia and the procedure is performed under local anaesthetic. Bone marrow biopsy has two aspects: aspiration of the liquid contents and fragments of the marrow called 'the aspirate' and a solid core of bone and marrow called the 'trephine'. The aspirate is spread onto a slide like a blood film and the cells, cell line ratios, precursors and cellularity can be observed. In urgent cases the preliminary result can be available within hours and later be sent for additional tests such as flow cytometry, cytogenetics, DNA analysis and fluorescence *in situ* hybridisation (FISH). The trephine result may take several days to become available and is stained immunohistologically, similar to organ or skin biopsy specimens. It provides a view of the marrow structure, architecture and cell or fibrotic content.

18 In those at high risk of CNS involvement, it is important to know whether there is evidence of disease in this area before starting therapy. Most traditional chemotherapy agents will not penetrate into the CNS, and additional treatment or a different regime will be given to those with CNS involvement.

Management

Short-term

Many patients with CLL will **never require treatment** [1]. This patient presents with transformation to high grade disease and is therefore a **candidate for chemotherapy** [2]. **Educate the patient** [3] with regard to the diagnosis and **prognosis** [4]. Check for exposure and **immunity to viruses** [5]. Prescribe **infection prophylaxis** [6] as per local guidelines and treat the thrush with **topical antifungals** [7]. Commence the **chemotherapy regime** [8], giving consideration to tumour lysis risk.

Long-term

Arrange **regular review** [9] for this patient, including examination for **lymphadenopathy, B symptoms** [10] and blood tests to monitor **FBE and lymphocytes** [11], **LDH** [12] and for haemolysis. If infections are recurrent, consider **immunoglobulin replacement** [13]. In the event of relapse, **further chemotherapy** [14] may be required. There may be consideration of **bone marrow transplantation** [15] in **eligible patients** [16]. For relapsed disease, consider enrolment in a **clinical trial** [17].

1 There is no evidence that commencing treatment in an asymptomatic patient will improve outcomes. Indications for treatment in CLL include 'B' symptoms, reduction in haemoglobin or platelets, bulky lymphadenopathy or rapid rise of lymphocytes. Chemotherapy is recommended for all patients with transformation to high grade lymphoma.

2 First-line therapy is determined by the patient's fitness and comorbidities, as well as the cytogenetics of the condition. In young patients, the aim is to use chemotherapy to achieve remission. In older patients the aim of treatment is to control symptoms. In CLL without transformation, therapy generally aims to be conservative, as treating too early and too aggressively may actually shorten life expectancy. In those with high grade lymphoma, chemotherapy is used to eliminate the high grade disease, but may not eliminate the underlying CLL.

3 Sensitively inform the patient of the diagnosis and the need for treatment. Involve a family member or friend in the discussion if appropriate. Provide written information for the patient to read in their own time. Allow time for questions to be answered.

4 Prognosis in this patient depends on many factors including age, cytogenetics and response to therapy. Remember, CLL is considered an incurable condition, although many patients will not die of CLL. Richter's transformation in an older patient with comorbidities may have a guarded prognosis. A minority of patients present with aggressive disease at transformation. This is usually associated with accumulation of a chromosome abnormality.

5 Every patient should be tested for hepatitis B, C and HIV before commencing chemotherapy. It is standard to also test for herpes virus (EBV, CMV and VZV) exposure, as these viruses can reactivate and cause clinical sequelae during therapy. Reactivation of hepatitis B is a particular risk of the immunosuppressive effects of some chemotherapeutic agents. Those with past hepatitis B exposure or infection are routinely given prophylactic antivirals.

6 All patients undergoing chemotherapy are given prophylaxis against the herpes viruses to prevent complications such as herpes zoster (shingles). Both the underlying haematological malignancy and the chemotherapy treatment increase the risk.

7 Topical antifungals should be initiated in all patients presenting with oral candidiasis. Left untreated, it can persist and progress to oesophageal candidiasis. This can result in malaise and poor oral intake. Both liquid and lozenge forms of topical treatment are commonly used.

8 In B-cell non-Hodgkin lymphoma, the current mainstay of first-line treatment is an anti-CD20 antibody combined with cytotoxic chemotherapy. The main anti-CD20 treatment used is called rituximab, an antibody also used in immunological, neurological and rheumatological conditions. The majority of patients with CLL and non-Hodgkin lymphoma will undertake their chemotherapy in an outpatient setting. Standard regimes involve infusion of cytotoxic treatment once every 3–4 weeks for 6–8 cycles in total. A semi-permanent CVAD is usually not required unless venous access is particularly difficult.

9 As CLL is usually incurable, the majority of patients will need to be monitored indefinitely. During chemotherapy patients are usually reviewed every few weeks to ensure treatment is tolerated and side-effects are managed.

10 Increasing lymphadenopathy or B symptoms may be indications of relapse and the need for re-treatment in the future.

11 If there are no other signs or symptoms, increasing lymphocyte count may not be an indication for re-treatment. Patients can be asymptomatic with lymphocyte counts of 30 times the upper limit of normal. However, if the lymphocytes double in several months this may be an indication for treatment. Evidence of persistent anaemia or thrombocytopenia indicating bone marrow failure (Binet stage C or Rai stage III–IV disease) is also an indication for treatment.

12 Rising LDH signals increased cell turnover and could be an early sign of relapse or transformation to high grade disease.

13 Many patients will meet the criteria for long-term immunoglobulin replacement due to low blood immunoglobulin levels and recurrent infections. This involves an IV infusion every 4–6 weeks. Hypogammaglobulinaemia occurs in up to half of patients, even without the immunosuppressive effects of treatment. Sinopulmonary infections are common. Those who have had chemotherapy treatment are more likely to then have T-cell deficiency, which can lead to viral and other opportunistic infections.

14 Some patients will relapse following a remission. Assessment of symptoms and discussion of the goals of treatment should be undertaken. If the remission has been long, they may receive the same chemotherapy again. In the case of relapse a short while after treatment, alternative agents need to be considered.

15 Both autologous and allogeneic transplants are used in CLL and non-Hodgkin lymphoma. The only potential cure for CLL is an allogeneic stem cell transplant.

16 Allogeneic bone marrow transplant carries a very high risk of treatment-related mortality. It is unlikely to be a consideration in the vast majority of patients with relapsed or refractory disease due to age and comorbidities. Observation and re-treatment when symptoms occur is appropriate for many. Autologous transplants are often indicated in those with high risk disease, to augment chemotherapy and ensure a deep remission.

17 Many current clinical trials focus on finding effective agents in treating the condition without causing side-effects or long-term complications. These are often termed 'targeted' therapies which select a mutation or marker on the malignant cells, leaving healthy cells unaffected. Immunotherapy is also increasingly used in haematological malignancies, mainly for relapsed disease.

CASE 33: Chronic myeloid leukaemia

History

- A **57-year-old male** [1] presents with **fatigue, poor exercise tolerance** [2], **early satiety** [3] and vague **abdominal discomfort** [4].
- There was no history of **fevers, sweats** or **weight loss** [5].
- **Easy bruising** [6] had been noted by the patient over the past few months.

- His medical history is significant for **gout** [7], including several recent flares.
- He has a past history of **obesity** [8], **type 2 diabetes mellitus and ischaemic heart disease** [9].
- There is no **family history** [10] of any blood disorders.

[1] Chronic myeloid leukaemia (CML) mainly occurs between the ages of 40 and 70, although it can occur at any age, including children. It is slightly more common in males. CML accounts for 15–20% of all adult leukaemias. With careful management, those with CML can anticipate a normal life expectancy.

[2] Fatigue is a common presenting symptom and is often due to a number of factors. These include anaemia, disease burden and cell turnover as well as cytokine release. Up to half of patients will be asymptomatic at diagnosis and the presence of CML will be seen incidentally on blood testing performed for other reasons.

[3] Early satiety refers to the feeling of being 'full' after eating only a small amount, rather than a full meal. This is a sign of splenomegaly, caused by the mechanical compression of the enlarged spleen on the adjacent stomach in the left upper quadrant of the abdomen. Nearly all patients with CML will have a degree of splenomegaly at diagnosis, and many will have massive splenomegaly. In some patients the massive spleen may weigh up to 5kg.

[4] Abdominal discomfort is also a sign of splenomegaly due to compression in the abdomen. There may be associated indigestion. Careful history is needed to separate a vague feeling of abdominal discomfort from the discrete left upper quadrant pain which could indicate a splenic infarct. This is a complication of massive or rapidly increasing splenomegaly. The white blood cells can accumulate so rapidly that the blood supply to the enlarging spleen is compromised, resulting in infarction. Ask about pleuritic

chest pain or shoulder tip pain which can indicate a splenic infarct in the area close to the diaphragm. Tenderness may occur over the lower sternum in some patients, due to the expanding bone marrow in this area.

[5] Symptoms of hypermetabolism of haematological malignancy include fevers, sweats and weight loss. An element of weight loss may also occur due to the abdominal discomfort and early satiety.

[6] Easy bruising, menorrhagia and epistaxis can occur in those with CML due to abnormal platelet function. This is despite the thrombocytosis that occurs with CML as the platelet function is abnormal.

[7] Acute gout can occur in patients with untreated CML. This is due to increased cell turnover, the by-products of which are broken down into uric acid, leading to high levels of uric acid in the blood. This can result in uric acid crystals depositing into joints, leading to gout.

[8] Obesity will make monitoring of spleen size as a marker of disease activity difficult. Obesity and associated complications may alter the choice of therapy in CML. Cardiovascular health is a key consideration in long-term treatment of CML.

[9] The presence of comorbidities such as diabetes, ischaemic heart disease and pulmonary disease need to be taken into account when deciding on treatment strategies.

[10] The abnormality of CML is caused by a somatic mutation, and therefore is not inherited.

Examination

- The patient **looks well** [1] and is afebrile.
- **Blood pressure and heart rate** [2] are normal.

- He has occasional **bruises** [3] to his forearms and shins.

- There is no **livedo reticularis** [4] and no sign of **erythromelalgia** [5].
- There is mild **conjunctival pallor** [6].
- Abdominal examination reveals a **spleen** [7] which is palpable 6cm below the costal margin without hepatomegaly.

- There are no signs of **chronic liver disease** [8].
- There is no **lymphadenopathy** [9] appreciated.
- The right great toe is swollen and tender, consistent with **gout** [10].

1 Unlike those presenting with acute leukaemia, patients presenting in chronic phase of CML will usually be well. The condition may have been diagnosed incidentally.

2 Massive splenomegaly and extramedullary haematopoiesis uncommonly can cause haemodynamic changes which can then lead to high output cardiac failure. Look for evidence of elevated JVP and pitting peripheral oedema. In those with advanced CML, release of cytokines can exacerbate this state.

3 Bruising may be present due to abnormal platelet function. Ask about any bleeding noted, such as epistaxis, haematuria and haematochezia.

4 Livedo reticularis is a reddish-purple mottled or lacy pattern that occurs on skin. It is associated with vascular micro-occlusion or poor venous flow and occurs in other myeloproliferative neoplasms. It can be diagnosed by biopsy of the area and is managed by treating the underlying disorder.

5 Erythromelalgia refers to pain, erythema and swelling due to vasomotor and vascular abnormalities. It most commonly occurs in the hands or feet. It is a key sign of the myeloproliferative neoplasms, most often seen in polycythaemia rubra vera or essential thrombocytosis. It is also seen in vascular and rheumatological disorders.

6 Conjunctival pallor may suggest the presence of anaemia.

7 The spleen lies between the 9th and 11th ribs and is not normally palpable. The tip of a normal spleen may be palpable rarely in very thin individuals on deep inspiration. In patients with myeloproliferative neoplasms such as CML, the spleen can be so massive it grows left to right across the abdomen and is palpated in the right iliac fossa. This is due to haematopoiesis (production of blood cells) occurring in the spleen, a process which in healthy individuals occurs in the bone marrow and is abnormal when occurring in the spleen. Ensure there is no peritonism and no focal tenderness suggestive of infarction. Auscultate in the left upper quadrant for a friction rub.

8 Cirrhosis could cause splenomegaly due to portal hypertension, with scarring of the liver that renders it small and impalpable. Less than a third of patients with CML will have hepatomegaly at diagnosis.

9 Lymphadenopathy and involvement of other extramedullary tissues is very uncommon, and is usually only seen in patients presenting in lymphoid blast crisis. The presence of lymphadenopathy could cause suspicion for a lymphoid malignancy (such as lymphoma).

10 Gout occurring in the great toe is referred to as podagra. This is the most common site of acute gout. Ask about pain in the knees and ankles. Examine the area for swelling and tenderness. Look for the presence of firm nodules consistent with the tophi of chronic gout.

Investigations

- FBE shows **elevated WCC** [1] with a mix of neutrophils, eosinophils, **basophils** [2] and **early granulocytes** [3].
- Blood film shows a **leucoerythroblastic picture** [4] with a mild **normocytic anaemia** [5] and mild **thrombocytosis** [6].
- There are no **blast cells** [7].
- The **LDH** [8] and **uric acid** [9] levels are elevated but creatinine is normal.
- **Vitamin B12** [10] level is normal.
- The **BCR-ABL fusion transcript** [11] is found in the peripheral blood but **cytogenetics** [12] are unable to be performed.

- Examination of the **bone marrow aspirate** [13] demonstrates **increased cellularity** [14] with **myeloid hyperplasia** [15] and no features of **blastic disease** [16].
- There is a **left shift** [17] with increased **megakaryocytes** [18].
- Cytogenetic examination of the bone marrow demonstrates the presence of the **Ph chromosome** [19].
- Abdominal ultrasound shows **moderate splenomegaly** [20] without hepatomegaly or local lymphadenopathy.

1 CML is a cancer of the white blood cells characterised by uncontrolled growth of the myeloid cells. It is classified as a myeloproliferative neoplasm (MPN), having common features with other MPNs, including cell proliferation and splenomegaly. The high white cells may be noted incidentally on routine bloods and may be the only evident abnormality. Lymphocytes will usually be normal or low, as these are not part of the myeloid lineage of cells.

2 Absolute basophilia is seen in nearly all patients with CML. Basophilia is uncommon in other haematological conditions so the presence in high numbers is very suspicious for CML. Basophilia may have adverse prognostic significance.

3 Early granulocytes refer to immature cells such as promyelocytes and myelocytes. These have been produced from the myeloid stem cell and are ready to differentiate or mature further into neutrophils, monocytes, eosinophils and basophils. The abnormal cells are pushed into the peripheral blood, leading to increased numbers of granular cells on the FBE. The granulocytes usually appear morphologically normal in early disease. Chemically and functionally, the neutrophils and other myeloid cells of CML are abnormal.

4 The leucoerythroblastic blood film refers to immature red cells and white blood cells in higher than expected numbers. It is a term describing the appearance of the overall blood film, rather than a diagnosis. It can be seen in myeloproliferative neoplasms, malignant infiltration of the bone marrow, bleeding and haemorrhage and acute haemolysis.

5 Myeloid cells overproliferate in the bone marrow, leading to decreased production of red cells. Patients may present with anaemia or normal haemoglobin. The lack of severe anaemia may help to differentiate from other MPNs such as myelofibrosis. If nucleated red cells or tear drop cells are noted, this is more consistent with myelofibrosis as an alternative diagnosis.

6 The platelet count in CML may be normal or elevated. Thrombocytopenia indicates advanced disease, or that another MPN is more likely than CML. For example, the presence of splenomegaly and thrombocytopenia is more likely to be seen in myelofibrosis than CML. Platelet function is abnormal.

7 The presence of blast cells in the peripheral blood is still consistent with a diagnosis of CML but this portends a poor prognosis. This reflects the presence of advanced (accelerated phase or blast phase) disease. This should be quantified and confirmed on bone marrow biopsy.

8 Elevated LDH reflects the turnover of cells, or cell death. This occurs in CML due to the markedly increased production of myeloid cells combined with the premature apoptosis and reduced lifespan of the ineffective cells.

9 Elevations in LDH and uric acid can be an indication of tumour lysis syndrome. This diagnosis would be supported by elevations in serum potassium, creatinine and phosphate, with a secondary hypocalcaemia. The elevation in uric acid is likely to be contributing to episodes of gout in this patient.

10 Vitamin B12 deficiency can cause haematological effects such as megaloblastic anaemia, neutrophil abnormalities, leucopenia and thrombocytopenia. Levels should be checked in any patient presenting with a blood film abnormality. In contrast, patients presenting with CML often have very high vitamin B12 levels. This is due to an increase in the vitamin B12 binding proteins in MPNs.

11 Translocation of chromosomes 9 and 22 leads to the Philadelphia (Ph) chromosome. A gene on chromosome 22 called *BCR* fuses with a gene on chromosome 9 called *ABL*. *BCR-ABL* can phosphorylate tyrosine residues, which can activate a cascade of proteins leading to increased cell cycle division. The BCR-ABL protein inhibits DNA repair, which can lead to further abnormalities. CML was the first cancer to be linked to a specific chromosome abnormality. A minority of cases of acute lymphoblastic leukaemia (ALL) will demonstrate the presence of the Philadelphia chromosome. The BCR-ABL transcript is usually detected by sensitive techniques such as FISH or PCR.

12 Karyotyping of the 9:22 chromosome translocation is usually successfully performed on the bone marrow aspirate cells. However, it may be not able to be obtained from the peripheral blood. A karyotype is taken from cells in metaphase and due to small numbers of myeloid cells in the peripheral blood, the sample may be inadequate.

13 Although the diagnosis can be obtained from the blood film and peripheral blood, the bone marrow examination is an important test. It is an easier way to obtain cytogenetic results, to assess for blastic transformation and to review the overall cellularity and marrow function.

14 The increased cellularity is consistent with CML due to the excess of granulocyte precursors in the marrow. In chronic phase, the granulocyte pattern seen in the bone marrow aspiration is similar to the peripheral blood. Normal marrow has 'fat spaces' which contain adipose cells thought to contribute to the haematopoietic microenvironment, but in hypercellular marrow this space is greatly reduced.

15 Myeloid hyperplasia: there may also be evidence of marrow fibrosis in long-standing disease, which decreases the space available for healthy haematopoiesis. This demonstrates the link with other MPNs such as myelofibrosis.

16 Peripheral blast cells upon diagnosis of CML would be very concerning for advanced disease or an alternative diagnosis such as acute leukaemia. Inexperienced scientists may mistake basophils or abnormal neutrophils for blast cells, as they can be similar in appearance.

17 Left shift is a common term used in reporting of blood films and is associated with multiple different aetiologies. It refers to the presence of immature leucocytes and neutrophils within the peripheral circulation in increased amounts. This can occur in CML as well as infection, trauma and inflammation.

18 Megakaryocytes are usually increased but may be smaller and appear atypical. These are the platelet-producing precursor cells in the bone marrow.

19 The Philadelphia chromosome produces an oncoprotein which makes the cells behave in a malignant fashion. The cells are adherent to the bone marrow and resistant to apoptosis.

The Ph chromosome is only found in blood and bone marrow cells; it will not be detected in other cells in the body. As it is not present in eggs or sperm, it will not be passed on from parents or to children.

20 Splenomegaly is common in MPNs such as CML. This is mainly due to ineffective haematopoiesis in the bone marrow resulting in haematopoiesis occurring elsewhere in the body, such as the spleen. Ultrasound may show evidence of recent or previous infarction of the spleen.

Management

Immediate

Tumour lysis risk [1] should be minimised by increasing **fluid intake** [2] and commencing **allopurinol** [3]. Consider using **hydroxyurea** [4] until the WCC normalises. Give analgesia for splenic pain.

Short-term

Commence an oral **tyrosine kinase inhibitor (TKI)** [5]. The patient should be linked in with a haematologist and **undergo regular review** [6] at least monthly, initially. Ensure the medication is **tolerated** [7] and **education** [8] is provided. Offer **psychological support** [9].

Long-term

The aim of therapy is to remain in **remission** [10]. Untreated, CML can progress from **chronic phase** [11] to **accelerated phase** [12] and to **blast phase** [13]. In those who remain in remission, the metabolic complications of therapy and cardiac risk factor identification and surveillance are of utmost importance. In those who present in **advanced phase** [14], an **allogeneic stem cell transplant** [15] should be planned in **eligible patients** [16] if a **suitable donor** [17] is available.

1 The risk of tumour lysis syndrome (TLS) may be overlooked in those treating CML, as there is not the measurable tumour burden of solid organ malignancies or the blast cells of acute leukaemia. TLS is more likely to occur in accelerated or blast phase CML receiving high dose chemotherapy.

2 Increasing the fluid intake of the patient, orally if possible or intravenously, assists with preventing renal dysfunction due to the cell turnover, by improving glomerular filtration and renal perfusion.

3 Allopurinol is a xanthine oxidase inhibitor used to prevent the production of uric acid which can occur due to the high cell turnover in CML. Allopurinol competitively inhibits xanthine oxidase, the enzyme responsible for the conversion of hypoxanthine and xanthine to uric acid. Production of new uric acid is therefore decreased; however, it does not break down existing serum uric acid.

4 Hydroxyurea is a medication used to reduce peripheral white cell count. It is an antimetabolite chemotherapeutic agent prescribed in many MPNs as well as sickle cell anaemia. It disrupts the DNA replication process of abnormal cells, resulting in increased apoptosis in the peripheral circulation. It has no effect on the bone marrow production of the

abnormal cells and therefore no effect on the underlying disorder.

5 Tyrosine kinase inhibitors are an example of targeted therapy rather than traditional cytotoxic chemotherapy. TKIs are usually well-tolerated by patients and are taken orally, once or twice daily. There is generally a requirement for continued therapy and it will be intended for most patients to take the medication for the rest of their life. TKIs revolutionised the treatment of CML which prior to this therapy was an often fatal condition treated with cytotoxic chemotherapy and curable only by bone marrow transplant. TKIs are able to switch off the deregulation of tyrosine kinase that causes the pathogenesis of CML.

6 The use of an oral medication to treat this form of leukaemia means that continued patient compliance must be ensured. It is more difficult to monitor daily oral therapy than with IV or subcutaneous treatment which is given in a ward or chemotherapy day unit. Complacency can occur in those who feel well and are able to live a normal life. The FBE should be monitored and progress is assessed by tracking the BCR-ABL transcript level. Cytopenias can occur with treatment. Ensure the patient has an up-to-date prescription and supply of medication.

7 Side-effects of TKIs should not be a barrier to prescribing appropriate therapy and are a major cause of avoidable non-compliance. There are several generations of therapy so those who are intolerant or resistant to one drug should promptly be prescribed a different agent. Each agent has a different side-effect profile and this is taken into account when prescribing for individual patients. For example, the TKI nilotinib is generally avoided first-line in those with cardiovascular comorbidities or vascular risk factors. Lack of patient compliance due to medication side-effects can lead to resistance or relapse.

8 Education should be provided with regard to the potentially life-threatening but treatable nature of the condition, the side-effects of treatment and the importance of follow-up. Ensure those of childbearing age are educated regarding the effects of treatment. In general, patients should not become pregnant or father children on TKIs and should be counselled on appropriate contraceptive use. Breastfeeding should also be avoided in those on TKIs. In those diagnosed at a young age, careful planning is needed if parenthood is desired and a period off treatment in order to facilitate may be achievable in those in long-term remission.

9 Although many patients are now able to achieve a normal life expectancy despite a CML diagnosis, it is still a significant shock to receive this diagnosis. Provide contact details for the local leukaemia or cancer support service.

10 Many patients are able to stay well in chronic phase indefinitely with oral TKIs. Remission is defined as:
- haematologic – normal blood counts including normal basophils
- cytogenetic – undetected Ph chromosome on bone marrow aspiration and trephine
- molecular – reduction/absence of BCR-ABL in peripheral blood and marrow.

If a patient remains in a deep, stable remission for many years, a medication-free remission can be discussed with the treating haematologist. Some patients do not achieve remission with TKIs, often due to drug resistance, side-effects or poor compliance.

11 Chronic phase is the first phase of CML and the aim is to keep patients in this phase. Patients are generally asymptomatic, and granulocyte and platelet counts should be close to normal. Blast cells in the bone marrow are <10%. Chronic phase may continue for decades in compliant patients with good cytogenetics and compliance. These patients will have a life expectancy similar to the general population.

12 The definition of accelerated phase varies, but usually refers to the presence of 10–19% blasts in the bone marrow. It is also defined by high blood basophils, thrombocytopenia that is not due to therapy, progressive splenomegaly and increasing WCC. TKIs may be suitable to treat a patient in accelerated phase and may be enough to achieve remission; however, this is less likely to occur compared with those in chronic phase. An allogeneic stem cell transplant should be considered in patients in accelerated phase if a suitable donor is found and remission is not achieved.

13 Blast phase refers to the evolution to an acute leukaemia type of condition. By definition this is the presence of >20% blasts in the bone marrow. Prior to the use of TKIs, this was the expected evolution of a patient approximately 3–5 years after diagnosis of CML. If a patient transforms to blast crisis it will be fatal unless they are eligible to undergo allogeneic stem cell transplantation. The blasts can be phenotyped to either lymphoid or myeloid blast cells, which is important as the type of blast crisis portends different chemotherapeutic treatment. Initial treatment of blast phase generally involves the intensive cytotoxic therapy given to patients with acute leukaemia.

14 Accelerated or blast phase CML portends a poor prognosis and allogeneic stem cell transplantation (alloSCT) following remission is likely to be offered. Morbidity and mortality rates remain high and the patient needs to be informed of risks and benefits prior to the transplant. Without the transplant, the CML is likely to progress through this phase. Prior to the use of TKIs an allograft was the only chance to cure the condition.

15 Despite the name, a bone marrow transplant (stem cell transplant) can occur with peripherally collected stem cell using a procedure similar to blood donation. Harvest from actual bone marrow in the iliac crests is rarely used these days. The donor-related discomfort and morbidity is low with peripheral collection. The patient is given a 'conditioning' regime of chemotherapy and sometimes whole body radiotherapy to ablate their bone marrow. Following this, the donor stem cells are infused into the patient like a blood transfusion. Immunosuppressive medications are given before and after the donor stem cells are given, to prevent bone marrow graft rejection.

16 In order to undergo an alloSCT, the patient must be aged <70 (at some centres the cut-off may be at age 65), have minimal comorbidities and be psychologically ready to undergo the transplant. They must have adequate social support and be willing to comply with the intense procedure and rigid follow-up.

17 An HLA-matched sibling is the preferred donor for an allograft. In those without siblings or without matched siblings, an unrelated HLA-matched living volunteer donor will be sought. There is a worldwide bone marrow donor registry with good participation rates in Europe and the USA. A third donor option is a single or double umbilical cord blood STC, mostly suitable for children and small adults due to the small numbers of cells obtained from this method. Some centres perform allografts using a 'haploidentical' (half-identical) donor, such as the patient's parent or adult child.

CASE 34: Haemolytic anaemia

History

- A **23-year-old** [1] **male** [2] of **Greek** [3] heritage presents with a **1-day history** [4] of **jaundice** [5] and **lethargy** [6] after eating a **bean-based meal** [7] at a vegetarian restaurant.
- He has also had intermittent **abdominal pain** [8] and noted that his **urine is very dark coloured** [9].
- He also experienced a fever yesterday but has not had a recent **infection** [10]. He is otherwise usually well with no previous jaundice.

- He last **travelled overseas** [11] one year ago to a non-tropical area which did not require **anti-malarial prophylaxis** [12].
- He does not **inject recreational drugs** [13] or partake in risky **sexual activities** [13].
- He has not recently taken any **prescribed or over-the-counter medications** [14] or **supplements** [15] and has not had a recent **blood transfusion** [16].
- He has no **family history** [17] of a similar illness.

1 Glucose-6-phosphate dehydrogenase (G6PD) deficiency is a congenital defect and can present in patients at all ages. This patient may have not been exposed to an offending agent or may have had minor exposure not resulting in a clinical syndrome. Low level haemolysis can be self-limiting and may not have been noted by the patient.

2 G6PD deficiency is an X-linked disorder and will be present in all males with an affected X chromosome. Heterozygous females may demonstrate clinical G6PD deficiency due to lyonisation (random X chromosome inactivation). It is very rare for females to be homozygous (two gene mutations) for G6PD deficiency.

3 G6PD deficiency is most commonly seen in those with African, Mediterranean, Asian, South American or Middle Eastern ancestry. G6PD deficiency is common in populations where malaria is or was endemic, as it may confer protection against severe malaria. Up to 10% of those of African origin are at risk of the most common type of G6PD deficiency. This condition is the most common congenital enzyme deficiency syndrome and occurs in around 200–400 million people worldwide. There are over 100 different mutations and genetic variants causing the condition.

4 An acute haemolytic crisis is the most common presentation of G6PD deficiency. It may also present as neonatal jaundice or chronic haemolytic anaemia. G6PD is an enzyme in the hexose-monophosphate pathway, responsible for generating nicotinamide adenine dinucleotide phosphate (NADPH). An acute crisis is precipitated by increased oxidative stress caused by an offending agent. Acute haemolysis usually occurs 24–72 hours after ingestion of the offending substance. This overwhelms the red cell supply of NADPH. Alternatively, if there is long-term exposure to the offending agent in small doses, the patient can have undetected chronic compensated haemolysis without ill effect.

5 Jaundice is a common presentation of haemolysis due to prehepatic bilirubin elevation (unconjugated bilirubin). With moderate–severe haemolysis the jaundice will be obvious to the patient or their family; however, a careful history may retrospectively reveal episodes of mild jaundice which was imperceptible to the patient at the time. Mild jaundice can also be a presenting feature of some infections, or acute hepatitis.

6 Due to the rapid reduction in haemoglobin available to carry oxygen to tissues, the patient may present with fatigue, lethargy and general malaise. Up to a third of the circulating red blood cells may be destroyed and effectively removed from the circulation, resulting in a large reduction in oxygen-carrying ability.

7 Acute haemolysis after ingestion of 'fava beans' occurs in two types of G6PD deficiency and appears to be one of the most common presentations aside from infection. The term 'fava beans' is a category referring to many types of bean such as broad beans. It is not exactly known which component of the bean causes oxidative damage.

8 Abdominal pain or acute back pain can occur in episodes of haemolysis due to the hyperbilirubinaemia and associated gall bladder tension. Rarely, the abdominal pain will be due to splenomegaly. Ask about episodic body or joint pain, as a sickle cell crisis may present similarly.

9 Dark urine is due to haemoglobinuria and may be due to increased urobilinogen. It is not due to bilirubin. The urine can appear as red, brown or black.

10 Infection is the most common precipitant of haemolysis in those with G6PD deficiency. It is thought that white blood cells release oxidative compounds during phagocytosis and apoptosis which cause oxidative stress to erythrocytes.

Infectious microbes known to cause oxidative haemolysis in G6PD-deficient individuals include influenza, hepatitis viruses, *E. coli*, B-haemolytic strep and *Salmonella*.

11 A history of travel to tropical countries may point towards infection as a cause for the haemolysis. This is more likely to cause extravascular haemolysis and is associated with parasites as well as more common infections such as mycoplasma (cold agglutinin haemolysis) and EBV infection. Malaria should be particularly noted, as up to a quarter of patients with *Plasmodium falciparum* malaria can present with severe haemolysis. Blood group A patients are most at risk for severe overwhelming haemolysis, while those with type O blood group are relatively protected.

12 Many of the agents commonly used for antimalarial prophylaxis can exacerbate G6PD. The main drugs implicated are primaquine and chloroquine. Ironically, the populations with higher rates of G6PD deficiency usually have higher rates of exposure to malaria which may increase the likelihood of conferred immunity.

13 Injecting drugs and unprotected sexual intercourse (especially male to male) are risk factors for acute hepatitis B or C which can present with acute liver failure resulting in a similar clinical picture. It is often wise to ensure the patient is asked these sensitive questions without family, their partner or friends present. Ask about a past history of hepatitis virus infection. Consider whether the patient is from an ethnic background in which hepatitis B is endemic.

14 Intentional or unintentional paracetamol overdose can cause acute hepatitis. Ask about paracetamol use including duration, dose and frequency. Check the serum paracetamol level if overdose is suspected; this can be processed rapidly in most laboratories. Medication history should specifically include all prescribed medications as well as those available from pharmacy or supermarket shelves.

15 Supplements can cause acute hepatitis or haemolysis due to high doses of ingredients which are not strictly regulated by the food or medication industries. Specifically ask about over-the-counter medication and supplement use.

16 Acute intravascular haemolysis can occur after the receipt of an ABO group mismatched blood transfusion (for example, blood type A is given to an O group recipient) or blood which is infected with bacteria. This will immediately present with signs of acute haemolysis, including pain and fever. Delayed transfusion reaction can also occur up to two weeks post transfusion. This is due to the formation of an antibody against a red cell antigen which the patient lacks. In most patients this reaction is self-limiting but some may present with fever and severe haemolysis.

17 G6PD deficiency is an inherited X-linked disorder although there may be no known history in other family members. There are many different pathogenic mutations, most of which are point mutations. Haemolysis is also associated with many other inherited conditions, the most common being hereditary spherocytosis (particularly in Europeans).

Examination

- The patient looks **unwell** [1].
- He is **jaundiced** [2] with marked **scleral icterus** [3].
- Mucous membranes are **pale** [4].
- He is **tachycardic** [5] with a regular rhythm and mild **hypotension** [6].
- There is no **rash** [7].
- There is no **lymphadenopathy** [8], and no **hepatomegaly** [9] or **splenomegaly** [10] is appreciated.
- There are no signs of **chronic liver disease** [11].

1 There are a number of reasons for the patient to appear generally unwell including:
- sudden loss of a large amount of the oxygen-carrying haemoglobin
- listlessness resulting from fever
- the sallow appearance of jaundice and pallor.

2 Jaundice is usually visible on the skin when the bilirubin level exceeds around 40–50µmol/L. It may be detectable at lower levels in the sclera. This may be the presenting feature that alerts the patient to receive medical attention.

3 Scleral icterus refers to the yellow appearance of the eyeball due to increased bilirubin levels. It can be best visualised in natural light by lifting the patient's top eyelid and asking the patient to look downwards. This exposes a large amount of the sclera for examination.

4 The anaemia may result in pallor of the skin, palmar creases and conjunctiva. This may be best appreciated in the conjunctiva or mouth as it will be less affected by the coexisting jaundice in the skin.

5 Severe anaemia can result in haemodynamic instability and compromise. The body has a remarkable ability to compensate by increasing red cell production by up to fivefold and increase the delivery of oxygen to tissues. However, there is a point beyond which the body is unable to compensate and this depends partly on the patient's cardiovascular fitness. Haemolysis can cause rapid destruction of blood cells, causing a clinical picture that is similar to acute blood loss. In severe cases hypovolaemic shock can occur.

6 It is likely that young patients will be able to compensate until an acute blood loss of about 30% of the blood volume in less than 12 hours. Beyond this point, the patient will begin to show signs of shock, including hypotension. This can result in inadequate perfusion of red cells to organs. There may be evidence of hypoxia, diaphoresis and even anxiety and confusion beyond this point. Initiation of intravenous fluid replacement should occur urgently. This may be in the form of IV saline until a blood transfusion is ready.

7 Rash may be present if the presentation is due to infection (such as malaria or dengue) rather than acute haemolysis. G6PD deficiency is not associated with rash. Look for the petechiae of thrombocytopenia, present in other (often life-threatening) causes of haemolysis.

8 Lymphadenopathy may be due to infection and will be transient. Malignant lymphadenopathy (such as lymphoma) is associated with immune dysregulation and autoimmune haemolytic anaemia. If lymphadenopathy is present, ask

the patient when they first noted it, as the chronicity of the abnormal lymph nodes would mean infection is less likely.

9 The presence of hepatomegaly would be more consistent with chronic liver disease or a chronic haemolytic anaemia causing hepatosplenomegaly.

10 The spleen is the major organ involved in destruction of the red blood cells. Blood flows through the spleen and it is able to test which red cells remain viable. Older and diseased cells will not be able to re-enter the circulation through the sinusoidal wall of the organ and will therefore be destroyed. This, as a chronic process, can result in splenomegaly. In autoimmune types of haemolytic anaemia, the red cells are primarily destroyed in the spleen.

11 Look for palmar erythema, bruising on the limbs, spider naevi on the chest, gynaecomastia, caput medusae or the presence of ascites. These are signs of chronic liver disease.

Investigations

- FBE shows **normocytic anaemia** [1] with marked **reticulocytosis** [2].
- Blood film reports **polychromasia** [3], macrocytosis (reticulocytosis) and **spherocytes** [4].
- 'Bite cells' are also present on the film but there are no **Heinz bodies** [5].
- **Bilirubin** [6] and **LDH** [7] are elevated.
- The **haptoglobin** [8] is undetectable.
- The laboratory notes that the **plasma is positive for haemoglobin** [9].
- **Direct antiglobulin test** [10] (Coombs test) is negative.
- **Malaria thick and thin films** [11] are negative.
- **Creatinine** [12] is normal.
- Urinalysis demonstrates the presence of **haemosiderin** [13] without **leucocytes or nitrites** [14].
- Ultrasound of the abdomen demonstrates no **gallstones** [15], normal **liver architecture** [16] and normal spleen size.
- **Testing for G6PD deficiency** [17] is not performed.

1 Normocytic anaemia suggests haemolysis or haemorrhage. Anaemia will occur if the haemolysis cannot be compensated by the increase in reticulocyte production. Normal red cell lifespan is around 120 days, after which red cell destruction occurs and the cells are removed via the reticuloendothelial system. In states of haemolysis, red cell survival may be just days. In acute haemolysis (or haemorrhage) the haemoglobin level may be initially normal due to the reduction in total blood volume and the delay in dilutional increase in plasma volume.

2 Reticulocytosis is a sign of increased red cell production and is one of five key tests which should be requested when suspecting haemolysis. The other tests are: LDH, bilirubin, haptoglobin and direct Coombs test. An otherwise healthy bone marrow will markedly increase the production of red cells and a large number of reticulocytes will be released into the peripheral circulation. Levels should be monitored during the recovery phase of haemolysis.

3 Polychromasia refers to multiple different colours and shades of red blood cells. This is due to the increased

reticulocytosis and red cells of differing stages of maturity being viewed with different shades of red, purple and blue cytoplasm.

4 Spherocytes are dense, dark cells which have lost the central pallor of normal red blood cells. These occur in hereditary spherocytosis (a rare inherited condition) and haemolytic anaemia. If seen on a blood film, an investigation for other features of haemolysis should occur.

5 Heinz bodies are seen within red blood cells on the blood film. They are specific inclusions within the red cells which are composed of denatured and precipitated haemoglobin which has been metabolised from damaged cells. It is unusual to see Heinz bodies with a functional spleen, as the filtering mechanism of the spleen will remove the denatured haemoglobin effectively from the circulation.

6 Bilirubin will be elevated in haemolysis due to metabolism of red cell components into protoporphyrin and then into bilirubin. The majority will be unconjugated. Levels of bilirubin of 40–90μmol/L are consistent with haemolysis.

Higher levels warrant investigation into alternative or additional causes.

7 Lactate dehydrogenase is released in red cell damage and is increased in states of high cell turnover. An elevated LDH in any patient should prompt consideration of further investigation for haemolysis as a cause.

8 Haptoglobin is a protein which takes free haemoglobin out of the circulation and into the spleen to be cleared. When there are high levels of free haemoglobin in the blood, haptoglobin is consumed and measured levels will be suppressed. The reticuloendothelial system removes the haptoglobin-haemoglobin complexes from the bloodstream. Haptoglobin may be high in those with inflammatory illness, and low or suppressed in those with liver disease who are unable to produce the protein.

9 Blood plasma is usually a clear to yellow colour when separated from the red blood cells. In intravascular haemolysis, even small amounts of lysed red cells can stain the plasma so it will appear pink macroscopically. This is a clue to the presence of intravascular haemolysis which may be noted early in the laboratory. The amount of haemoglobin can be quantified but the presence of pink in the plasma itself is usually abnormal and should prompt further investigation.

10 The direct antiglobulin test (DAT) (Coombs test) is positive in cases of autoimmune haemolytic anaemia (AIHA). There are also many causes for false positives. AIHA is then further divided into 'warm' and 'cold' types which have different causes and treatments. The DAT will be negative in haemolytic anaemia caused by oxidative haemolysis, as it is not caused by an antibody produced by the body against its own cells.

11 Malaria is diagnosed by examination of the whole blood under the microscope. The 'thick' film is a drop of blood on a slide which allows visualisation of the presence of parasites. The 'thin' film is used to appreciate finer detail and determine the species of parasite.

12 Acute haemolysis can be toxic to renal tubules and cause acute renal failure. Those with chronic renal failure are less likely to be able to compensate and more likely to have increasing creatinine levels. In those with renal failure, metabolic acidosis may further increase the haemolysis.

13 Haemosiderin will be present in those with intravascular haemolysis. Urine haemoglobin is broken down in the kidneys to form haemosiderin. This may be seen for up to weeks post an acute haemolytic event as the renal tubular cells shed the haemosiderin. A Prussian blue stain will positively identify urinary haemosiderin.

14 Leucocytes and nitrites in the urine can indicate infection as a precipitant for the haemolysis in a patient with G6PD deficiency. Infection can also cause haemolysis in healthy individuals; however, this is rare and usually only with severe sepsis such as meningococcal or pneumococcal septicaemia.

15 Gallstones can occur due to high levels of pigment (bilirubin). This will be seen on abdominal ultrasound. Those with disorders leading to chronic haemolysis, such as hereditary spherocytosis, commonly have multiple gallstones.

16 Ultrasound imaging is very useful to exclude intrinsic pathology affecting the liver. Liver architecture will be normal in acute haemolysis due to G6PD deficiency. Abnormalities of the liver may be seen in hepatitis.

17 Assessment of G6PD activity may not be useful during an acute attack. False negatives are common due to the older red cells with the highest levels of deficiency being haemolysed during the acute phase and therefore being physiologically excluded from the testing. In addition, reticulocytes and young erythrocytes which are increased during periods of haemolysis have a relatively high concentration of G6PD, again leading to near normal levels.

Management

Immediate

Consider a **transfusion** [1] of **packed red blood cells** [2], determining **the risks** [3] and benefits for this patient. Maintain hydration to **protect renal function** [4]. Give analgesia for the **abdominal pain and paracetamol for fever** [5].

Short-term

Reassure the patient [6]. Commence the patient on **folic acid** [7]. Give prophylaxis against **thrombosis** [8]. Monitor **haemolysis markers** [9] until normalised.

Long-term

Once the patient has recovered from the acute episode, send formal **testing for G6PD deficiency** [10]. The patient should be educated with regard to **avoiding offending agents** [11]. **Offer screening** [12] to family members. Ensure there is a **follow-up blood test** [13] organised.

1 Blood transfusion is indicated if:
- the patient is decompensated or haemodynamically compromised
- the patient has comorbidities such as unstable angina or severe pulmonary disease
- the rate of haemolysis is rapid, or
- there are symptoms of decreased organ perfusion.

The amount of blood required to be transfused depends on the patient's age, ongoing likelihood of destruction, and comorbidities. Children are more likely to require a transfusion than adults. The general aim is to keep the haemoglobin level above 70–80g/L. Those with cardiac comorbidities need to keep the Hb above 100g/L to prevent demand ischaemia. Following an acute intravascular haemolytic event, haemoglobin levels can rapidly fall as the haemoglobin released from the cells is cleared from the circulation.

2 A blood transfusion is given as preserved donated packed red blood cells which have been separated from whole blood. The donor blood is machine cross-matched with the recipient's blood. Red cells can be stored for up to 42 days before being used. Red cell transfusion will not be sufficient to replenish iron stores, and iron replacement is required in addition.

3 Complications of blood transfusion include haemolytic reaction, febrile reaction, volume overload, infection (rare), alloimmunisation (development of antibodies) and thrombophlebitis at the cannula site. Frequent blood transfusions can result in iron overload conditions. Blood donors are carefully screened and tested to reduce the risk of infection transmission, particularly in respect of bloodborne viruses. Tropical infections such as malaria and West Nile virus can be transmitted and this is also reduced by donor screening. Blood is now universally leucodepleted (the white cells removed).

4 Adequate hydration will improve flow through the glomeruli and renal tubules to protect against deposition of red cell breakdown products causing renal damage. If diagnosis is delayed, the patient may be at risk of acute tubular necrosis. Monitor renal function along with the haemoglobin level.

5 The patient should receive supportive care to assist with recovery. Paracetamol to lower fever can quickly result in increased comfort and provide an analgesic effect. Paracetamol is usually safe to prescribe despite the jaundice, as liver function itself is usually unaffected.

6 The sudden presentation of jaundice and the related symptoms would be very alarming for the patient, particularly upon the first episode. Educate the patient regarding the self-limiting nature of the condition.

7 Patients with all types of haemolytic anaemia should be supplemented with folic acid. It is a key 'building block' of the red blood cells and without adequate stores the haematopoiesis will be ineffective, resulting in poor red cell survival. Ensuring adequate iron stores is also important.

8 There is an association between haemolytic anaemia and thrombosis. The exact mechanism is unknown but may be due to circulating antiphospholipids or free haemoglobin which has been released from damaged cells. Ensure hospitalised or immobilised patients receive chemical thromboprophylaxis.

9 There is no specific treatment for haemolysis associated with G6PD deficiency aside from removing and avoiding the offending agent. It is usually self-limiting once the older cells with low levels of G6PD have been destroyed and removed from the circulation. The younger erythrocytes and reticulocytes formed and released into the circulation usually have sufficient amounts of G6PD to prevent ongoing haemolysis despite ongoing ingestion or infection.

10 G6PD deficiency can be tested using quantitative or qualitative methods. Screening tests are useful, especially when treatment with an oxidant medication is urgently required. However, this must be followed with a confirmatory test. Ideally testing is performed at least 3 months after an acute episode. Specific mutation testing is not useful in sporadic cases as the exact mutation may not be known.

11 Medications causing G6PD exacerbation include:
- antimalarials – primaquine, chloroquine, quinine
- sulfonamides – sulfasalazine, dapsone, co-trimoxazole
- antibiotics – nitrofurantoin and quinolones such as ciprofloxacin
- aspirin in large doses
- other drugs including naphthalene, probenecid and vitamin K analogues.

Some offending agents can be given safely in small doses to those with G6PD deficiency. In large enough doses, some agents (such as dapsone and naphthalene) can cause haemolysis in those with normal G6PD due to overwhelming NADPH. The susceptibility to each drug varies considerably amongst individuals.

12 Newborn testing is not usually performed in western countries but does occur in populations with a high rate of the enzyme defect. PCR can be used if a specific mutation is known. It may be prudent to suggest screening of family members prior to starting offending medications such as antimalarials.

13 It is very important to ensure a full blood examination is checked approximately one week and again several weeks after the episode to ensure haemoglobin stabilises and further haemolysis is not occurring. Check the haemolysis markers (LDH, bilirubin, reticulocytes). Ensure iron stores are replete.

CASE 35: Haemophilia

History

- A **19-year-old** [1] **Caucasian** [2] **male** [3] presents with **sudden onset pain** [4] and **swelling** [5] in his **elbow** [6].
- There is no recent history of **trauma** [7] to the area.
- **Range of movement** [8] of the joint is limited.
- He has had no **fevers or sweats** [9] and does not otherwise feel unwell.
- He gives a history of **previous joint bleeds** [10] without any history of **mucosal bleeding** [11].
- There is no history of **liver disease** [12] and he does not take any **anticoagulant medications** [13].
- He has a **normal diet** [14] with no abdominal symptoms or dyspepsia.
- There is no **family history** [15] of bleeding disorders.

[1] The majority of haemophilia is inherited, affecting patients throughout their lifespan. It is a chronic condition requiring multidisclipinary management from diagnosis due to the absence or very low levels of factor VIII in the body. In very rare cases haemophilia can be acquired, due to an autoantibody, mostly occurring in the elderly.

[2] The prevalence of haemophilia A is the same throughout the world with minimal variation amongst people of different races. It affects approximately 1 in 7000 live male births.

[3] The genes that regulate the production of factor VIII and IX are found on the X chromosome. Congenital haemophilia is an X-linked dominant condition. Haemophilia occurs in females only in rare cases, although heterozygous females may experience mild symptoms.

[4] Blood in the synovial space is acutely and intensely painful. There may be a prodrome of stiffness followed by sudden onset warmth in the joint, prior to the onset of pain. Some patients may experience tingling or a sensation of joint tightness during the prodrome. Ask how long the pain has been present for and whether it is new pain.

[5] Tissue swelling occurs at the site of bleeding and in enclosed spaces can compress local structures and cause complications such as compartment syndrome.

[6] Those with haemophilia can bleed into any part of the body; however, the most common sites are muscles or joints. Large joints such as ankles, knees, hips, shoulders and elbows are the most often affected. Ask the patient about previous bleeds and where they have tended to occur. Ask whether they have had muscle, ocular or organ bleeds. Those with severe haemophilia usually begin to have joint and soft tissue bleeds from toddler age as they start to become active.

[7] Severity of bleeding correlates with the level of factor VIII activity and in severe haemophilia, bleeding occurs with little

or no provocation. Normal factor VIII levels are between 50 and 150%. 100% factor VIII activity is measured as the level in pooled plasma from many different patients, representing the average factor level. Those with severe haemophilia will have baseline factor VIII levels of <1% from birth.

[8] Loss of range of movement can occur acutely due to blood in the joint. However, if there is a history of recurrent joint bleeding the patient may have chronic arthropathy and reduced function. Ask whether the joint can be fully straightened normally or if there is a pre-existing arthropathy. Compare the joint to the unaffected side.

[9] A major differential is septic arthritis, and in those without a clear history of a bleeding disorder it can be difficult to differentiate. Ask about fever, sweats, fatigue or whether they feel generally unwell. Note whether there are raised inflammatory markers.

[10] A positive personal history of joint bleeds points towards a congenital bleeding problem or haemostatic deficiency. Bleeding into joints and muscles is seen in coagulation factor deficiencies. It is less likely to be seen in those with platelet function disorders or thrombocytopenia.

[11] Mucosal bleeding can occur in those with haemophilia but is not a common manifestation. Mucosal bleeding usually suggests the presence of thrombocytopenia, as platelets assist with forming the primary haemostasis. Haematuria can occur, but is also less common. Occasionally, mild haemophilia patients are diagnosed post dental extraction which is uncomplicated initially but persistent bleeding occurs several hours later. This occurs in haemophilia due to the primary haemostasis being adequate in forming the initial clot, then it loses effect and the defective intrinsic coagulation pathway is inadequate to maintain haemostasis.

[12] Liver disease is an important cause of abnormal coagulation due to a number of causes:

- impaired absorption of vitamin K leading to decreased synthesis of vitamin K-dependent coagulation factors (II, VII, IX, X)
- dysfibrinogenaemia
- reduced levels of factor V
- impaired removal of activated clotting factors
- thrombocytopenia due to decreased platelet stimulation production (thrombopoietin)
- hypersplenism from portal hypertension leading to platelet sequestration and thrombocytopenia.

13 The use of anticoagulant therapy such as warfarin or antiplatelet medications should be clarified. Haemarthrosis can occur in those with supratherapeutic INR levels associated with warfarin use.

14 Deficient intake of vitamin K or vitamin C can cause bruising and bleeding. The fat-soluble vitamin K is required as an essential cofactor for carboxylation and conversion to

vitamin K epoxide which is reduced to vitamin K epoxide reductase. This is important for the vitamin K-dependent factors II, VI, IX, and X and the anticoagulants protein C and S. Vitamin C causes bleeding in a very different pathway due to its requirement for collagen synthesis and stabilisation. Collagen is a key structural protein which is needed to form multiple tissues including blood vessels. Defective collagen leads to loss of tissue and vessel structure and subsequent bleeding. It also leads to impaired wound healing.

15 Despite haemophilia having a clear inheritable genetic cause, up to one-third of hereditary haemophilia cases will have no family history of bleeding disorders. This is likely to be due to mutation in the index patient or the maternal carrier of the disorder. Ask about family history in detail, including both males and females. Ask about previous generations including grandparents, aunts and uncles.

Examination

- The patient looks **distressed due to pain** [1] and is holding his elbow.
- He is **afebrile** [2].
- The elbow area is not **erythematous and local lymphadenopathy** [3] is not present.
- There is no **break to the skin or discharge to the area** [4].
- The **elbow circumference is 4cm larger** [5] than the contralateral side.
- There are no **other joints** [6] acutely affected; however, **reduced range of movement** [7] is noted in the contralateral elbow.
- He has a **yellow bruise** [8] to his left knee and no **petechiae** [9].
- Oral examination reveals no **wet purpura** [10] or **mucosal bleeding** [11].
- There is no evidence of **muscle bleeding** [12].
- The abdomen is **soft and non-tender** [13].
- His **weight is 80kg** [14].

1 Acute intra-articular bleeding usually results in rapid and intense pain. Blood within the narrow joint space causing synovial distension is very irritating to the local sensory nerves. Muscle spasm is associated. The pain is also due to compression on local structures within the joint space causing a degree of ischaemic necrosis.

2 A fever may indicate septic arthritis. It could also occur in a very large bleed or indicate an infected haematoma less acutely.

3 Erythema and local lymphadenopathy may indicate infection in the area.

4 A break in the skin or discharge would suggest infection could be a cause of the patient's symptoms rather than bleeding. Take a swab of the discharge if present.

5 It is useful to measure the circumference of a joint affected by haemarthrosis and compare to the other side. This can objectively define the presence of swelling due to bleeding and be used to assess recovery from the acute event. This can be performed in the larger joints such as knee,

ankle and elbow. This should be documented in the clinical notes.

6 Examine other joints for evidence of bleeding. Common sites include the contralateral elbow, shoulders, wrists, hips, knees and ankles. Children often present with bleeding in the weight-bearing joints, i.e. ankles and knees.

7 Reduced range of movement and stiffness, without pain, in other joints is indicative of chronic haemophilic arthropathy due to previous recurrent bleeds.

8 Yellow-coloured purpura indicates that particular bruise is at least a day old. This may indicate recurrent issues with bleeding such as a coagulation disorder.

9 Petechiae would occur in a qualitative or quantitative platelet disorder, as opposed to a coagulation system disorder.

10 Wet purpura are 'blood blisters' on the oral mucosa or tongue. They are more associated with severe thrombocytopenia than haemophilia. However, bleeding can occur from the nose, in the oral cavity or from the gums.

11 Mucosal bleeding and bleeding due to small cuts is usually minimal, as platelet function is intact.

12 Spontaneous or traumatic bleeding into muscles can occur and result in haematoma formation in the area. If bleeding is extensive it can cause compression on local structures resulting in compartment syndrome. This is most likely in the lower leg and forearm. The most commonly affected muscles in haemophilia are the quadriceps, iliopsoas muscles and the muscles of the arm.

13 Retroperitoneal haemorrhage or visceral bleeding is a major cause of morbidity and potential mortality in patients with bleeding disorders and must not be missed. Abdominal haematoma formation must be considered in any haemophilic patient presenting with abdominal pain. Rarely, haematomas can form in the bowel wall. Without effective coagulation, bleeding in these compartments can continue to spread, causing large haematomas.

14 The patient must be accurately weighed in order to dose the factor replacement. This should be recorded in the clinical history for future reference.

Investigations

- FBE is **normal** [1].
- Coagulation studies demonstrate a **normal INR and PT** [2] with a **prolonged aPTT** [3].
- **LFTs** [4] are normal.
- **Ultrasound** [5] of the elbow joint reveals a haematoma and the presence of a **pseudotumour** [6].

- **Joint aspiration** [7] is not performed.
- Factor VIII level comes back as **<1%** [8] of normal.
- **Factor IX** [9], **factor XI** [10] and **von Willebrand** [11] testing are normal.
- Genetic analysis of the factor VIII gene reveals heterozygosity for the **intron 22 mutation** [12].

1 It is important to ensure platelet levels are normal as significant thrombocytopenia may exacerbate bleeding. A drop in haemoglobin can occur with a large bleed, such as a large intramuscular haematoma.

2 The prothrombin time (PT) evaluates extrinsic and common pathways of the coagulation system. It involves mixing plasma with thromboplastin and calcium to identify deficit or antagonism of factors II, V, XII and X. The INR was introduced to standardise the PT measurement across different laboratories using different reagents. In those with a deficiency in factor VIII or IX, measurement of the PT and INR will not be affected.

3 The activated partial thromboplastin time (aPTT) is a measurement of the intrinsic coagulation system. It is measured as the time taken for the plasma to form a fibrin clot, measured in seconds. Prolonged aPTT can indicate deficiencies in factors VIII, IX, XI and XII.

4 Liver disease is an important cause of bleeding, due to reduced production of procoagulants and anticoagulants. It is also important to consider the prevalence of hepatitis viruses in patients with haemophilia due to the previous high risk of bloodborne virus transmission with frequent factor replacement. This is seen in older patients as the risk is low in the present day.

5 The diagnosis of haemarthrosis can usually be made clinically, although imaging may be performed to assist with confirming a bleed. This is especially useful in those with recurrent bleeds to determine whether there is a new event. Plain radiography may show local soft tissue swelling and can

rule out fractures to the area. Those with severe haemophilia and recurrent bleeds may have abnormal-appearing joints at baseline with previous damage to cartilage and bone. Ultrasound is a non-invasive method to help identify a joint effusion, which in context would suggest a haemarthrosis. It can also evaluate surrounding structures and is cost-effective to perform. CT can detect acute blood deposition and MRI will detect haemosiderin deposited post bleeding episode.

6 A haemophilic pseudotumour is a benign, cyst-like structure which is formed after a large bleed in the area. The blood is walled off from the surrounding tissue by the formation of a fibrous structure. In the long term, there may be expansion of the pseudotumour which can result in compression on surrounding tissues. Those occurring in bones can erode adjacent bone tissue.

7 Joint aspiration, which would be useful to diagnose the differential of septic arthritis, is not appropriate in those suspected of having haemarthrosis due to haemophilia. This is likely to exacerbate bleeding without clear diagnostic benefit.

8 Severe haemophilia is defined as baseline factor levels of <1%. Those with factor levels of 1–5% have moderate haemophilia and this factor level is just enough to protect against the severity of disease seen with severe haemophilia. These patients are at risk of significant haemorrhage with medical procedures, surgery and trauma but are less likely to have spontaneous bleeds. Patients with mild haemophilia have a baseline factor level of 6–30% and may not present until adulthood if not haemostatically challenged; this may be with post-procedure or post-surgical bleeding.

9 Factor IX deficiency is haemophilia B and occurs in 1 in 25 000 male births. It is phenotypically identical to haemophilia A. It is critical to confirm the patient has haemophilia B rather than the more common haemophilia A, and to ensure the correct factor replacement is used (i.e. factor IX).

10 Factor XI deficiency (haemophilia C) is very rare, seen predominantly in those of Ashkenazi Jewish heritage. Bleeding tendency tends to be less severe than that of haemophilia A or B, even in those with factor XI levels of <5%.

11 Von Willebrand disease is the most common bleeding disorder and affects males and females equally. It is caused by a deficiency in von Willebrand factor, which can be either quantitative or qualitative. The deficiency affects platelet adhesion and causes a secondary deficiency of factor VIII. There are three main types of von Willebrand disease which have very different mechanisms and bleeding phenotypes; haematology input is recommended to distinguish between the types.

12 In severe haemophilia A this is the most common genetic mutation. Between 20 and 30% of haemophilia A cases are caused by a spontaneous mutation and therefore will have no family history of bleeding.

Management

Immediate

The patient needs to be **urgently** [1] discussed with the **haematology team** [2], who may need to liaise with the local **haemophilia treatment centre** [3]. He should be given **analgesia** [4] and **tranexamic acid** [5]. Severe factor VIII deficiency is best treated with **factor VIII concentrate** [6] with guidance from the specialty team regarding **dosing** [7]. This patient should not be given DDAVP [8].

Short-term

The patient may need **further doses of factor replacement** [9]. He should be reviewed by a **haemophilia-specific physiotherapist** [10]. Follow up to ensure **resolution of symptoms** [11].

Long-term

The patient needs to be registered on the **bleeding disorder registry** [12] and issued with an **emergency information card** [13]. He should be linked in with the local **haemophilia treatment centre** [14] and be tested for **factor inhibitors** [15]. He may be offered **prophylactic factor replacement** [16] and be educated on **self-treating at home** [17]. There may be the opportunity to be enrolled in a **clinical trial** [18]. Information about **genetic counselling** [19] should be provided to the patient and **his family** [20].

1 Delay in treatment can result in increased joint destruction and chronic sequelae. It is crucial to avoid this increase in morbidity.

2 Specialist advice should be sought to determine the best treatment for this patient. The ideal method of factor replacement, product used, number of doses and target plasma factor VIII level should be determined by a clinician experienced with haemophilia patients. For example, if the patient presents with haematuria, the advice may be to monitor rather than initiate factor replacement, as the subsequent clots formed when haemostasis is restored can result in blockage of the ureters.

3 The haemophilia centre may keep details on the patient's baseline factor levels, previous treatment and the particular type of treatment needed. Some patients have developed inhibitors to factor treatment, which requires the use of a different product and will make standard products ineffective.

4 Haemorrhage into a joint is extremely painful. If the patient is known to a haemophilia centre, advice may be given regarding previous analgesic regimes and tolerance. Some patients may have developed chronic pain and have previously tolerated large opioid doses.

5 Tranexamic acid is an antifibrinolytic medication. It may be helpful as the sole treatment of mild bleeding episodes and can be used in conjunction with factor replacement in significant bleeds. Its role is in stabilising the clot to enhance haemostasis and reduce the risk of re-bleeding.

6 Factor replacement can be made from human plasma concentrates or be in recombinant form. The recombinant form is most commonly used today and there are newer longer-acting products which require less frequent dosing. The use of human plasma concentrates has resulted in transmission of bloodborne viruses such as hepatitis B and C and HIV. These viruses are more commonly seen in older haemophilia patients who received frequent products in the era of poorer screening practices, in which up to 80% of patients were infected with one or more bloodborne viruses. Factor replacement can be given intermittently or as a continuous infusion.

7 Dosing depends on the severity of the bleed and the patient's weight. In mild haemorrhage (epistaxis, gum bleeding) the aim is usually to maintain factor level at 30%. Moderate haemorrhage (muscle, joint bleed) may require a factor level closer to 50%. In severe haemorrhage (major trauma, major surgery, intracranial events, advanced haemarthrosis, GI bleed) factor levels of 80–100% should be targeted, and this may involve a continuous infusion. Overdose of factor replacement results in risk of thrombosis.

8 Those with mild or moderate haemophilia may be able to use DDAVP (vasopressin). This is not suitable for those with haemophilia B or severe haemophilia A. It is an alternative way of increasing the plasma VIII level in those with mild disease by initiating factor VIII release from endothelial cells. It is associated with an antidiuretic action and hyponatraemia, so care is needed in the elderly or those with cardiac or renal dysfunction.

9 Further doses of factor replacement should be discussed with the specialist haematology team. In moderate–severe bleeding a continuous infusion of factor replacement may be needed, with regular testing of the serum factor VIII level to target the ideal factor VIII level.

10 Recurrent haemorrhage into joints or muscles causes long-term disability due to arthropathy and contractures. Repeated joint bleeds can result in permanent damage and subsequent loss of mobility.

11 Bleeding into a joint and the resulting damage and inflammation increases the risk of further bleeding into the same joint. This is referred to as a 'target' joint. This can result in chronic synovitis and disability.

12 Registration on a bleeding disorder registry allows ready access to the patient's details by healthcare professionals working with bleeding disorder patients. The bleeding disorder registry includes patients with inherited and acquired haemophilias, von Willebrand disease, platelet function disorders and other rare bleeding disorders. It includes details of the patient's specific condition, any inhibitors to factor replacement, historical weight and preferred treatment product.

13 An emergency card or medical alert bracelet should be carried by the patient. This gives information to bystanders and medical practitioners in an emergency. An emergency card can also provide the patient with emergency contact numbers. This should also alert first responders and emergency clinicians to seek specialist advice before emergency procedures such as arterial blood gas sampling, invasive line insertion and lumbar punctures.

14 Haemophilia is a chronic disorder which needs to be managed by an MDT. This includes doctors, nurse practitioners, physiotherapists, social workers, chronic pain practitioners, dentists, genetic counsellors and psychologists. The key to management of haemophilia is prevention of bleeds, but if they occur, ensuring early recognition resulting in prompt initiation of treatment to preserve joint function. Many centres will follow up haemophilia patients on a yearly or twice-yearly basis to review management, assess for complications of the disorder and test for the presence of factor inhibitors.

15 Alloantibodies to the infused factor concentrate can develop post treatment. This results in loss of efficacy of the treatment and necessitates the use of alternative products. It is important to recognise the presence of inhibitors and this is one of the most serious complications of haemophilia.

16 Patients with severe haemophilia may be offered prophylactic factor replacement. This is given 2–3 times a week by the patient, usually at home. The patient needs to be reliable, compliant and willing to administer the treatment. As factor replacement is given intravenously, this requires rigorous education, and permanent venous access devices may be required.

17 As soon as a bleeding episode is suspected, those who are willing and able to can administer the first dose of factor replacement at home. This will immediately assist with minimising the bleed and can also reduce the amount of treatment needed. The patient should be instructed to then seek further advice from the haemophilia centre or ED.

18 There is increasing research into newer drugs and gene therapy which may provide a cure for haemophilia, or reduce the need for prophylaxis. Gene therapy is also an emerging and interesting treatment being researched.

19 A patient with haemophilia will pass on the gene to his daughters. They will become obligate carriers and this has implications for their subsequent children. A son of a male with haemophilia cannot have the disorder as he will receive a Y chromosome from his father.

20 The diagnosis has implications for family members including any sisters. If a female carries the gene for haemophilia on one of her chromosomes, she will not have haemophilia, but will be a carrier for the disorder. There is a 50% chance of passing on the genes to one of her sons, who will then be born with haemophilia. There is a 50% chance one of her daughters will be a carrier for haemophilia.

CASE 36: Hodgkin lymphoma

History

- A **23-year-old** [1] female presents with a 2-week history of **drenching night sweats** [2] and **pruritus** [3].
- This is associated with **loss of 6kg of weight** [4] over the **past 3 months** [5].
- Over the past week she has noted a **gradually enlarging lump** [6] on the right side of her neck.

- She has not had recent **upper respiratory tract symptoms** [7] and has not **travelled overseas** [8] previously.
- She has not noted any **dyspnoea or chest pain** [9].
- Her past history is significant only for appendicectomy and **'glandular fever' infection** [10] 2 years ago.
- She is a **non-smoker** [11] and has **one child** [12].

[1] Hodgkin lymphoma presents in a bimodal age distribution, mostly found in teenagers or young adults with a second peak incidence after age 50 years. It is more common in the Caucasian population and higher socioeconomic groups.

[2] 'B symptoms' such as night sweats and fevers occur in advanced or aggressive lymphoma. The name originates from the use of the Ann Arbor staging system which assigns the letter 'B' to the presence of these symptoms, as opposed to 'A' which refers to no symptoms. B symptoms are a negative prognostic factor in Hodgkin lymphoma. Pel–Ebstein fever is the intermittent fever of Hodgkin lymphoma which can occur over days or weeks and occurs in about 30% of patients.

[3] Pruritus occurs in around a quarter of patients and can be very severe. It is often classically associated with increased symptoms after drinking alcohol. Consumption of alcohol can also induce significant pain at the site of lymphadenopathy.

[4] Weight loss is an additional B symptom which is thought to be even more significant prognostically than night sweats. Some chronic infections such as TB may cause weight loss.

[5] Classic Hodgkin lymphoma often progresses slowly, and patients may in hindsight recognise symptoms which have been present for weeks to months prior to diagnosis.

[6] Cervical lymphadenopathy is the most common presenting sign and occurs in up to two-thirds of patients. Ask about how long the patient has noted the lymphadenopathy. It is very common to present with cervical lymphadenopathy that has been waxing and waning. Other sites of lymphadenopathy which may be self-detected by patients include axillary or (less likely) inguinal lymphadenopathy.

[7] Infections can cause transient palpable lymphadenopathy. This includes common respiratory viruses, infectious mononucleosis, cytomegalovirus, HIV primary infection, adenovirus or streptococcal infection. There may be significant delay in the diagnosis of Hodgkin lymphoma in young patients, as transient cervical lymphadenopathy due to viral infection is common, and malignant diagnoses are unexpected in this age group.

[8] Infections which are more common in returned travellers and can cause lymphadenopathy include toxoplasmosis or rubella. TB can also present with fever, sweats, weight loss and a mass.

[9] Dyspnoea or chest pain can suggest the presence of a mediastinal mass which is a common presentation in those with Hodgkin lymphoma. These masses can grow slowly and in well-compensated patients may not be noted until a large size. A mass may be noted incidentally on chest radiography performed for other reasons.

[10] Glandular fever refers to the Epstein–Barr virus (EBV) infection. Over 90% of adults have been exposed to EBV in their lifetime. Hodgkin lymphoma is associated with EBV infection (in up to 50% of cases) and immunosuppressed states, such as those with HIV. In those who have lived overseas, ask whether they have had rheumatic fever.

[11] Cigarette smoking is associated with an increased risk of Hodgkin lymphoma. It is thought that there is an interaction between EBV and smoking to further increase this risk. This is likely to have a stronger impact on older patients and those with a long smoking history. Complications of treatment for Hodgkin lymphoma are increased in those who smoke. Smoking is also associated with other head and neck malignancies which may present with weight loss, cervical lymphadenopathy and sweats, generally in those above the age of 50.

[12] It is important to take a thorough social history when a diagnosis of malignancy is suspected. Involve the social work team early. Enquire as to possible childcare arrangements.

Examination

- The patient appears **pale** [1] and slightly **cachectic** [2] with no evidence of a **rash** [3].
- Temperature is **37.9°C** [4] and there is a mild **tachycardia** [5].
- There is a **2 x 2cm rubbery, fixed mass** [6] in the right anterior cervical area.
- A similar mass is found in the **axilla** [7].

- Examination of the scalp, ears and **oropharynx is normal** [8] and **breast examination** [9] reveals no lump.
- There is no hepatomegaly or **splenomegaly** [10]. There is no inguinal lymphadenopathy appreciated.
- Heart sounds are dual with **no added sounds** [11].

1 Pallor is likely to be due to anaemia. This may be evident on examination of the face. With the patient's permission, check the conjunctiva for pallor and compare the anterior rim to the deep rim of the palpebral conjunctiva of the lower eyelid.

2 Cachexia refers to the loss of muscle and/or fat mass due to illness. There may be evidence of sunken cheekbones or loose skin on the abdomen. Significant cachexia is more likely to occur in advanced malignancy and in the elderly. Weight loss is due to the increased metabolic demands of malignancy and may be due to loss of appetite associated with hepatosplenomegaly or the disease itself.

3 Many types of infection can present with rash. Hodgkin lymphoma is not associated with a rash, even in those with pruritus. Scratch marks may be noted in those with significant pruritus. Some patients may have non-specific areas of erythema associated with febrile episodes.

4 There is a low grade fever. Fever could be caused by a viral infection. However, it can also be a pathological sign of a lymphoproliferative condition caused by release of cytokines from the malignant cells. This is associated with night sweats and raised inflammatory markers. Ask whether the patient has measured their temperature at home. Ask how often they have noticed the fever and whether it is continuous or intermittent.

5 Tachycardia can occur due to the increased metabolic demand of the disease or due to the low grade fever. Rule out infection or pulmonary embolism as a cause for tachycardia, as both are increased in haematological malignancy. Care needs to be taken in those with tachycardia and a mediastinal mass which can cause compression on the heart and mediastinal structures.

6 Note the size of the lymph nodes, whether they are soft or hard and whether there is tenderness. Palpate whether it appears to be an enlarged single lymph node or a group of lymph nodes 'matted' together. Note whether the mass is irregularly shaped or smooth, and if it is fixed to surrounding structures. Ensure the mass is not soft and subcutaneous, which would be more consistent with a benign lipoma.

7 Location of abnormal lymph nodes is important. Axillary or supraclavicular lymphadenopathy is very suspicious for underlying malignancy and should be investigated. In the submandibular or inguinal areas, small and sometimes transient lymphadenopathy may be seen, and may reflect chronic dental or lower limb infection rather than malignancy.

8 Oropharyngeal erythema or exudate, or tonsillitis may be an infectious cause of cervical lymphadenopathy with fevers. In older patients, especially those with a history of smoking or chronic alcohol use, the oropharynx and tongue should be examined for malignant lesions.

9 Breast examination should be done in a female who has been found to have axillary lymphadenopathy. This should be performed bilaterally. Offer a chaperone while performing the examination.

10 It is important to know whether the spleen is involved, although this should be confirmed on imaging. Involvement of the spleen may occur prior to haematogenous spread throughout the body so is noted when staging the patient prior to therapy.

11 Ensure the patient has no murmurs, especially in this patient with fever and tachycardia. Rheumatic fever or infective endocarditis can cause fevers and weight loss in young people. It is also important to recognise any cardiac abnormalities prior to treatment in Hodgkin lymphoma. Examine the cardiovascular system thoroughly if the patient is suspected of having a mediastinal mass; signs of a pericardial effusion or even tamponade may be elicited.

Investigations

- Full blood examination and film shows a mild **normochromic normocytic anaemia** [1] with **eosinophilia** [2], **lymphopenia** [3] and **thrombocytosis** [4].
- **ESR and LDH** [5] are elevated.
- **EBV IgG is positive** [6] but **IgM is negative** [7]. HIV serology is negative.
- **Cardiac** [8] and **pulmonary function** [9] testing is normal.

- **PET scan** [10] demonstrates avid and enlarged lymph nodes in **two separate groups** [11] **above the diaphragm** [12] with no bone marrow involvement.
- Axillary **biopsy** [13] **under ultrasound guidance** [14] shows the characteristic **Reed–Sternberg cells** [15] on the background of inflammatory infiltrate.
- It is consistent with **nodular sclerosing** [16] Hodgkin lymphoma.
- **Bone marrow aspirate and trephine** [17] is normal.

[1] This anaemia is likely to be an anaemia of chronic disease, which is uncommon in a young female who is otherwise healthy. It is unusual to have bone marrow involvement in early stage disease causing anaemia due to infiltration of the marrow. If bone marrow involvement does occur it can cause anaemia or thrombocytopenia. Ask about other causes of anaemia such as significant menorrhagia. Ensure iron stores are replete.

[2] Eosinophilia is common in Hodgkin lymphoma and is part of the pathologic process by providing cellular ligands for receptors. It may be associated with a survival advantage depending on the histological subtype of the disease. Many patients will also have a neutrophilia.

[3] Lymphopenia is usually seen in advanced disease. There is an association with cell-mediated immunity. Lymphopenia as an isolated finding is non-specific and may be associated with viral infections. It is not a specific finding of lymphoma.

[4] Thrombocytosis can be found in reactive conditions or acute haemorrhage. In Hodgkin lymphoma patients usually present with normal or increased platelet counts. Thrombocytopenia occurs in very late disease with marrow infiltration.

[5] ESR is elevated in patients with infections or malignancy due to high levels of immunoglobulins or fibrinogen as acute phase reactants. CRP may also be elevated. ESR can be useful as a marker to monitor disease progress and is also included in prognosis scoring systems at diagnosis. LDH is elevated in around a third of patients at diagnosis as a marker of cell turnover.

[6] The presence of EBV IgG suggests past infection and conferred immunity. Those with previous EBV infection have a threefold increased risk of developing Hodgkin lymphoma, although overall numbers are low and EBV infection is common in the general population. Those who have been diagnosed with EBV infection do not need specific screening for Hodgkin lymphoma.

[7] Current EBV infection would be suggested by a positive IgM and negative IgG, although there can be cross-reactivity

with other infections. The IgG will be negative as immunity will not yet have developed during the acute infection. Acute EBV infection can cause transient, tender cervical lymphadenopathy, weight loss and sweats.

[8] Cardiac function must be assessed prior to the use of anthracycline chemotherapy. This may be in the form of an echocardiogram, or a nuclear medicine scan assessing formal ejection fraction.

[9] Pulmonary function must be assessed prior to the use of bleomycin chemotherapy. Doses may be reduced in those with underlying lung disease, or this medication may be omitted altogether.

[10] F-fluorodeoxyglucose (FDG) PET scanning is a mainstay of diagnosis and staging of malignancies, especially lymphoma. Rapidly dividing (i.e. malignant) cells take up large amounts of glucose for their cellular activities. The full body PET scan measures radiolabelled glucose infused into the patient and taken up into tissues. Metabolically active tissues such as the brain, heart and liver have physiologically elevated uptake of the FDG marker. Uptake into malignant or potentially malignant sites is compared to the uptake in liver and mediastinum as internal controls. It can be used to detect whether lesions seen on plain CT scanning are metabolically significant or benign.

[11] Hodgkin lymphoma usually spreads from a single lymph node group via lymphatic channels to adjacent nodal groups. Therefore it is common for nodal groups that are located close together to be involved. It is unusual to have non-contiguous spread to distant sites without involvement of the nodal groups in between.

[12] Location and number of groups of abnormal lymph nodes are important in staging. Stage I indicates involvement in only one lymph node area, e.g. isolated unilateral cervical lymphadenopathy. This patient has stage II disease, as they have two separate nodal groups involved on the *same* side of the diaphragm. This could be one group of right-sided cervical nodes and a group of mediastinal nodes. Stage III involves nodal groups above and below the diaphragm, i.e. a cervical group and an inguinal group. If the spleen is

involved in stage III disease it is referred to as stage IIIS. Stage IV disease indicates involvement outside of the lymph node groups. This includes bone marrow, liver, testes, lung and other skeletal sites. However, if extranodal disease is purely an extension of localised disease it is not upstaged but the letter 'E' is added to the stage, e.g. stage IIE. In all cases the stage is followed by the letter A (absence of symptoms) or B (presence of symptoms). Symptoms include fever, loss of >10% body weight and night sweats. The patient in this case would be classified as stage IIB.

13 The preferred type of biopsy in lymphoid malignancies is an excision biopsy of an entire lymph node. This allows the architecture to be appreciated. A fine needle aspirate (FNA) of an affected lymph node is frequently inadequate and non-diagnostic. A proportion of patients will require more than one biopsy before diagnosis is made. It is not uncommon to have non-diagnostic samples, even if a core biopsy is taken. Biopsy should be taken for histology, formalin fixed for haematoxylin and eosin (H&E) stain and immunohistochemical staining. If lymphoma is suspected, the biopsy needs to be prepared and sent for flow cytometry analysis in addition.

14 Superficial nodal groups can be biopsied under local anaesthesia. Usually this is done with radiological guidance to ensure the correct node is sampled and local structures are not at risk. Ultrasound is used to locate lymph nodes in the cervical, inguinal and axillary regions. Deeper nodes,

such as in retroperitoneal and abdominal regions, may require CT guidance. Mediastinal and chest nodes can be difficult to access and in some cases bronchoscopy and endobronchial ultrasound is used. Surgical excision is used for deep abdominal nodes which are inaccessible by imaging guidance due to local structures such as bowel.

15 Reed–Sternberg cells are large binuclear cells with prominent 'owl-eyed' nuclei. They resemble a macrophage-like cell. They are often difficult to find in the biopsy specimen, as they comprise just 1–2% of the tumour cells. Other cells in the biopsy specimen include lymphocytes and eosinophils.

16 Nodular sclerosing Hodgkin lymphoma is the most common type in young people and portends a favourable prognosis. Histology classically demonstrates nodules of abnormal tissues partitioned by bands of collagen. Lymphocyte-depleted Hodgkin lymphoma is the least common and portends a poor prognosis; however, it only occurs in 1% of cases.

17 Bone marrow aspirate and trephine is not required in patients with limited stage disease and a normal FBE. It is reasonable to perform in this patient with prominent B symptoms. Involvement of lymphoma in the bone marrow will result in a higher stage of disease (stage IV) and additional cycles of chemotherapy.

Management

Short-term

Tell the patient the **diagnosis** [1] and educate regarding **treatment options and prognosis** [2]. Discuss with the patient and their family about **fertility preservation** [3]. Arrange to commence **chemotherapy** [4] and for **regular review** [5] during the treatment. Refer for **radiotherapy** [6] if indicated. **Psychological and social work support** [7] should be offered to all patients.

Long-term

Relapsed or refractory disease may be amenable to **further treatment** [8]. Hodgkin lymphoma has a high rate of cure and survivors should have long-term follow-up to monitor for treatment-related problems. Late treatment effects can include **infertility** [9], ongoing **infection risk** [10], **secondary malignancy** [11], **cardiac disease** [12], **lung damage** [13] and **hypothyroidism** [14].

1 Ensure the diagnosis is delivered in a sensitive manner. With the patient's permission, have supportive family or friends present for the discussion. Allow an appropriate amount of time for the discussion. Organise a follow-up review with opportunity for the patient and family to ask additional questions.

2 Overall the cure rate for Hodgkin lymphoma is around 85% of patients. This is dependent on age, stage of disease, comorbidities, histology and response to treatment. Discuss the use of chemotherapy and the importance of maintaining compliance with treatment.

3 Fertility preservation must be discussed prior to commencing treatment and appropriate collection and storage should be offered. Infertility can occur due to chemotherapy or radiotherapy. Current treatment approaches are generally fertility sparing so appropriate contraception during treatment should be discussed and utilised. Female fertility preservation in the form of ovarian tissue or egg storage is often difficult to access and impractical with the urgency of commencing treatment.

4 Treatment for Hodgkin lymphoma usually commences with chemotherapy and may also involve radiotherapy in some patients with bulky disease. The use of surgery is not usual. Standard first-line chemotherapy involves 2–6 cycles of IV cytotoxic therapy. With high cure rates now achievable for many patients, the long-term toxicity of treatment is now a concern and must be balanced against the likelihood of cure.

5 Regular review must be organised during treatment. Watch for respiratory symptoms or cardiac symptoms, which can indicate serious adverse effects of chemotherapy. Assess for peripheral neuropathy prior to each treatment, which is a complication of a commonly used chemotherapy. Ensure the patient is psychologically coping with therapy.

6 Radiotherapy is commonly used in Hodgkin lymphoma, generally after the planned chemotherapy is complete. Indications include:
- single site of disease, after two cycles of chemotherapy (as opposed to 4–6 cycles)
- bulky disease (larger lymph nodes at diagnosis), or
- single site of residual disease after chemotherapy.

Radiotherapy is given by specialised radiation oncologists using ionising radiation delivered to the specific area by a linear accelerator. The radiation dose is measured in grays (Gy) and is divided in fractions (sessions) – i.e. a patient may receive a total of 20Gy in 10 fractions.

7 Hodgkin disease frequents affects young healthy people who are just beginning their adult lives. It often interrupts work and/or study, for a period of 4–6 months or more. Social workers can assist with ensuring financial support is available during this period and assist with recommending appropriate childcare arrangements. The vast majority of treatment will be given as an outpatient. The chemotherapy regime used for Hodgkin disease almost always results in alopecia (hair loss) which can have an underestimated impact on patients. Encourage smoking cessation in those who are currently smoking, to protect against cardiac and lung damage and infection.

8 For those who do not respond to the standard treatment, options include:
- escalating the chemotherapy to alternative (often more intense) regimes
- using targeted therapies such as anti-CD30 antibodies or PD-L1 inhibitors
- chemotherapy plus additional radiotherapy or autologous stem cell transplantation.

Allogeneic stem cell transplantation is used in a minority of patients with relapsed or refractory disease.

9 Males can experience transient or permanent azoospermia or low sperm quality. Women may experience loss of menstrual periods which can resume after treatment. Some women go into early menopause with treatment. Offer gynaecology review to affected women.

10 Hodgkin lymphoma can be associated with a profound immunodeficiency, even after successful treatment. This is primarily due to a defect in T-cell response. This can lead to an increase in viral infections such as herpes zoster.

11 Radiotherapy to the chest area increases the risk of lung cancer and breast cancer. Newer techniques and increased awareness of the harmful effects of radiotherapy in young patients have decreased the risk in the past 30 years. Smoking should be discouraged and regular breast screening should be carried out. Alkylating chemotherapy agents can increase the risk of AML. There may also be an increased risk of second malignancy in Hodgkin lymphoma patients due to the impaired T-cell surveillance. This persists even after disease remission.

12 Anthracycline chemotherapy is associated with cardiac failure. A baseline ejection fraction should be obtained prior to starting treatment, and dose-adjusted or alternative therapy should be used in those with pre-existing cardiac impairment. Radiotherapy to the chest is associated with coronary artery disease as a late effect.

13 Bleomycin chemotherapy and radiotherapy are both associated with lung fibrosis. Baseline pulmonary function testing should be performed prior to treatment. Respiratory symptoms developing during treatment should be promptly assessed and if persisting or severe, the patient should undergo high resolution CT scanning. Bleomycin will be dose-reduced or omitted if there are lung infiltrates.

14 Up to a third of patients treated for Hodgkin lymphoma are at risk of developing hypothyroidism as a late effect. This is more pronounced in those who have received radiotherapy above the diaphragm. The development of hyperthyroidism, thyroid nodular disease or secondary thyroid cancer is less common. Thyroid function should be reviewed at least yearly.

CASE 37: Idiopathic thrombocytopenic purpura

History

- A **27-year-old female** [1] presents with **blood blisters** [2] in her mouth and a **pinprick erythematous rash** [3] to her feet.
- She also has had two prolonged episodes of **epistaxis** [4] within the last few days and noted gum bleeding post flossing.
- She has noted **spontaneous bruising** [5] on her arms.
- She has otherwise been well with no **weight loss or night sweats** [6] and no **arthralgias or other rashes** [7].

- She has a **normal diet** [8] with no **excess alcohol intake** [9], is on **no medications** [10] and has not been exposed to any **anticoagulants** [11].
- She previously had a pregnancy with normal delivery with **no excess bleeding** [12].
- She has not suffered from **menorrhagia** [13].
- She also had a previous **uncomplicated tonsillectomy** [14].
- There is no **family history** [15] of bleeding.

[1] Younger patients are less likely to have an intrinsic marrow disorder such as the myelodysplastic syndrome which mostly occurs in older people. If other cell lines are affected, aplasia or haematological malignancy may be considered. Idiopathic thrombocytopenic purpura (ITP) is most common in women, usually between age 15 and 50, and is a diagnosis of exclusion. It can also occur in children and usually follows a viral infection.

[2] Wet purpura refers to 'blood blisters' inside the mouth and on the oral mucosa. They are usually a late sign of severe thrombocytopenia which requires urgent medical attention. They usually appear when the platelet count is below 10 x 10^9/L.

[3] The appearance of a petechial rash strongly suggests thrombocytopenia. It tends to be most prominent in the lower limb (such as on the top of the feet) due to increased hydrostatic pressures. The rash will be non-blanching.

[4] Mucosal bleeding is common.

[5] Spontaneous bruising is not necessarily pathological. Clarify whether this has been for years, or whether it is just recent. A long history of simple bruising is common and alone can be benign, especially occurring in healthy women of childbearing age. A more sudden and recent history of bruising suggests a new cause for the problem. Large or widespread bruising in unusual sites is likely to have a sinister cause.

[6] The presence of weight loss and night sweats should alert consideration of the possibility of underlying leukaemia or lymphoma. ITP is most strongly associated with chronic lymphocytic leukaemia or Hodgkin lymphoma. It could also

indicate rheumatological disease in a young woman, such as systemic lupus erythematosus (SLE). Sweats may be a sign of infection causing thrombocytopenia but infection is unlikely to cause significant weight loss.

[7] Arthralgias and rashes may indicate an underlying autoimmune cause such as lupus. Joint pain, such as that of a haemarthrosis, would be very unusual in a patient with thrombocytopenia: this is more likely to occur in those with coagulation factor deficits.

[8] Diet and any history of malabsorption should be noted. Ask about dysphagia or discomfort after eating. Inadequate dietary intake or absorption of vitamin C or vitamin K can cause bleeding.

[9] Heavy alcohol use contributes to thrombocytopenia in two main ways:
- alcohol is a direct toxin to platelets and reduces the lifespan in the circulation
- excess alcohol consumption over a long period can lead to cirrhosis with portal hypertension and congestive splenomegaly, leading to pooling and sequestration of platelets in the spleen.

[10] Medications causing bleeding include chemotherapeutic agents, antimicrobials, NSAIDs, diuretics, anti-epileptics. Ask about previous or long-term use of steroids such as prednisolone, including inhaled corticosteroids for respiratory conditions, which can cause purpura due to impaired connective tissue. The use of inhaled medications is often overlooked in a medication history.

[11] Ensure she is not taking anticoagulant medication such as aspirin and other antiplatelet agents, warfarin, DOACs or heparin. Recent exposure to heparin (unfractionated,

but also low molecular weight heparin, e.g. enoxaparin) should alert the clinician to the possibility of heparin-induced thrombocytopenia (HIT). This is a life-threatening complication caused by formation of an autoantibody directed against endogenous platelet 4 (PF4) and heparin. Despite the progressive thrombocytopenia, the patient is at high risk of arterial and venous thrombosis due to the large complexes depositing in vessels. It should be suspected if:

- platelet count falls between 5 and 10 days post heparin exposure
- the platelet count falls >50% to a nadir of not less than 20
- there is new thrombosis despite thrombocytopenia, and
- there is no other concomitant, more likely cause for the thrombocytopenia.

If HIT is suspected, heparin should be ceased immediately and laboratory investigations for HIT should be ordered on recommendation of the haematology team.

12 Personal history of previous excess of bleeding is crucial here, to differentiate between congenital or acquired disorder. This patient has successfully had two significant events which challenge the body's haemostatic mechanisms – a normal vaginal delivery and a tonsillectomy without bleeding. A history of bleeding may point towards a congenital condition or deficiency such as von Willebrand disorder or haemophilia (more commonly in males). Inherited platelet production and function disorders are rare.

13 Menorrhagia can indicate an issue with haemostasis and in young healthy females may be the only challenge of haemostasis the patient is exposed to. Ask about duration of menstrual bleeding and the number of sanitary products required on 'heavy' flow days.

14 A tonsillectomy is a relatively common procedure in children so it is a good idea to specifically ask whether the patient has undergone this procedure previously when enquiring about bleeding history. Other procedures to ask about include other surgical procedures, dental extractions and any previous trauma.

15 Family history of bleeding is also very important here. This leads to consideration of the possibility of inherited bleeding disorders such as von Willebrand disorder or haemophilia.

Examination

- The patient **looks well** [1].
- She has **non-palpable purpura** [2] on her shins and forearms.
- There is a fine **petechial rash** [3] to bilateral lower legs.
- She has **wet purpura** [4] to her tongue and roof of her mouth and petechiae in the mouth.
- She has no **facial rash** [5].
- Abdominal examination reveals no **splenomegaly or hepatomegaly** [6].
- There is no **lymphadenopathy** [7].
- The **chest is clear** [8] to auscultation.
- She has no **joint erythema, swelling or bogginess** [9].
- **Ophthalmoscopy** [10] is normal.

1 Immune thrombocytopenia may be preceded by a viral illness; however, patients with ITP are usually systemically well. Young patients are often frustrated at staying in hospital with dangerously low platelet counts while feeling well. A differential diagnosis of a purpuric or petechial rash which must not be missed is meningococcal septicaemia and in this case the purpura occurs due to disseminated intravascular coagulation. The patient with meningococcal sepsis will appear *unwell* with the condition.

2 Purpura refers to the purple/black/red 'bruise'-like appearance of the breakage and leakage of small blood vessels under the skin. They are most commonly found on the skin but can also occur on mucosal surfaces (such as in the mouth) and on the surface of organs. They may appear black or very dark red in colour. There is no blanching on the application of pressure. A formal way to test this is to place a glass slide on the skin and press down – the colour will remain and be seen through the glass. Palpable purpura may occur in vasculitic conditions (such as Henoch–Schönlein purpura).

3 Petechiae form due to the same pathological process as purpura, but are very small (1–2mm in diameter) and often appear to be a non-blanching rash. They can occur due to thrombocytopenia but also vasculitic conditions, nutritional deficiency, conditions of abnormal collagen formation and due to medications. Examples of petechial rashes which do blanch include the exanthem of a febrile illness, telangiectasia and allergic rashes.

4 Wet purpura are small blood-filled vesicles which are found on the lips, palate and buccal mucosa. The term 'wet purpura' can also refer to the general mucosal bleeding – from nose, mouth and gums – that occurs with severe thrombocytopenia.

5 It is unusual to see a petechial rash on the face. The presence of a malar or 'butterfly' rash across the temporal area of the face may raise concern for underlying SLE.

6 The presence of splenomegaly raises concerns for an underlying lymphoproliferative disorder such as CLL. Despite the peripheral platelet destruction that occurs in ITP, the spleen is not usually enlarged in idiopathic cases that are not associated with an underlying disorder. Hepatomegaly may occur in those with a lymphoproliferative disorder or chronic liver disease, both of which can cause low platelet counts.

7 Small, tender cervical lymphadenopathy may indicate a recent viral infection as the precipitant of ITP. It could also occur in EBV or acute HIV. Large, smooth, fixed lymph nodes in areas such as the axilla or supraclavicular region may point towards malignancy as a cause for the thrombocytopenia.

8 The chest should be examined for signs of infection. In those with suspected rheumatological disease, auscultate the heart and lungs for serositis: namely, a pleural or pericardial effusion.

9 Signs of arthritis in a young female point towards the consideration of autoimmune or rheumatological causes for the ITP.

10 Ophthalmoscopy should be performed to ensure there is no evidence of fundal haemorrhage occurring due to the thrombocytopenia.

Investigations

- FBE shows **normal haemoglobin and WCC** [1].
- There is severe **thrombocytopenia** [2].
- Blood film shows rare platelets which are **large in size** [3] and there is no **platelet clumping** [4].
- There are no **schistocytes** [5] or **blasts** [6].
- **LFTs** [7] are normal.
- **B12 and folate** [8] stores are replete.
- **Coagulation studies** [9] including fibrinogen and D-dimer are normal.
- An **ANA is weakly positive** [10] and anti-DNA antibodies are negative.

- Viral serology is negative for **hepatitis C and HIV** [11].
- *Helicobacter pylori* [12] testing is negative.
- **Urine B-hCG** [13] is negative.
- Abdominal ultrasound demonstrated a **normal sized spleen** [14] and no features of **liver cirrhosis** [15].
- **Bone marrow aspiration and trephine** [16] shows **plentiful megakaryocytes** [17] and no excess of blasts.
- **Antiplatelet antibodies** [18] are not found in the serum.

1 The commonest cause of thrombocytopenia is suppression of the bone marrow or decreased production of cells by the bone marrow. Causes of this include chemotherapy, marrow infiltration, aplastic anaemia and leukaemia. This is usually manifested as a reduction in red and white cell production in addition to reduction in platelet production. This is not evident in this patient. Autoimmune haemolytic anaemia can be associated with immune thrombocytopenia in rare cases (Evans syndrome). Immune neutropenia can also occur in parallel.

2 Platelets are anuclear cells involved in primary haemostasis and produced by megakaryocytes in the bone marrow. Platelets form from fragmentation of the cytoplasm of the megakaryocytes and each megakaryocyte can give rise to thousands of platelets. Once released from the bone marrow, platelets are filtered by the spleen before being released into the circulation where they have a lifespan of 7–10 days. In ITP an autoantibody is formed against a protein on the platelet membrane. It is phagocytosed by macrophages in the reticuloendothelial system. This primarily occurs in the spleen. The platelet is destroyed along with the autoantibody. The lifespan of the platelet is reduced to just hours and this overwhelms the compensatory production by the bone marrow.

3 The platelets produced in individuals with ITP are very healthy and functional, unlike in the thrombocytopenia of intrinsic marrow disorders, such as leukaemia or the myelodysplastic syndrome. This usually results in less bleeding than in those with thrombocytopenia due to a primary marrow disorder.

4 The results of an FBE are normally determined by machine counting. The machine is unable to analyse an accurate platelet count if the cells are clumped, which can occur due to poor storage or certain conditions. A low platelet count will usually be verified by the laboratory scientist or haematologist by looking at the blood film and counting the platelets manually.

5 Schistocytes, or fragments, indicate red cell haemolysis. This, in combination with thrombocytopenia, would be concerning for a diagnosis of a life-threatening condition called thrombotic thrombocytopenic purpura (TTP). In TTP the red cells are sheared and fragmented upon flowing past intravascular platelet thrombi. Schistocytes may also indicate the presence of haemolytic uraemic syndrome.

6 The presence of blasts on a peripheral blood film is abnormal and suggests the myelodysplastic syndrome or acute leukaemia. The blood film must be reported immediately by an experienced scientist or haematologist in any patient presenting with severe thrombocytopenia to ensure a diagnosis of acute leukaemia (i.e. TTP) is not missed. A haematologist may not be available immediately (especially after hours), but all laboratories will have a scientist available who should be called directly and requested to look at the blood film as a matter of urgency.

7 LFTs may be useful if the thrombocytopenia is suspected to be due to liver disease, splenomegaly or chronic viral infection. Cirrhosis and chronic liver disease can cause thrombocytopenia due to decreased thrombopoietin production. LFTs may be abnormal in hepatitis B or C infection. This would usually be demonstrated by increased aminotransferases and/or low albumin but there may also be evidence of a cholestatic picture.

8 B12 deficiency can be a rare cause of thrombocytopenia. Thrombopoiesis (and myelopoiesis) is ineffective in B12 deficiency resulting in reduced numbers and functionally abnormal platelets in severe deficiency.

9 Performing coagulation studies is crucial in a patient with evidence of bleeding and thrombocytopenia. An elevated INR or aPTT will occur in coagulation factor defects. It is also an important tool to rule out the presence of disseminated intravascular coagulation (DIC).

10 Autoimmune causes should be considered in a young woman presenting with acute thrombocytopenia. A weakly positive ANA is non-specific but negative anti-DNA antibodies is reassuring for ruling out lupus.

11 Chronic viral infections such as hepatitis C and HIV can cause thrombocytopenia due to multiple factors including immunogenicity, bone marrow suppression, decreased production of thrombopoietin and functional hypersplenism. The patient should be informed prior to HIV serology being tested.

12 *Helicobacter pylori* infection has been associated with chronic immune thrombocytopenia. Guidelines vary as to whether this should be tested in all new patients, or for refractory cases with GI symptoms. There have been reports that *H. pylori* eradication can cause remission of ITP.

13 ITP is one of many causes of thrombocytopenia in pregnancy and should be differentiated from gestational thrombocytopenia. Pregnancy-associated life-threatening conditions such as the haemolysis, elevated liver enzymes and low platelet count (HELLP) syndrome, DIC and microangiopathic processes must be ruled out. Before treating a woman of childbearing age, it must be ensured that she is not pregnant. This has implications for the use of second-line agents and must be discussed with the patient.

14 The spleen normally contains a third of the platelets in the periphery; however, in those with massive splenomegaly the spleen may contain up to 90% of the platelets, resulting in thrombocytopenia in the circulation. The spleen is not usually enlarged in adults presenting with ITP, but this occurs slightly more commonly in children with ITP.

15 Liver cirrhosis is a cause of thrombocytopenia due to portal hypertension and congestive splenomegaly leading to pooling of platelets in the spleen. There may also be a reduction in production of precursors required for platelet production and survival.

16 Bone marrow aspiration and trephine is usually only performed in those >60 years of age, or those not responding to therapy. In older patients there is greater suspicion for an underlying myelodysplastic syndrome (uncommon in younger age groups) or a lymphoproliferative disorder such as lymphoma. In younger patients, if there are no abnormal features on history, examination or investigation and there is response to immunosuppression, the diagnosis can be made without a bone marrow biopsy.

17 The increase in megakaryocytes indicates that production of platelets from the bone marrow is normal. This suggests the platelets are being destroyed in the circulation prematurely. The most likely cause is due to an immune process. In those with splenomegaly, it is likely the platelets are being pooled in the spleen.

18 There are several important surface proteins involved in platelet-specific autoimmunity. The lack of measurable antiplatelet antibody in the serum does not preclude the diagnosis of ITP. Platelets also express ABO and HLA class I antibodies. Generally, testing for a specific antibody does not change management and is rarely performed in clinical practice.

Management

Immediate

Platelet transfusion [1] is not indicated as the patient is not bleeding. Commence **tranexamic acid** [2]. Provide **reassurance** [3] to the patient.

Short-term

In children the condition often spontaneously remits; however, this is unlikely in adult patients. The patient should be started on **immunosuppressive therapy** [4], usually in the form of the steroid prednisolone. Some patients are given **intravenous immunoglobulin (IVIg)** [5]. **Close monitoring** [6] and follow-up is required in the immediate period, as relapse is common. **Proton pump inhibitors** [7] and infection prophylaxis should be used in those receiving high dose corticosteroids.

Long-term

Some patients will have a durable remission with normal platelet counts. However, in others the aim may be to simply maintain a **safe platelet count** [8]. In those who are refractory to initial therapy, options include alternative **steroid-sparing agents** [9] or the **anti-CD20 rituximab** [10]. **Splenectomy** [11] may offer the chance of a long-term cure in those who are eligible. **Thrombomimetics** [12] are available for those who are refractory or ineligible for splenectomy. Some patients may go on to develop an **underlying cause** [13] for the immune thrombocytopenia.

---

1 In ITP, platelet transfusion is not indicated unless there is major bleeding or the patient is at significant risk of bleeding. Those with single digit platelet counts are usually monitored in hospital but not given platelets unless indicated. If donor platelets are transfused in patients with ITP, these platelets will also be coated with the antiplatelet antibody and sequestered by the spleen, resulting in rapid destruction. In those who are bleeding, platelet transfusion in conjunction with immunosuppression and IVIg can retain platelets in the circulation at a level sufficient to cease the bleeding.

2 Tranexamic acid is a synthetic inhibitor of fibrinolysis, acting to reduce clot breakdown. It blocks the lysine binding sites of plasminogen (fibrin clot dissolving molecule). It can be given orally or intravenously, or made into a paste to use as a mouthwash. It should be used initially to reduce the superficial bleeding during periods of severe thrombocytopenia. Continued use on platelet recovery will contribute to thrombotic risk.

3 The presence of bleeding and a petechial rash can be extremely concerning for the patient. Providing basic education regarding the aetiology and expected prognosis of ITP should be reassuring to the patient. Impress upon the patient the importance of adhering to management and follow-up to prevent complications.

4 Response to immune suppression is the best diagnostic test for ITP. Corticosteroids, such as prednisolone or dexamethasone, are usually first-line therapy.

5 Intravenous immunoglobulin is a plasma-derived blood product containing donated human proteins and immunoglobulins, in particular IgG. It is prepared from pools of donor plasma and may contain proteins from thousands of

donors, providing a broad spectrum of antibodies. IVIg can be used for a number of autoimmune conditions. It is usually well tolerated, with the main side-effect being a self-limiting post-infusion headache.

6 Many patients respond well to therapy and platelet increment occurs quickly. However, this response can be lost and the patient may require re-induction therapy with high dose immunosuppression. In those who respond, immunosuppression should be weaned slowly to prevent relapse.

7 Proton pump inhibitor use is indicated in those who are being treated with high dose steroids. Steroid use is associated with GI bleeding and perforation.

8 Some patients will have a sole episode of ITP and remain in remission, but this is not the reality for most patients. Ideally remission will be achieved with a platelet count over $150\,000 \times 10^9/L$, which is the normal range for most laboratories. The risk of significant haemorrhage increases with platelet counts of $<20\,000 \times 10^9/L$ and many clinicians will elect to treat patients at this level. In some patients, platelets of $50\,000–100\,000$ is more achievable and safe than using additional immunosuppressive agents to aim for the normal reference range. Comorbidities, the need for anticoagulation for other medical conditions, severity of previous bleeding and high risk occupations should be taken into account.

9 Additional immunosuppressive agents are sometimes added in those with a poor response to lower doses of corticosteroids, or who relapse when the steroid dose is reduced. Steroid-sparing agents include azathioprine, mycophenolate mofetil, ciclosporin or cyclophosphamide.

10 CD20 is a molecule seen on B lymphocytes. The use of the anti-CD20 therapy results in prolonged B-cell depletion. Side-effects include infusion reactions and long-term immune suppression effects.

11 Splenectomy may be indicated in those with ITP which is not responding to immunosuppression or in those without a durable response. It often has a curative effect in these patients. Prior to the availability of tolerable steroid-sparing agents, splenectomy was a common second-line treatment of ITP. Splenectomy can be performed laparoscopically or with open surgery. The effect of splenectomy (if successful) can be seen rapidly and results in platelet levels rising to double the upper limit of normal, given the compensatory thrombopoiesis due to the splenic destruction of platelets. The major risk of splenectomy is overwhelming bacterial sepsis. This risk is mitigated by registration with the splenectomy registry, vaccination against encapsulated organisms and influenza, and long-term antibiotic prophylaxis.

12 Thrombomimetic medications are structurally dissimilar to the hormone thrombopoietin but act by stimulating the receptor for thrombopoietin. To simplify, this can be compared to the action of erythropoietin (EPO) on red cells, although *in vivo* the comparison is not so straightforward. These medications (given orally or subcutaneously) since their development several years ago have put many patients into remission who achieved inadequate response to corticosteroids. However, there may be concerns with the lack of knowledge with regard to long-term sequelae including bone marrow fibrosis, thrombotic complications and possible stimulation of malignancy.

13 Long-term follow-up may reveal the development of criteria-proven SLE, B-cell malignancies, antiphospholipid syndrome or HIV. Treatment of the underlying disorder is most appropriate in these situations.

CASE 38: Iron-deficiency anaemia

History

- A **37-year-old female** [1] of **Caucasian ethnicity** [2] presents with **fatigue, lethargy** [3] and **decreased exercise tolerance** [4].
- Her history is significant for being 6 months **postpartum, currently breastfeeding** [5] and being diagnosed with **coeliac disease** [6].
- She is **menstruating** [7] intermittently and has not had **changes in her appetite** [8] or **bowel habit** [9].
- She has no symptoms of **gastritis** [10].
- Prior to pregnancy, she partook in **regular jogging** [11] and was a **blood donor** [12].
- She takes **no regular prescribed medications** [13].
- She avoids gluten but otherwise follows a normal **diet** [14].
- There is no history of any previous **surgical procedures** [15].

1 Iron-deficiency anaemia (IDA) is very common in women of menstruating and childbearing age and may affect up to a quarter of females in this age group. Pregnancy causes an increased physiological demand for iron in the body. Menstruation increases the loss of iron from the body. Children are at risk during periods of rapid growth and in neonates who are rapidly expanding their red cell population in the first year of life.

2 Ethnicity is very important to note in those presenting with anaemia. Inherited haemoglobinopathies (such as sickle-cell anaemia) and disorders of haemoglobin synthesis (such as thalassaemia) are uncommon in Caucasian individuals. Thalassaemias are seen in those from South East Asia, the Mediterranean and Middle East.

3 In gradual onset anaemia, symptoms are often insidious and non-specific. The patient may complain of weakness, headaches and palpitations. Older patients or those with comorbidities may present with symptoms of angina pectoris, cardiac failure or confusion.

4 The main function of red cells in the circulation is to carry oxygen to tissues and return carbon dioxide to the lungs. Anaemia reduces the oxygen-carrying capacity of the erythrocytes. This will result in a shift of the haemoglobin-oxygen dissociation curve to the left. Dyspnoea on exertion is a common symptom at low haemoglobin levels.

5 During pregnancy and lactation there is a significant increase in iron demand. Approximately 1mg of iron is required per day to maintain normal stores; however, up to 20mg per month of iron may be lost due to menstruation and up to 1000mg additional iron may be required during a pregnancy to maintain stores.

6 The body already has a limited ability to absorb iron, and coeliac disease may perpetuate this. Coeliac disease is associated with malabsorption of nutrients, including iron

and vitamin B12. Dietary iron is absorbed in the duodenum. Malabsorption or poor intake of iron is rarely a stand-alone cause for iron deficiency. In developing countries, iron deficiency is common due to a cereal- and vegetable-based diet, or due to the presence of parasites causing chronic GI damage.

7 Recommencement of menstruation combined with breastfeeding results in a high requirement for iron intake. Chronic blood loss in the form of menorrhagia (a loss of >80ml of blood per cycle) is a key cause of iron deficiency for women. It can be difficult to quantify blood loss in a cycle. Ask about number of sanitary products used per day. Clarify how many days the patient menstruates, and which days are 'heavy' in flow.

8 Pica refers to the presence of unusual dietary cravings and may occur in those who are deficient in minerals and vitamins such as iron, calcium, zinc, vitamin C, vitamin D or thiamine. The person is attracted to consuming non-nutritive substances such as dirt, paints, clay, paper or glue. It is more common in children, pregnant women or those with coeliac disease.

9 The most common cause of IDA, especially in those aged >50, is GI tract bleeding. Each millilitre of blood loss can result in the loss of 0.5mg of iron. Ask about bleeding noted when passing stool. Clarify whether the blood is bright (lower tract) or dark (upper tract) and whether it is on the toilet paper only (superficial) or mixed into stool (higher tract). Ask whether there is pain associated with the bleeding.

10 'Gastritis' is a broadly used term referring to gastric inflammation and symptoms of nausea, burning acid reflux, delayed gastric emptying and bloating. It may indicate the presence of gastric erosions or ulcers which can contribute to GI blood loss.

11 Intense running or jogging can contribute to anaemia via 'march haemolysis'. This is when the red cells break down due to repetitive traumatic contact between the feet and hard surfaces. Athletes are also at risk of iron deficiency due to inadequate iron intake, iron losses in sweat, upregulation of hepcidin due to inflammation, low grade GI bleeding and haemodilution.

12 Regular blood donation can cause anaemia in those who are at risk. It is routine to check haemoglobin levels with a fingerprick test prior to donation; however, iron levels are not routinely measured prior to donation. Whole blood donation can result in a loss of up to 250mg of iron, so donations are only permitted once every 3 months to ensure stores are replenished between donations.

13 Patients should be specifically asked about the use of over-the-counter medications and supplements. Many patients will be taking vitamin and mineral supplements which are widely available from pharmacies, healthcare stores and supermarkets. Ingestion of vitamin C will be helpful for iron absorption. Use of proton pump inhibitors is common in the general population and can result in impaired nutrient absorption due to reduced gastric acid secretion. Use of NSAIDs or corticosteroids can precipitate anaemia and iron deficiency due to GI bleeding.

14 Dietary habits should be asked about, clarifying whether the patient is following a restrictive diet or avoiding certain foods. Differentiate between vegetarian (no meat), vegan (no animal products) and pescetarian (fish or seafood as the only source of meat) diets. Consideration needs to be given to both the iron content of foods and the proportion of iron able to be absorbed from that food. Haem iron (from animal sources) is bound to haemoglobin and myoglobin and is more efficiently absorbed into the body. Non-haem iron absorption is prone to being inhibited by consumption of oxalates, phytates, calcium and tannins.

15 Recent surgery can contribute to anaemia or iron deficiency due to blood loss during the procedure and increased requirements in the recovery phase.

Examination

- The patient looks **pale** [1], with pallor to her **mucous membranes** [2].
- She is **haemodynamically stable** [3], with a normal heart rate and blood pressure.
- Radial pulse is **strong and regular** [4] and her hands feel warm and **well perfused** [5].
- There is no **skin atrophy** [6] or **koilonychia** [7].
- There is **angular stomatitis** [8] without **glossitis** [9].
- There is no **frontal bossing** [10] or **lymphadenopathy** [11].
- There is no evidence of **bruising or petechiae** [12].
- Dual heart sounds are auscultated, with **nil added heart sounds** [13].
- There is no **abdominal tenderness** [14], and **rectal examination** [15] is unremarkable.

1 Pallor can suggest the presence of anaemia in fair-skinned patients. This is not a reliable sign in those with pigmented or dark skin. If family members or friends are present, it may be useful to ask whether the patient appears pale compared with usual.

2 Pale mucous membranes are often a more reliable sign with less confounding variables than simply assessing skin colour. Look at the palmar creases and nail beds on the hands. Check the conjunctiva of the eyes and the lips and inside of the mouth for pallor. Pallor may be present in haemoglobin levels <90g/L.

3 It is likely this anaemia has developed gradually, allowing for an increase in plasma volume and establishment of compensatory mechanisms. These include:
- shift in haemoglobin-oxygen dissociation curve
- redistribution of blood flow
- compensatory increase in cardiac output.

4 Palpation of a weak or thready pulse may occur in severe anaemia. In older patients, anaemia can contribute to exacerbations of atrial fibrillation which can present as an irregular heartbeat.

5 In those with severe anaemia or acute blood loss, the skin (particularly in the extremities) may be cold and/or clammy. This is usually associated with a weak pulse and measurable hypotension.

6 Skin atrophy can occur with anaemia. Thinning of the hair may also be noted by the patient.

7 Koilonychia refers to spoon-shaped nails and is associated with iron deficiency as a cause for anaemia.

8 Angular stomatitis refers to sores on the side of the mouth. It is due to iron or vitamin B deficiency.

9 Glossitis usually refers to both the sign of a red, erythematous and smooth surface as well as the symptom of a painful tongue. It is most commonly associated with pernicious anaemia (autoimmune B12 deficiency) but can occur with iron or vitamin B deficiencies.

10 Skeletal changes such as frontal bossing are associated with thalassaemia, another cause of microcytic anaemia. Thalassaemia is an inherited condition in which one or more haemoglobin genes are faulty, causing defective haemoglobin synthesis. Many patients will be diagnosed in childhood, although those with mild thalassaemia may not be diagnosed until pregnancy or other physiological challenges later in life.

11 Lymphadenopathy can be due to malignancy (such as lymphoma) or infection (such as infectious mononucleosis). This is an important clue to the underlying aetiology of the anaemia.

12 Abnormal bruising or the presence of petechiae suggests a coexisting thrombocytopenia with the anaemia. This could suggest a primary bone marrow problem. Look at the lower limbs for petechiae, the forearms for bruises and in the mouth for petechiae and purpura.

13 If compensation is yet to occur, the patient may have signs of a hyperdynamic circulation. These signs include

tachycardia, bounding pulse or a systolic flow murmur. There may be cardiomegaly in chronic cases or signs of congestive cardiac failure. Look for an elevated JVP and observe the waveforms. In acute blood loss the neck veins may be unfilled and therefore flat when supine.

14 Palpable abdominal tenderness can occur due to bloating and discomfort of malabsorption syndromes or coeliac disease. Tenderness may occur in those with a gastric or duodenal ulcer, or a GI malignancy.

15 Rectal examination should be performed to exclude GI blood loss. This is most important in males and in patients over the age of 50 presenting with anaemia. Rectal examination can detect anal or rectal lesions; and the colour of the stools (looking for frank blood or dark melaena) can be assessed in this way.

Investigations

- FBE shows a **low haemoglobin** [1] with slightly **raised platelet** [2] levels.
- **Reticulocytes** [3] are increased.
- The **blood film** [4] shows **microcytic, hypochromic** [5] cells with **anisocytosis** [6] and mild **poikilocytosis** [7].
- There is **polychromasia** [8].
- The **MCV** [9] is slightly low and the **distribution of red cell distribution widths (RDW)** [10] is high.

- Iron studies reveal a very **low ferritin** [11] and **transferrin saturation** [12].
- **Serum iron levels** [13] are normal.
- **Haemolysis markers** [14] are negative, **haemoglobin electrophoresis** [15] is normal and **thyroid function** [16] is normal.
- **Erythropoietin (EPO)** [17] level is elevated.
- **Bone marrow biopsy** [18] is not performed.
- **Faecal occult blood** [19] test is negative and *Helicobacter pylori* **serology** [20] is negative.

1 The definition of anaemia is a haemoglobin level below the reference range for the laboratory. Age and gender are taken into account. The WHO defines anaemia as Hb <130g/L for men and <120g/L for non-pregnant women. The lower limit of the reference range is 110g/L for pregnant women due to the dilutional effect of increased plasma volume in this state.

2 Iron deficiency is commonly associated with a reactive thrombocytosis but the causative mechanism is not clear. It may be an adaptation to increase coagulation in those with chronic blood loss.

3 Reticulocytes are immature erythrocytes and can be used as a marker of erythrocyte production. They are large in size and hyperchromic. A normal bone marrow will respond to anaemia by increasing the reticulocyte count due to stimulation by erythropoietin. If the reticulocytes are not raised in anaemia, this is an inappropriate response and suggests lack of erythropoietin or a bone marrow disorder. It can also indicate lack of substrates such as vitamin B12 or folate.

4 The blood film is a very important investigation in

haematological conditions and most haematologists are trained to be able to decipher the film themselves, as are some laboratory scientists.

5 In IDA, the synthesis of haemoglobin is abnormal. This results in small red cells (microcytic) which contain reduced amounts of haemoglobin (hypochromic). Microcytic anaemia can occur in other disorders such as thalassaemia, sideroblastic anaemia and anaemia of chronic disease. If thalassaemia is suspected, a haemoglobin electrophoresis should be ordered. Ask about ethnicity and whether there is a family history of anaemia.

6 Anisocytosis refers to red blood cells of varying and unequal sizes. In IDA this is likely due to the presence of small microcytic red blood cells, as well as large reticulocytes within the smear. This is measured in the RDW (red cell distribution width) reported on the FBE count, which will be elevated.

7 Poikilocytosis refers to red blood cells of varying shape. This occurs due to a number of processes including fragmentation (e.g. in haemolysis or DIC), in megaloblastic anaemia (oval-shaped cells) or if the cells appeared teardrop-shaped (in thalassaemia or myelofibrosis). In iron deficiency, erythroid production is ineffective in response to high levels of stimulation from EPO, resulting in unusual and inconsistent morphology.

8 Polychromasia refers to the colour of the red blood cells and reflects the increase in the number of reticulocytes. The blue-grey colour of reticulocytes is due to the ribosomal content.

9 The mean corpuscular volume (MCV) is a very useful test to differentiate between types of anaemia. The red cells are measured by a machine and the size of each red blood cell is measured on a distribution curve which is used to calculate the mean size. It is a general reflection in the increase or decrease in the patient's population of red cells as a whole, but does not reflect small populations of abnormally sized cells. Common causes for a low MCV (microcytic cells) include iron deficiency and thalassaemia. In thalassaemia the MCV can be very low (>3 standard deviations below the mean). Common causes for a high MCV (macrocytic cells) include vitamin B12 or folate deficiency, liver disease, excess alcohol, thyroid disease and myelodysplasia.

10 The RDW measures the difference between the size of the largest red cell and smallest red cell. In normal marrow production of red cells they should be of fairly equal size. In IDA there will be small red cells (microcytic) and large cells seen due to the reticulocytosis. In thalassaemia, the cells will be microcytic but the RDW will usually be normal, which reflects the uniform population of small cells.

11 Ferritin is the most useful test to reflect iron stores. It, however, is an acute phase reactant and can be increased in inflammation, malignancy, infection and liver disease. Iron deficiency is the main cause of low ferritin, and ferritin levels below 15g/L is diagnostic of iron deficiency. In cases where ferritin may be falsely elevated, the soluble transferrin receptor assay (sTfR) may be used to aid in diagnosis. sTfR is elevated in iron deficiency and not affected by the presence of inflammation.

12 Transferrin saturation is a percentage, measured by dividing the serum iron level by the total iron-binding capacity (TIBC). A result of 30% means that 30% of the available binding sites are being occupied by iron. Transferrin molecules can contain up to two atoms of iron and deliver iron to tissues which have the receptors for transferrin. In the bone marrow, transferrin delivers iron to erythroblasts where it is then used to synthesise haemoglobin. Transferrin is also used to transport iron released from haemoglobin in the macrophages which have broken down old red blood cells for recycling.

13 Measuring iron levels in the serum may not be a useful marker for iron deficiency. The majority of iron in the serum is bound to transferrin and not 'free'. It is also present as myoglobin in muscle and in cells in the body. Levels can fluctuate significantly and follow a diurnal pattern. Iron levels are low in systemic inflammatory conditions (such as the

differential diagnosis of anaemia of chronic disease) and may not be depleted in iron-deficient states. Most of the body's iron is stored in the red cells, and is recycled and reused upon red cell apoptosis.

14 Haemolysis markers include bilirubin, LDH, haptoglobin, reticulocytes and direct Coombs test. In this patient the reticulocytes are high, but if the other parameters are normal it is unlikely haemolysis is present.

15 Haemoglobin electrophoresis is a blood test performed in the laboratory to detect the presence of different chains of haemoglobin. The use of gel electrophoresis can separate the different haemoglobins due to the unique charge of each chain resulting in a different speed of migration along the gel. It is most useful in detecting thalassaemia or sickle-cell disorders.

16 Hypothyroidism can cause anaemia due to impaired production of red blood cells. Hypothyroidism in a young woman is most commonly due to autoimmune thyroiditis (Hashimoto's). The anaemia of thyroid dysfunction is usually macrocytic.

17 Erythropoiesis (production of red blood cells) is stimulated by the hormone EPO, therefore an appropriate response in times of anaemia is to increase EPO synthesis. 90% of EPO is produced in the kidney, in response to hypoxia detected in the kidneys. This stimulus and subsequent EPO production leads to the formation of new vessels, synthesis of transferrin receptors and increased iron absorption due to downregulation of hepcidin. EPO stimulates erythropoiesis by increasing the production of precursor cells required to produce red blood cells.

18 Bone marrow aspiration is the gold standard assessment of tissue iron stores. The Prussian blue stain will show decreased iron in the macrophages, or in severe cases a total absence. This is not required in the vast majority of patients in whom the diagnosis is straightforward.

19 The faecal occult blood test is a sensitive but not specific test to perform to investigate for GI bleeding. The patient provides a stool sample and a small amount is tested. Oxidation of the test area by the presence of haemoglobin will be detected if haemoglobin is present. False positives can occur with meat ingestion. Three separate tests are recommended to increase the sensitivity of the test.

20 *Helicobacter pylori* infection is associated with peptic ulceration which can cause anaemia due to GI bleeding. If serology is positive, the infection should be eradicated to prevent GI symptoms, ulceration and in some cases malignancy. Presence of *H. pylori* infection is also associated with poor iron absorption.
Should a gastroscopy be done, one may also see pharyngeal webbing. A pharyngeal web is associated with Plummer–Vinson syndrome, a cause of chronic IDA. It is also associated with coeliac disease. It is typically associated with odynophagia.

Management

Short-term

Determine whether the patient will benefit from a **blood transfusion** [1]. Along with implementation of **dietary strategies** [2], the patient should be prescribed iron to increase her stores. If **tolerated** [3], oral iron supplements are first-line and are available in a number of **preparations** [4]. Oral iron replacement should be continued for a **therapeutic period** [5]. For those who **fail to respond** [6] to oral therapy and for **special circumstances** [7], **parenteral iron infusions** [8] are available.

Long-term

The patient may need to be prescribed iron supplementation during periods of increased demand or iron loss. **Education** [9] should be provided to the patient.

---

[1] An anaemia that is of gradual onset is usually well tolerated compared to sudden blood loss, and a transfusion may not be required if the cause of the anaemia is able to be corrected. Red cell transfusion will not be sufficient to replenish iron stores and iron replacement is required in addition.

[2] In those with frank iron deficiency, dietary supplementation is unlikely to be effective enough to reverse the deficiency. Consumption of iron-containing foods should be increased, whilst avoiding foods and beverages that inhibit absorption.

[3] Side-effects of oral iron replacement include nausea, diarrhoea or constipation and abdominal pain. The iron can result in dark-coloured stools. Be cautious in those with chronic GI blood loss: oral replacement may mask further blood loss.

[4] If a patient is troubled by side-effects from oral iron, a different preparation may be of benefit. Ferrous sulphate is the most common preparation, with additional options being ferrous gluconate or ferrous fumarate. A trial of a lower dose or intermittent dosing (every other day or once weekly) may be effective in correcting the deficiency while improving tolerability.

[5] Reticulocytosis begins to occur in 72 hours after commencing supplementation. A haemoglobin rise of 20g/L every 3 weeks should be the aim. However, iron supplementation should be continued for at least 3–6 months after the haemoglobin has corrected, to ensure stores are replenished.

[6] The main reason for failure of oral therapy is poor compliance. Oral replacement may also be inadequate in those with severe GI losses, malabsorption or in those with chronic inflammatory conditions. Oral iron therapy should not be taken at the same time as calcium supplements and simultaneous ingestion of tea (tannins) and some cereals (phytates) will reduce absorption, so they should be avoided.

Ascorbic acid (vitamin C) aids absorption and is included in many commercially available supplements. Patients may fail oral therapy because of ongoing blood loss, mixed deficiency (folate or vitamin B12) or another cause for the anaemia (e.g. malignancy, thalassaemia or chronic disease).

[7] Parenteral replacement can be used in patients on dialysis and in some malignancies. Recent studies have shown parenteral iron replacement improves symptoms and functional capacity in those with chronic heart failure and iron deficiency, independent of the presence of anaemia.

[8] Parenteral iron replacement can be in IV form and will not make the haemoglobin rise any faster than with oral replacement. IM iron replacement is rarely used now and is not recommended due to permanent skin staining at the site of administration. Parenteral iron supplementation is usually given under close supervision as there is a risk of reaction, including anaphylaxis, in select patients.

[9] A large part of the management of iron deficiency is avoidance of precipitating factors. Educate the patient with regard to their individual risk factors and negotiate strategies to minimise these risks. Arrange follow-up to recheck the haemoglobin and iron studies and ensure compliance to therapy is maintained.

CASE 39: Multiple myeloma

History

- A **62-year-old** [1] **male** [2] presents to a hospital emergency department with **nausea, muscle cramping and reduced urine output** [3] .
- He reports feeling **fatigued** [4] and having **lost weight** [5] over the past **six months** [6] but exact history is difficult due to **confusion** [7] .
- Medical history is significant for **type 2 diabetes mellitus** [8] for which he takes an **oral hypoglycaemic medication** [9] .

- He has also been taking regular paracetamol and **NSAIDs** [10] for new **lumbar back pain** [11] .
- It is noted he had two **chest infections** [12] this winter which is unusual for him.
- There is no history of **abnormal bleeding** [13] .
- Surgical history is significant for recent **carpal tunnel** [14] release.

[1] Multiple myeloma is a disease of the older adult, with peak incidence being between the ages of 60 and 70 years. Less than 2% will be diagnosed before the age of 40.

[2] Myeloma is slightly more common in men than women. It is twice as common in those of African origin compared to Caucasian or Asian origin.

[3] These are symptoms of renal failure. Nausea is likely to be due to the uraemia which can also lead to anorexia, vomiting and altered mental status. Muscle cramps are a symptom of hyperphosphataemia and hyperkalaemia of renal failure. Reduced urine output is concerning for oliguric renal failure due to multiple myeloma.

[4] Fatigue may be due to anaemia from bone marrow infiltration. It may also be due to the underlying disease process, or from slowly progressing undiagnosed renal failure.

[5] Weight loss is due to the hypermetabolic activity of the disease process. This often occurs gradually and may not be noted by the patient. If the patient is unable to quantify the weight loss, ask whether their clothes feel loose or whether they've tightened their belt recently. Ask family or friends present if they have noted weight loss. Pay attention to loose skin folds on examination.

[6] There are a number of metabolic abnormalities which could contribute to confusion in this patient including uraemia, hypercalcaemia of myeloma, anaemia and hypoglycaemia due to accumulation of oral hypoglycaemics in renal failure.

[7] Multiple myeloma is a neoplasm caused by accumulation of abnormal plasma cells in the bone marrow. It is thought to develop over a period of time and almost all cases originate from the precancerous monoclonal gammopathy of unknown significance (MGUS). This patient

may have had myeloma for many months and has only presented acutely with the symptoms of renal failure.

[8] This patient may have a background nephropathy due to his T2DM. Previous renal function testing should be sought from his local GP. The background history of diabetes is significant in a malignancy such as multiple myeloma, as a large part of the treatment involves intermittent high doses of oral corticosteroid (such as dexamethasone) and this can cause difficulties in glycaemic control.

[9] It is likely the oral hypoglycaemic will need to be stopped in this time of acute renal failure. Insulin may need to be used to control the blood sugars, especially in the context of steroid use.

[10] The use of NSAIDs to control the back pain is likely to be further contributing to his renal failure. The acute tubular damage and necrosis induced by the combination of dehydration, hypercalcaemia and abnormal protein deposition is exacerbated by the use of NSAIDs.

[11] Back pain is reported to be one of the most common symptoms in patients with new diagnosis of multiple myeloma, occurring in up to 70%. This may be due to undiagnosed lytic lesions or crush fractures, or due to bone marrow infiltration. The abnormal plasma cells can secrete factors which activate osteoclasts. This results in bone breakdown, leading to lytic lesions, hypercalcaemia and bone pain.

[12] Infection occurs in multiple myeloma patients due to reduced functional immunoglobulins. This is called 'immunoparesis'. Those with hypogammaglobulinaemia are more susceptible to infection with encapsulated bacterial organisms. The absence of the antibody results in decreased response to polysaccharide antigens such as in the bacterial

cell wall, leading to limited ability to phagocytose and kill the bacteria. Respiratory and urinary infections are common. Infection may also be due to neutropenia (from marrow infiltration) or abnormal cell-mediated immunity.

13 Thrombocytopenia is usually only seen in advanced disease and may contribute to bleeding. However, the myeloma paraprotein can interfere with platelet function and coagulation factors in the absence of thrombocytopenia and

consequently cause bleeding and bruising. Uraemia can also lead to platelet dysfunction and increased bleeding.

14 Carpal tunnel syndrome is relatively commonly seen in the general population. However, in a patient with myeloma this history is concerning for a complication of myeloma called secondary amyloidosis. Ask about other symptoms of peripheral neuropathy or cardiac failure as amyloidosis can affect the peripheral nerves and cardiac function.

Examination

- The patient looks unwell and is **hypertensive and tachycardic** [1].
- There is **pallor** [2] to the palmar creases but **no bruising** [3] is seen on the limbs.
- **Asterixis** [4] is not present.
- There is no **macroglossia** [5].
- **Jugular venous pressure** [6] is elevated.

- The **chest is clear** [7] to auscultation and **cardiovascular examination** [8] reveals tachycardia with no other abnormalities.
- No **lymphadenopathy** [9] is appreciated.
- **Palpation of the thoracolumbar spine** [10] reveals tenderness between L3 and L5.
- Urine dipstick reveals **protein** [11].

1 Tachycardia may be due to compensation in oxygen delivery due to anaemia, dehydration due to poor oral intake, or an early sign of infection. Those with acute kidney injury may present with hypotension or hypertension, depending partly on the underlying cause and their volume state.

2 Pallor is likely due to anaemia. In some patients, anaemia may be the initial clue to the underlying bone marrow disorder. In hindsight, this patient may have been anaemic for months prior to presenting acutely.

3 Bruising may occur due to coagulopathy or abnormal platelet function which can occur in myeloma or uraemia. Bruising is also rarely a sign of hyperviscosity syndrome which can occur with high paraprotein levels.

4 Asterixis may be present in those with uraemia. It is elicited by asking the patient to flex their hands back towards their face in an outstretched position. Upon holding this position for at least 20 seconds, a jerky flapping tremor may be noted. A similar sign can be elicited in those with hypercapnia.

5 Macroglossia refers to the presence of a large, thickened tongue which would be concerning for the presence of amyloidosis. This occurs due to extracellular deposition of fibrillar insoluble proteins.

6 Elevation in JVP is a sign of fluid overload. The chest should be examined for crepitations and the lower limbs for peripheral oedema. Fluid overload may be noted by the patient around the abdomen or in the face.

7 Examine the chest to elicit signs of fluid overload and infection, which can occur due to the immunoparesis of multiple myeloma. A pleural friction rub is associated with uraemia.

8 Findings on cardiovascular examination may include a pericardial friction rub due to anaemia, signs of fluid overload due to renal failure or signs of cardiac failure due to amyloidosis. These signs include raised JVP, displaced apex beat due to cardiomegaly, and added heart sounds or a systolic murmur.

9 Uncommonly, multiple myeloma can cause lymphadenopathy due to infiltration of the lymph nodes. More commonly lymphadenopathy in the context of a plasma cell disorder is due to a lymphoproliferative disorder such as lymphoplasmacytic lymphoma (Waldenström's macroglobulinaemia) or a plasmablastic lymphoma. These may have overlap with myeloma but have different treatment strategies.

10 Palpable bony tenderness may be elicited in patients with crush fractures or plasmacytomas of myeloma. Gently press the fist against each vertebrae, if possible, assessing the patient's reaction to the movement.

11 Proteinuria, albuminuria or nephrotic syndrome can occur due to a number of causes in myeloma including amyloidosis, paraprotein deposition, and a membranoproliferative glomerulitis occurring in response to the paraprotein.

Investigations

- FBE demonstrates a **normochromic normocytic anaemia** [1] with a **mild neutrophilia** [2] and **normal platelet count** [3].
- The blood film shows **red cell rouleaux** [4].
- There are no **blasts** [5] or **plasma cells** [6] seen.
- The **ESR** [7] is markedly elevated.
- UEC shows an **elevated urea** [8] and a markedly **elevated creatinine level** [9].
- Estimated glomerular filtration rate is **8ml/min** [10].
- **Corrected calcium** [11] is markedly elevated.
- **Albumin** [12] is below the normal range; however, the patient's **total protein** [13] is elevated.
- **Beta-2 microglobulin and LDH** [14] are elevated.

- Further analysis demonstrated an **IgG kappa paraprotein of 42g/L** [15] with markedly **elevated kappa free light chains** [16] but normal lambda free light chains.
- Kappa free light chains are found on **urinalysis** [17].
- Testing of the serum immunoglobulin levels shows an **elevated IgG level but low IgA and IgM** [18].
- **Skeletal survey** [19] reveals **lytic lesions** [20] in the lumbar spine.
- **Bone marrow aspiration and trephine** [21] demonstrates an excess of plasma cells with normal **cytogenetic analysis** [22].
- **Congo red stain** [23] is negative.
- **NT-proBNP and troponin** [24] are normal.

---

[1] Anaemia is due to decreased red cell production in the infiltrated bone marrow. The abnormal plasma cells crowd the bone marrow, halting production of normal blood cells. The anaemia is usually normocytic or macrocytic. A myeloma screen should be performed in patients presenting with an unexplained macrocytosis.

[2] Mild neutrophilia may be reactive due to the patient being unwell and due to the dehydration of acute renal failure. This patient could also be presenting with infection (such as urinary tract or respiratory) in the context of being immunosuppressed due to the malignancy. Neutropenia (low neutrophils) occurs in advanced disease.

[3] In late stage disease, patients can be very thrombocytopenic due to severe marrow infiltration. This is exacerbated by cytotoxic chemotherapy agents.

[4] Red cell rouleaux refers to 'stacking' of the red blood cells. This can reflect an increase in plasma fibrinogen (an acute phase reactant), immunoglobulins or proteins in the blood. It is associated with an increased ESR (erythrocyte sedimentation rate) by definition. Rouleaux is common in myeloma but can occur in infection and other malignancies.

[5] Patients with multiple myeloma will not have blasts in the circulation as this is not a myeloid condition. The malignant plasma cells of myeloma are a mature haematological cell, whereas blasts are very immature forms.

[6] In rare cases, patients can present with plasma cells in the peripheral blood. This is very abnormal and is referred to as plasma cell leukaemia. It presents with features of both acute leukaemia and multiple myeloma. Despite systemic chemotherapy it has a very poor prognosis.

[7] The erythrocyte sedimentation rate is a measure of the rate of red cells falling (sedimenting) in a tube in one hour.

A very high ESR suggests serious infection, autoimmune conditions or malignancy. In myeloma, the ESR is raised due to the presence of a serum paraprotein causing increased plasma viscosity.

[8] Elevated urea is a consequence of the acute renal failure and is likely to be a cause for the patient's presenting symptoms. It is not directly related to the myeloma itself.

[9] The elevated creatinine suggests the patient is in renal failure. This may be due to dehydration or hypercalcaemia. It may also be directly due to the myeloma and there are two main mechanisms for this. The serum free light chain can deposit in the kidney, causing mechanical obstruction. This is referred to as 'cast nephropathy' and 'myeloma kidney' and is only likely to occur in patients who secrete free light chains. Less commonly, the patient may have secondary amyloidosis, an abnormal protein which can deposit in the renal tissue causing nephropathy including nephrotic syndrome.

[10] This patient is in acute renal failure. Up to 50% of myeloma patients will have a degree of acute kidney injury at diagnosis. Severe kidney injury requiring consideration of dialysis occurs in <5% of patients with myeloma.

[11] Serum calcium is increased in some patients due to resorption of bone. Serum calcium must be measured upon suspicion of a plasma cell disorder. Evidence of hypercalcaemia indicates tissue damage and is an indication for treatment of symptomatic myeloma. It is useful to consider the acronym CRAB in relation to evidence of tissue damage: hyper**C**alcaemia, **R**enal failure, **A**naemia, **B**one disease.

[12] Low serum albumin can be a sign of advanced disease. Albumin is a key prognostic factor and is used in scoring systems to calculate staging at diagnosis.

13 This patient is presenting with a protein-albumin gap. In the serum, there are many types of proteins present in small amounts with differing functions. Albumin is one protein that is commonly able to be measured on laboratory tests and makes up a large proportion of protein in the serum. When there is a large gap between the amount of total protein and the major protein albumin, it is suspected that an abnormal 'paraprotein' is making up the difference.

14 Beta-2 microglobulin is a molecule that sits on the surface of lymphocytes and plasma cells. As it is excreted by the kidneys it is also elevated in renal failure. It is used as a prognostic marker, reflecting the presence of large numbers of plasma cells. It is necessary to calculate the International Staging System (ISS) in myeloma. LDH is a marker of the abnormal cell turnover.

15 A paraprotein is a monoclonal immunoglobulin produced by malignant plasma cells. The abnormal plasma cells produce paraproteins which are abnormal immunoglobulin light chains. The paraprotein is also referred to as the 'M protein'.

16 Immunoglobulins are Y-shaped molecules made up of two 'heavy chains' and two 'light chains' of protein. They can normally be measured in very low levels in the serum and as they are filtered by the kidneys, can be present in slightly higher levels in those with abnormal renal function. The light chains are divided into two classes – kappa and lambda. In myeloma, the light chains produced by the abnormal plasma cells are not paired with the heavy chains and are released into the circulation. The abnormal 'free light chains' can be measured in the serum in sometimes very high levels. Some patients have purely light chain only multiple myeloma and do not have a serum paraprotein detectable.

17 Urinalysis in patients with multiple myeloma may show increased protein, a paraprotein, or abnormal levels of free light chains. This is known as the Bence Jones protein in the urine. Light chains are usually filtered across the glomerulus and reabsorbed by proximal tubular cells. In myeloma, this reabsorptive capacity is overwhelmed.

18 There are five main classes of immunoglobulins – IgG, IgA, IgM, IgD and IgE – all with slightly different functions. A 'polyclonal' mixture of immunoglobulins is made in a normal immune response to bind foreign antigens such as bacteria and viruses. These are made from thousands of different plasma cells. However, in multiple myeloma, identical 'monoclonal' immunoglobulins are made by the abnormal cells, and other immunoglobulins will be suppressed. Testing of the three most prevalent immunoglobulin classes in the serum usually reveals an elevated abnormal Ig and suppressed residual classes. IgG myeloma occurs in about 50–60% of cases.

19 A skeletal survey is a full body X-ray, usually taken of the skull, spine, ribs, pelvis and long bones of the arms and legs. Increasingly, skeletal survey is being performed as a low dose CT which is more sensitive to abnormalities. Other imaging modalities that may be used include MRI (for early bone changes and soft tissue deposits) and PET-CT scans. Imaging may be particularly important in cases of smouldering myeloma, where there is potential to detect early bone lesions which would indicate prompt initiation of therapy rather than observation.

20 Lytic lesions have a 'punched-out' appearance on X-ray. They can occur anywhere in the skeletal system. Lytic lesions are caused by activation of osteoclasts due to high levels of RANKL (receptor activator of nuclear factor-KB ligand) produced by the pathological plasma cells. Despite the lesions, the serum alkaline phosphatase (ALP) is usually normal, unless there is a pathological fracture.

21 Normally, plasma cells will comprise <5% of the cells in the bone marrow. Patients with MGUS or smouldering myeloma may have 5–10% plasma cells in the bone marrow. Those with IgG or IgA MGUS have a 1% chance of developing myeloma per year and have been shown to have reduced survival compared to controls, despite MGUS being considered a 'precancerous' condition. Accumulation of additional genetic changes increases the risk of and accelerates the progression to overt myeloma. Malignant myeloma cells may contain in excess of 30 different somatic mutations.

22 Cytogenetics or analysis of chromosomes may be predictive of patient outcome. It is used to guide prognosis and treatment choices. Almost all malignant myeloma cells will demonstrate aneuploidy (more or less than the normal 46 chromosomes).

23 Amyloid deposition in tissues has a particular histologic appearance. To confirm the presence of the abnormal protein, Congo red stain is added to the tissue and it is viewed under polarised light microscopy. The tissue will have apple-green birefringence if positive for amyloid.

24 Testing a troponin level and brain natriuretic peptide (BNP) are easily available tests which can assist with screening for the presence of cardiac amyloid. They should be interpreted in the context of the clinical history and comorbidities. If the troponin or BNP are positive, an echocardiogram or preferably a cardiac MRI should be ordered.

Management

Immediate

Start **intravenous hydration** [1] with normal saline while monitoring fluid status and **urine output** [2]. Seek advice from the renal team as this patient may need **dialysis** [3] in the short term. If the hypercalcaemia does not respond to fluids, give a **bisphosphonate** [4].

Short-term

Commence **steroid** [5] therapy once the investigations are complete. The patient should start **chemotherapy** [6] as soon as it is available. This patient is a **candidate** [7] for, and should undergo an **autologous stem cell transplant** [8]. Commence **infection prophylaxis** [9] and prescribe **analgesia for bone pain** [10]. Offer **social work and pastoral care** [11] referral.

Long-term

The patient's prognosis depends partly on **renal recovery** [12]. The patient may need a **maintenance therapy** [13], which may involve a **clinical trial** [14]. Commence regular **bisphosphonate infusions** [15]. Consider a further **stem cell transplant** [16] if eligible. Consider whether **radiotherapy** [17] is needed. **Monitor regularly** [18] for tolerability of treatment and signs of relapse.

[1] Aggressive hydration may assist with removal of casts and light chains as well as improving the hypercalcaemia. It will also assist with preventing tumour lysis upon treatment commencement.

[2] Urine output has a prognostic impact and those with good urine output may be less likely to need dialysis. In the immediate phase, a strict fluid balance chart should be kept, detailing intake and output.

[3] Some patients with severe renal dysfunction due to myeloma kidney require dialysis in the short term and a proportion of these will go on to be dialysis-dependent. The renal team will be able to advise on indications for dialysis and conservative options to improve function and prevent complications. Indications for dialysis may include:
- persistent fluid overload
- anuria or oliguria
- uraemic signs and symptoms
- GFR <5ml/min
- refractory acidosis, hyperkalaemia or hyperphosphataemia.

[4] Intravenous fluids should be the first step in treatment of hypercalcaemia of malignancy but it may not respond to fluid alone. Care needs to be taken in this patient with renal dysfunction and specialist or pharmacy advice should be sought with regard to dosing and rate of administration.

[5] Steroids, such as dexamethasone, are the backbone of treatment for multiple myeloma. Malignant plasma cells are very susceptible to the effects of steroids and can improve hypercalcaemia and inflammation around bony tumours very rapidly.

[6] First-line treatment for untreated multiple myeloma in the UK is usually protease inhibitor-based, a combination of subcutaneous bortezomib, oral thalidomide and oral dexamethasone given weekly.

[7] Those who are very elderly or have significant medical comorbidities such as severe cardiac failure will not be able to undergo a stem cell transplant (SCT). Patients with minimal comorbidities who are well into their 70s may still be eligible for reduced intensity transplant. Autologous SCT is still performed in patients undergoing dialysis.

[8] An autologous SCT is performed in two parts. Firstly, the patient's stem cells are collected from peripheral blood, frozen and stored for the transplant. This is usually performed as an outpatient, utilising injections of growth factor (G-CSF) to stimulate bone marrow production. Then the patient is admitted to hospital for high dose chemotherapy to obliterate the remaining cells in the bone marrow. The frozen stem cells are thawed and infused back into the patient to 'repopulate' the bone marrow. The role of the autologous SCT is not to cure the patient; it is to create a deeper response to treatment.

[9] All patients on chemotherapy should be prescribed medications to prevent viral, bacterial and fungal infections depending on the chemotherapy protocol, local risk factors and patient risk factors. Particular infections being prophylaxed against include shingles, *Pneumocystis jirovecii* pneumonia (PJP) and fungal lung infection. For those with significant immunoparesis and recurrent bacterial infections, infusions of IV immunoglobulin may be required. Infection needs to be treated promptly.

[10] Bony disease has the potential to impact markedly on the quality of life of a myeloma patient. Crush fractures and plasmacytomas of the bone can be exquisitely painful. Some respond poorly to first-line and traditional analgesia. Radiotherapy should be considered for symptomatic management in those with persistent pain. Consider referral to a pain specialist for refractory pain.

11 Although treatments have improved markedly over the last decade, myeloma remains an incurable condition. Overall median survival is approximately 5–7 years with symptomatic disease. The renal dysfunction portends an even more guarded prognosis. Multiple myeloma is not a well-known or -understood condition amongst the general population so education and information is the key. Support should be offered to both patient and family, including written information about the aetiology, symptoms and treatment of myeloma.

12 There is a correlation between renal dysfunction and poor overall survival. The life expectancy for patients on dialysis is around 10% over 3 years. Those who recover their renal function, however, have a similar prognosis to those without kidney injury.

13 Although myeloma is treatable, it is rarely curable and will almost invariably relapse. The aim of the initial treatment and autologous SCT is to be able to put the patient into a deep treatment-free remission. Treatment resistance can also occur over time.

14 There are many novel and new agents involved in the treatment of myeloma. Treatment regimes change rapidly, even over a few years. Enrolment in a clinical trial may be considered upfront at diagnosis, or upon relapse post SCT. A trial may involve treatment with one novel medication, or involve a potentially synergistic agent combined with standard chemotherapy.

15 Bisphosphonates are a class of drug used to treat osteoporosis called osteoclast inhibitors. They are used in most patients with myeloma to 'coat' the surface of the bones and protect from damage due to myeloma. They are usually given IV once per month. Side-effects include flu-like symptoms, renal dysfunction and the potentially serious osteonecrosis of the jaw.

16 Some patients may be eligible for a second autologous SCT, or in rare cases an allogeneic transplant. Given the median age of patients and the significant end-organ damage that can be associated with myeloma, the majority of patients will not be eligible to undergo an allogeneic transplant due to high treatment-related mortality.

17 Radiotherapy is used to treat specific areas, rather than to control or cure the multiple myeloma. It may be considered in those with symptomatic bony disease, bulky tumours, areas of acute pain or in impending spinal cord compression. It may be used as a short course and can be repeated when needed.

18 Presence of disease is monitored by serial measurement of the paraprotein, serum free light chains, renal function, serum calcium and full blood count. In those with bony disease, imaging is usually performed after a specific treatment or upon diagnosis of relapse.

CASE 40: Venous thromboembolism

History

- A 42-year-old **female** [1] presents with a 4-day history of **right calf swelling** [2] and a 1-day history of **pleuritic chest pain** [3].
- This is not associated with **fever or cough** [4], including no **haemoptysis** [5].
- There was no **trauma** [6] to the leg.
- She has not been **immobile** [7] but has recently returned on a **long-haul flight** [8] from Australia.
- She has not been **hospitalised or had surgery** [9] recently.

- There is no history of **malignancy** [10] or **ischaemic heart disease** [11].
- She has had two previous **normal pregnancies** [12] and no previous **miscarriages** [13].
- She is now on the **combined oral contraceptive pill (COCP)** [14].
- She does not take any **other medication** [15] and is a **non-smoker** [16].
- **Family history** [17] is significant for an aunt who had a large pulmonary embolus.

[1] Venous thromboembolism (VTE) is slightly more common in females of reproductive age. This is due to a number of common precipitating factors, including oral contraceptive use, pregnancy and hormone replacement.

[2] Unilateral calf swelling raises the possibility of a deep venous thrombosis (DVT). It is important to differentiate between a thrombus of the deep venous system and the superficial venous system, as risk of progression and treatment options are different. Common sites for DVT include the peroneal, anterior and posterior tibial, popliteal, femoral and iliac veins.

[3] Pleuritic chest pain is described as a sharp, stabbing pain occurring in the inspiratory and/or expiratory phase of breathing. It is exacerbated by coughing, sneezing and deep breathing. It is caused by inflammation of the nerve receptors on the parietal pleura, which are not present on the visceral pleura. Inflammation near the diaphragm can refer to the shoulder or neck.

[4] Rule out infective symptoms suggesting an alternative diagnosis such as pneumonia. Pneumonia can cause chest pain but is usually associated with other symptoms, or risk factors such as immunosuppression.

[5] Haemoptysis can occur in pulmonary embolism, but also pneumonia, bronchiectasis, lung carcinoma, TB and congestive cardiac failure. Ascertain whether the blood is bright, dark, streaky or in clots and whether the sputum is purulent or frothy. If haemoptysis is present on history, it is critical to ensure the blood is coming from the lower respiratory tract and being coughed up. Nasal mucosal bleeding can track down the back of the throat and present as haemoptysis, but the causes of this will be very different.

[6] A history of trauma could suggest another cause for the leg swelling such as fracture or muscle strain. This may warrant different imaging, such as a plain X-ray, to make a diagnosis.

[7] Immobility is associated with a higher risk of DVT. The Wells criteria for pulmonary embolism include bed rest for at least 3 days or recent major surgery as positive risk factors. Activation of the calf muscles is required to assist with venous return from the lower limb and is reduced in immobility.

[8] Prolonged air travel is associated with an increased risk of VTE due to immobility, dehydration (often exacerbated by alcohol ingestion) and frequently poor positioning of the lower limb causing mechanical compression of the venous system.

[9] Up to half of DVT and pulmonary embolism (PE) events occur after hospitalisation. This risk can remain for weeks after the admission. Most hospitals have stringent guidelines on the use of chemical thromboprophylaxis in patients admitted to their service. This may be advised to continue post discharge in high risk individuals, such as post-surgical (especially joint replacement) patients. Surgery is associated with increased risk of VTE, especially in those with prolonged anaesthetic times (resulting in extended venous stasis) and those in whom thromboprophylaxis is not administered due to perceived bleeding risk. Some centres use elasticated stockings to reduce VTE; however, evidence for this method is poor.

[10] Malignancy is consistently associated with VTE due to production of tissue factor and procoagulants. Risk may also be increased due to local obstruction by tumour, the use of chemotherapy, increased use of intravascular lines and relative immobility. Those with brain, pancreatic, renal and

ovarian carcinoma and myeloproliferative neoplasms are particularly at high risk.

11 The presence of previous ischaemic heart disease could suggest myocardial ischaemia is a more likely cause for the chest pain. This, along with PE, is a diagnosis not to be missed. The pain of myocardial ischaemia is likely to be constant, left-sided or central, described as 'crushing' and referring to the shoulder, neck or down the arm. Although presentations in patients vary, this differs from the pleuritic chest pain of a pulmonary embolism.

12 Pregnancy is a very high risk state for VTE, but a lack of VTE during previous pregnancies does not rule this out as a current diagnosis. There is a five- to sixfold increase in relative risk of thrombosis during pregnancy, and VTE occurs in 1 in 1500 pregnancies. The risk is highest in the third trimester and postpartum period.

13 A history of miscarriages suggests concern for the antiphospholipid syndrome. Antiphospholipid syndrome is a diagnosis defined as the occurrence of venous thrombosis, arterial thrombosis or recurrent miscarriage plus detection of a persistent antiphospholipid antibody. It may involve a circulating lupus anticoagulant as a primary condition, or be secondary to SLE. Catastrophic antiphospholipid syndrome is a life-threatening condition characterised by small vessel thrombosis, DIC, acute haemolytic anaemia, multi-organ failure and acute respiratory distress syndrome. Patients with the antiphospholipid syndrome should be anticoagulated indefinitely with warfarin therapy, and a higher INR than standard may need to be maintained.

14 The use of oestrogen therapy such as the oral contraceptive pill or hormone replacement therapy increases plasma levels of factors II, VII, VIII, IX and X and reduces antithrombin levels. This is clinically significant in those on high dose therapy and lower risk in those on the low dose oral contraceptive pills. There is increased use of low dose hormone replacement therapy due to the known thrombotic risk.

15 Other medications that are associated with increased risk of VTE in susceptible individuals include certain chemotherapy agents (tamoxifen, lenolidomide), antipsychotics, glucocorticoids, antifibrinolytics and testosterone.

16 Smoking may be associated with multiple causes for the chest pain, including pneumothorax, lung malignancy and pneumonia. Smoking can increase the risk of VTE, pulmonary embolism and arterial thromboses such as cerebral events.

17 A positive family history of venous thromboembolism may indicate an inheritable cause increasing the risk of VTE in this individual. Ask whether there is a family history of leg clots or clots of the lungs. Ask whether there has been sudden death with unexplained cause in the family which could suggest pulmonary embolism as a cause. Ask whether any of the events in family members were unprovoked before the age of 50 and whether they were recurrent or life-threatening. The cause may be measured and diagnosable (e.g. factor V Leiden mutation) and able to be screened for, or it may be a combination of inherited factors that cannot be identified.

Examination

- The patient is diaphoretic and is **tachypnoeic** [1] at rest.
- Oxygen saturation is **95% on air** [2].
- There is no **peripheral cyanosis** [3].
- Heart rate is **115bpm** [4] and regular.
- Respiratory rate is 28, **BP is 110/70mmHg** [5] and she is **afebrile** [6].
- **Cardiorespiratory examination** [7] is normal.

- **Examination of the lower limb** [8] reveals the right calf is 5cm larger than the left calf with unilateral non-pitting oedema and localised tenderness.
- There is no **cellulitis** [9] and she does not have evidence of varicose veins.
- **Homans' sign** [10] is positive.
- Her **weight** [11] is 60kg.

1 Pulmonary embolism causes a V/Q mismatch due to obstruction of the pulmonary blood supply causing lack of perfusion to an area of lung tissue despite adequate ventilation. This results in dyspnoea and hypoxia but can correlate poorly with the radiological signs. Dyspnoea may be significant for the patient with peripheral emboli but not be noted by a patient with a saddle embolus.

2 In a young non-smoker this is relative hypoxia; however, she may be reasonably comfortable at this level without requiring supplemental oxygen. Correlate this finding with the respiratory work and effort.

3 Cyanosis is usually a late sign of right heart failure in a massive pulmonary embolism.

4 Tachycardia is common and is usually sinus rhythm. The presence of tachycardia is part of many diagnostic criteria. Those who are susceptible may go into atrial fibrillation. Bradycardia or broad complex tachycardia is a sign of right heart strain and imminent potential for cardiogenic or obstructive shock.

5 Blood pressure is very important to monitor in the immediate phase post diagnosis. Hypotension should be corrected with IV fluid and persistent hypotension is a sign of impending obstructive shock associated with right heart failure.

6 Low grade fever (up to 37.5°C) can occur in patients with pulmonary embolus. A high fever may indicate other pathology such as pneumonia or cellulitis of the leg causing the presentation.

7 Cardiac examination findings in pulmonary embolism can include signs of pulmonary hypertension such as loud pulmonary component of the second heart sound, palpable P2 and parasternal heave. There may be dullness to percussion of the lungs consistent with pleural effusion, decreased breath sounds or rales in the chest. In rare cases signs of right heart failure can include a third heart sound or jugular venous distension.

8 Clinical suspicion of DVT is high in those with unilateral leg or calf swelling, unilateral pitting oedema or tenderness along the calf vein. Objective evidence can be documented by measuring each calf at set point below the tibial tuberosity. The presence of superficial collateral veins may be observed in some patients.

9 Cellulitis is often the main differential and can be difficult to distinguish clinically from a DVT. Look for erythema on the skin, a break in the skin or discharge from the area. Pain is likely to be significant. Local lymphadenopathy may be palpated such as in the inguinal area.

10 Homans' sign is elicited by asking the patient to flex the calf at the ankle and assessing whether pain is present. It may be used to increase suspicion of a clinically relevant DVT. However, the DVT needs to be confirmed on imaging.

11 It is important to know the approximate weight of the patient when starting anticoagulation or seeking anticoagulation advice from a specialty team. Low molecular weight heparin (LMWH) is dosed based on weight and renal function. The direct oral anticoagulants (DOACs) do not have proven efficacy in obese patients so should not be used in these patients. Specialty advice should be sought for the use of both LMWH and DOACs in patients >120kg.

Investigations

- An **ECG** [1] shows sinus tachycardia without any voltage changes.
- FBE is unremarkable, with a **normal WCC** [2] and **platelet count** [3].
- **UEC** [4] is normal, **liver function** [5] tests are normal and **B-hCG** [6] is negative.
- Coagulation testing shows a **normal INR and aPTT** [7].
- D-dimer [8] is elevated and **troponin** [9] is normal.
- **Chest X-ray** [10] is normal.

- A **Doppler ultrasound** [11] of the lower limb demonstrates a thrombus in the **peroneal vein** [12] extending to the level of the **popliteal vein** [13].
- **CT pulmonary angiogram** [14] shows a **segmental pulmonary embolus** [15] with a small **pulmonary infarction** [16].
- Further **thrombophilia testing** [17] reveals the patient is **heterozygous** [18] for the **factor V Leiden** [19] mutation with no other **inheritable mutations** [20] found.

1 The ECG is abnormal in many patients with PE but this may be as non-specific as sinus tachycardia. There may be right axis deviation or evidence of right heart strain. The classic ECG sign is S1Q3T3, a pattern indicating right heart strain and an incomplete RBBB. Alternatively, the ECG may reveal other causes of chest pain, such as myocardial ischaemia or pericarditis.

2 A normal white cell count may assist with ruling out infection as a cause for pleuritic chest pain. An elevated WCC can be non-specific and occur as a reaction to infection, infarction or ischaemia. A vastly elevated WCC could suggest a haematological malignancy such as CLL or CML as an underlying cause for the thrombosis.

3 It is important to know that the platelet count is normal before starting anticoagulation, as thrombocytopenia will increase the risk of clinically significant bleeding. In contrast, a very high platelet count should prompt investigation for an underlying myeloproliferative disorder such as polycythaemia rubra vera or essential thrombocythaemia.

4 Knowledge of the creatinine clearance is important to choose the most suitable anticoagulant for this patient. In renal impairment, enoxaparin needs to be dose-reduced and in severe renal impairment direct oral anticoagulants (DOACs) are contraindicated. Warfarin is safe even in patients with end-stage renal failure and on dialysis.

5 An abnormality in liver function would preclude the use of a DOAC for anticoagulation in this patient and should be tested prior to treatment commencement in all patients. New derangement of transaminases in an unstable patient with pulmonary embolism can occur due to hypotension and liver ischaemia.

6 It must be established whether a woman is pregnant before starting anticoagulation. LWMH and unfractionated heparin are safe in pregnancy. Warfarin has a potential to be teratogenic and the DOACs are not proven to be safe in pregnancy so should be avoided. LMWH is the treatment of choice in pregnancy but must be stopped 24 hours prior to delivery. This would need to occur under the monitoring of a haematologist.

7 It is routine to check baseline coagulation markers prior to starting anticoagulation. An elevated aPTT prior to starting therapy should prompt investigation for antiphospholipid syndrome, specifically the presence of a lupus anticoagulant or acquired inhibitor. A shortened aPTT may be seen in acute thrombosis due to activation of the clotting factors.

8 D-dimer is a reflection of the increased fibrin breakdown products in the circulation when a newly formed thrombus is present. D-dimer is useful to rule out DVT or PE in patients with a low likelihood of venous thromboembolism. This may prevent unnecessary imaging in low risk patients. It can also assist with ruling out the presence of a new thrombus at a site of previous VTE in a scan with equivocal findings. D-dimer does not correlate with severity of clot. It should not be used as a positive diagnostic test alone.

9 A troponin leak can occur in those with pulmonary embolism resulting in right ventricular (RV) dilation and right heart strain. It is a reasonable prognostic marker. In those presenting with chest pain and an elevated troponin, thorough history and examination is required to differentiate between non-ST elevation myocardial infarction (NSTEMI) and PE.

10 Chest X-ray is usually normal in cases of pulmonary embolism; in fact, a normal chest X-ray in a patient with severe dyspnoea is suggestive of a PE. Positive findings reported by experienced radiologists can include:
- a 'bronchial cut-off' sign due to the obstruction
- oligaemia, which refers to a decrease in local perfusion
- a wedge-shaped area indicative of pulmonary infarction, or
- evidence of pulmonary artery dilation in massive PE.
Despite these signs, pulmonary embolism cannot be diagnosed on X-ray. Chest X-ray is a useful test in clinically stable patients to rule out pneumonia (local consolidation), pleural effusion, pneumothorax, cardiomegaly and a widened mediastinum.

11 Doppler ultrasound is the investigation of choice for thrombus of the venous system. It is non-invasive and involves no radiation; however, it requires the use of a specialist radiographer called a sonographer and may not be available after hours in some centres. Ultrasound cannot differentiate between acute and chronic clots. If ultrasound is not available, the next best investigation is a CT venogram. This may need to be used if a patient is particularly obese or has a lack of skin integrity (e.g. coexisting cellulitis or burns). An MRI is an alternative in these cases; however, expense and lack of availability are likely to be a barrier to use.

12 The peroneal vein is a deep vein in the calf and a thrombus in this area is called a 'distal' DVT. Distal DVTs are

associated with lower risk of propagation to a pulmonary embolism and are almost always suitable for outpatient therapy. Many clinicians will elect to give a short course of anticoagulation in those without ongoing risk factors, particularly if bleeding risk is elevated.

13 Knowledge of a thrombus in the popliteal vein is important because it is classified as a 'proximal' DVT, despite the popliteal vein ending 'below the knee'. Proximal DVTs portend a far higher risk of being symptomatic and causing pulmonary embolus. They are also associated in many studies with a higher risk of recurrence.

14 If there is clinical suspicion of pulmonary embolism, definitive imaging should be undertaken. Computed tomography pulmonary angiography (CTPA) uses fine slices of the lungs and an injection of contrast dye to demonstrate filling defects in the pulmonary arterial supply. CTPA is more useful than ventilation perfusion scintigraphy (V/Q) if the baseline CXR is abnormal, and is often more widely available (particularly outside usual hours) than a V/Q scan. There is a requirement for adequate glomerular filtration to tolerate the contrast load. V/Q scan is a nuclear medicine test which demonstrates areas of the lungs which are being ventilated but not perfused; a PE occurs due to mechanical obstruction of blood supply.

15 The location of the pulmonary embolism may assist with determining the monitoring of the patient that is required. A central pulmonary embolism is more likely to portend a higher risk of haemodynamic compromise. This includes a saddle embolus (within the bifurcation of the pulmonary trunk) or including at least one main pulmonary artery. A lobar embolism refers to involvement of at least one lobar artery at the most proximal end of the thrombus. More distal clots are reported as segmental or subsegmental emboli. The location is not the only factor which determines the patient's clinical state: a patient with a segmental pulmonary embolus may be hypoxic and hypotensive, while some patients with near saddle emboli may be haemodynamically stable.

16 A wedged-shaped opacity on a chest X-ray or CTPA is suspicious for an area of pulmonary infarction. The shape of the area reflects the pattern of vascular supply. It is unusual to have an infarction in lung tissue as it is supplied by two vascular systems with anastomoses: the pulmonary vascular system and the bronchial vascular system.

17 The merits of testing for an underlying inheritable mutation depend on the presence of other risk factors and clinician preference. Up to a third of VTE cases may be attributed to an inherited mutation. Identifying the presence of a genetic risk factor may add more clinical information for management.

18 In normal development, one copy of a gene is inherited from the mother and one from the father. Mutations can occur in one or both of the genes present in an individual. A mutation in one gene results in a heterozygous state, and in both genes is referred to as homozygous. A non-mutated gene is referred to as 'wild type'. Heterozygotes for factor V Leiden deficiency have 4–8x increased risk of VTE. Homozygous state is rare, but those affected have a 100x increased risk of VTE compared with wild type.

[19] Factor V Leiden is an abnormal factor V molecule caused by a point mutation. It affects the cleavage site on the activated molecule. In the UK, the mutation is present in 1 in 20 individuals of European origin and is autosomal dominant. Those with the mutation are at increased risk of cerebral venous thrombosis, and females are at risk of recurrent pregnancy loss. It is suggested that the gene has persisted in the population due to a survival advantage, possibly because of protection against bleeding, such as postpartum haemorrhage.

[20] Other genetic mutations leading to a hypercoagulable state include:
- deficiency of protein C or S, vitamin K-dependent natural anticoagulants that are also depleted by a number of medical conditions, including VTE and pregnancy
- point mutation in the prothrombin gene
- deficiency or reduced activity of antithrombin.

Less common inherited causes of thrombotic tendency include increased homocysteine levels and an impaired fibrinolysis system or dysfibrinogenaemia. Those with a non-O blood group (e.g. blood group A, B or AB) have a higher risk of VTE due to higher plasma levels of von Willebrand factor (vWF) and factor VIII.

Management

Immediate

Consider supplemental oxygen therapy, aiming for saturations >95%. Monitor the **vital signs** [1] and if hypotensive give **intravenous normal saline** [2]. Prescribe **analgesia** [3] for the pleuritic pain.

Short-term

Commence **anticoagulation** [4], considering risks and benefits of the **currently available medications** [5].

Long-term

The patient should continue anticoagulation for at least **3 months** [6]. She should consider **alternative contraceptive options** [7]. She must inform all **treating medical practitioners** [8] that she is on anticoagulation. If anticoagulation is ceased, she should give consideration to **prophylaxis in high risk situations** [9]. She should be educated regarding reduction in **transient risk factors** [10].

[1] Those with large PEs and right heart strain should have 24 hours of continuous cardiac monitoring, looking for bradycardia or ventricular arrhythmias. Blood pressure should be checked regularly and the patient moved to a resuscitation area if systolic is <90mmHg.

[2] Intravenous fluids are the first therapy that should be given in those with hypotension. IV fluids improve cardiac output; however, care needs to be taken in those with RV dilation, as this will worsen with aggressive filling.

[3] Pleuritic chest pain can cause significant morbidity and in some cases is the barrier to discharge after stabilisation and initiation of appropriate management. Paracetamol is usually a safe first-line choice. NSAIDs, if tolerated, are often a preferred agent for the ischaemia-related nerve pain. A short course of opioid-based medication may be required. The pain will resolve within a week in most patients; persistence beyond this time frame should prompt investigation for alternative causes.

[4] Initial choice of anticoagulation depends on the extent of thrombosis, clinician preference and the patient's clinical state. Many patients with pulmonary embolus will initially commence on low molecular weight heparin (LMWH).

Compared to standard (unfractionated) heparin, LMWH has the advantages of ease of administration (subcutaneous vs. IV), good bioavailability and predictable dosing, and longer half-life in plasma.

[5] The DOACs have revolutionised treatment of thrombosis, and in the majority of patients they will be a safe option. The alternative is the traditionally used warfarin. Contraindications to DOAC use include:
- morbid obesity of >130–150kg
- CrCl <15–25ml/min
- severe liver dysfunction
- very high bleeding risk requiring immediate reversal.

The main advantage of DOACs is the predictable dosing with variations in food and medication administration.

[6] This patient has had a provoking factor of a long-haul flight on the background of two risk factors in factor V Leiden heterozygosity and oestrogen-based contraception. Duration of anticoagulation is generally 3 months for a provoked VTE with a removable risk factor, and 6 months or more for unprovoked or permanent risk factor. This may be dependent on patient preference and the clinician. Many patients will be advised to continue anticoagulation indefinitely if there is a permanent risk factor.

7 A discussion should be had regarding alternative contraception. However, it is usually safe to continue hormone-based medications whilst being anticoagulated. It is preferred that she not continue a systemic oestrogen-based contraception in the absence of anticoagulation. Local hormonal therapy such as intrauterine devices (IUDs) are considered safe.

8 The use of anticoagulation is not a contraindication to elective procedures but the treating practitioner must be informed. This includes dental procedures. In most cases warfarin or DOACs can be safely stopped prior to a procedure, with bridging treatment using LMWH or standard heparin in high risk patients.

9 Patients with a previous PE may be advised to use a preventive dose of anticoagulation, such as enoxaparin or low dose DOAC, prior to and after long-haul flights. They must have prophylaxis during hospital admissions and peri-operatively. Some intermediate–high risk patients receive prophylaxis during pregnancy and for 6 weeks postpartum.

10 Risk of VTE can be reduced by keeping hydrated, avoiding immobility and bed rest. Maintaining a healthy weight should be encouraged.

CASE 41: Cellulitis

History

- An **80-year-old** [1] male presents with a **two-day history** [2] of a **unilateral** [3], red, swollen, painful [4] **lower limb** [5] associated with **fever and malaise** [6].
- This has occurred after he sustained a **small graze** [7] on his left shin the week before.
- The leg has not had exposure to **soil, river or sea water, nor animal bites** [8]. The pain is worse on touching the red area, but is not described as excruciating nor excessive.

- The patient reports no recent **air travel, periods of immobility or recent surgery** [9]. The patient has a history of eczema and T2DM. There is no history of immune compromise, burns, tattoos or injecting drug use.
- The patient has had **three similar episodes** [10] within the past two years, for which he received **courses of antibiotics** [11] from his GP.
- The patient reports **no allergies** [12].

[1] There is no age or gender preponderance for cellulitis; however, extremes of age can develop more severe illness.

[2] Cellulitis is the infection of superficial layers of skin. It develops over hours to days. If it develops very rapidly, or if there is pain that is unexpectedly severe, this may suggest necrotising fasciitis is present. Necrotising fasciitis is a severe, destructive inflammatory process which affects the deeper layers of dermis, subcutaneous fat and tissues and the deep fascia. Two types exist: type 1 is polymicrobial and tends to occur postoperatively, or in patients who are diabetic or immunocompromised; type 2 is caused by Group A *Streptococcus pyogenes*. Although necrotising fasciitis is rare, it has a high mortality rate and is a medical emergency.

[3] Cellulitis is predominantly unilateral. The presence of bilateral symptoms should prompt investigation for mimics of cellulitis, including leg oedema, varicose eczema, lipodermatosclerosis, vasculitis and venous thromboembolism.

[4] The symptoms of cellulitis include dolor (pain), rubor (redness), tumor (swelling) and calor (heat). There may be blisters, superficial haemorrhage or lymphadenopathy. The area is often well-demarcated, diffuse and erythema spread can be tracked. Presence of a well-circumscribed raised fluctuant area should prompt suspicion for underlying abscess.

[5] Most cellulitis occurs on the lower limbs, presumably due to being a frequent site for skin trauma. Another important site is the periorbital region, and post-septal cellulitis (orbital or retro-orbital involvement is an ophthalmic emergency).

[6] Systemic features of fever and malaise are common, and can occur before the classical symptoms and signs of cellulitis. In a patient with fever and no clear source, consider early cellulitis in the differential diagnoses.

[7] Trauma predisposes to cellulitis, as does any condition providing a portal of entry for organisms through the skin barrier. Other conditions include eczema, bites, burns, ulcers or fungal infections such as tinea. Lifestyle risk factors of injecting, piercings or tattoos also predispose to skin and soft tissue infections. Medical comorbidities such as diabetes, vascular disease, obesity and immunocompromised state, including hepatic or renal impairment, also predispose to cellulitis.

[8] History taking should include an assessment of potential exposures. Atypical organisms as a cause of cellulitis should be considered if there is exposure to river (*Aeromonas* spp.) or seawater (e.g. *Vibrio vulnificus*), spas or pools (*Pseudomonas aeruginosa*), exposure to animals, fish or reptiles, and soil. Animal bites can cause cellulitis from other organisms such as *Pasteurella* (cat bites) and *Capnocytophaga* (dog bites). History will also identify whether there is a risk of tetanus exposure requiring booster vaccination.

[9] These important negatives point away from the alternative diagnosis of venous thromboembolism. Risk factors for VTE include immobility, long-haul flights, malignancy, pregnancy, recent surgery, haematological disorders, antiphospholipid syndrome and some hormonal medications.

[10] Previous episodes of cellulitis increase the risk of another episode, likely due to a combination of persistent risk factors as well as local tissue damage from inflammation associated with the infection.

[11] In the setting of recurrent cellulitis, the response to prior courses of antibiotics may give a clue as to the causative organism, and help guide antibiotic therapy. If episodes do not resolve then consider resistant organisms.

[12] Allergy status is essential to clarify, in order to ensure safe antibiotic prescribing.

Examination

- The patient is alert and appears well. He is pyrexial with a temperature of 38.4°C, but other observations are **within normal limits including heart rate and blood pressure** [1].
- He is overweight with a **BMI of 36** [2] and uses a **walking stick** [3].
- There is a well-demarcated area of erythema on the left anterior shin, **marked with a pen, but spreading beyond the margins** [4].
- The erythema is also **tracking linearly along the lower limb, and unilateral left inguinal lymphadenopathy is present** [5].

- The erythema is warm to touch but there is no significant exudate nor **features of necrosis** [6], and the patient reports it is painful but not excruciating.
- The erythema does not **overlie any joints** [7]. The patient has full range of movement of the knee and ankle joints.
- The overlying skin is eczematous bilaterally. A small penetrating wound is visible in the centre of the area of erythema, but there are **no associated blisters, bullae or abscesses** [8].
- There is **associated swelling with unilateral mildly pitting oedema** [9]. Examination of other organ systems was unremarkable.

1 It is important to establish whether the patient is demonstrating signs of sepsis, as deterioration can happen very quickly. Sepsis may indicate bacteraemic complication, but can happen with severe infection and exotoxins (toxic shock syndrome). Fever is not always present, and the patient may be hypothermic or normothermic despite being septic. Increased respiratory rate, low oxygen saturations, low blood pressure (such as systolic BP <90mmHg), altered mental state, low urine output and mottling or duskiness of the skin are all features of sepsis.

2 Obesity is a risk factor for cellulitis, but also a number of other comorbidities. Taking the opportunity to discuss strategies for self-management of obesity should be considered in a non-judgemental manner as part of the holistic care of this patient.

3 The presence of a gait aid identifies opportunity to discuss the patient's mobility. Is this stick a new aid since the development of cellulitis, or is it a sign of impaired mobility and frailty that can be assessed and optimised whilst an inpatient, to help reduce the risk of further accidents causing skin trauma and wounds? Assessment by physiotherapy, occupational therapy and podiatrist may be useful.

4 There are three mechanisms of extension of erythema. The first is seen with horizontal spread along the tissue planes, as seen here. Marking the area of erythema with a pen is a practical way of monitoring the spread of infection, although not an accurate correlation with severity. It should be done with the patient's permission, and care taken not to damage broken or inflamed skin.

5 The second mechanism of extension is seen with lymphangitis, i.e. the spread of infection along the regional lymphatic vessels. This can be visualised as tracking erythema. Inguinal lymphadenopathy is often present on the side of the infection, and can occur prior to the development of erythema.

6 The third mechanism of extension is vertical extension across tissue planes, such as is seen with necrotising fasciitis or particularly aggressive cellulitis. Features of necrosis include dusky, purplish or black areas of tissue, but fasciitis may not be visible as the infection extends along the fascial plane more rapidly than extension to the skin surface. Therefore, absence of visual features of necrosis does not exclude necrotising fasciitis if there are other features of concern, such as excessive pain or signs of sepsis. Likewise, a lack of severe pain does not exclude necrosis, especially in a patient with diabetic neuropathy or chronic inflammatory changes that can impair the pain response.

7 The presence of wounds, erythema or pain overlying a joint should be monitored carefully, and further arthrocentesis or imaging considered if there is concern for complications of septic arthritis or osteomyelitis. Additionally, cellulitis overlying a joint will cause pain on movement, and can further restrict mobility. Examination should include assessment of joint movement to identify these complications.

8 Features of suppurative infection point towards *Staphylococcus aureus* as a likely causative organism, and antibiotics should be targeted towards this. Clues to a resistant strain such as methicillin-resistant *Staphylococcus aureus* (MRSA) include patient's demographics (e.g. nursing home residents), prior growth, known colonisation status, recurrent exposure to healthcare settings (e.g. hospitalisations, dialysis), or failed resolution of a previous infection to antibiotics that would be expected to effectively treat susceptible *S. aureus*. If abscesses are present, surgical drainage or aspiration may be useful and samples sent for culture.

9 Oedema may be due to acute inflammation and/or chronic venous insufficiency, including from previous inflammatory trauma in the setting of previous episodes of cellulitis, or from other intercurrent conditions such as cardiac failure. When examining it is important to note that applied pressure can be painful for the patient, and adjust your examination accordingly. If there are concerns over an underlying disease process contributing to the presentation, e.g. cardiac failure with fluid overload, this should also be treated to aid with resolution of cellulitis.

Investigations

- Blood tests are performed including an **FBE** [1] showing raised white cells with neutrophilia, **CRP** [2] which is raised, **renal and liver function tests** [3] which show stage 3 chronic kidney disease similar to previous results and normal liver function, and an **HbA1c** [4] which shows suboptimal glycaemic control.
- A **D-dimer** [5] is not performed.

- **Blood cultures** [6] are performed which are negative.
- **Wound swab** [7] is not performed and previous swabs are reviewed, showing mixed growth only.
- An **ultrasound scan** [8] rules out a deep vein thrombosis.
- No further imaging such as **X-ray, CT or MRI** [9] is performed.

[1] A full blood examination is expected to be abnormal in cellulitis, with raised white cells, predominantly neutrophils. In some cases, low white cells can indicate severe sepsis or underlying immune compromise. There may also be thrombocytosis associated with the acute inflammatory response.

[2] C-reactive protein is expected to be raised, although there is a lag time, meaning that testing very early in the disease process may yield lower than expected or falsely normal levels. In a patient diagnosed with cellulitis, a normal CRP, particularly if the erythema is bilateral, should prompt a search for an alternative diagnosis. It is important to note that CRP is not specific for infection, and may be raised in other conditions such as thrombophlebitis or venous thromboembolism.

[3] Renal and liver function tests will help identify whether there is end-organ damage from sepsis, and aid with guiding appropriate antibiotic therapy and doses. It is important, as in this case, to identify what the baseline renal and liver function are.

[4] An HbA1c, or glycated haemoglobin, gives an indication of diabetic control over the prior 3 months. A result of >7% indicates suboptimal diabetic control.

[5] D-dimer is a good 'rule-out' test for VTE, with good negative predictive value in low risk patients. In this case, however, an active infective process is likely to produce a false positive D-dimer result and therefore the test is of little utility.

[6] Blood cultures are positive in only around 10% of cases of cellulitis, but if positive can help guide antibiotic therapy.

Group A streptococcus accounts for a large proportion of cases of culture negative cellulitis.

[7] Wound swab should never be done on an intact skin in cellulitis or chronic wound which does not look infected. Wound or tissue cultures are negative in around 70% of cases, and if positive, clinical judgement must be taken to distinguish between colonising and pathological bacteria. Prior swabs may be helpful, for example if *S. aureus* has been grown from purulent tissue, and can help guide subsequent antibiotic choice. If drainage of abscesses is performed, pus samples should be sent for microbiological analysis.

[8] Ultrasound scan can be useful for Doppler imaging of leg veins in ruling out venous thrombosis as a differential diagnosis, and can also assist with identification of suspected abscesses, but should not be routinely ordered if the clinical diagnosis of cellulitis is obvious. Keep in mind that ultrasound scans require direct pressure on the area, which can be particularly painful with cellulitis. Appropriate analgesia should be given to the patient prior to the scan.

[9] The diagnosis of cellulitis is predominantly based on history and examination, and imaging has a limited role. X-ray is suitable for bony imaging but not soft tissue and is therefore not clinically useful. CT can, however, be useful in differentiating between superficial and deep cellulitis, and can identify complications associated with cellulitis including abscesses, myositis and fasciitis. If necrotising fasciitis is suspected, however, CT should not delay definitive management with surgical debridement. MRI will provide further information on myositis and osteomyelitis but is unlikely to have additional clinical value in uncomplicated cellulitis.

Management

Short-term

Commence on **empiric intravenous antibiotics** [1] and change to **oral antibiotics when clinically appropriate** [2]. Consider the use of **outpatient IV antimicrobial therapy** [3] if the patient requires a longer period of intravenous antibiotics but is systemically well. Monitor for signs of deterioration from sepsis which may require resuscitation with **fluids and inotropes** [4]. Prompt surgical review is essential if symptoms or signs suggestive of **necrotising fasciitis** [5] occur. Elevate the patient's leg and provide appropriate **analgesia** [6]. Commence blood glucose measurements and aim to **improve glucose control** [7]. Commence **low molecular weight heparin** [8] for VTE prophylaxis whilst not mobilising. Instigate treatment and education to improve **skin condition** [9]. Involve **multidisciplinary team** [10] including diabetes specialist, physiotherapy, occupational therapy and podiatry, and liaise with the patient's GP on discharge.

Long-term

After resolution of the acute episode, it is important to help the patient **reduce their risk of future episodes of cellulitis** [11]. **Prophylactic antibiotics** [12] may help problematic cases.

[1] Local antimicrobial guidelines should be consulted for empiric and directed therapy. Narrow-spectrum penicillins to cover *Streptococcus* spp. should be used, with additional staphylococcal cover in the event of purulent infection. Previous swabs may be useful; for example, evidence of colonisation with MRSA would prompt addition of appropriate cover. If necrotising fasciitis is suspected, the empiric antibiotic regimen must also cover Gram-negative and anaerobic bacteria including *Clostridia*. Addition of lincosamides for antitoxin effect may be beneficial.

[2] The decision to change to oral antibiotics depends on a number of factors including resolution of pyrexia, haemodynamic stability and the ability to use an antibiotic with good cover for *Streptococcus* and *Staphylococcus* with good penetration into soft tissue. The erythema of cellulitis is not a good indicator of improvement, as it persists, often maturing to a darker red colour before fading.

[3] Outpatient intravenous antimicrobial therapy can help with early discharge home for particular patients who are well but need prolonged courses of IV therapy. This service includes regular nursing visits and scheduled medical reviews to monitor progress and initiate alternative management strategies, if required.

[4] In the setting of signs of sepsis, early intervention is essential. The 'sepsis six' bundle – blood cultures, fluid bolus, lactate measurement, measurement of urine output, oxygen therapy if <94% and antibiotics within an hour – is a widely used approach to resuscitation. Blood pressure not responding quickly to fluid bolus requires early escalation, consideration of inotropes, +/– HDU/ICU review to provide support and maintain adequate organ perfusion whilst sepsis resolves and antibiotics work.

[5] Definitive management of necrotising fasciitis warrants urgent surgical review and debridement in theatre, and this should not be delayed if this diagnosis is suspected. Antibiotic therapy is not sufficient to manage this condition.

[6] Analgesia is important for patient comfort and to facilitate earlier mobilisation and reduce the rate of complications from immobility. Analgesia should start with simple measures such as paracetamol and NSAIDs, unless contraindicated such as with renal impairment. Stronger opioid-based analgesia may be required, but care should be given to renal and liver function, as well as monitoring for drowsiness or hypotension from such drugs which can cause complications in the unstable septic patient.
Elevating the leg can help with pain management and can reduce oedema.

[7] Improving glycaemic control will help with control of the acute infection, and in the long term will help reduce risk of recurrence. Involvement of pharmacist, diabetes educator and endocrinologist may be useful. The patient should also be assessed for complications of diabetes, and receive advice on secondary prevention and other strategies such as foot care in the presence of diabetic neuropathy.

[8] Reduced mobility, localised oedema and inflammation increase the risk of venous thromboembolism. The use of LMWH as prophylaxis against VTE is important and should continue until the patient is mobilising normally.

[9] Immediate treatment of fungal infections and dry skin should be initiated. It is also important to discuss a skin care regimen with the patient including cleaning, creams and dressings. The patient may benefit from a Dermatology review and Wound Care/Tissue Viability nurses, and longer-term input from district nurses can be very helpful.

[10] Physiotherapist and occupational therapist input will help the patient with mobility and functional status, in the short and long term. Involving the GP in ongoing

care is essential, as they will be the mainstay of support for the patient on discharge. A timely, succinct but thorough discharge outlining management is ideal, with a phone call to discuss any specific follow-up recommendations.

11 Cellulitis can often recur, particularly in cases affecting the lower limbs. Episodes can lead to chronic inflammatory changes with lymphoedema, requiring management with compression bandages and elevation of the legs. The patient should also be educated on their individual risk factors and ways to self-manage these; for example, weight loss if obese, improved glycaemic control if diabetic.

12 Once other factors have been addressed and improved as much as possible, patients who still suffer from 3–4 episodes per year can be considered for prophylactic antibiotics with narrow-spectrum penicillins. The benefit of this needs to be weighed up against the risk of side-effects from prolonged antimicrobial therapy, including GI upset, *Clostridioides difficile* infection and antimicrobial resistance.

CASE 42: Gastroenteritis

History

- A 55-year-old man presents with colicky **lower abdominal pain associated with nausea, vomiting and diarrhoea** [1].
- The symptoms began **36 hours previously** [2], and the patient has had 10 bowel motions over the past 12 hours, initially large volume and watery, but now smaller volume with small amounts of **fresh blood** [3]. He also feels feverish, is not tolerating fluids, and feels light-headed.
- **Past medical and surgical history** [4] is unremarkable including no history of diabetes, immune deficiency nor GI disorder, including no previous diarrhoeal illness.
- The patient does not take any regular **medications** [5] such as steroids, immune therapies and has not had any recent courses of antibiotics within the last 6 months.

- **Travel history** [6] is unremarkable, with no travel abroad recently, and no obvious exposure to unsanitary water supplies or rural farm areas.
- He received full courses of childhood **vaccinations** [7] and has also been fully immunised against typhoid and hepatitis A.
- He has not **consumed** [8] raw seafood, unheated cooked rice or unpasteurised dairy products, but reports consuming chicken from a restaurant three days prior to presentation and has otherwise eaten the same food as his well partner.
- The patient works in a **care home** [9] as a chef, but reports no colleagues or residents are unwell.
- There have been no reported outbreaks in the local area according to the **public health** [10] information.

[1] The symptoms of gastroenteritis include vomiting and/or diarrhoea, and are often associated with other features including nausea, abdominal pain, cramps and fever. Features that raise concern include clinical evidence of severe dehydration, bloody stools, severe abdominal pain, weight loss or prolonged symptoms.

[2] The incubation period of infectious gastroenteritis is frequently short, and the timing of infection can give an idea of the potential pathogen, particularly if there is a suspected exposure. Toxin-mediated gastroenteritis, such as enterotoxin-producing *Staphylococcus aureus*, often manifests within about 6 hours of exposure, but should be considered if within 18 hours of suspected exposure. Other bacterial infections such as *Bacillus cereus* have short incubation times of 1–6 hours, whereas others may become symptomatic around 12–72 hours after exposure. Viral infections (overall the most common cause of infectious gastroenteritis), such as rotavirus or norovirus, have short incubation periods. A longer duration of symptoms should raise suspicion for protozoal infections; however, non-infectious causes become more likely.

[3] The features of diarrhoea can give a clue to the underlying pathogen. 'Secretory' diarrhoea is watery and non-bloody, and is associated with organisms that produce exotoxins such as *S. aureus*, *B. cereus* and *Vibrio cholerae*. Other organisms may directly invade the bowel mucosa or secrete cytotoxins, such as *Campylobacter*, *Shigella* and

enterohaemorrhagic strains of *Escherichia coli*. These can cause bloody diarrhoea and systemic upset. *Salmonella* may cause both these presentations.

[4] Past medical history can elicit clues as to whether this presentation is infective in nature, and whether the patient is at particular risk of severe disease. Differentials for this presentation include non-infectious GI conditions such as diverticulitis, inflammatory bowel disease, and a new presentation of bowel malignancy. The short duration of symptoms, presence of fever and usual good health are more suggestive of an acute infectious process. Red flag symptoms for underlying pathological processes, such as unintentional weight loss, melaena or fresh rectal bleeding, should be explored. Immunocompromised state raises the possibility of opportunistic infections and more severe infections. The elderly and pregnant are also at increased risk of complications.

[5] Medication history can identify whether patients are at increased risk of opportunistic or severe infections from immune-modulating medications. Recent or multiple courses of antibiotics should raise suspicion of *Clostridioides difficile* as a cause of presentation. As dehydration and acute kidney injury are a risk, note should be taken of concurrent nephrotoxin use, including non-steroidal anti-inflammatories for pain relief.

6 Travel history can give valuable clues as to whether this is traveller's diarrhoea, a common illness that can manifest during travel or shortly after return from areas where particular organisms such as *Shigella, Campylobacter, Giardia, Salmonella typhi* and enterotoxigenic *E. coli* are found.

7 Travel vaccination history, such as immunisation against hepatitis A and typhoid, is helpful to know.

8 The majority of GI infections are food- or waterborne, and are contracted via the oral or faecal–oral route, therefore it may be possible to identify a particular exposure of a potential infectious agent. Unheated cooked rice, and uncooked seafood or meats such as chicken pose particular risks; other less common but important exposures include ingestion of unpasteurised dairy products, contaminated eggs or travel to an area with inadequate sanitation.

9 The patient's occupation is important to ascertain; in this case, working in a care home may have exposed him to particular organisms such as norovirus, but also identifies the risk he may pose on return to work of passing on his infection if not fully recovered.

10 If there is suspicion of a particular source of an outbreak of infectious gastroenteritis, it is useful to review local public health information to identify if there are any warnings on current outbreaks.

Examination

- On examination, the patient is febrile at 38.3°C and appears **dehydrated** [1] with a pulse of 106bpm and BP of 100/68mmHg.
- He has slightly cool peripheries but is not mottled or jaundiced, and does not have a **rash** [2].
- The patient is of normal body habitus and does not appear **cachectic** [3].
- The **abdomen** [4] is not distended and although there is mild tenderness in the lower abdomen, there is no localised guarding, severe pain, nor any rebound tenderness. No masses are palpable.
- **Rectal examination** [5] reveals no masses, and liquid stool with a small amount of mixed fresh blood.
- Other systems examination is normal including **neurological examination** [6].

1 It is important to assess the fluid status of the patient, from clinical examination looking for dry mucous membranes, and from vital signs including tachycardia and hypotension, as well as urine output and general mentation. This assists with assessing for red flags for the severity of the infection.

2 A rash, if present, can assist with diagnosis. *S. typhi* can be associated with rose spots on the trunk. Diarrhoea associated with viruses can also manifest as exanthems. Mottling of the skin suggests hypovolaemia or sepsis and should raise concern for severe disease. Jaundice is indicative of hepatitis, and should prompt examination for features of acute liver failure and consideration of acute viral hepatitis as the causative organism.

3 Weight loss can occur in the setting of severe or prolonged illness, due to increased catabolism or malabsorption, and should also prompt significant concern for parasitic causes or non-infectious inflammatory and neoplastic causes.

4 Abdominal examination can reveal features of concern, such as diffuse pain suggestive of peritonitis, or localised tenderness suggestive of cholecystitis, appendicitis or other focal infection. Severe abdominal pain is a red flag for severe disease, including perforation of a viscus as a complication, and if present should prompt consideration of detailed imaging and consult with surgical specialists. Palpable masses should also raise concern for complex intra-abdominal abscess or an alternative diagnosis such as malignancy.

5 Rectal examination is not routinely required but can be helpful to assess for alternative diagnoses such as rectal malignancy and for assessment of bloody stools. The presence of stool with mixed fresh blood suggests there is haemorrhagic colitis rather than external bleeding that may occur from external haemorrhoids.

6 Neurological findings can occur in specific infections such as invasive *Listeria monocytogenes* infection, or with rarer conditions such as scombroid poisoning, a toxin-mediated condition caused by bacterial overgrowth on fish, which can present with features of histamine poisoning similar to anaphylaxis. Presentation with seizures, jaundice, hypertension, oligoanuria and petechiae may represent the uncommon but severe complication of enterohaemorrhagic *E. coli* (serotype 0157:H7) (also known as Shiga toxin-producing *E. coli*) infection with haemolytic uraemic syndrome, especially in children.

Investigations

- **Blood tests** [1] demonstrate normal haemoglobin and raised white cells with a mild neutrophilia. Renal function shows a slightly raised creatinine with an eGFR of 65ml/min/1.73m^2, and potassium is slightly low at 3.0mmol/L. CRP is slightly raised. Liver function and lipase are normal.

- A **blood gas** [2] demonstrates normal pH and lactate.
- **Stool** [3] microscopy, culture and sensitivity (MCS) as well as PCR testing identifies *Campylobacter jejuni*.
- **Blood cultures** [4] are negative.
- **Abdominal X-ray** [5] is normal, and no other radiological investigations are performed.

[1] A full blood examination may be normal, or may demonstrate increased peripheral white blood cells. It does not help to differentiate between the potential causes of the gastroenteritis, nor between infective and non-infective inflammatory diseases. It may also demonstrate a raised haematocrit consistent with dehydration. If volume depletion is present, there may be electrolyte abnormalities such as hypokalaemia and metabolic acidosis, and acute renal impairment may occur. C-reactive protein may be raised; liver function tests should be normal, but if there is evidence of deranged function with a hepatitis picture, then further testing for synthetic function with coagulation and albumin measurements is important, and directed testing for viral hepatitis considered.

[2] A blood gas contains useful information on acid–base balance, including whether the presentation is severe enough to cause a metabolic acidosis with contributors of sepsis and lactic acidosis from dehydration. A normal pH and lactate are reassuring.

[3] Stool samples should be considered if findings are likely to impact on management. Stool microscopy and cultures are indicated in the presence of severe disease, immunocompromised state or bloody stools, and protracted clinical course. Microscopy can identify erythrocytes in addition to leucocytes, which can be raised in infections caused by *Shigella*, *Campylobacter* or *Salmonella*. Ova, cysts and parasites may be visualised and can be present if the gastroenteritis is caused by a protozoal infection. Many laboratories will perform a multiplex PCR to rapidly identify common organisms. *C. difficile* testing should be requested, particularly if there has been a prior history, or recent antibiotic use, although the test can remain positive for some time after recent treatment, and interpretation of positive results should therefore weigh up the likelihood of recurrent infection.

[4] In the febrile, hypotensive patient, blood cultures should be performed to identify whether bacteraemia is contributing to the presentation. Typhoid fever may be complicated by *Salmonella typhi* bacteraemia and can be associated with seeding to other distant sites in the body, necessitating specific directed therapy. The majority of patients will have no growth on blood cultures.

[5] In the absence of significant abdominal pain it is unlikely that radiological investigations will yield useful information. Abdominal X-ray can identify the presence of emerging bowel obstruction, particularly in the patient with increasing abdominal pain, distension, lack of flatus and vomiting. If severe abdominal pain is present, CT of the abdomen should be considered which can identify presence of bowel perforation, toxic megacolon (which can be associated with *C. difficile* colitis), intra-abdominal abscesses or other differential diagnoses including appendicitis. There may be radiological features of pseudomembranous colitis associated with *C. difficile* colitis.

Management

Short-term

If admitted to hospital, the patient should be managed with appropriate **contact precautions** [1]. The main focus of management of acute gastroenteritis is **rehydration** [2] and electrolyte replacement. **Symptomatic relief** [3] may be required. **Usual medications** [4] with potential to worsen hydration status or symptoms should be reviewed. **Low molecular weight heparin** [5] should be considered for patients admitted to hospital. Empirical **antimicrobial therapy** [6] may be considered if features of severe diseases are present, with early switch to directed antimicrobial therapy if an organism requiring ongoing treatment is required. In addition, in severe disease, specific treatment of complications such as organ support may be required.

Long-term

Recovery is usually fairly rapid without significant sequelae, although some patients may develop a postinfectious irritable bowel syndrome or other **complications** [7] at a later date. Patients should be given advice on **reducing risk of recurrence** [8] depending on their risk factors, such as provision of travel advice, hand hygiene instructions and vaccination advice. In particular cases, liaison with **public health** [9] may be required if the organism is notifiable.

[1] Patients with enteric infection require contact precautions, which include thorough hand hygiene before and after patient contact, as well as use of gloves and gown when likely to touch the patient or patient's surroundings. This assists with reducing the spread of infection from the patient to the healthcare provider and subsequently to others.

[2] For most patients, oral rehydration with added electrolytes is sufficient; however, if there is evidence of significant dehydration, renal impairment, intolerance of oral intake or other markers of severe disease then IV rehydration with electrolyte replacement may be required. Usually, hypovolaemic hypotension will respond to rehydration but in very severe cases, assessment by a critical care specialist may be required to consider inotropic support.

[3] Symptoms of nausea, abdominal pain and fever may be relieved by use of anti-emetics and analgesia. Care should be taken to avoid the use of anti-inflammatories in the context of renal impairment and gastritis. Anti-motility agents may be considered for mild disease but should be avoided in the patient with fever or bloody diarrhoea, due to increased risk of severe disease.

[4] Medication reconciliation is important for any patient admitted to hospital, and consideration given to temporarily withholding regular medications. Antihypertensives and other nephrotoxic agents such as anti-inflammatories should be reviewed carefully. Patients on steroids may have underlying adrenal suppression and consideration should be given to stress dosing whilst unwell.

[5] Dehydration, acute inflammation and reduced motility all represent risk factors for venous thromboembolism, and patients admitted to hospital should be considered for prophylaxis with LMWH and compression stockings.

[6] Antibiotics are not routinely recommended for treatment of gastroenteritis. They may be considered for patients who have severe disease or who are immunocompromised who are more likely to benefit from treatment than suffer side-effects of antimicrobials. Clinical features that may prompt treatment include very frequent stools with significant volume depletion, features of invasive bacterial infection with bloody stools and fever, and those with significant underlying health problems. Empirical therapy is usually with a fluoroquinolone or azithromycin if fluoroquinolone resistance is suspected, if tolerating oral therapy, or with a broad-spectrum cephalosporin intravenously if not tolerating oral therapy. If a pathogen is identified, directing therapy towards likely or confirmed susceptibilities is ideal to complete a course of treatment. Of importance, Shiga toxin-producing *E. coli* should not be treated with antimicrobials due to an increased risk of haemolytic uraemic syndrome.

[7] Postinfectious IBS may occur in some patients, whereby an episode of infectious gastroenteritis triggers the onset of irritable bowel symptoms. The aetiology is uncertain but may relate to changes in gut motility and composition in gut flora. Another recognised complication is of Guillain–Barré syndrome, a disorder of acute progressive muscle weakness frequently triggered by an infection, of which *Campylobacter jejuni* infection is the most commonly identified.

[8] The mainstay of preventive advice is maintaining good hand hygiene and sanitary practices. Specific risk factors, such as travel to areas where traveller's diarrhoea may be contracted, can be addressed by vaccinations and food hygiene. Some infections such as *C. difficile* have the potential to recur, particularly if risk factors of future antimicrobial use persist. These patients should be counselled to avoid unnecessary antibiotic exposure and to re-present for assessment if symptoms recur, particularly with significant diarrhoea and abdominal pain.

[9] Specific organisms are notifiable to public health, such as *C. jejuni*, *Norovirus* and toxin-producing *E. coli*. This is to ensure that clusters of cases are identified and potential outbreaks limited. In addition, it is important to ensure that those in higher risk occupations, such as this patient who is a chef at a care home, are cleared of infection before going into an environment where they may pose a risk to others.

CASE 43: HIV/AIDS

History

- A **36-year-old male** [1] presents with a 4-week history of increasing breathlessness and dry cough, on a background of 4 months of weight loss and swollen lymph glands. He also notes the presence of a purplish nodular rash on his shins which has been present for the same time.
- His GP has referred him to the Infectious Diseases clinic with a concern that he may have a new diagnosis of human immunodeficiency virus/acquired immune deficiency syndrome (**HIV/AIDS** [2]) and that these may represent **AIDS-defining illnesses** [3].
- His **past medical history** [4] includes anxiety and depression, mechanical lower back pain and a previous syphilis infection treated with penicillin 7 years ago, when he recalls also **being unwell** [5] with fevers and lymphadenopathy for a few weeks.
- The patient reports no **allergies** [6].
- His **medications** [7] include regular fluoxetine, and as required diazepam for anxiety. He also takes paracetamol and codeine for his back pain.

- His social history and **risk factors** [8] for HIV/AIDS are explored: he is a non-smoker, drinks 4–6 units of alcohol most days and has previously injected drugs, but not within the past 10 years. He has no tattoos and has never had a blood transfusion. He is Caucasian, lives in the UK, and has no family history of HIV.
- His **sexual history** [9] includes a current male partner with whom he has had protected sexual intercourse on an exclusive basis for the past 6 years. However, prior to this he has had unprotected sexual intercourse with both male and female partners. His last check for sexually transmitted infections was 7 years ago, 2 weeks after his last unprotected sexual encounter.
- At this time HIV and viral hepatitis (B and C) testing were negative, treponemal serology indicated acute syphilis infection which was treated, but he did not attend **follow-up testing** [10] nor undergo hepatitis B immunisation.

[1] First identified in the 1980s, HIV/AIDS affects around 37 million people worldwide, with a slightly higher male prevalence compared to female. Rates and epidemiological risk vary by region, with most cases obtained via sexual transmission, in addition to vertical transmission and via bloodborne mechanisms such as needle sharing.

[2] HIV retrovirus establishes chronic infection and predominantly affects CD4 T cells. Clinical manifestation can vary from the asymptomatic patient with incidental diagnosis, through presentation with acute HIV infection prodrome, to presentation at a later stage with evidence of immunodeficiency. If left undiagnosed and untreated after initial infection, the CD4 T-cell count depletes over the years, resulting in a state of compromised immune function. Non-specific constitutional symptoms may then occur, including weight loss, sweats and generalised lymphadenopathy, but most patients with HIV have few symptoms prior to development of AIDS.

[3] AIDS is defined as HIV infection that has advanced to a stage with a CD4 cell count of <200 cells/µl, or the presence of an AIDS-defining condition, including

opportunistic infections with recurrent bacterial infections, invasive candidiasis, *Cryptococcus* infection, Kaposi sarcoma, *Pneumocystis jirovecii* pneumonia, *Mycobacterium* infection, herpes viruses and lymphomas. Advanced HIV is the term given when the CD4 count has dropped below 50 cells/µl.

[4] Past medical history can identify particular comorbidities that can impact on prognosis and treatment decisions. Previous tuberculosis raises the possibility of latent TB that can reactivate, viral hepatitis B and C co-infection with HIV increases the likelihood of, and speed of progression of chronic liver disease complications. Existing cardiovascular disease or risks can be worsened by HIV or antiretrovirals. There is also an increased risk of malignancy, therefore systemic enquiry should be thorough to identify red flag symptoms for occult malignancy. Previous history of sexually transmitted infections (STIs) should be asked about, as concurrent infections with HIV are common. In women, obstetric and gynaecological history should include whether cervical smears are up to date and whether any previous abnormal smears have been identified, in addition to clarifying previous and current obstetric history, contraceptive

use and pregnancy planning. Psychiatric history is important to clarify.

5 A patient who contracts HIV may develop symptoms of acute HIV infection around 2–4 weeks after exposure, although many are asymptomatic. Known as the acute retroviral syndrome, symptoms tend to be constitutional, with fever, sore throat, myalgia and lymphadenopathy the most common symptoms, and symptoms tend to correlate with HIV viraemia if tested for. Painful ulcers affecting the mucocutaneous surfaces may also occur, and rarer symptoms include GI upset, headache and aseptic meningitis. This syndrome usually self-resolves and may go uninvestigated.

6 Allergy status is important to clarify, predominantly to be able to select appropriate antimicrobials for treatment of opportunistic infections. In addition, specific testing may be required prior to certain medications, including checking for G6PD deficiency in patients being treated with dapsone or primaquine for *Pneumocystis jirovecii* infections, and HLA testing prior to commencing the antiretroviral abacavir, as HLA-B*57:01 type is associated with abacavir hypersensitivity reaction.

7 Antiretrovirals, used to treat HIV, are a group of medications with high potential for drug–drug interactions. A thorough medication history is essential, including asking about use of over-the-counter medications, contraceptives and recreational drugs. The majority of drug interactions occur via induction or inhibition of hepatic metabolism, and are particularly seen with protease inhibitors and non-nucleoside reverse transcriptase inhibitors. Resources to assist with medication choices and adjustments include online interaction checkers, and the involvement of a specialist pharmacist is also recommended.

8 Risk factors for exposure to HIV include sexual activity, of which particular practices are deemed high risk due to the increased likelihood of viral transmission. These include receptive oral sex, penetrative anal sex and the coexistence of other STIs associated with ulcers. Other risk factors include IV drug use and tattoos with shared needles, needlestick injuries from patients known to have HIV with detectable viral load, blood transfusion from unscreened blood, and vertical transmission from mother to child.

9 Sexual history is important to explore, as this can help identify the potential exposure, risk of having exposed other partners to the virus, and identify the need to test for other sexually transmitted infections.

10 Standard HIV testing usually consists of a combination of an antigen/antibody assay and if indicated, a viral load measurement. During early HIV infection, testing may be negative. HIV antigen testing can be done to identify the p24 antigen, a protein from the HIV viral core, and can allow detection of early HIV infection prior to seroconversion. Serology can also be measured but will be negative until seroconversion occurs, and it is recommended to have follow-up serological testing. Hepatitis B and C serology status should also be concurrently tested. It is also recommended for syphilis testing to be rechecked after completion of treatment to ensure that titres are reducing, indicating successful treatment.

Examination

- On general inspection, the patient appears **thin** [1] but generally well and is **haemodynamically stable** [2] with blood pressure 116/72mmHg, heart rate 84bpm, and he is **pyrexial** [3] with a temperature of 38.3°C.
- He appears to be **oxygenating** [4] suboptimally at rest with peripheral saturations of 94% on air, but desaturates quickly to 83% on mobilising. He appears tachypnoeic on mobilising with respiratory rate of 22 breaths per minute.
- On further examination, the patient has non-tender cervical and axillary **lymphadenopathy** [5].
- Chest examination demonstrates occasional quiet crackles but otherwise normal air entry. **Cardiac, abdominal, joint and genitourinary examination** [6] are otherwise normal.
- **Small purplish nodules** [7] are evident on the shins bilaterally.
- **Mental state examination** [8] reveals that the patient is oriented to time, place and person, and cognition appears normal, but he is tearful and anxious.

1 Weight loss can occur during the chronic HIV stage of the disease, as part of the constitutional symptoms seen before developing AIDS. As HIV is associated with increased risk of malignancy, occult cancer should be considered in the differential.

2 Most patients are haemodynamically stable at the time of their diagnosis of HIV/AIDS; however, if they have advanced immune suppression, and if they present with a severe opportunistic infection, then they may be critically unwell. Their capacity to respond to worsening infection is also impaired by immune suppression and should be factored into decision-making about escalation of care to involve intensive care.

3 The presence of a fever suggests infection as the most likely cause of the presentation, and should trigger evaluation of the patient for potential opportunistic infections. Non-infective causes of fever, including malignancy, should also be considered.

4 *Pneumocystis jirovecii* (previously *P. carinii*) pneumonia (PJP) is an opportunistic infection, and can occur in HIV-infected patients with low CD4 count (<200 cells/μl) who are not on prophylaxis. This atypical fungus manifests with gradually worsening respiratory symptoms of non-productive cough and dyspnoea, in addition to fever, weight loss and fatigue, usually over a period of about 3 weeks. On examination, hypoxia is often present, and exercise-induced oxygen desaturation is particularly suspicious for infection with PJP.

5 Patients with HIV may develop generalised lymphadenopathy during the chronic HIV stage, prior to development of severe acquired immune deficiency (AIDS). The enlarged lymph nodes tend to examine as mobile, rubbery and painless and are usually found symmetrically in the cervical and axillary lymph node areas. Lymphoma, *Mycobacterium avium* complex (MAC) and tuberculous mycobacterial infections, toxoplasma and human herpesvirus-8 related diseases should be considered in the differential list for lymphadenopathy in patients with advanced stage disease.

6 A thorough examination is important to identify other complications of HIV/AIDS and immune suppression, looking for features of opportunistic infections. There may also be features of comorbid conditions that can accompany chronic HIV infection, thought to be due to chronic inflammation or immune activation. These include cardiovascular disease, malignancies, cognitive impairment and metabolic bone disease such as osteoporosis.

7 Kaposi sarcoma are vascular tumours associated with human herpesvirus 8, and can have cutaneous and visceral involvement. They present as small purplish nodules when found cutaneously. A biopsy should be obtained to assist with diagnosis, and can help differentiate from the other important differential of bacillary angiomatosis caused by *Bartonella* infection. It is important to stage the extent of disease, looking for visceral and lymph node involvement.

8 Assessment of current and pre-existing mental health is essential. HIV significantly increases the risk of neuropsychiatric complications, ranging from delirium, depression and mild cognitive impairment to substance abuse, dementia and HIV-associated mania. These are due to the HIV infection itself, as well as medication side-effects and psychosocial factors that increase the patient's vulnerability to psychiatric illness. Early involvement of a psychologist can be beneficial to help the patient process their diagnosis and its implications, and regular mental health screening should form part of long-term care.

Investigations

- **Blood tests** [1] are performed, including a full blood examination showing leucopenia and anaemia, with normal renal and liver function and a mildly raised C-reactive protein.
- An **arterial blood gas** [2] demonstrates mild hypoxaemia, a chest X-ray shows diffuse non-specific alveolar changes, and a CT chest shows ground-glass changes bilaterally. Respiratory secretions are obtained and pneumatoceles are visualised, confirming the diagnosis of PJP.
- **HIV testing** [3] is performed including serology, which is positive. Further testing identifies a raised HIV viral load, and CD4 count of 180 cells/μl.

- **Antiretroviral resistance testing** [4] demonstrates no resistance, and HLA-B*57:01 is not present.
- A full **sexually transmitted infection screen** [5] is completed, which shows that the patient has had previous hepatitis C which has spontaneously cleared, but has not had previous exposure to hepatitis B and is non-immune. Gonorrhoea and chlamydia testing are negative, treponemal serology does not suggest active syphilis infection, and there are no features suggesting current herpes simplex virus infection, genital warts or lymphogranulomata venereum. Biopsy of the cutaneous nodules confirms the diagnosis of Kaposi sarcoma.

1 Cytopenias are common with chronic HIV infection, with leucopenia, particularly lymphopenia, anaemia and thrombocytopenia found in a large proportion of patients with low CD4 count. Chronic kidney disease can occur due to HIV nephropathy, and should be evaluated thoroughly to identify contributing factors and risk for progression. Abnormal liver function may indicate opportunistic infection or malignancy with hepatic involvement, or may be present

due to coexistent chronic viral hepatitis infection. Renal and liver functions are important to identify as this will impact on choice of antiretroviral (ARV) therapy.

2 Evaluation of the severity of any underlying respiratory disease includes an arterial blood gas to accurately evaluate hypoxaemia and the alveolar-arterial oxygen gradient, which is typically widened in PJP infection. Radiological imaging will be of benefit to further evaluate suspected PJP infection, as well as other concurrent opportunistic infections. Chest X-ray is often normal in initial stages, but may then progress to typical features of diffuse infiltrates throughout the interstitium or alveoli. High resolution CT of the chest showing ground-glass attenuation in a patchy or nodular pattern is suggestive of PJP. Definitive diagnosis of PJP is most easily made by PCR analysis of induced sputum; microscopic analysis of sputum may also demonstrate the pneumocystis.

3 HIV serology will be positive at this stage of the illness, and viraemia detectable. Whilst early HIV infection is typically associated with significant viraemia, with RNA levels frequently >100 000 copies/ml, the viral load tends to drop into the thousands and settles into a steady state by about 6 months. A detectable viral load is generally considered to represent potential for person-to-person transmission.

Undetectable viral loads, on the other hand, as can be achieved with ARV therapy, are associated with extremely low risk of transmission, as identified in a landmark study (undetectable = untransmissible).

4 Drug resistance genotype testing is essential to perform in order to identify the appropriate ARV regimen. If the source of the HIV infection is known, any known drug resistance or risky behaviours, such as non-compliance, will increase the likelihood of the patient's HIV genotype displaying ARV-resistant mutations. Resistance to non-nucleoside reverse transcriptase inhibitors is most common, compared to mutations conferring resistance to integrase inhibitors and protease inhibitors.

5 Full screening for other STIs is essential, to allow directed treatment, including the use of particular antiretrovirals if hepatitis B is also present.

Management

Short-term

The immediate management of the patient who presents with a new diagnosis of chronic HIV infection includes **counselling** [1] the patient of their diagnosis, **initiating antiretroviral treatment** [2], and managing acute complications from opportunistic infections and concurrent sexually transmitted infections. HIV is a **notifiable disease** [3] and the local public health body should be contacted, who will then initiate contact tracing. The patient should also be advised about their **responsibilities** [4] with regard to notifying future sexual partners, the specifics of which vary depending on local jurisdiction.

The patient should receive input from the **multidisciplinary HIV team** [5] including specialist HIV nurses, HIV pharmacist, psychologist, social work and peer support groups; both in the short and longer term.

Long-term

Regular reviews with the specialist HIV team should be conducted initially, to establish complications from commencing ARV therapy, including drug side-effects, as well as complications from **immune reconstitution syndrome** [6]. The importance of **compliance** [7] with ARV therapy should be highlighted each visit, and the patient evaluated for **complications** [8] associated with chronic HIV infection and long-term side-effects associated with specific ARV therapy, including advice on screening for malignancy and osteoporosis, and immunisations.

It is also important to be aware of the use of **pre-exposure prophylaxis (PrEP)** [9] and **post-exposure prophylaxis (PEP)** [10].

1 Communicating the diagnosis of HIV to a patient must be done sensitively, by an experienced person, and with supports made immediately available. Care should be taken to maintain confidentiality, and may extend to not sharing the diagnosis with other health professionals, depending on patient wishes.

2 It is increasingly recognised that ARV therapy brings morbidity benefits when commenced earlier, and the current standard of care is to commence ARV therapy at or close to diagnosis, regardless of CD4 count. Specific clinical scenarios where earlier ARV therapy is indicated include young age, pregnancy, concurrent active TB or hepatitis B, and HIV-positive patients in serodiscordant relationships – i.e. with an

HIV-negative partner. Check local guidelines for eligibility to commence ARV therapy. In the presence of an opportunistic infection, guidelines tend to recommend starting ARV within 2 weeks, unless there is known to be evidence of cryptococcal or tuberculous meningitis.

3 The local public health board should be advised of the new diagnosis, and the patient informed that they will be contacted to initiate contact tracing. Contact tracing can be initiated by the patient if they wish to contact potential partners themselves, or can be performed by the public health jurisdiction with the aim of maintaining maximum confidentiality to the patient whilst still identifying and screening those at potential risk.

4 The patient should be advised of the potential for HIV transmission to others, and advised regarding avoiding risky behaviours such as needle sharing, unprotected sexual activities, and of recommendations to achieve adequate HIV control in pregnancy to reduce the risk of vertical transmission. Early HIV infection is associated with high infectivity due to the significant viral load. Depending on the location of the patient, specific legal responsibilities may exist with regards to informing sexual partners of HIV status, which usually exist if the patient has detectable viral load and has unprotected sexual intercourse.

5 Involvement of the multidisciplinary team is of significant importance. Individual patient needs may necessitate occupational therapy and physiotherapy input; social work input can be particularly useful, and the involvement of specialist HIV nurses invaluable to help patients engage and come to terms with their diagnosis. A dedicated HIV or infectious diseases pharmacist is important to identify the appropriate ARV regimen for the patient, identify potential interactions with other medications, and educate the patient on their particular medications. Input from psychologist or psychiatrist can be very helpful, and a number of peer support groups frequently offer peer support particularly around the time of diagnosis.

6 Immune reconstitution inflammatory syndrome (IRIS) occurs in a number of patients who commence ARV treatment. In the early time frame after commencing ARV therapy, there is immune restoration through a rapid rise in CD4 cell count, leading to a paradoxical reaction in response to subclinical infections. IRIS is usually seen in patients with AIDS who commence ARV, although *M. tuberculosis* may become unmasked even with CD4 counts with nadir >200 cells/µl. The main risk factor for developing IRIS is low CD4 count or high viral load. Management includes continuation of ARV therapy and treatment of the opportunistic infection, and in severe cases glucocorticoids may be used.

7 Medication compliance is essential. To facilitate this, the patient should be offered the regimen easiest for them to comply with. Resistance can occur rapidly, as the HIV virus multiplies rapidly and is prone to replication error, meaning mutations can occur quickly in the setting of even short periods of non-compliance. This can lead to treatment failure and the need to use more complex, more toxic ARV therapeutic regimens.

8 With the increasing efficacy of antiretrovirals, life expectancy is much better than previously expected; however, patients with HIV are at increased risk of a number of chronic comorbid conditions, thought to be due to chronic inflammation, in addition to effects from ARV medication. Patients should be screened for underlying and new cardiovascular disease, metabolic bone disease, malignancies, liver and renal dysfunction and cognitive deficits, and worked up as required.

9 Pre-exposure prophylaxis (PrEP) refers to the use of ARV in an HIV-negative person at high risk of contracting HIV, and has been shown to significantly reduce the risk of this. Individuals should be counselled about the benefits of PrEP, and educated about the need for excellent compliance, as well as the potential side-effects of these medications, in order to make an informed choice.

10 Post-exposure prophylaxis (PEP) may be considered for individuals who have had recent high risk exposure to HIV. Example scenarios include the healthcare worker who has had a needlestick injury from an HIV-positive patient with high viral load, and the individual who has had unprotected receptive anal sex with a partner either known to be HIV-positive with detectable viral load, or with unknown HIV status. PEP regimen will depend on local guidelines, patient preference, and whether drug resistance is known or suspected. PEP is usually given for 4 weeks, unless the source is subsequently confirmed to be HIV-negative.

CASE 44: Infective endocarditis

History

- A 58-year-old woman presents with a **six-week** [1] history of **lethargy, malaise, night sweats and a low-grade fever** [2].
- She reports mild breathlessness which has worsened over the past two weeks, but has **no neurological symptoms, and no joint or abdominal pains** [3].
- She is usually well but is under regular review by cardiology for a '**leaky heart valve**' [4] identified on echocardiography after a routine check-up picked up a cardiac murmur two years previously.
- The patient is not immunocompromised and does not have a **history of rheumatic fever, congenital heart disease or previous endocarditis** [5].

- She has had no **recent dental procedures** [6] or other **risk factors** [7] such as recent surgery, prosthetic cardiac valves, endovascular grafts, metalware and indwelling venous or urinary catheters.
- Her only medication is hormone replacement therapy and she has not had **any recent antibiotic treatment** [8].
- There is no history of **allergy** [9], and no history of **IV drug use or overseas travel, nor exposure to farms or abattoirs** [10].

[1] Onset of infective endocarditis can be widely variable, ranging from a rapid, aggressive illness with fulminant cardiac failure (acute endocarditis) to a more insidious onset with non-specific systemic symptoms, as in this case (subacute endocarditis). The timeline and urgency of presentation can be a clue to the underlying organism, with more aggressive organisms such as *Staphylococcus aureus* causing a rapid deterioration in symptoms, compared to the more insidious onset seen with other less aggressive organisms.

[2] Symptoms may also vary widely, although 90% of patients have a fever on presentation, often accompanied by systemic symptoms including weight and appetite loss and malaise. Fever of unknown origin is a common presentation of subacute bacterial endocarditis. Absence of fever is more common in the elderly, or after pretreatment with antibiotics. Cardiac murmurs are a common finding. Differential diagnosis should also include other causes of a prolonged fever, including TB, occult non-cardiac infections, haematological or solid organ malignancies and connective tissue disorders.

[3] It is important to identify complications of infective endocarditis, which occur due to valvular destruction, embolisation or seeding of infected material to distant sites. Breathlessness and peripheral swelling suggest a degree of valvular cardiac failure. Embolisation to the coronary arteries can occur, causing myocardial infarction. Neurological symptoms may occur due to septic emboli to the cerebral vasculature, causing focal neurology and mimicking a stroke. Abdominal pain may occur due to emboli to the spleen or renal vasculature; joint pain can suggest seeding with subsequent septic arthritis or osteomyelitis, and ischaemic

limb occurs from arterial occlusion. Mycotic aneurysms occur from infection which occurs at an arterial wall, often as a result of seeding from endocarditis, and can manifest as pulsatile swellings where an artery lies. The patient is at risk of intracranial haemorrhage if this occurs at cerebral arteries.

[4] Pre-existing valvular disease is a risk factor for infective endocarditis, and this history should increase the suspicion of infective endocarditis in the undifferentiated presentation.

[5] A history of rheumatic fever is also important to elicit, as rheumatic heart disease may be present but asymptomatic. Other risk factors include structural congenital heart disease, mitral valve prolapse, degenerative heart disease, hypertrophic cardiomyopathy and a past history of infective endocarditis.

[6] The patient may not report dental problems, but poor dentition and caries are risk factors for endocarditis with viridans streptococci, and the teeth should always be examined for caries, periodontitis and root abscesses. Recent dental procedures are also important to note. Referral for formal dental review is important if problems are identified, and a plan for treatment made to reduce risk of recurrence.

[7] Both bioprosthetic and mechanical cardiac valves (including transaortic valvular replacement) and intracardiac devices (pacemakers, implantable defibrillators, closure devices) constitute foreign material and therefore form a focus for organisms to adhere to during haematogenous travel. The presence of foreign material with endovascular grafts, metalware from joint replacement and indwelling urinary and venous catheters also pose risks.

Other non-cardiac risk factors include malignancy or instrumentation of the GI or genitourinary tracts, which can predispose to haematogenous translocation of organisms.

8 Recent antibiotic therapy is important to note, as this may have temporarily suppressed infection, masked symptoms and contributed towards organism resistance, and may make organism culture more difficult.

9 It is important to elicit allergy status, as treatment for infective endocarditis frequently requires prolonged courses of antibiotics. If an antibiotic allergy is elicited, the nature of this allergy or drug reaction should be explored in more detail, and if appropriate, antibiotic desensitisation should be considered to allow optimal treatment.

10 Social history will identify risk factors and potential exposures to specific organisms. Intravenous drug use is a significant risk factor due to the potential for direct inoculation of skin pathogens into the bloodstream, frequently under unclean conditions. Endocarditis associated with IV drug use is more frequently associated with tricuspid and pulmonary valve involvement than other precipitants, is often caused by *Staphylococcus aureus* and may be complicated by recurrent emboli to the lungs causing pulmonary abscesses. Travel and exposure history will help identify other potential causative organisms, for example Q fever caused by *Coxiella burnetii* from farm exposure, or brucellosis from abattoirs.

Examination

- The patient looks pale but is not breathless at rest. **Vital signs** [1] show pulse oximeter reading of 97% on air, regular pulse rate at 86bpm, respiratory rate of 18 breaths per minute and blood pressure of 128/78mmHg. She has a low grade fever of 38.1°C. Her weight is 68kg with a BMI of 22kg/m^2.
- **Examination of hands** [2] shows dry, cracked skin. Two splinter haemorrhages are seen in the proximal plate of her left fourth finger, but no other peripheral or ophthalmic **stigmata of infective endocarditis** [3] are seen. Examination of the mouth demonstrates dental caries but no mucosal petechiae.

- **Cardiac examination** [4] reveals a 3/6 pansystolic murmur, loudest at the apex and radiating to the axilla. Heart sounds are regular and pulse is of normal character. There are no signs of cardiac failure with clear chest to auscultation, normal JVP and no peripheral oedema.
- **Targeted examination** [5] shows no neurological deficits and soft and non-tender abdomen. Palpation of joints, including percussion of the vertebrae, is not painful.

1 Initial assessment should identify whether the patient is haemodynamically stable or not. Acute endocarditis with severe valvular dysfunction or sepsis can cause significant haemodynamic instability and necessitates urgent intervention with source control and valvular surgery.

2 Examination of the skin, particularly the hands and feet, can identify sources of pathogen entry. If intravenous drug use is suspected, needle track marks may be seen around injecting sites and infected veins may be seen with evidence of overlying thrombophlebitis and hardened vessels to palpation.

3 Immunological phenomena include splinter haemorrhages on hand and foot nails, Osler nodes, Roth spots and glomerulonephritis. Splinter haemorrhages may occur due to nail trauma but are more likely to be distal, therefore linear haemorrhages seen more proximally close to the nail bed are more suspicious for infective endocarditis. Osler nodes are tender, reddish-purple lumps found on the digits. Roth spots are retinal haemorrhages, usually with a pale centre, seen on fundoscopy. These phenomena are more likely to occur in subacute endocarditis than acute, due to the length of time until the patient presents. Embolic

phenomena occur in about 30% of patients, and produce symptoms and signs dependent on the site that they embolise to. Petechiae may be seen in the oral or conjunctival mucosa. Janeway lesions are painless ecchymoses on the palms and soles. It is important to regularly examine for evidence of new emboli until the infection is under control, and new neurological deficits, abdominal pain or joint pain should be investigated thoroughly with a high index of suspicion.

4 Cardiac examination frequently reveals a murmur, and in this case the features are suggestive of mitral regurgitation with a pansystolic murmur loudest at the apex. Complications of severe mitral regurgitation should be identified and may include atrial fibrillation and signs of cardiac failure such as dullness to percussion and reduced breath sounds at the lung bases from pleural effusion, pulmonary crepitations, raised JVP and peripheral pitting oedema.

5 Examination should include assessment for embolic complications of infective endocarditis, including neurological deficits from cerebral emboli, splenomegaly, left upper quadrant pain or flank pain from splenic or renal infarction, and features of ischaemic limb such as being cold and painful to touch, pale or purple, and pulseless. Vertebral osteomyelitis from haematogenous seeding should be examined for by percussing down the vertebrae to elicit

tenderness. If present, this should prompt further imaging to evaluate.

Investigations

- **Blood tests** [1] show a mild leucocytosis and microcytic anaemia on full blood count, with a moderately raised CRP and ESR.
- Liver and renal function are normal. **Urinalysis** [2] is normal.
- Three sets of **blood cultures** [3] are obtained with aseptic technique, at 6-hour intervals, prior to antibiotic therapy, which are all positive for *Streptococcus mitis* [4] sensitive to penicillin.
- **Serology** [5] for *Coxiella burnetii* and *Bartonella* is not performed.

- An **electrocardiogram** [6] demonstrates normal sinus rhythm without conduction disturbance.
- **Transthoracic echocardiography** [7] reveals stable, moderate mitral regurgitation without evidence of vegetations. A transoesophageal echo identifies a small vegetation on the mitral valve.
- **Duke criteria** [8] are fulfilled with two major criteria and three minor criteria.

[1] Blood tests are generally non-specific but may show anaemia and raised inflammatory markers of raised leucocytes, CRP and ESR. Renal and hepatic dysfunction can occur as a complication of infective endocarditis. Glomerulonephritis is commonly associated with endocarditis.

[2] Microscopic haematuria may identify glomerulonephritis, seen by the presence of blood on dipstick. If present, a sample of urine should be sent for phase-contrast microscopy and checked for presence of proteins. Active urinary sediment may be seen with immune complex glomerulonephritis, causing the presence of dysmorphic red cells and red cell casts.

[3] Blood cultures should be obtained prior to starting antibiotic therapy to maximise yield, using an aseptic technique to reduce the risk of skin contaminants and false positive cultures. Especially in the setting of subacute bacterial endocarditis, increased sampling of blood for culture increases the likelihood of identifying the causative organism, as there tends to be a continuous low density bacteraemia. If the patient is severely septic or unstable, empirical therapy should not be delayed after obtaining at least two initial sets of blood cultures, but in the stable patient with subacute presentation, maximising yield before antibiotic therapy is beneficial.

[4] The most common causative organisms are *S. aureus* and *Streptococcus viridans*. *S. mitis* is in viridans groups of streptococci. Other viridans groups include *S. anginosus/S. constellatus/S. intermedius* group, *S. sanguinis* group, *S. mutans* group and *S. salivarius* group. Injecting drug users are at higher risk of *S. aureus* as a cause, whereas endocarditis in patients with prosthetic valve involvement may be caused by coagulase-negative staphylococci such as *S. epidermidis*. Isolation of *Streptococcus gallolyticus* suggests seeding from

the GI tract and should raise concerns for bowel malignancy; likewise, enterococcal endocarditis can occur due to genitourinary disorders. Culture-negative endocarditis can occur due to pretreatment with antibiotics, insufficient blood culture sampling, or because of the nature of the causative organism. The 'HACEK' organisms are fastidious organisms accounting for about 5% of endocarditis, requiring prolonged culture, and include *Haemophilus* spp., *Actinobacillus*, *Cardiobacterium*, *Eikenella* and *Kingella kingae*.

[5] A number of other organisms may require serology for diagnosis, including *Coxiella*, the causative agent of Q fever, *Bartonella* (from cats and dogs), and in at-risk patients, *Brucella*. Fungal endocarditis, especially with *Candida* spp., may not be cultured easily and requires an index of suspicion in immunocompromised patients or those with long-term IV access.

[6] Electrocardiography can identify complications of endocarditis, such as atrial fibrillation as a complication from mitral regurgitation, and conduction disturbances such as prolongation of the PR interval, or higher degrees of heart block, that can raise the suspicion of endomyocardial infection or abscess involving the sinoatrial node, as may be seen with aortic root abscess. A normal ECG does not exclude endomyocardial complications.

[7] Echocardiography is recommended urgently in all patients with clinical suspicion of infective endocarditis; within 24 hours if possible. This includes patients with bacteraemia with a suspect organism such as *S. aureus* or *Candida* spp. If echocardiography is negative, but suspicion remains high 7–10 days later, this should be repeated. If previous valvular dysfunction is known, an assessment as to whether this has worsened is essential. Sensitivity of transthoracic echocardiography (TTE) ranges from 70–80%, with transoesophageal echocardiography 90–100%. Current

recommendations are for transthoracic echo as first-line, then proceed to transoesophageal echo if TTE is negative but there is high suspicion, or if TTE is of poor quality or positive. If a vegetation is seen, this confirms endocarditis. A vegetation consists of a collection of fibrin, platelets and small colonies of the microorganism.

8 Modified Duke criteria helps with diagnosis of infective endocarditis: clinical diagnosis requires the presence of two major, one major and two minor, or five minor criteria. Major criteria are met if there is:
- ≥2 positive blood cultures with a likely organism, and
- evidence of endocardial involvement on echocardiogram.

Minor criteria include fever >38.0°C; predisposing cardiac condition or IV drug use; immunological phenomena; positive blood culture, serology or echocardiography not fulfilling major criteria; RNA analysis.

Management

Short-term

The patient is diagnosed with **native valve endocarditis** [1]. Empirical **IV antibiotic therapy** [2] is commenced, and then rationalised to a penicillin-based regimen after the blood cultures demonstrate a susceptible organism. A **peripherally inserted central catheter** [3] is inserted for longer-term antibiotic therapy once treatment is established and the patient is stable. The patient is reviewed by a **multidisciplinary team** [4] inclusive of Cardiology, Infectious Diseases and Cardiothoracic specialists, with the decision taken for conservative management with antimicrobial therapy. She is examined daily for new **complications of infective endocarditis** [5] and valvular deterioration, but remains stable. **Dental review** [6] is performed and orthodontic treatment implemented for dental caries. **Prophylaxis for venous thromboembolism** [7] is given.

An assessment of suitability for **home-based antimicrobial therapy** [8] is made, including input from the MDT: physiotherapy, occupational therapy and dietitian. Blood tests are performed for the duration of therapy and the patient undergoes **weekly medical review** [9].

Long-term

The patient is educated on ways to minimise a further episode of infective endocarditis, and on symptoms that should prompt early review. The patient is advised to discuss **antimicrobial prophylaxis** [10] with her healthcare providers for planned procedures in case this is required. The patient is advised regarding long-term cardiology follow-up with regular echocardiography to monitor for worsening valvular function, and for early cardiothoracic referral if required.

1 Infective endocarditis carries a high mortality if untreated; therefore treatment is essential. Native valve endocarditis describes endocarditis affecting the patient's original heart valves, compared with prosthetic valve endocarditis (PVE) which affects bioprosthetic or mechanical heart valves. Treatment of these differs, as the presence of foreign material with PVE makes source control much more difficult. Expert opinion should be sought at an early stage with PVE.

2 Empirical antibiotic therapy should be commenced, taking into account local and regional microbiology and guidelines, but usually directed against *S. aureus* and viridans streptococci. Once the causative organism is identified, targeted antibiotic therapy should be commenced. The regimen and duration of treatment is dependent on the organism, as well as left- or right-sided involvement of the heart, but it is usually given for 4–6 weeks. There are high quality guidelines to help guide treatment. Glycopeptides and aminoglycosides may form part of antibiotic treatment; care should be taken to monitor therapeutic drug levels. Complications of therapy, including with baseline and serial

audiology assessments and renal function, should also be monitored. Antibiotic toxicities and allergies are common, occurring in up to 40% of patients, and may occur after several weeks of treatment; a high index of suspicion should be maintained.

3 As the patient frequently receives multiple doses of antibiotics per day, for several weeks, establishing good vascular access is essential. The insertion of a peripherally inserted central catheter (PICC) can provide more reliable access, as it remains in for longer, and can be placed in a location that reduces the chance of accidental removal. As the catheter also constitutes foreign material, it is important to time insertion at a point when the infection is under control so that further haematogenous seeding to the catheter is unlikely to occur. Other complications of PICCs include local infection at the site of insertion and venous thrombosis.

4 Endocarditis requires a multispecialty approach, with Cardiology and Infectious disease specialists involved at a minimum to establish the best approach. Surgical input is important to gauge whether surgery or conservative therapy is most appropriate. Other complications will require the involvement of other specialties depending on the specific pathology, such as Neurology, Vascular surgery, Neurosurgery and Orthopaedics.

5 A number of situations may prompt the need for surgery in order to control disease and limit complications. Early surgery in serious disease gives a greater chance of survival. Indications include large size of vegetations, endocardial abscess or paravalvular involvement, cardiac failure due to valvular incompetence, recurrent embolism, and endocarditis not otherwise responding to treatment such as persistent bacteraemia (>7 days). Careful serial assessment and liaison with Cardiothoracic specialists is essential to time surgery. Intra-operatively, tissue should be sent for Gram stain and culture, with enough sample stored for additional analysis if identifying the organism is proving difficult.

6 The opportunity should be taken whilst the patient is in hospital to address potential sources of infection; particularly with regard to dental and skin care. In the setting of an organism that hints at underlying malignancy (e.g. *S. gallolyticus*), appropriate investigations should also be organised, such as colonoscopy or CT imaging.

7 Venous thromboembolism prophylaxis is important to consider, as patients are frequently less mobile with an inflammatory process. In the patient who is likely to undergo cardiothoracic surgery, it is important to liaise closely if the patient is on any anticoagulants, particularly longer-acting ones at therapeutic doses, as this may delay urgent surgery. VTE prophylaxis should be judiciously administered in those with mycotic aneurysms identified.

8 In patients who are clinically stable, with established therapy and who are compliant with treatment, outpatient antibiotic therapy can be considered. Assessment by physiotherapy, occupational therapy and social work can identify any potential issues. Outpatient therapy then requires liaison between pharmacy staff to provide antibiotics, nursing staff to administer at home or in a daily clinic, and medical staff to perform regular reviews. Using this approach provides patient autonomy and reduces economic cost of care for these patients who require prolonged therapy.

9 Blood tests should be performed regularly, usually weekly, to monitor for antibiotic toxicity. This can manifest as cytopenias and renal or hepatic impairment, and if detected, should prompt review of antibiotic therapy and a decision made about continuation or switching therapy. Blood cultures should be performed daily in cases of *S. aureus* endocarditis until sterile, i.e. no organisms are grown; they should also be performed if a further fever occurs, and at 4–6 weeks following completion of therapy to document that the episode has been cured, or to identify ongoing infection.

10 The patient is at increased risk of a further episode of endocarditis, and should be advised regarding ways to reduce her risk, including dental and skin care. Knowing the symptoms and presenting early can also improve outcomes in recurrent cases. Antibiotic prophylaxis is recommended for high risk dental procedures involving manipulation of the gingival tissue, periapical region of the teeth, or with perforation of the oral mucosa: in high risk patients such as those with recurrent endocarditis, or those with prosthetic valves, grafts or closure devices. The patient should be encouraged to notify healthcare providers of their history of endocarditis to ensure prophylaxis is discussed in accordance with up-to-date guidelines.

CASE 45: Malaria

History

- A 25-year-old medical student presents **10 days after returning** [1] from a 3-month elective trip to **rural Tanzania** [2].
- She reports a week of **fevers and rigors** [3] associated with lethargy, confusion and breathlessness.
- Her **past medical history** [4] is unremarkable, and she is not immunocompromised or pregnant.
- Her **medications** [5] include antimalarial prophylaxis, which she reports inadequate adherence with, as well as oral contraceptive pills. She has no allergies. She reports minimal alcohol use and is a non-smoker.

- She sought **travel advice** [6] and received all recommended vaccinations including hepatitis A, typhoid, measles and influenza vaccinations.
- **During her travels** [7] she stayed in rural villages and ate carefully, cooking all food and boiling water. She did not consume unpasteurised dairy products or uncooked meat. She had no specific farm contact but was exposed to domestic animals and birds, and sustained mosquito bites despite taking precautions including using mosquito nets at night. She did not engage in high risk sexual activities, intravenous drug use or tattooing.

1 The incubation period for malaria is usually around 2 weeks from inoculation by an infected *Anopheles* mosquito, but can be longer. These sporozoites travel to the liver rapidly, later emerging into the bloodstream to infect red blood cells and causing symptoms as the erythrocytes rupture. The incubation period may be longer in patients who have been taking antimalarials incompletely for prophylaxis, and in those with a degree of immunity from prior malaria exposure. It is therefore important to consider malaria as a cause for fever in a returned traveller for up to a year after return from an endemic region.

2 Malaria occurs in tropical regions, where the *Anopheles* mosquito which carries the malaria parasite lives, with the majority of malaria occurring on the African continent. There are five main species; *Plasmodium falciparum, P. vivax, P. ovale, P. malariae* and *P. knowlesi*. Falciparum malaria is mostly found in sub-Saharan Africa and accounts for most cases and deaths. *P. vivax* is the next most prevalent, particularly outside of Africa, but *P. knowlesi*, increasingly seen in areas of Southeast Asia, is also of importance. It is important to check the known epidemiology of all regions travelled to.

3 The symptoms of malaria range from fever and chills, to lethargy, nausea, vomiting, diarrhoea, joint and muscle aches, headaches and coughing. Severe malaria can occur with all species, but predominantly with *P. falciparum*, and is diagnosed with any of the following complications: severe anaemia, renal impairment, severe jaundice, bleeding, reduced conscious level, seizures, severe weakness, pulmonary oedema with hypoxia, hypoglycaemia, acidosis or shock. A parasite load of >2–5% in the blood is generally

classified as severe malaria. Uncomplicated malaria occurs at lower levels of parasite load, without accompanying clinical complications of severe malaria.

4 Groups who are at increased risk of malaria include pregnant women, as well as those who are visiting friends and relatives (VFR). The latter group often have had immunity to malaria through previous exposure in their native countries, which then wanes on spending time away from endemic areas. They therefore are at increased risk of severe disease upon return to their native country, as frequently they fail to take adequate precautions or prophylactic medications. Children are also at increased risk of severe infection. The presence of other medical conditions can worsen outcomes, particularly if there is underlying cardiac, renal or hepatic dysfunction. Patients with immune deficiency, such as HIV and asplenia, are at increased risk of severe disease, and along with all patients with underlying health conditions should be counselled to travel with a copy of their health record, sufficient supplies of medication, travel insurance, and a knowledge of how to access local medical services when travelling.

5 A medication history should include all prescribed medications, including compliance to these, in addition to those bought over the counter and including herbal remedies, which may interact with prescribed medications to reduce efficacy or increase toxicity. Antimalarial compliance should be carefully assessed, as these should be started prior to travel, continued diligently during exposure in endemic areas, and depending on the antimalarial, continued for a specific period of time after leaving the area. Intolerance and severe side-effects often lead to discontinuation of malarial prophylaxis. An allergy history is important to evaluate, to assist with subsequent treatment choice.

6 It is recommended that all travellers undergo travel consultation to advise on potential health risks, and undertake strategies to minimise these. Advice will take into account the geographical area, planned duration of travel, individual traveller risks, and potential exposures such as time spent in rural areas with inadequate sanitation and accommodation. Strategies include pre-travel vaccination, discussion about ways to minimise risk including hand and food hygiene, avoidance of outdoor exposure at dawn and dusk when the *Anopheles* mosquito feeds, use of mosquito nets and appropriate clothing, and prophylactic medications. Antimalarials are important to consider in malarial regions, and a choice made based on traveller risk for particular side-effects, as well as local antimalarial resistance patterns.

It is essential to educate the traveller on the importance of medication compliance, but also that it is impossible to eliminate all risk, and therefore travellers should be educated on which symptoms are warning signs that should prompt urgent medical attention.

7 A thorough travel history is essential in the febrile returned traveller, to identify risk of exposure to specific organisms from particular risky activities, and using a timeline to identify likely incubation periods. This should include history of exposure to running and stagnant water (e.g. malaria from mosquito colonies around stagnant water), exposure to undercooked or potentially contaminated food (e.g. hepatitis A, *Campylobacter*, *Escherichia coli*, *Shigella*), to wildlife or unpasteurised foods (e.g. brucellosis), and high risk sexual activity or potential for injection of contaminated blood (e.g. viral hepatitis, HIV).

Examination

- On examination, the patient is **febrile** [1] at 40.2°C, tachycardic at 104bpm and tachypnoeic at 28 breaths/minute, with blood pressure of 80/64mmHg. Peripheral oxygen saturations are normal.
- She looks **unwell** [2], with cool peripheries and delayed capillary refill time of 4 seconds.
- She has **pale conjunctivae** [3] and slightly **yellow sclera** [4].
- She is **oriented** [5] to time and place, and has not witnessed seizure activity nor focal neurological deficits.
- There are no **rashes, petechiae, mucosal bleeding or features of thrombosis** [6].
- **Cardiorespiratory examination** [7] is otherwise normal.
- Abdominal examination reveals **splenomegaly** [8].

1 Fever is common, and can occur cyclically depending on the life cycle of the parasite, with *P. knowlesi* every 24 hours, *P. falciparum*, *P. ovale* and *P. vivax* every 2 days, and *P. malariae* every 3 days. Non-immune patients, those who have had multiple inoculations, and those early on in their infection are more likely to have daily or irregularly spaced fevers. In the non-immune, fevers can be very high and can occur alongside tachycardia, and in children febrile convulsions may occur. It is important to consider other causes for fever, particularly if parasite load is low, as this suggests a concurrent infection. Of note, hypothermia may occur if the patient is profoundly shocked.

2 Patients with severe malaria can deteriorate rapidly, and early signs should be identified and responded to. Shock can manifest with impaired perfusion and hypotension, and may progress rapidly to organ dysfunction. A capillary refill time >3 seconds suggests early evidence of shock, and in conjunction with cool peripheries and a systolic blood pressure of <80mmHg should prompt rapid escalation of care and commencement of IV antimalarial therapy.

3 Pale conjunctivae are a feature of anaemia. In those who live in areas where malaria is endemic, it is usually multifactorial and can be a chronic finding, particularly in

children. In those who have not had prior exposure to malaria, acute anaemia may occur. This is predominantly caused by haemolysis and destruction of erythrocytes due to the malarial illness. The type of malaria impacts on the likelihood of developing severe anaemia: *P. falciparum* affects all stages of erythrocytes and multiplies rapidly, therefore has the highest propensity to causing severe anaemia. *P. vivax* and *P. ovale* affect reticulocytes only, whilst *P. malariae* affects all erythrocytes but multiplies at low levels, therefore these malarial types are much less likely to cause severe anaemia.

4 Jaundice can occur in both uncomplicated and complicated falciparum malaria. Mild jaundice is reasonably common, occurring due to haemolysis. Severe jaundice can occur due to a combination of haemolysis as well as direct liver injury from hepatocyte damage and cholestasis, and represents a poorer prognosis.

5 The patient should be examined carefully for features of cerebral malaria, including disorientation, reduced conscious state and seizure activity. Focal neurological deficits may occur rarely, such as hemiplegia, ataxia and aphasia. Neuro-ophthalmic signs, including nystagmus and gaze deviation, may also be present in a small number of cases. Cerebral manifestations are more likely to occur in children, pregnant women, the elderly, and in those with specific conditions such as HIV, asplenia and malnutrition. Cerebral malaria requires urgent treatment, with very high mortality rates if left untreated.

6 Rash is not a common feature of malaria, and if present should be characterised to assist with finding an underlying cause. Coagulopathy may occur in patients with severe falciparum malaria, with a small proportion developing disseminated intravascular coagulation (DIC). Petechial rash can occur in the presence of thrombocytopenia and DIC, and may be accompanied by mucosal bleeding, and oozing at sites of trauma such as cannulation or catheterisation. Thrombosis is another complication of DIC. Alternative pathologies such as meningococcal meningitis, dengue fever,

typhoid fever, measles and viral haemorrhagic fevers should be considered in the febrile returned traveller with rash.

7 Examination of the cardiac and respiratory systems may reveal complications associated with severe malaria, as well as identify features suggestive of concurrent infections in the returned traveller. Non-cardiogenic pulmonary oedema can occur in both uncomplicated and severe malaria, with uncertain pathogenesis, manifested as widespread crepitations. Focal crepitations are more suggestive of a concurrent pneumonia and should prompt investigation for this.

8 Splenomegaly is common in patients with acute malaria, in addition to those who live in endemic areas. In a setting of multiple episodes of malaria, the spleen may then become small due to infarcts during illness.

Investigations

- **Blood tests** [1] are performed: a full blood examination shows a low haemoglobin of 105, mild thrombocytopenia at 115 but is otherwise normal. Renal function and electrolytes are normal. Liver function tests demonstrate a bilirubin of 48µmol/L but is otherwise normal. Coagulation testing is normal.
- **Glucose level** [2] is low at 2.1mmol/L.
- An arterial **blood gas** [3] is performed which shows normal oxygenation and a slightly raised lactate of 2.2mmol/L with a mild concurrent acidosis.
- **Urinalysis** [4] is unremarkable.

- **Blood microscopy** [5] is performed, and demonstrates malaria parasites.
- Malaria **antigen test** [6] is positive.
- **Concurrent tests** [7] including blood cultures, urine cultures, dengue serology, influenza and hepatitis are sent, and are all negative.
- A **chest X-ray** [8] is normal.
- **Lumbar puncture** [9] and other neurological investigations are not performed.
- An electrocardiogram shows normal sinus rhythm with no prolongation of the QT interval. A screening test demonstrates no evidence of **G6PD deficiency** [10].

1 FBE often shows mild anaemia, although haemoglobin can be particularly low in severe falciparum malaria. Thrombocytopenia is often present and whilst usually mild, can also be severe, predisposing to bleeding. White cells are frequently within the normal range, and if raised should prompt review for alternative sources of infection. Renal function is frequently impaired in patients who have severe malaria, caused by hypovolaemia, haemolysis and erythrocyte sequestration affecting blood flow to the kidneys. Bilirubin may be raised due to haemolysis and high levels indicate severe malaria. Coagulation testing may show evidence of DIC with low fibrinogen and abnormal clotting profile.

2 Hypoglycaemia is common in severe malaria, and is associated with worse outcomes. It occurs due to increased consumption of glucose, alongside inhibited gluconeogenesis. It can also occur due to the use of IV quinine, during the treatment of malaria.

3 A blood gas can provide useful information, including an accurate representation of oxygen levels in the patient with hypoxia from acute respiratory distress syndrome. An

assessment of acid–base balance is also extremely useful, with the presence of severe acidosis prognosticating poorer outcomes. Acidosis can occur due to the presence of lactate production from circulatory insufficiency or microvascular occlusion.

4 Urine microscopy is routinely performed in specimens sent for culture. Severe malaria can be complicated by intravascular haemolysis, causing dark-coloured urine as a result of the presence of pigments from haemoglobin. This can manifest as a positive urine dipstick for the presence of blood, but the absence of red blood cells on microscopic analysis. 'Blackwater fever' is a syndrome caused by significant intravascular haemolysis with very dark urine, and is associated with renal failure and DIC.

5 Blood samples should be sent for examination in an experienced laboratory, using light microscopy to look at Giemsa-stained blood smears. This can allow for identification of the malaria parasite and the level of parasitaemia density calculated, although lower levels of parasites make diagnosis harder. A thick film lyses erythrocytes, so parasites are visualised independently, and aids with identification of the presence of malaria parasites. A thin film keeps red blood cells intact, allowing easier identification of the species. A single negative thick/thin film is insufficient to exclude malaria, and at least three are recommended, more if the diagnosis of malaria is highly suspected.

6 Rapid diagnostic tests can be helpful, particularly in areas where access to experienced laboratories is limited. Antigen tests can help identify if malaria is present, but are most sensitive at identifying *P. falciparum*; therefore a negative test does not exclude malaria, particularly if another species is epidemiologically more likely.

7 Differential diagnoses are important to consider, particularly in the febrile returned traveller, based on epidemiological risk factors. Investigations should include common infections such as influenza, pneumonia and urinary tract infections, but also other vector-borne diseases such as dengue, chikungunya and Zika virus. Serology for HIV and viral hepatitis should be considered, as well as rare infections such as leptospirosis, particularly in the presence of renal failure and jaundice. Blood cultures should be performed to look for alternative, or concurrent bacteraemia, including typhoid fever. If haemorrhagic features are present in the skin

and mucous membranes, consider viral haemorrhagic fevers in the patient who has travelled to at-risk areas.

8 A chest X-ray is useful to provide a baseline, and to identify features suggestive of acute respiratory distress syndrome. These tend to show diffuse, non-specific, widespread opacities. X-ray may also identify patients with superimposed or concurrent bacterial lung infections, to help direct additional therapy.

9 Analysis of the CSF may be useful if there are features suggestive of cerebral malaria. Opening pressure and CSF analysis are often normal; however, there may be slightly raised protein and cell count and slightly low glucose levels. This test is most useful to evaluate differential diagnoses of viral encephalitis. Imaging with CT may show evidence of oedema or watershed infarcts, and EEG usually shows non-specific abnormalities.

10 Patients with glucose-6-phosphate dehydrogenase (G6PD) deficiency are at risk of severe haemolysis if treated with primaquine and tafenoquine. This may form a part of treatment of relapsing malaria species (*P. vivax* and *P. ovale*), in addition in some scenarios to reduce transmission of *P. falciparum*, and screening should be performed if there is a likelihood of needing to use primaquine.

Management

Short-term

Resuscitate[1] the patient as required, in an appropriate setting with assistance from Intensive Care. Commence **antimalarial therapy**[2] and **monitor**[3] blood pressure and glucose, and perform cardiac monitoring when using IV antimalarial therapy. Consider whether **adjunctive therapy**[4] is required. Directed therapy may be required for specific **complications of malaria**[5]. Careful consideration should be given to **risk of venous thromboembolism**[6]. In patients with severe complications, **early involvement of appropriate specialist teams and the multidisciplinary team**[7] is essential to aid longer-term recovery.

Long-term

After immediate management, assess whether treatment is required to prevent **malaria relapse**[8]. **Biochemical and parasitaemic recovery**[9] of patients with severe malaria should be assessed. Patients who have been critically unwell may benefit from rehabilitation. In the patient with cerebral malaria, assess for **neurological sequelae**[10] and provide appropriate support. **Public health notification**[11] may be required, depending on jurisdiction. **Opportunistic travel advice**[12] should be provided.

1 In the patient with shock, hypoxia, reduced consciousness or other evidence of organ dysfunction, resuscitation using basic principles should be initiated. Urgent glucose replacement should be given in the setting of severe hypoglycaemia, and IV fluids to address hypovolaemic hypotension. Early involvement of the Intensive Care team is essential, to provide inotropic and ventilator support if required, as well as the high intensity of monitoring required for patients with severe malaria, whose mortality risk is highest in the first 24 hours of presentation.

2 Antimalarial therapy should be started urgently in the presence of severe malaria and cerebral malaria. The treatment of choice for severe or cerebral malaria is parenteral artemisin or quinine, including in pregnant women in any trimester. However, Infectious diseases specialist advice should be sought, to identify whether the patient is likely to be at risk of resistant malaria acquisition, based on the geographical area. In patients with uncomplicated malaria, and with severe malaria once clinically stable, switch to oral antimalarials for the remainder of therapy.

3 Patients treated with IV quinine are at risk of hypoglycaemia due to quinine stimulating secretion of insulin. Cardiac monitoring may be required in patients at risk of developing prolonged QT interval, with subsequent risk of arrhythmias. It is important to liaise closely with an experienced pharmacist to identify potential interactions and toxicities, particularly in patients with comorbidities who are on other medications and in those receiving adjunctive therapy.

4 Adjunctive therapy should be considered in cases of severe malaria. IV broad-spectrum antibiotics should be commenced to cover for concomitant bacteraemia. Paracetamol can help with symptomatic fever and pain.

5 Directed therapy may be required, including blood transfusion in patients with severe anaemia, blood products if required to treat severe bleeding associated with thrombocytopenia or DIC, benzodiazepines to treat seizures associated with cerebral malaria, and renal replacement therapy in the setting of significant renal impairment.

6 All patients who are hospitalised with malaria should be considered for prophylaxis against VTE, due to increased risk associated with immobility, inflammatory state and, frequently, recent travel. In patients with DIC, there is a risk of both bleeding and thrombosis, and discussion with Haematology specialists is recommended to provide individualised recommendations.

7 Infectious disease specialists should be consulted from admission in the patient suspected of having malaria. Depending on the severity of disease and the nature of complications, additional input may be required, particularly from Intensivists, Haematology and Renal specialists. Input from the MDT is essential, in particular pharmacists, but also for severely unwell patients, early rehabilitation with physiotherapy, occupational therapy and dietitian involvement is of benefit.

8 *P. ovale* and *P. vivax* have a dormant phase in the malaria parasite life cycle, meaning they have the potential to relapse months later when these hypnozoites reactivate. This phase is absent in the *P. falciparum*, *P. knowlesi* and *P. malariae* life cycles, therefore relapse is not a problem. Relapsing species should receive additional treatment with primaquine or tafenoquine to kill the dormant parasites.

9 Patients should have their parasite count monitored twice a day until clinically stable, then daily until the parasite counts are negative. In severe malaria, it is recommended to check FBE and microscopy for malaria at weekly intervals for four weeks after completion of oral therapy, to check for recrudescence of parasites as well as delayed haemolysis from artemisin use.

10 Those with malaria complicated by cerebral manifestations should be evaluated for longer-term neurological sequelae, including focal neurological deficits, impaired hearing and cognition, and epilepsy. Rarely, cerebral malaria can be followed by an autoimmune encephalitis that is steroid-responsive. Affected patients should be assessed for requirement and eligibility for neurorehabilitation, and should be linked in with an appropriate healthcare provider for long-term follow-up. It is important to evaluate the impact of chronic consequences on the patient's mental status, and offer appropriate psychological and psychiatric help, if required.

11 Malaria is generally notifiable to local public health authorities, who may elect to contact members of the travel party who may also have been exposed to mosquito bites, to advise on symptoms of malaria. In non-endemic areas, where the *Anopheles* mosquito is unable to survive, transmission to other people is not an issue.

12 It is important to provide the patient with pre-emptive travel advice on how to protect themself on return to malarial areas, particularly in those who are visiting friends and relatives and those who have had previous exposure and therefore prior immunity. In particular, advice on methods to avoid mosquito bites is important, as well as encouragement to seek travel advice. Other specific advice may be warranted; for example, for the patient who regularly donates blood, there are frequent restrictions, and the patient should be directed to seek advice from official blood collection centres.

CASE 46: Meningoencephalitis

History

- A **34-year-old** [1] woman presents with a **12-hour history** [2] of a **severe, generalised headache with confusion and lethargy** [3] but no history of rash, seizures or arthritis.
- **Past medical history** [4] includes previous splenectomy after a car accident, but she has no history of diabetes or immunosuppression, and she takes no regular medications.
- There is **no past history of previous meningitis** [5], **no history of acute or recurrent herpes simplex virus (HSV) 1 and 2 ulcers** [6], and no history of **neurosurgical devices nor sinusitis** [7].
- The patient is an ex-smoker but reports alcohol intake of up to ten units per day. There is no **history of recent travel, exposure to rivers or lakes, nor a history of exposure to ill people** [8].
- The patient does not report **allergies** [9] and reports receiving the **Haemophilus influenzae, meningococcal and pneumococcal vaccinations** [10] within the past 5 years.

[1] The epidemiological features of meningoencephalitis vary depending on the organism. *Neisseria meningitidis, Streptococcus pneumoniae* (the most common bacterial cause in adults), *Staphylococcus aureus* and coagulase-negative *Staphylococcus* may cause meningoencephalitis at any age, whereas older adults and neonates are more susceptible to *Listeria monocytogenes* and Gram-negative bacilli infections. *Haemophilus influenzae* type B is now much less likely to be seen in the young due to good vaccination coverage, but should be considered in adults presenting with meningoencephalitis. Healthcare-associated bacterial meningitis tends to be caused by *Staphylococcus* and Gram-negative bacilli, especially following invasive neurosurgical procedures. The most common cause of encephalitis is herpes simplex virus, but other pathogens should be considered based on recent travel and immune status.

[2] Patients with bacterial meningitis tend to present soon after symptom onset, usually within 24 hours, and are generally quite unwell at presentation. Subacute presentation may occur with particular organisms such as *Cryptococcus gattii, C. neoformans* and tuberculous meningitis. These presentations may occur in uncontrolled or undiagnosed HIV-infected patients.

[3] Fever, neck stiffness or nuchal rigidity, and change in mental state are the classical features of bacterial meningitis, although <50% present with all three features. Fever is present in almost all patients. Headache is a frequent symptom and is usually severe; altered mental status is present in >75% of patients and can range from lethargy to coma. Photophobia, nausea and vomiting are common. Seizures and focal neurologic deficits can occur, particularly with *Listeria* meningitis, whereas a petechial non-blanching rash or arthritis may occur with *N. meningitidis*. Encephalitis is characterised by fever and neurological symptoms and signs, rather than signs of nuchal rigidity.

[4] Past medical history can identify risk factors for developing meningoencephalitis. Asplenia increases the risk of infection with encapsulated organisms such as *S. pneumoniae, H. influenzae* and *N. meningitidis*. Immunocompromised states also increase the risk, including HIV, steroid use, diabetes mellitus, post-transplant states on immunosuppressive therapies, pregnancy, alcoholism, injecting drug use, and malignancy.

[5] A history of recurrent bacterial meningitis occurs most commonly in patients who have a condition that breaches the meninges, such as middle ear disease or skull fractures. Recurrent severe invasive bacterial infections should also prompt a search for underlying immune deficiencies, such as terminal complement deficiency.

[6] Herpes simplex virus-1 (HSV-1) is estimated to infect two-thirds of the world's population, as chronic infection follows acute infection, and the virus becomes latent within neural ganglia. Reactivation may occur and cause a number of presentations, including most commonly oral, ocular and genital ulceration, and less commonly encephalitis, meningitis and severe organ disorders. A fine balance between host immunity and pathogen virulence means that immunocompromised hosts are more likely to experience reactivation, but immune-competent hosts are also at risk for intermittent reactivation of the infection. Although primary HSV-1 infection is most likely to cause systemic infection, recurrent ulcers can suggest a viral rather than bacterial aetiology for presentation with meningoencephalitis, and aciclovir should be commenced. HSV-2 is most likely to cause recurrent genital ulceration, and can also cause recurrent

episodes of meningitis, also known as Mollaret's meningitis. Overall, HSV encephalitis has high rates of morbidity and mortality.

7 Neurosurgical devices (e.g. shunts, deep brain stimulators or external ventricular drains) provide a direct portal of entry for organisms into the central nervous system, as do local infections of the sinuses, middle ear and mastoids, or in the event of trauma. Other portals of entry include nasopharyngeal colonisation causing bloodstream infection, or other sources of bacteraemia such as endocarditis, which then result in invasion of the CNS.

8 Potential exposures should be sought to assist with identifying the most appropriate tests for diagnosis of the underlying organism, such as exposure to current outbreaks or individuals known to have an active infection. In addition, travel to areas with endemicity for *N. meningitidis* (e.g. sub-Saharan African countries) is important to clarify, as well as exposure to mass gatherings such as the Hajj pilgrimage, where unintended exposure may occur.

9 Allergy status is imperative to clarify, particularly as most initial empirical therapeutic approaches use penicillin or cephalosporin-based regimens. If there is concern regarding hypersensitivity, the exact nature of the reaction should be identified urgently, and a decision made regarding which antimicrobial groups are safe to use.

10 Asplenic patients are at particular risk from infections by encapsulated organisms, particularly *S. pneumoniae*, *N. meningitidis* and *H. influenzae*. Vaccination against these pathogens are highly advised for patients without spleens as well as other at-risk individuals. Inclusion of the pneumococcal vaccination on the childhood immunisation schedules has significantly decreased rates of invasive pneumococcal disease including pneumococcal meningitis; however, a shift has been seen with an increase in cases caused by serotypes not included in the vaccine. It should be remembered that although vaccination is important, it does not exclude the possibility of these diseases and thus there should be a uniform approach to assessment, diagnosis and treatment of the patient presenting with suspected meningoencephalitis.

Examination

- The patient appears unwell and is **disoriented to time and place** [1] . She opens her eyes to voice but struggles to follow commands. There is no focal neurological deficit.
- She is pyrexial with a **temperature of 38.6°C** [2] . The remaining vital signs are otherwise normal with blood pressure of 128/70mmHg, heart rate 84bpm and respiratory rate 16 breaths/minute.
- Photophobia is present. **Meningeal irritation** [3] is demonstrated, with nuchal rigidity present with both passive and active flexion of the neck. Kernig and Brudzinski signs are negative.
- **Examination of other organ systems** [4] is unremarkable, with no swollen joints or **rashes** [5] present.

1 Altered mental status is important to identify, and can be characterised by the Glasgow Coma Scale, although changes may be more subtle. It may occur as a general symptom of meningoencephalitis, but particular complications such as hydrocephalus or seizures should also be considered. Focal neurological deficits can occur, with significant deficits of aphasia or hemiparesis in up to 20% of patients with bacterial meningitis, and in smaller numbers, coma and cranial nerve palsies. *Listeria* meningitis may present with rhombencephalitis, characterised by ataxia, nystagmus and cranial nerve palsies. The predominant symptom of encephalitis is the acute change in mental state, and it should be considered in any patient with this presentation.

2 Sepsis may be the presentation, particularly in invasive meningococcal or pneumococcal disease. It is important to remain alert for signs of early sepsis or septic shock, and to respond quickly and appropriately should sepsis develop.

3 Meningeal irritation should be assessed, with nuchal rigidity demonstrated when the patient is unable to touch their chin to the chest with passive or active flexion of the

neck. Specific tests to demonstrate meningism include Kernig's sign, where difficulty is seen when attempting to fully extend the knee whilst the hip is flexed to 90°, and Brudzinski's sign, where attempted passive neck flexion causes spontaneous hip flexion. It should be noted that although specificity is high for these manoeuvres, sensitivity is low.

4 Other organ involvement can occur, signalling severe disease with seeding. There may be sinusitis, pneumonia, septic arthritis or endocarditis concurrently. In particular, *N. meningitidis* is associated with complications of arthritis. Swollen joints should be assessed with fluid aspiration and culture if possible, as this will dictate the length of treatment, if positive.

5 Rash is often thought to be a significant feature of meningitis, but its absence does not rule it out, nor is its presence pathognomonic. *N. meningitidis* is associated with a characteristic rash with petechiae and palpable purpura, occurring in up to a quarter of patients with meningitis, but rashes may also appear maculopapular.

Investigations

- **Blood tests are performed** [1] showing an elevated WCC with left shift and reduced platelets. Electrolytes demonstrate a mild hyponatraemia and coagulation studies are normal. C-reactive protein is moderately elevated.
- **Two sets of blood cultures** [2] are obtained prior to initiating antimicrobial therapy which are positive for *N. meningitidis* at 24 hours.
- A **lumbar puncture** [3] is performed and a **raised opening pressure is noted** [4].
- **Analysis of the cerebrospinal fluid** [5] identifies raised lactate, raised protein, low glucose, raised white cell count with neutrophils accounting for 85% of the cells and a small number of **erythrocytes** [6].
- **Gram stain** [7] shows Gram-negative diplococci and a **rapid diagnostic test** [8] for *S. pneumoniae* antigen is negative, as is PCR for **herpes simplex virus** [9].
- A **CT head** [10] performed after the lumbar puncture is normal.

[1] Blood tests should include full blood count and CRP, which would be expected to show elevated white cell count, although leucopenia may occur with severe infections. Thrombocytopenia may also be seen. Electrolyte measurements may demonstrate hyponatraemia, found in up to 30% of patients, but this is usually mild. Glucose should be measured, in order to correlate with CSF measurements. Abnormal coagulation studies may represent DIC.

[2] Blood cultures are frequently positive and should be obtained in addition to cerebrospinal fluid cultures, prior to antimicrobial treatment if possible. Meningococcal infections are less likely to yield positive blood cultures, particularly after antimicrobials have been administered.

[3] Lumbar puncture is essential unless contraindicated, and is likely to yield important information. This is particularly the case if done prior to commencing antimicrobials, although definitive treatment should not be delayed whilst waiting for this test. Relative contraindications include patients with bleeding tendencies, including suspected DIC, localised infection over the lumbar spinal area or suspected spinal abscess, significant haemodynamic instability, and those where there is a possibility of mass lesion or raised intracranial pressure (ICP). Patients in whom raised ICP is suspected should undergo CT of the brain prior to lumbar puncture, as detailed below.

[4] Opening pressure should be measured in the lateral decubitus position, and monitored in conditions such as cryptococcal meningitis, where raised intracranial pressure is related to complications of hearing and visual loss. Opening pressure tends to be raised in bacterial meningitis. In the patient with raised opening pressure and depressed neurological status, discussion with neurosurgical colleagues is recommended to identify those who would benefit from ICP monitoring and directed treatment.

[5] Cell count, microscopy and culture yield important information. A raised CSF lactate is more consistent with bacterial meningitis. Other characteristic findings in bacterial meningitis include a low CSF glucose, low CSF to serum glucose ratio and a raised CSF protein. CSF pleocytosis (increased white cell count) is non-specific and can occur in bacterial and viral meningitis, but predominant neutrophilia can suggest bacterial causes rather than viral.

[6] The presence of red blood cells should be noted. In a 'champagne tap' with no erythrocytes, the presence of white blood cells is indicative of infection. However, if there are erythrocytes present from either a traumatic lumbar puncture, or from subarachnoid or intracerebral haemorrhage, a false-positive elevation of CSF white blood cells can occur. To account for this, for every 500–1000 erythrocytes, one white blood cell can be discounted, and the remaining white blood cell count should be interpreted instead.

[7] Gram stain should be requested urgently and positive results phoned through to the treating clinician. If there is a concern for cryptococcal, tuberculous or eosinophilic meningitis, this information should be included and specific stains used for diagnosis. If Gram-positive diplococci are seen, pneumococcal infection is suggested; meningococcal if Gram-negative diplococci, *Listeria* if Gram-positive coccobacilli and *H. influenzae* if small Gram-negative coccobacilli. If Gram stain is negative, but the CSF findings are otherwise consistent with bacterial meningitis, empirical therapy should be continued.

[8] Bacterial antigen testing in the serum and urine tend not to be useful although pneumococcal antigen testing on CSF, and sometimes urine, may be useful when antimicrobials have already been given. Meningococcal PCR from serum and CSF samples can also provide a diagnosis with rapid turn-around time, and are especially useful when antimicrobials have been given prior to cultures.

[9] Testing for herpes simplex virus (HSV) is done using a nucleic acid amplification test on CSF. These can be negative early in the course of the illness, and thus testing should be repeated if there is clinical suspicion that HSV is the causative agent. In conjunction with a normal MRI, a negative HSV PCR is usually sufficient to exclude this cause of viral encephalitis.

10 Decisions around imaging are related to the potential for abnormalities that can predispose to cerebral herniation from lumbar puncture and removal of CSF. CT head should be performed prior to lumbar puncture if specific risk factors are present, such as being immunocompromised, or in patients with a known pathology affecting the central nervous system, and those with recent seizure, focal neurological deficit or papilloedema. In the diagnosis of viral encephalitis, MRI is particularly useful, as specific findings can assist with diagnosis of particular organisms; for example, limbic and temporal involvement seen with herpes simplex encephalitis.

Management

Short-term

Commence **empirical IV antibiotics** [1] and **dexamethasone** [2] – preferably after appropriate cultures have been obtained, but within 60 minutes of arrival at hospital or beforehand if identified in the **community** [3]. Change to **targeted therapy** [4] if an organism is identified, using initial Gram stain results to guide therapy early. Commence appropriate **isolation precautions** [5]. Commence **supportive management** [6] with fluids and monitor the patient carefully for complications such as septic shock, septic arthritis, DIC or acute respiratory distress syndrome. Refer for review by Intensive Care team. Administer **prophylaxis** [7] against VTE if appropriate, and provide adequate analgesia to the patient. Involve the **multidisciplinary team** [8] including physiotherapy, occupational therapy and dietitian.

Long-term

Notify Public Health [9] of the diagnosis if required. Contact tracing will take place, and some patients and close contacts may be offered antibiotics for **nasopharyngeal clearance** [10]. The **prognosis** [11] for many patients includes long-term neurological sequelae and they should be supported with rehabilitation on their journey to return to the community. Functional and cognitive assessments may be required, in addition to specific tests – e.g. for hearing assessments – and the patient may require ongoing support to return to previous occupation, or be supported in accessing financial assistance in the event they cannot.

1 Early empirical therapy is important, preferably within 60 minutes of arrival at the healthcare facility. Local guidelines will be of use, particularly in the recommendations for antimicrobials in the context of local susceptibility patterns, but should encompass the likely organisms for the individual patient as well as having appropriate penetration into the CSF. Most antimicrobials will need to be given intravenously. An example regimen would be high dose ceftriaxone, 2g 12-hourly, to achieve adequate penetration into the CNS. If there is a risk of *Listeria*, penicillin should be added due to intrinsic resistance of this organism to cephalosporins. In areas where the prevalence of ceftriaxone-resistant pneumococci is over 1%, vancomycin should also be added. Antivirals should be commenced to cover herpes simplex encephalitis if this is suspected, with IV aciclovir at appropriate doses to penetrate the CSF.

2 The use of dexamethasone is recommended, which has been shown to improve outcomes in bacterial meningitis caused by *S. pneumoniae* and *H. influenzae*, and reduce the risk of severe hearing loss in *Streptococcus suis* meningitis. Dexamethasone is not shown to provide benefit in meningococcal meningitis, nor in neonates less than a month old, and should be stopped if viral meningoencephalitis is diagnosed. Corticosteroids should be continued in bacterial meningitis caused by *S. pneumoniae*, *H. influenzae* type B, *S. suis*, and in tuberculous meningitis and eosinophilic meningitis.

3 In the patient with suspected meningococcal meningitis assessed in the community, a dose of ceftriaxone or benzylpenicillin should be administered, depending on availability. There is increasing resistance of *N. meningitidis* to benzylpenicillin and in the hospital setting cephalosporins with adequate CSF penetration are first-line, with benzylpenicillin added for *L. monocytogenes* cover.

4 Targeted therapy is essential once the organism is identified, as the antimicrobial regimens required to penetrate cerebrospinal fluid may bring adverse effects. In addition, empirical therapy may not adequately cover some organisms. If Gram-positive cocci resembling staphylococcus, Gram-positive diplococci or positive pneumococcal antigen are found, vancomycin should be added to ensure MRSA or penicillin/cephalosporin-resistant *S. pneumoniae* isolates are covered. Once an organism and susceptibility has been identified, an individualised regimen can be instigated, with advice from Infectious diseases teams recommended.

5 Patients with suspected bacterial meningitis should be placed in droplet isolation, specifically for containment of *N. meningitidis* and *H. influenzae*. This involves the use of standard precautions plus private room if possible, and use of standard facemasks when within 1 metre of the patient.

6 Septic shock is important to identify early and is frequently present in the setting of meningococcal meningitis. There is evidence that IV fluids confer improved neurological outcomes if given early in areas with high mortality rate, in addition to treatment of hypotension. In addition to signs of haemodynamic instability, features of sepsis in meningococcal disease have been reported to include leg pain and features of peripheral vasoconstriction, such as cold peripheries and mottling of the skin. Hypotension may occur due to reduced intravascular volume or shock. Alternatively it may occur in the setting of adrenal haemorrhage and subsequent acute hypoadrenalism, the Waterhouse–Friderichsen syndrome typically caused by *N. meningitidis*. Given the significant risk of deterioration, it is advised to seek Intensive Care support, and many places will preferentially take care of patients with bacterial meningitis in a high dependency or intensive care setting.

7 Prophylaxis against VTE should be considered carefully, especially if the patient is demonstrating features consistent with DIC. Mechanical prophylaxis with thromboembolic stockings is reasonable, but the benefit of LMWH at prophylactic doses should be weighed up against bleeding risk, acknowledging that DIC increases the risk of both clotting and bleeding.

8 Multidisciplinary assessment, including physiotherapy and occupational therapy input, is essential, and for some patients psychologist input and neurorehabilitation will be of benefit. Social work input may be required, particularly in patients who have residual neurological deficits and who require long-term support.

9 The causative organism may require notification to the local or national Public Health authority. Local requirements should be checked and notified as required. Public Health departments will then investigate and commence the process of contact tracing to identify at-risk contacts, to ascertain if they have become infected, and to offer clearance antibiotics if felt at risk.

10 Patients with *N. meningitidis* who have been treated with benzylpenicillin only, and those with *H. influenzae* not treated with ceftriaxone, ciprofloxacin or cefotaxime, require antibiotics for nasopharyngeal clearance of the organism. In addition, close contacts of patients with *N. meningitidis* and *H. influenzae*, including exposed staff, should be offered clearance antibiotics whether or not they are vaccinated.

11 Meningoencephalitis carries a risk of significant morbidity and mortality. The mortality risk increases with age, and is higher amongst meningitis cases due to *S. pneumoniae* and *L. monocytogenes*, as well as in patients who present late, or who are immunocompromised. Neurological deficits are common but most are transient. Rates of 10% of long-term neurological sequelae are reported, which mostly consist of impaired hearing, speech or cognition, and motor or cranial deficits.

CASE 47: Osteomyelitis

History

- A **55 year-old man** [1] presents with **lower back pain, radiating to the groin and associated with fevers and night sweats** [2].
- The pain began **six days ago** [3], is gradually worsening and is exacerbated by movement.
- He reports no **neurological symptoms** [4], including no loss of bladder or bowel function.
- **Past medical history** [5] includes hypertension, mild osteoarthritis and type 2 diabetes complicated by peripheral neuropathy and end-stage renal failure, for which he receives haemodialysis three times a week via a left arteriovenous fistula.

- He has no cardiac, orthopaedic or other prostheses *in situ*, and has no history of endocarditis, recent trauma or **tuberculosis** [6].
- His medications include insulin, antihypertensives and oral electrolyte replacement, but he is on no immune suppressive therapy. He has no **allergies** [7].
- The patient is an ex-smoker, consumes alcohol within recommended limits, has never injected drugs and has not **travelled** [8] abroad within the past five years.

[1] Whilst osteomyelitis can affect all ages, most cases of vertebral osteomyelitis occur in older adults, affecting men more commonly than women. Long-bone osteomyelitis is seen most often in children, generally affecting the bone adjacent to the growth plate.

[2] Symptoms include localised pain, swelling and occasionally an overlying wound or sinus tract; for example, if complicating a diabetic or venous ulcer. The pain may radiate to surrounding structures or may be referred, if spinal column and nerve roots are involved, and is often worse on movement or palpation. Systemic symptoms such as fever, sweats and rigors may be present.

[3] Osteomyelitis may present acutely, over days to weeks, or may be insidious. Chronic osteomyelitis occurs over months or even years, may manifest with intermittent flares, and is associated with bone necrosis and sometimes a sinus tract.

[4] The presence of neurological symptoms is a red flag for patients presenting with back pain from any cause, and in the setting of osteomyelitis, raises concern for concurrent epidural abscess from posterior spread of the infection. A careful history should be taken to identify any early symptoms of radiculopathy, motor or sensory deficit, and loss of control of bladder or bowel function. If present, urgent imaging and consideration of Neurosurgical input are required.

[5] A number of risk factors predispose to developing osteomyelitis by either non-haematogenous or haematogenous spread. Direct spread of infection can occur from chronic wounds, such as diabetic, arteriovenous or pressure ulcers in the presence of peripheral vascular disease or peripheral neuropathy, or acute events such as from surgical procedures or traumatic injuries. The presence of underlying prostheses increases the risk of developing osteomyelitis. Distant spread of infection via the haematogenous route is more likely when there are risks of introducing infection into the bloodstream, including IV drug use, haemodialysis and patients with intravenous catheters. A history of endocarditis or prosthetic valves raises concern for recurrence as a source for osteomyelitis. Other groups of patients at increased risk include immunocompromised patients and patients with sickle-cell anaemia.

[6] Tuberculosis is an uncommon cause of osteomyelitis, but should be considered as a potential cause in patients with epidemiological risk factors, including a previous personal history of TB, current or past residence in an endemic area and cohabitation with a person known to have active TB.

[7] Duration of treatment of osteomyelitis is relatively long compared to other infections. Thus a thorough history to assess allergy and intolerance to antibiotics is important, to assist with deciding on the best antimicrobial and ensuring the patient is able to tolerate the regimen for extended periods.

[8] Travel history can identify whether the patient is at risk of particular pathogens from exposure, including multi-drug-resistant organisms, TB or other uncommon pathogens such as *Brucella*.

Examination

- On examination, the patient looks well with a mild pyrexia of 38.1°C. Blood pressure is 140/90mmHg and other **vital signs** [1] are normal.
- Mobility is limited by pain and there is **tenderness** [2] on palpation of the lumbar region, particularly the L2 vertebra, but no overlying skin erythema or sinus tract formation is noted.
- **Neurological examination** [3] reveals that power and coordination are objectively normal, reflexes are normal and no sensory level deficit is elicited. There is reduced sensation to light touch and proprioception in both feet in keeping with the

patient's known peripheral neuropathy. Perianal sensation is intact.
- **Cardiorespiratory examination** [4] is normal with no murmur auscultated, and there are no peripheral stigmata of endocarditis.
- **Abdominal examination** [5] reveals a soft, non-tender abdomen without palpable bladder.
- **Skin examination** [6] reveals dry skin but no ulcers or fungal infections. His arteriovenous fistula has marks consistent with current use, and a small area of erythema around a recent needle mark.

[1] The patient will usually be haemodynamically stable, and presentation with sepsis syndrome from underlying osteomyelitis is not common. Fever may be present, but about half will be afebrile. If the patient is hypotensive or displaying features of septic shock, it is important to treat this in the first instance before pursuing dedicated investigations for osteomyelitis.

[2] In the case of vertebral osteomyelitis, examination of the spine may reveal bony tenderness to palpation at the site of the infection, and the patient's mobility may be impaired due to pain. Paraspinal muscles may also be tender or in spasm. The presence of flank pain, or pain on extension of the hip, suggests possible psoas abscess complicating the infection. Osteomyelitis involving non-vertebral sites may not be overly tender to palpate, particularly if there is concurrent peripheral neuropathy, such as may be present in a diabetic foot ulcer complicated by osteomyelitis.

[3] A thorough neurological examination must be performed, to provide a baseline evaluation and to objectively assess reported symptoms. This will help identify whether there is radiculopathy or spinal cord compromise present, occurring as a consequence of epidural abscess or vertebral fracture. A digital rectal examination may be required to assess for anal tone and perineal sensation.

[4] Examination of the cardiovascular and respiratory systems may reveal signs of infection elsewhere that may

represent a source for seeding of a pathogen to bone. In particular, it is important to evaluate for signs of infective endocarditis such as splinter haemorrhages or new cardiac murmurs.

[5] Abdominal examination may identify an intra-abdominal or genitourinary source of infection. Splenic and renal infarcts from emboli from endocarditis may cause pain on palpation, or there may be features suspicious of liver abscess such as right upper quadrant pain. A palpable bladder raises suspicion for spinal cord compression with subsequent bladder dysfunction.

[6] There may be clues to the source of infection on examination of the skin, as breach of this organ provides a path for organisms to enter the bloodstream and seed to the bone. Dry skin or wounds should be evaluated, particularly any wounds associated with poor healing such as ulcers of diabetes or vascular insufficiency. There may be needle tracks or infected injection sites in the skin of an IV drug user; similarly there may be erythema or discharge around indwelling vascular devices or at sites of IV access such as an arteriovenous fistula in a haemodialysis patient. Suspected osteomyelitis complicating a diabetic foot ulcer can be hard to identify on external examination, but there may be increased erythema, discharge, evidence of a soft tissue collection, or a sinus tract.

Investigations

- **Blood tests** [1] show slightly raised white cells with a neutrophilia, and a raised CRP. Renal function demonstrates significantly raised creatinine consistent with end-stage renal failure, and normal electrolytes. Liver function is normal and blood

glucose is within target limits for the patient's diabetic control.
- Blood and urine **cultures** [2] are sent prior to antibiotics but do not grow an organism.
- A lumbar **X-ray** [3] does not show evidence of acute fracture.

- An **MRI** [4] of the lumbar spine demonstrates features consistent with osteomyelitis and no evidence of epidural abscess.
- A **CT-guided biopsy** [5] is performed and bone samples sent for bacterial, mycobacterial and fungal culture in addition to histopathological analysis.
- *Staphylococcus aureus* [6] is cultured, resistant to penicillin but susceptible to flucloxacillin. A swab of the area of erythema overlying the recent haemodialysis access point also grows *S. aureus*.
- Apart from a transthoracic echocardiogram which does not demonstrate features suggestive of infective endocarditis, no **other imaging or microbiological analysis** [7] is performed.

1 Full blood count often shows a raised WCC, usually neutrophilic, in the context of acute osteomyelitis, but may be normal in chronic infection. Platelets may be raised as part of the acute phase reaction, in addition to CRP. Erythrocyte sedimentation rate is usually elevated and may serve as a sensitive biomarker of disease activity. It is important to know the patient's baseline renal and liver function, as this will affect the choice and dosing of antimicrobial therapy, particularly in the patient with end-stage renal function on haemodialysis. In addition, a number of antibiotics can cause liver dysfunction, particularly in cumulative doses over a prolonged course of treatment. Achieving good glycaemic control is also an important part of treating the diabetic patient with an infection.

2 It is important to obtain cultures for microbiological analysis prior to administering antibiotics, if possible. Blood cultures may be positive in patients who have haematogenous osteomyelitis, but about half will not culture an organism. If a suspect organism is grown from blood cultures, this can reduce the requirement to obtain biopsy for culture. Urine culture may identify a potential organism such as enteric Gram-negative organisms or *Pseudomonas aeruginosa*. If *Staphylococcus aureus* is grown in urine, this suggests bacteraemia with spill into the urinary tract. In the patient with epidemiological risk factors for TB, dedicated staining for acid-fast bacilli and extended mycobacterial culture can help identify this pathogen. In patients with suspected chronic osteomyelitis complicating a wound, swab of the wound is unlikely to assist with directed therapy, as differentiating between colonising and pathogenic organisms is difficult.

3 X-ray is unlikely to be helpful in acute osteomyelitis, although it can help with identifying complications such as vertebral collapse, alternative diagnoses such as a metastatic lesion, or underlying arthritic disease. There may be changes seen in chronic osteomyelitis, with early changes demonstrating soft tissue swelling, followed by periosteal thickening, osteopenia and lytic changes, and sclerosis.

4 Magnetic resonance imaging is the most sensitive imaging modality for osteomyelitis, and can demonstrate bone marrow oedema early in the infection. A classic pattern is the involvement of an intervertebral disc with signal changes in the inferior end-plate of the vertebral body above, and the superior end-plate of the vertebral body below. It can also characterise complications such as epidural abscess and paraspinal involvement. Specific features on MRI may raise suspicion of tuberculosis as the causative organism, and can assist in guiding directed culture and treatment.

5 Microbiological diagnosis should be obtained if possible, to guide definitive management. In patients where blood cultures are negative, or where a culture result does not suggest the primary causative organism, direct sampling of infected bone is recommended. Radiologically guided biopsy with CT is ideal, with samples then sent for bacterial, fungal and mycobacterial culture as well as histological analysis, which typically demonstrates necrotic bone with features of resorption and inflammation. If cultures are negative, for example in a patient partially treated with antibiotics, the use of nucleic acid diagnostics such as 16S rRNA identification can help identify the organism.

6 Vertebral osteomyelitis is most commonly caused by *S. aureus*, with other potential microbes including *Streptococcus* spp., Gram-negative bacilli, coagulase-negative *Staphylococci*, *P. aeruginosa*, and less commonly fungal infections such as *Candida* or *Aspergillus* in the immune-compromised host. Tuberculosis and *Brucella* should be considered in patients with epidemiological risk factors. Whilst most cases of vertebral osteomyelitis are monomicrobial, patients with risk factors for non-haematogenous osteomyelitis may have either a monomicrobial or polymicrobial cause for their infection.

7 Investigations should be performed if a systemic infection is suspected. Identification of *S. aureus* should always prompt concern for infective endocarditis, and a transthoracic echocardiogram performed as a minimum, although the presence of a likely mechanism of haematogenous introduction in this patient via the arteriovenous fistula, and absence of bacteraemia, makes this less likely. The presence of Gram-negative bacilli may prompt imaging of the urinary tract, and a suspicion of TB should prompt a chest X-ray with other directed imaging as appropriate. If epidemiology suggests an alternative pathogen, such as *Brucellosis* or fungal infection, consider directed investigations, including an assessment of underlying immune status.

Management

Short-term

Admit the patient to hospital for observation, investigation and treatment. Provide analgesia and prophylaxis for **venous thromboembolism** [1]. Determine appropriate **antimicrobial therapy** [2] based on microbiological cultures. Initiate additional investigations if required, depending on the pathogen identified. **Educate** [3] the patient, including potential **complications** [4] and prolonged **duration of treatment** [5] if required. Ensure appropriate **specialist medical teams** [6] are involved, including Renal, Surgical and Endocrinology. Involve the **multidisciplinary team** [7] early including physiotherapy, occupational therapy and pharmacy, and consider the role of outpatient antimicrobial therapy.

Long-term

The patient should be monitored regularly until they complete their treatment. Signs of **treatment failure and recurrence** [8], and risk factors for this, should be addressed. Notably, pain may persist despite treatment and **pain management** [9] should be prioritised, in addition to an assessment of the patient's physical and psychological status, with regular liaison with the patient's primary care practitioner and involvement of community multidisciplinary services as required.

[1] Risk factors for VTE in the patient with osteomyelitis include an inflammatory state and significantly impaired mobility as a result of their pain. Patients with severe vertebral osteomyelitis at risk of neurological impairment may be advised to limit their motion, and in some cases are advised bed rest. Prophylaxis against VTE is particularly important, and patients should be considered for mechanical and pharmacological prophylaxis.

[2] Ideally, antimicrobial therapy should not be started until the organism is identified, allowing directed therapy based on susceptibilities. If the patient is unwell with sepsis or has evidence of neurological deficit, then empirical antimicrobial therapy can be given, using local guidelines to assist with choice of antimicrobials, and providing cover for common organisms including *S. aureus*, *Streptococcus* spp. and Gram-negative bacilli.

[3] It is important to involve the patient in conversations about their treatment options, and to educate them about their condition to facilitate informed decision-making. Given the risk of serious complications, potential need for operative management and requirement for prolonged antibiotic therapy, it is important that the patient receives careful explanation and is given frequent opportunity to ask questions and receive updates on their progress.

[4] The potential complications of osteomyelitis depend on its site, with vertebral osteomyelitis having the potential for local extension into nerve structures and surrounding tissue. Patients with wound-associated osteomyelitis and those with metalware in or adjacent to the affected bone can have issues with source control and the patient should be counselled about the indications for surgery. The patient should also be educated about the potential for antibiotic side-effects as well as the risk of treatment failure and recurrence of infection.

[5] The duration of antimicrobial therapy depends on the organism, site and other factors involved in achieving source control. Patients with vertebral osteomyelitis are often treated with parenteral and/or oral antibiotics for a minimum of six weeks; local and national guidelines should be consulted to help guide decision-making. In the setting of non-haematogenous osteomyelitis, achieving source control by successful debridement of infected bone tissue can allow for significantly shortened duration of postoperative antimicrobial therapy. If full debridement is not successful, a longer course of antimicrobials is required. In the setting of a patient with infected metalware complicating osteomyelitis, there may be a requirement for surgical exchange of the hardware, with duration of antimicrobials dependent on the strategy and outcome.

[6] In such complex infections, it is important to liaise with appropriate specialists early in the patient's management. For patients with vertebral osteomyelitis, assessment by Neurosurgery is useful and imperative if there is neurological deficit, for consideration of neurosurgical intervention to stabilise the spine prior to significant neurological impairment. Orthopaedic Surgery can provide advice on management of suspected infected metalware. Interventional Radiology can provide opinion and assistance with obtaining suitable specimens for culture. Patients with diabetes are likely to benefit from involvement of Endocrinology and Diabetes specialists, to enable peri-operative glucose management as well as providing advice on improved longer-term management of their diabetes. Other specialist teams, such as the Renal service for the patient on dialysis, Addiction Medicine services for the patient who intravenously injects drugs, Cardiology for evaluation of potential endocarditis, amongst others, may be helpful.

[7] The MDT can provide essential support, including physiotherapy and occupational therapy assessments to assist

with mobility and activities of daily living; social work to help access financial aid if the patient is unable to work due to their symptoms; dialysis nurses for the patient on haemodialysis; and pharmacist to assist with dosing and therapeutic drug monitoring as required. Outpatient antimicrobial therapy is often helpful to provide at-home treatment as parenteral therapy is frequently required.

8 There is a risk of recurrence of the infection during treatment, or after ceasing antimicrobials. Generally the patient is monitored for clinical symptoms and signs of infection recurrence, alongside biochemical markers for inflammation and objective measurement of fevers. Risk factors for future osteomyelitis should also be addressed, such as skin condition, vascular access, IV drug use and diabetes, and the patient counselled about the importance of management and mitigation of these risks for future health.

9 With pain often being a predominant symptom, adequate analgesia is essential, using simple analgesia including paracetamol. NSAIDs and opioids should be used with caution, particularly with renal impairment. Non-pharmacological methods of analgesia should be explored, and Pain specialist involvement may be useful. Finally, the psychological impact of chronic pain must be recognised, and patients supported early if their pain does not resolve. Close liaison with community services to provide longer-term treatment is essential in the holistic care of these patients.

CASE 48: Pneumonia

History

- A **75-year-old woman** [1] presents with a **three-day history** [2] of **purulent cough, rigors and vomiting** [3] .
- She reports greenish sputum with **rusty-coloured streaks of blood** [4] , but no overt haemoptysis.
- The cough was initially dry, associated with rhinorrhoea, and is painful with **sharp left-sided chest pain, worse on inspiration** [5] .
- The cough is occasional and does not occur in **paroxysms or prolonged bouts** [6] .
- The patient feels mildly **breathless at rest** [7] and reports a mild headache.
- The patient has a past history of hypertension for which she takes an antihypertensive, but has **no risk factors** [8] such as underlying lung disease nor immune deficiency, and does not take steroids or other immune-suppressing medications.
- The patient is an **ex-smoker** [9] , drinks in moderation and does not use illicit drugs.
- **Potential exposures are explored** [10] : she is a retired secretary, lives in her own home by herself, owns a cat and a dog but no birds, and has not travelled locally or overseas, especially to tropical areas. It is the winter season, and apart from some influenza cases, there are no known unusual local outbreaks currently reported. She reports no unwell contacts nor recent hospital admissions, but does have a 2-year-old grandson who visits regularly.
- She has not had **influenza or pneumococcal vaccinations** [11] in the past 5 years. She has no allergies.

[1] The elderly are at increased risk of respiratory infection due to reduced immune response, higher rates of chronic lung disease, reduced lung capacity to clear infection, and higher rates of comorbidities that predispose to pneumonia. Most deaths from pneumonia in high income countries occur in the elderly.

[2] Pneumonia tends to present acutely, although in some patients it can occur as a secondary complication following a viral infection, and therefore it is important to get an accurate history of symptomatic evolution over time.

[3] The typical symptoms of pneumonia include respiratory symptoms of cough, mucopurulent sputum, haemoptysis on occasion; and systemic symptoms including fever, rigors, headache, appetite loss and vomiting.

[4] Although not specific, rusty-coloured streaks of blood in sputum can suggest *Streptococcus pneumoniae*. Frank haemoptysis can occur with pneumonia, but differential diagnoses should be considered, including pulmonary embolism, pulmonary infarction, lung abscess, pulmonary tuberculosis and underlying malignancy.

[5] Sharp chest pain worse on deep inspiration or coughing is classic for pleuritic chest pain, and this may be felt locally or referred to the shoulder tip. It occurs due to pain caused by friction of the two inflamed pleural membranes against each

other. Differential diagnoses for pleuritic chest pain are similar to those for haemoptysis.

[6] Whooping cough, caused by *Bordetella pertussis*, is seen in areas where immunisation rates are suboptimal, or in patients who have waning immunity, such as the elderly. It is associated with classic paroxysmal coughing bouts with laryngospasm, which can last for weeks.

[7] Dyspnoea is an important symptom which can be particularly distressing for patients. Although it is subjective, it can be used to help gauge how quickly the patient's symptoms have progressed, and also to assess response to therapy such as oxygen supplementation. In the breathless patient, it is important to be mindful that talking can exacerbate their symptoms, and to tailor history-taking accordingly.

[8] A number of conditions predispose to developing pneumonia, including the more obvious respiratory diseases such as asthma, chronic obstructive pulmonary disease, bronchiectasis and cystic fibrosis, but also other diseases and medications which affect the immune system, such as diabetes mellitus, malignancy, frailty, alcohol, corticosteroids, immunosuppressants and chemotherapy.

[9] Smoking impairs mucociliary clearance and neutrophil function, and predisposes to pneumonia. It is also important

to assess smoking history for likelihood of pre-existing or undiagnosed lung disease. This should be quantified as 'pack years', where a pack year is counted as smoking a pack of twenty cigarettes each day for a year. If identified on history, patients who smoke should be offered nicotine replacement therapy during their inpatient stay and assistance with smoking cessation, including referral to inpatient and outpatient services.

10 History should include an assessment of potential exposures to identify likely organisms. Whilst respiratory viruses, including influenza, are a common cause of pneumonia overall, especially in young children, frequently detected bacterial organisms include *S. pneumoniae* in all age groups, *Mycoplasma pneumoniae* and *Chlamydophila pneumoniae* in younger patients, whereas the elderly are more likely to be infected with non-typable *Haemophilus influenzae*. Recent hospital admission or nursing home residents should be assessed as potential hospital-acquired pneumonia, which is associated with different pathogens. Patients with previous stroke or neuromuscular conditions are predisposed to aspiration pneumonia. Occupational history is important: certain workplaces increase the likelihood of certain organisms such as *Coxiella burnetii* (Q fever) in farm and abattoir workers. Exposure to birds, especially recently imported birds, would increase the likelihood of *Chlamydophila psittaci*. Travel history, both domestic and international, is particularly important. Cruise ship travel increases the likelihood of contracting all contagious organisms, but particularly *Legionella pneumophila*, which is associated with water storage facilities. Assessing for outbreaks in the area of travel or residence, using real-time reporting sources such as with the Centers for Disease Control, are very useful. TB should be suspected in patients who have travelled to or come from endemic areas.

11 Annual influenza vaccination is recommended to reduce the risk of influenza and death in the elderly and at-risk. Pneumococcal vaccinations are recommended every 5 years in at-risk populations to reduce the incidence of invasive pneumococcal disease.

Examination

- The patient appears breathless at rest and is on **oxygen at 2L/minute via nasal prongs** [1] with a pulse oximeter reading of 91%.
- She does not appear **confused** [2].
- She does not appear centrally or peripherally **cyanosed** [3].
- Her heart rate is 96bpm, and blood pressure is 110/76mmHg. She is pyrexial at 38.3°C and is thin, with a **BMI of 18** [4].
- A sputum pot containing **thick green sputum** [5] is beside her; there are no inhalers or spacers seen.
- Respiratory effort is mildly increased with respiratory rate of 24 breaths per minute, but on **observation** [6] she is able to speak in full sentences without the use of accessory muscles. Trachea is central, chest expansion is equal and not hyperinflated on palpation.
- The sharp left-sided chest pain is **not reproducible on palpation** [7].
- Signs of **lobar consolidation** [8] are present. Percussion is resonant throughout apart from dullness in the lower third of the left chest posteriorly. On auscultation, vocal resonance in this area is increased and there are coarse crepitations in the lower left chest area.

1 Oxygenation is important to assess accurately, as hypoxia from pneumonia is a significant cause of morbidity and mortality. Pulse oximetry reading is a useful first measurement of oxygenation status, as it is simple, non-invasive, and can help guide initial oxygen therapy. Measurements can be spuriously low if peripheral perfusion or circulation is poor. Measurements of SaO_2 <92% should prompt an arterial blood gas for a more accurate assessment of oxygen status.

2 Disorientation and confusion are signs of delirium complicating the picture, which can occur as a result of a number of causes including sepsis, hypoxia and medications. It is a marker for severity and included within the CURB-65 score; delirium is associated with poorer outcomes and recognising this early is essential to minimise morbidity and mortality.

3 Cyanosis is generally caused by high levels of deoxygenated haemoglobin (central cyanosis of the lips and tongue) or vasoconstriction (peripheral cyanosis of extremities). If present, further assessment with arterial blood gases (ABGs) is required to determine whether this clinical finding is as a result of hypoxaemia.

4 Nutritional status is important to assess, as poor nutritional status can be a risk factor for more severe infections, whilst infections can worsen nutritional state. Hospitalised patients remain at risk of malnutrition, particularly if they are too unwell to eat or are delirious.

5 Examination of the sputum can yield useful information. It is important to know whether the patient chronically produces sputum, such as might be seen in one who smokes, or a patient with COPD or bronchiectasis; and if so, whether sputum characteristics have changed. A change in colour and consistency supports the diagnosis of respiratory infection; the presence of pink frothy sputum or frank blood may suggest an alternative diagnosis, such as pulmonary oedema or pulmonary embolism.

6 Observation of the patient can provide many clues: from identification of respiratory aids (oxygen, inhalers, spacer devices) to the respiratory effort required by the patient to ventilate. A simple way to gauge this is to observe how easily the patient performs usual tasks such as talking, walking and moving around the bed. Accessory muscle use is important to note, as this suggests increased respiratory effort and a sicker patient.

7 Examination of the area where the patient describes pain will help determine the origin, in addition to history. It is important to palpate the area where pain is experienced,

as reproducible pain may suggest a musculoskeletal cause rather than a pleural cause. Musculoskeletal chest wall pain also tends to be exacerbated by movement, and could be present in this patient as a result of muscle strain or coughing.

8 The classic signs of lobar consolidation include dullness to percussion, increased vibration sensation to tactile fremitus, crepitations and bronchial breathing at the area of consolidation. Bronchial breathing occurs due to turbulent airflow in large airways which is conducted easily to the chest wall and heard more harshly than vesicular breath sounds. There may be associated signs suggestive of pleural inflammation such as with pleural effusion, with stony dullness to percussion and reduced breath sounds, or a pleural rub, which manifests as a soft noise often described as 'treading on fresh snow'. Lobar collapse can manifest with unequal chest expansion, tracheal deviation and reduced breath sounds.

Investigations

- **Blood tests** [1] are performed, including a full blood count showing raised white cells with neutrophilia, CRP which is raised, renal function showing an acutely raised urea of 8mmol/L and normal liver function.
- An **arterial blood gas** [2] shows hypoxaemia in keeping with type 1 respiratory failure.
- A **CURB-65 score** [3] of 2 is calculated.
- Blood cultures are performed which are positive for *S. pneumoniae*, and **sputum culture** [4] grows *S. pneumoniae*.

- A **urinary pneumococcal rapid antigen test** [5] is positive for pneumococcal antigen.
- Atypical bacterial serology is not performed. A **nasopharyngeal swab** [6] is negative for all tested pathogens including *Bordetella pertussis* and *Influenza A, B*.
- A **chest X-ray** [7] shows **left lower lobar consolidation** [8] with a trace effusion. Other radiological investigations are not performed.

1 Full blood count with raised white cells, neutrophilia and raised CRP are expected, in keeping with acute bacterial infection. Low white cells can also be seen in severe infection. Acute impairment in renal function may indicate severe disease, with ensuing sepsis due to hypoperfusion. Renal and liver function are also important to take into account when deciding on appropriate antibiotics and doses.

2 An ABG is important to accurately gauge the degree of hypoxaemia, hypercapnia and acid–base status. Type 1 respiratory failure refers to hypoxaemia without hypercapnia; type 2 has both hypoxaemia and hypercapnia. In addition, this information can be used to calculate the Alveolar–arterial (A–a) gradient, which can help identify the cause of hypoxaemia. A normal A–a gradient in this setting suggests alveolar hypoventilation, whereas a raised A–a gradient suggests an alternative cause; for example, a ventilation-perfusion (V/Q) mismatch, right to left shunt or diffusion defect. Pneumonia may cause a V/Q mismatch because of a defect in ventilation due to consolidation.

3 Severity scores can be useful to help risk-stratify patients with pneumonia. A common, quick scoring system is the CURB-65 score, which scores 1 point for any of: confusion, urea >7mmol/L, respiratory rate >30/minute, systolic blood pressure <90mmHg or diastolic blood pressure <60mmHg, and age over 65 years. Patients with scores 0–1 can be considered for home treatment, 2 for hospital admission, and 3 or more to be managed in hospital as severe pneumonia. Other severity scores include CORB, PSI (Pneumonia Severity Index) and SMART-COP: these again help to risk-stratify patients to identify those at risk of severe disease earlier.

4 Sputum culture has low sensitivity; however, it should be routinely ordered to guide treatment. Deeply expectorated cultures must be obtained to avoid being salivary samples. Due to colonisation of the respiratory tract in certain conditions such as bronchiectasis, growth of an organism does not necessarily implicate pathogenicity. If there is a suspicion of TB, three induced sputum specimens should be obtained and sent for Ziehl–Neelsen stains and mycobacterial culture.

5 Urinary antigenic testing can be performed for pneumococcal and legionella antigens, which detects specific proteins shed by these organisms in the urine. These tests are rapid, and have high specificity. Serology can also be used to detect atypical infections with *C. pneumoniae*, *M. pneumoniae* and *Legionella* spp., but usually needs 'paired' samples.

6 Nasopharyngeal swabs are helpful for identifying causative organisms in children, or during influenza epidemics. This tests for common viruses and pertussis by PCR analysis. Rapid testing is often helpful for institution of respiratory contact precautions during influenza epidemics. Rhinovirus is a common cause of coryza and would not be expected to cause a significant lobar pneumonia.

7 Chest X-ray usually shows opacification in the area of pneumonia, although radiological findings often lag behind clinical symptoms and signs. Imaging is also helpful for information on whether the pneumonia is affecting single or multiple lobes, and whether effusions or abscess are present.

Chest X-ray should be repeated at around six weeks after resolution of the pneumonia, especially in high risk patients such as smokers and those with recurrent pneumonia in the same lobe, to ensure that changes have resolved; occasionally an underlying malignancy is diagnosed after initially being hidden by the infective changes. CT can be useful in further evaluation of complications such as rib fractures or abscess. Ultrasound may be helpful to assess complications such as effusions, particularly if drainage is considered. MRI is rarely required.

8 Some pneumonias cause specific patterns of infection, although not exclusively. *Staphylococcus aureus* tends to cause multilobar abscesses, whilst *Klebsiella* infections are more likely to involve the upper lobes. Upper lobar changes are also more often associated with pulmonary tuberculosis. Aspiration pneumonia commonly affects the right middle and lower lobes, as the right main bronchus is more vertical than the left, making it easier for aspirated material to enter.

Management

Short-term

Initiate appropriate **respiratory isolation measures** [1]. Optimise oxygenation using nasal prongs and humidified oxygen; escalate if breathing or oxygenation deteriorates, and involve critical care team early if there is a chance that the patient will deteriorate and require **additional respiratory support** [2] such as non-invasive or invasive ventilation. Considerations regarding appropriateness of **escalation of care** [3] should be made early and reviewed in line with the patient's progress. **Consult local antimicrobial guidelines and commence empirical antibiotics with appropriate cover** [4]. Ensure that microbiological tests are followed up and that antimicrobials are appropriately narrowed down if the organism is identified. Resuscitate with **intravenous fluids** [5] if there are signs of sepsis or acute kidney injury. Provide appropriate **analgesia** [6] to allow the patient to breathe and cough effectively. Administer prophylaxis against **venous thromboembolism** [7]. Utilise the **multidisciplinary team** [8]: physiotherapist to assist

with chest physio and breathing exercises, occupational therapist to assess activities of daily living, dietitian to assess nutritional status.

The patient should be assessed regularly for improvement and to identify **potential complications** [9] of pneumonia early. **Public health notification** [10] is required for some organisms.

Long-term

Discharge from hospital should be considered once the patient is clinically stable, including off oxygen therapy and mobilising safely. Chest X-ray should be repeated at 6 weeks to ensure resolution of radiological changes, and combined with a clinical review either by primary care or in a hospital clinic. **Preventive measures** [11] are important: influenza and pneumococcal vaccinations should be offered and the patient educated on good hand hygiene and methods to reduce transmission during the winter season.

1 Respiratory isolation measures are important tools to reduce the spread of particular infectious organisms. If influenza or TB is suspected, the patient should be placed in appropriate isolation until these infections are excluded, or a quarantine period has been completed. Hand hygiene and personal protective equipment are essential.

2 There are a range of options for providing oxygen therapy, and early recognition of the deteriorating patient who will need advanced ventilation to maintain oxygenation is essential. If a patient is not responding to ward-based measures and supplemental oxygen, early review by Intensive Care team is needed for invasive ventilator support.

3 A discussion around escalation of care, resuscitation and any limitations is important, particularly with a patient who may deteriorate and require invasive treatments like ventilation, or those who may develop impaired ability to consent, such as with delirium or drowsiness. This empowers the patient to communicate their wishes, and enables a discussion around which interventions would be likely and unlikely to optimise outcomes.

4 Cultures should be obtained prior to commencing antibiotics if it is possible to do so without delaying treatment. Antibiotics should cover the most likely pathogens, which vary with local outbreaks and resistance patterns. Most regimens will cover *S. pneumoniae* plus a Gram-negative cover if severe, hospital-acquired or aspiration pneumonia.

5 IV fluids should be administered to the patient early in the context of sepsis, and should be considered in the more well patient if a clinical reason exists such as acute kidney injury. In milder cases, oral hydration may be adequate, but hydration status should be assessed regularly. Inotropic support may be needed in the shocked patient.

6 Analgesia is important to help the patient breathe, cough and move easily. This will assist with sputum clearance, reduce the risk of complications such as deep vein thrombosis, and accelerate the patient's recovery. Options include paracetamol, NSAIDs and opiates, which should be used with caution in patients at risk of drowsiness and respiratory depression.

7 As with any hospitalised patient, consideration of prophylaxis against VTE with mechanical prophylaxis (stockings) and chemical prophylaxis (LMWH) is important to reduce the morbidity and mortality of this hospital-associated complication.

8 Input from the MDT is important. The patient will benefit from chest physiotherapy and input from occupational therapy to assess functional status and home set-up. Nutritional assessment by dietitian should also be offered.

9 Pneumonia can be associated with local complications such as para-pneumonic effusion, empyema, lobar collapse, lung abscess and pneumothorax; and systemic complications including acute renal failure, invasive disease as with pneumococcal meningitis, delirium and thromboembolic disease. These may occur during hospital stay or after discharge.

10 Public health notification is required for certain organisms including *Haemophilus influenzae b*, influenza, invasive pneumococcal disease, legionellosis, melioidosis, psittacosis and TB. Consult local guidelines for information on how to report.

11 Preventive measures are important to reduce the risk of further episodes of pneumonia. In addition to influenza and pneumococcal vaccinations, the patient should be educated on symptoms of pneumonia, including signs of sepsis, and advised to seek medical attention early. Avoidance of ill persons, such as the unwell grandson in this case, should be discussed, and the importance of good hand hygiene emphasised. Smoking cessation should be addressed if relevant, as should nutritional and dental care.

CASE 49: Septic arthritis

History

- A **72-year-old** [1] male presents with a one-day history of a **swollen, painful left knee associated with fever and restricted movement** [2] of the joint.
- His past medical history includes **type 2 diabetes mellitus and osteoarthritis** [3] affecting the hands, feet and knees.
- He reports no recent penetrating trauma, joint surgery or injections, no skin or **chronic joint infections** [4] and does not have any **prosthetic joint replacements** [5] or indwelling devices.
- His medications include metformin, rosuvastatin, paracetamol and celecoxib; he has not had any recent courses of **antibiotics** [6]. He is a non-smoker and non-drinker who has never injected drugs.
- **Travel history and sexual history** [7] are unremarkable and he is fully immunised, including pneumococcal vaccination.

[1] Septic arthritis can affect all ages, but is most common in the elderly, immunocompromised, children or premature neonates.

[2] Septic arthritis usually develops quickly, causing an acutely painful monoarthritis, tending to affect joints with good vascular supply to the metaphyses such as the knee (over 50% of cases), hip, shoulder, ankle, wrist, or occasionally multiple joints. Intravenous drug users may develop septic arthritis of the sternoclavicular joint. The majority, about 80%, develop pain, swelling, warmth and restricted movement of the joint.

[3] Risk factors for septic arthritis include older age, pre-existing joint disease such as gout, pseudogout, osteoarthritis, rheumatoid arthritis or Charcot arthropathy, immunosuppressed status including diabetes, recent joint surgery or intra-articular injection particularly with steroids, IV drug use, indwelling catheters or other potential sources for bacteraemia, and skin or soft tissue infection including ulcers.

[4] The most common route for pathogenesis of septic arthritis is via haematogenous spread, leading to suppuration within the joint space. Occasionally, spread can occur from direct inoculation from a penetrating wound, and rarely from extension from neighbouring infection such as chronic osteomyelitis, whereby infection can transcend the bony cortex and expel pus into the joint.

[5] Prosthetic joint infection is of particular concern. An early prosthetic joint infection typically occurs during the implantation, and is usually caused by *S. aureus*, Gram-negative bacilli, or polymicrobial infection. Early prosthetic joint infection usually presents acutely in a similar manner to native septic arthritis, with joint pain, erythema, warmth, effusion and fever. A patient with the above clinical features and a recent history of surgery should raise strong suspicion

for likely prosthesis infection. In delayed-onset prosthetic joint infection, occurring 3–12 months post-surgery, a more indolent course tends to be seen, usually with joint pain, implant loosening and frequently no fever. Causative organisms include coagulase-negative staphylococci, enterococci or *Propionibacterium* spp. Late-onset prosthetic joint infection tends to occur in a similar manner to most septic arthritis, due to haematogenous seeding, with similar organism profile. Complications include dislocation of the prosthesis and the requirement for removal of the prosthesis for source control.

[6] Recent antibiotic use may mask symptoms or cause a more indolent course as well as negative culture results. The indications for antibiotic use can identify potential organisms, for example streptococcal infection with recent treatment for pneumonia or gonococcal infection with treatment for STIs.

[7] Particular recent exposures can help guide clinical suspicion of the underlying organism and appropriate tests. History of recent animal bites, STIs and travel to areas with potential exposure to Lyme disease, *Mycobacterium tuberculosis*, and other pathogens is important to elicit. Immunisation status is important, particularly in children, and pneumococcal vaccination status is useful to note, although most cases of *Streptococcus pneumoniae* septic arthritis tend to be caused by non-vaccinable serotypes.

Examination

- The patient is **pyrexial** [1] with a temperature of 38.2°C, and has a tachycardia of 108/minute, normal blood pressure and respiratory rate.
- His left knee appears **swollen and red** [2] compared with the right knee, and is warm and painful to touch. An effusion is palpable, and movement of the knee is painful and restricted with both active and passive movement.
- The **overlying skin** [3] is tense but intact and there is no evidence of overlying cellulitis or of lesions elsewhere on the body.
- **All other joints** [4] are normal and non-tender to examine.
- **Examination of other organ systems** [5] is unremarkable.

[1] Patients are often pyrexial, although older adults may be afebrile. Many manifest with tachycardia. It is important to ascertain whether there are signs of haemodynamic compromise pointing towards sepsis as a complication. The diagnosis in infants and neonates tends to be more subtle, and there may be evidence of septicaemia, cellulitis, fever without a clear infective focus, or evidence of discomfort such as reduced use of the involved limb or distress at being picked up. Diagnosis in older children can also be difficult, and a new limp should raise concerns. Pain can be referred, on occasion mimicking intra-abdominal or pelvic pathology, e.g. with referred pain from sacroiliac joint septic arthritis.

[2] The septic joint is generally swollen and warm, although this may be more difficult to identify in particular joints such as the hip or spine. The joint tends to be painful, and usually an effusion is present. The pain and effusion often restrict the motion of the joint through both active and passive motion.

[3] It is important to examine skin condition, to identify potential unseen inoculation sites as well as evidence of sinus tracts. Old scars can give clues as to previous prosthetic joint surgery, and overlying cellulitis can give a clue as to the source or potential organism. Examination of the skin elsewhere in the body is important, to identify other rashes such as may occur with disseminated gonococcal or meningococcal infection.

[4] A fifth of patients with septic arthritis develop oligoarthritis or polyarthritis, particularly those who have a predisposing systemic condition such as rheumatoid arthritis or sepsis. If multiple joints appear to be involved, a viral, reactive arthritis or an inflammatory arthropathy become more likely than a bacterial arthritis.

[5] Examination should be thorough and signs of underlying infective endocarditis identified if present, as this may represent a source of haematogenous seeding of the joint. A high index of suspicion should be maintained if there are particular risk factors such as injecting drug use.

Investigations

- Blood tests are performed showing **raised inflammatory markers** [1] with raised white cells and CRP. Renal and liver function are normal, and HbA1c shows adequate diabetes control.
- **Blood cultures** [2] are performed, which are negative.
- **Imaging** [3] is performed: knee X-ray demonstrates features of osteoarthritis and ultrasound confirms the presence of an effusion.
- **Aspiration of synovial fluid** [4] is performed and **analysed** [5] with cell count and differential, crystal assessment under polarising microscope, and undergoes Gram stain and microbiological culture, finding evidence of purulent synovial fluid consistent with septic arthritis.
- *Pseudomonas aeruginosa* is **cultured** [6].
- No other examination of **synovial tissue** [7] is undertaken.

[1] Abnormal inflammatory markers such as raised WCC, CRP and ESR are common but not diagnostic of infection. Differentials include an inflammatory arthritis such as might be seen with a flare of gout or rheumatoid arthritis, and similar results would be expected in these conditions. Other differentials include a haemarthrosis, and raised inflammatory markers would be less likely in this instance.

[2] Two sets of blood cultures should be obtained, prior to antibiotic treatment. Blood cultures are positive in about 50% of cases, if the septic arthritis has occurred as a consequence of haematogenous seeding.

[3] Radiography may be normal in the early stages of septic arthritis, but frequently an effusion can be seen as well as

underlying bone and joint disease. If later in the disease process, there may be evidence of cartilage or subchondral bone destruction with narrowed joint space or bony erosions. Ultrasound is useful, particularly if effusions are not particularly large, to guide joint aspiration. Larger joints that yield difficulty in assessment of presence of effusion, such as sacroiliac joints, can benefit from imaging with CT or MRI; these modalities can provide more detailed information if underlying osteomyelitis is also suspected.

4 Aspiration of synovial fluid should be performed with aseptic technique. This can be carried out without radiographic guidance if the effusion is amenable and easy to access, but some joints may require radiographic guidance to safely access the fluid with asepsis, or may require surgical washout in theatre, such as the hip joint. The exception to this is if prosthetic joint infection is suspected, in which case aspiration of synovial fluid should not be attempted, and early Orthopaedic and Infectious Diseases opinions sought with a view to surgical washout in theatre.

5 Synovial fluid analysis is crucial to diagnosis. Gross appearance of the synovial fluid can be opaque or purulent if leucocyte count is high, suggestive of infection or inflammation. A haemorrhagic appearance is more suggestive of a haemarthrosis from trauma or coagulopathy. If the WCC is significantly raised (e.g. >2000 cells/µl), this is suggestive of an inflammatory or septic arthritis, or both; the counts are typically very high in septic arthritis, >20 000/µl or even higher if the causative organism is *S. aureus*. A lower

WCC is more consistent with non-inflammatory conditions such as trauma or osteoarthritis. The presence of crystals can suggest the presence of gout or pseudogout, but does not exclude a septic arthritis, therefore microbiological cultures should still occur. If no crystals are present and culture is negative, then diagnosis and further investigations are reliant on history and clinical suspicion. Treatment as septic arthritis may be prudent, and consideration given to mycobacterial or fungal culture among other investigations.

6 Septic arthritis is usually monomicrobial, frequently caused by *Staphylococcus aureus* which tends to spread via haematogenous seeding and adherence to the synovium. Other pathogens include *Streptococcus pneumoniae*, particularly in those with spleen disorders, Gram-negative bacilli, particularly in older, immunocompromised adults or IV drug users, *Neisseria gonorrhoeae* in younger adults or those with complement deficiency, and polymicrobial as a rare occurrence, usually in patients with penetrating wounds as the mode of seeding.

7 Biopsy of synovial tissue may be required for culture, if there is insufficient synovial fluid for diagnosis, if there is concurrent evidence of osteomyelitis, or if infection with a fastidious organism or mycobacterium is suspected. If gonococcal arthritis with *N. gonorrhoeae* is suspected, routine culture is insufficient and therefore specific culture for this organism should be requested from the laboratory. Nucleic acid amplification testing may be required to identify this organism. The patient should also be screened for STIs.

Management

Short-term

Provide **simple analgesia** [1] and antipyretics to the patient. The left knee joint should be drained via needle aspiration in the first instance but if the effusion reaccumulates and there is concern over **source control** [2], surgical drainage may be required. **Empiric** [3] systemic antimicrobial therapy should be commenced, then amended to targeted antipseudomonal therapy once this organism is identified and sensitivities confirmed.

Regular joint examination can assist with clinical **monitoring** [4] of the progression of the condition, alongside trends in inflammatory markers. **Duration** [5] of treatment should be considered alongside other clinical features such as bacteraemia or other complications such as endocarditis, and consideration given to the use of **outpatient antimicrobial**

therapy [6]. MDT involvement with physiotherapy and occupational therapy are essential. Inpatient care should aim to minimise the risk of **hospital-acquired complications** [7] with LMWH, glycaemic control, early mobilisation and aseptic technique for joint aspiration. If infection is not easily contained, liaison with surgical and orthopaedic colleagues is essential to establish whether **surgical intervention is required** [8].

Long-term

Once the acute episode of septic arthritis has resolved, it is important to educate the patient on their risk factors for **recurrence** [9] and provide advice on how to identify this early and seek medical advice accordingly. Close liaison with the patient's GP is important.

1 Analgesia is important to provide symptomatic relief to the patient, which will assist with examination, investigation and treatment of the septic arthritis. Improved pain control will also allow improved mobility and will assist with reducing risk of VTE from reduced mobility. Antipyretics will also assist with patient comfort.

2 Source control with removal of infected fluid from the joint is essential, as it is otherwise difficult for the infection to be expelled from this closed space. If easy to achieve, needle aspiration under aseptic technique can remove the infected synovial fluid; joints most amenable to this approach include the knee, wrist, ankle or elbow. Other joints are harder to achieve adequate drainage and may require arthroscopy or open surgical drainage in theatre. Joints with suspicion for foreign body should be explored surgically, as should joints with persistent effusion despite attempts at aspiration. If source control is not achieved adequately and in a timely manner, irreversible joint damage or osteonecrosis can occur.

3 Empiric antimicrobial therapy should be commenced once cultures are obtained. Local guidelines should be consulted and will cover most likely pathogens, particularly *Staphylococcus aureus*. Directed therapy should be initiated as soon as causative organisms are confirmed; daily review of antimicrobials should be undertaken to assess if current drug, dose and route remain the most appropriate. If cultures remain negative, an empirical therapy based on most likely and most serious infective organism is appropriate. Systemic therapy rather than intra-articular antibiotics is used, as adequate drug levels are achieved in the joint fluid, and serial joint injections carry a risk of iatrogenic infection.

4 Clinical assessment of swelling, erythema, pain, joint movement, systemic features such as fever, and reaccumulation of effusion will assist with following the progress of the infection alongside trends in inflammatory markers. If serial joint aspiration is performed, trends in cell counts, colony counts on culture, and overall appearance of fluid can also assist with monitoring response to treatment.

5 There is no specific consensus on the optimal duration of antimicrobial treatment for septic arthritis, and therefore duration will depend on clinical judgement, the causative organism and concurrent complications. Infections with concurrent endocarditis or bacteraemia, particularly with *S. aureus*, often require longer duration of treatment, with 2–4 weeks of IV therapy then oral therapy. Concurrent osteomyelitis or infection with pathogens that are difficult to treat often require longer courses of treatment.

6 Outpatient antimicrobial therapy may be required if there are complicating features requiring prolonged courses of antimicrobial therapy, and if the patient is suitable to undertake this treatment approach. A mobility assessment by physiotherapy and occupational therapy assessment will assist with identifying suitability for this.

7 The presence of an inflammatory process that reduces patient mobility increases the risk of VTE, and prophylaxis should be considered. Other hospital-acquired complications include pneumonia and iatrogenic complications of haemarthrosis or secondary joint infections; preventive measures should be enacted with early mobilisation and aseptic technique for joint aspiration with an experienced proceduralist, with radiological guidance as required.

8 Although around 90% of patients with septic arthritis achieve good recovery, a small proportion will have unsuccessful treatment of their septic arthritis, resulting in significant functional impairment, multiple surgical washouts, surgical prosthetic joint surgery, and at extremes patients may undergo amputation or die from infection. Mortality usually occurs in the presence of significant comorbidities such as advanced age, immunosuppression, disease of other organs, or in the presence of polyarticular arthritis, particularly due to *S. aureus*. IV drug use is also associated with poorer outcomes.

9 Underlying joint pathology such as gout, osteoarthritis or rheumatoid arthritis increases risk of recurrence, as does the presence of prosthetic material. The patient should be educated on any individual risk factors, and provided with advice on how to manage these risks, for example improved glycaemic control if they are diabetic. Advice on early symptoms and signs of recurrence should be given prior to discharge and a plan to access medical services outlined. A clear and timely discharge summary should be provided to the GP who will be involved with management of chronic pathological processes.

CASE 50: Urinary tract infections

History

- An **82-year-old woman** [1] presents with a **three-day history of dysuria and a one-day history of rigors, chills, vomiting and left flank pain** [2].
- She has **risk factors** [3] including recurrent urinary tract infections over the past 5 years but has no known history of kidney stones, renal transplant, neurogenic bladder, **urinary catheters** [4] or genitourinary operations.
- She is not known to be immunocompromised nor on any immunosuppressive medications. The patient was commenced on trimethoprim when the symptoms started, and a urine culture sent, but has **worsened despite this antibiotic treatment** [5].
- She resides in a care home, is not sexually active and has not travelled out of the country for over 10 years. Her medications include oral metformin for type 2 diabetes, propranolol for anxiety and citalopram for depression. She has no allergies.

[1] Urinary tract infections (UTIs) affect women more than men, presumed due to the shorter distance between the urethra and the anus, as well as the shorter distance for pathogens to travel up the urethra to the bladder. Pregnant women are another susceptible group, and are more likely to have recurrent bacteriuria and pyelonephritis than non-pregnant women. Asymptomatic bacteriuria is considered a medical concern in pregnant women, as up to a third will go on to develop a symptomatic UTI if not treated, which is associated with higher risk of pregnancy complications. Another important group is in renal transplant recipients, where UTIs are the most common infection post-transplant and are associated with rejection, impaired graft function and death.

[2] Cystitis refers to infection of the bladder and lower urinary tract, and classically presents with symptoms of dysuria, urgency and increased frequency of micturition, pain in the suprapubic region and haematuria. Pyelonephritis refers to infection of the upper urinary tract and kidneys, caused by bacterial ascent from the lower urinary tract, and may present with fever, nausea and vomiting, rigors, chills and flank pain or costovertebral angle tenderness. Prostatitis may present with pain in the pelvis or perineum. Signs of haemodynamic instability suggest septic shock in the context of urinary tract infection, usually as a result of systemic inflammatory response with development of abscess, or bacteraemia. In addition, specific populations may present with atypical symptoms: elderly patients may present with falls, undifferentiated fever or confusion, whilst patients with neurogenic bladder may present with increased spasticity or signs of autonomic dysreflexia with hypertension and bradycardia.

[3] Risk factors for UTIs include anatomical factors such as nephrolithiasis, previous genitourinary surgery, indwelling catheters and stents, cystocele and neurogenic bladder; physiological factors such as postmenopausal state, pregnancy; behavioural and psychosocial factors such as sexual intercourse including with a new partner, incontinence, cognition, use of particular contraceptives (spermicides, diaphragms); and systemic factors including immunocompromised state, diabetes mellitus, maternal history of UTIs and host genetics. Recurrent simple cystitis is common in women, particularly if the initial infection was caused by E. coli, with similar reasons as for UTIs in general. Host genetics are important to note, as there may be susceptibility of the host to specific pathogenic mechanisms displayed by bacteria like E. coli which bind to the uroepithelium.

[4] Bacteria commonly colonise long-term urinary catheters. Catheter-associated urinary tract infections (CAUTI) should be considered in catheterised patients only if systemic and/or genitourinary symptoms are present. CAUTI should not be assumed in the context of isolated bacteriuria or pyuria without accompanying symptoms. In fact, catheter specimens of urine should be collected only if genitourinary symptoms are present, and this information provided to the laboratory in order to assist with appropriate interpretation of results. Samples should be collected either after removing or replacing the indwelling catheter, and should not be collected from the catheter drainage bag.

[5] In a patient whose clinical state worsens despite treatment for UTI, consideration of multi-drug-resistant organism should occur. Risk factors for a multi-drug-resistant organism include previous resistant isolate or known colonisation, resident of a care facility or recent inpatient stay at a hospital or nursing home, travel to areas with known high rates of drug-resistant organisms, and recent exposure to antibiotics, particularly fluoroquinolones and broad-spectrum beta-lactam antibiotics.

Examination

- The patient appears slightly confused and is **disoriented to place** [1].
- She is warm to touch and **pyrexial at 38.4°C** [2].
- **Blood pressure is 130/80mmHg and heart rate is 84bpm** [3].
- On **abdominal examination** [4], mild suprapubic tenderness is present to gentle palpation, and tenderness is elicited at the left costovertebral angle to percussion.
- The bladder is not palpable, and **no other masses are palpable** [5].
- **Genitourinary examination** [6] shows vaginal atrophy and vaginal discharge with appearance of candidiasis. No other abnormalities are present throughout other organ systems.

[1] Elderly or otherwise vulnerable patients may present with fluctuating conscious state and may develop delirium. Screening for delirium can identify patients who may benefit from dedicated measures to reduce the morbidity and mortality associated with delirium. Importantly, altered mental status in the absence of other symptoms and signs of UTI should be investigated fully for other sources of infection. Asymptomatic bacteriuria, where bacteria are cultured but do not cause host infection, is common in the elderly and can lead to overdiagnosis of UTI, and thus overtreatment.

[2] Fever is suggestive of a complicated UTI rather than simple cystitis. Lack of fever does not exclude pyelonephritis, however, particularly in the elderly who may not mount a fever in the context of severe infection. A low index of suspicion should be maintained in the presence of other features of concern.

[3] Haemodynamic stability should be assessed, including early features of a systemic inflammatory response such as tachycardia. Any concurrent medications and their effects should be noted when evaluating haemodynamics, such as a blunted tachycardic response in the presence of beta blockers.

[4] Suprapubic tenderness is in keeping with cystitis, but may also represent urinary retention and the bladder should be percussed and palpated to identify whether retention is present. Pyelonephritis is suggested by the presence of costovertebral angle tenderness, particularly on percussion. Full abdominal examination should be undertaken to elicit features suggestive of an alternative diagnosis, such as appendicitis, hepatitis or diverticulitis. Pelvic examination may be useful in sexually active patients at risk for pelvic inflammatory disease, and in men with features suggestive of prostatitis, careful rectal examination may identify a tender or swollen prostate.

[5] Finding of an abdominal mass suggests the possibility of a renal or perinephric abscess, although focal tenderness is much more likely to be elicited than a palpable mass. The possibility of an underlying malignancy or other pathology should be considered in this setting.

[6] Genital examination is not specifically required for diagnosis of cystitis or pyelonephritis, but in the setting of recurrent UTIs it can identify treatable risk factors for recurrent cystitis, such as vaginal atrophy, and identify specific causes of symptoms of cystitis, such as candidal infection, of particular note in the diabetic patient.

Investigations

- **Blood tests** [1] are performed: a full blood examination shows raised neutrophils and thrombocytosis, renal function demonstrates a raised creatinine of 110µmol/L with corresponding eGFR of 45ml/min/1.73m², and a CRP is raised. Liver function and electrolytes are normal, and blood glucose level is raised at 9mmol/L.
- The **urine sample** [2] from the community shows mixed growth with large numbers of epithelial cells and commensal organisms. A dipstick urinalysis identifies leucocytes, erythrocytes and nitrites and a further urine specimen is sent for microscopy, culture and sensitivities.
- Two sets of blood cultures are sent prior to changing antibiotics, which are positive for **E. coli** [3] with **extended-spectrum beta-lactamase (ESBL) production** [4].
- A bedside **bladder scan** [5] shows post-void residual amount of 200ml of urine.
- **Imaging** [6] is performed: a renal tract ultrasound demonstrates a small renal abscess without complications of hydronephrosis or emphysema. A CT scan is performed with contrast 2 days later after renal function has improved, and demonstrates no calculi.
- **Sexually transmitted infection** [7] testing should be performed in at-risk patients.

1 Blood tests are useful to confirm raised inflammatory markers including white cells, particularly neutrophilia, thrombocytosis and raised CRP consistent with the acute phase reaction. Renal function should be noted carefully as this will help guide further investigations, including whether contrast should be administered, and treatment, including antibiotic dosing. Rapidly worsening renal function should also raise alarm bells for complications such as obstructive nephropathy, and warrants urgent investigation. Glycaemic control is important to note and control appropriately, and pregnancy test should be performed as clinically appropriate in women of childbearing age. Blood cultures are essential if features of sepsis are present.

2 Urinalysis is particularly useful in this setting and should be interpreted appropriately. Appropriate urine sampling is essential to ensure accurate results. Urine dipstick analysis testing should not be performed in the asymptomatic patient. Identification of leucocyte esterase suggests pyuria, and nitrites suggests the presence of Enterobacteriaceae, although false negative results can occur if infection is due to pathogens that cannot convert urinary nitrates to nitrite, such as *Enterococcus faecalis*. Urinalysis which is negative for both leucocyte esterase and nitrites has a high negative predictive value for UTI. When collecting samples for microscopy and culture, mid-stream sampling is important, excluding the initial stream which is usually contaminated by urethral contaminants. The presence of epithelial cells and mixed growth suggests poorly collected sample, and resampling indicated if ongoing symptoms. In care home residents, a mid-stream urine sample may be difficult to obtain; in-out urinary catheters or condom catheters may be used in this setting.

3 *E. coli* is the most common cause of simple cystitis as well as complicated UTI. Other common pathogens include *Pseudomonas* spp., Enterobacteriaceae (*Proteus, Klebsiella)*, Enterococci and staphylococcal infections including *Staphylococcus aureus* and *S. saprophyticus*. Risk factors for *Pseudomonas* include patients who have been exposed to healthcare facilities, or who have undergone surgery or instrumentation. Catheter-associated UTIs are caused by similar organisms to other UTIs and can be polymicrobial. The presence of *S. aureus* should be treated with importance and the potential for a concurrent bacteraemia from another source with overspill into the urinary tract considered. The presence of yeast such as *Candida* can be difficult to distinguish between sample contamination, colonisation or infection and should be interpreted in keeping with other clinical findings.

4 Drug resistance in urinary tract pathogens is increasing, particularly extended-spectrum beta-lactamase-producing pathogens. The presence of risk factors as previously described should raise concern for drug resistance, and antimicrobial treatment adjusted accordingly, including taking local resistance patterns into account. Analysing previous urine cultures can also identify whether drug-resistant organisms have previously been isolated in the patient, and if so, assumption of ongoing resistance is often appropriate whilst awaiting updated cultures.

5 A bladder scan is useful in identifying urinary retention, which may require urinary catheterisation, but also as an initial investigation to identify the presence of high post-void residual urine volumes that can predispose to UTIs. If present, the patient may benefit from referral for Urological input.

6 Imaging is not always warranted, and should be considered in systemically unwell patients, those who have persisting clinical symptoms despite appropriate treatment, and those where urinary tract obstruction is suspected. The main aim of imaging is to identify obstruction, renal calculi or a complication such as an abscess that requires intervention or source control. Renal tract ultrasound is useful to avoid contrast and radiation associated with CT. CT is more sensitive in identifying anatomical abnormalities, and can identify calculi, abscesses and haemorrhage easily. Renal perfusion changes require contrast administration.

7 Screening for STIs should be performed where indicated; gonorrhoeal and chlamydia urine PCR is easy to collect. Additional testing for syphilis, HIV and viral hepatitis (B and C) may be offered.

Management

Short-term

Initial management should include **resuscitation** [1] with IV fluids and inotropes as required. **Antimicrobial therapy** [2] should be initiated early, preferably after collection of urine and blood cultures, taking into account potential antimicrobial susceptibilities and in consultation with local guidelines and experts, and with appropriate de-escalation once culture and sensitivities are returned. Specific **urinary tract abnormalities** [3] should be assessed and managed appropriately. **Urological opinion** [4] may be required. In the presence of **delirium** [5], management should include minimising distress and morbidity associated with this complication. Appropriate measures for escalation of care [6] should be considered, particularly in this care home resident, and discussion with patient and family members prioritised in addition to use of existing documents such as Advanced Care plan. **Analgesia** [7] and **venous thromboembolism prophylaxis** [8] are essential components of care. Once improving, assessment by **multidisciplinary team** [9] including physiotherapist, occupational therapist and dietitian are important to assist with return of baseline functioning prior to discharge home.

Long-term

Discharge from hospital should be considered once the patient is clinically stable. Advice on **symptom recurrence** [10] should be provided, including when to seek medical assistance. **Education** [11] to the nursing home on assisting with accurate mid-stream urine sampling may assist with early diagnosis in future episodes. **Follow-up urinalysis** [12] may be considered in specific circumstances. **Preventive measures** [13] may be considered which are patient-dependent.

[1] Resuscitation is essential for the patient in septic shock, which can develop rapidly in the context of UTI as the source. If haemodynamic instability is present, IV fluids should be trialled, followed by inotropes if no response. The patient should be reviewed by ICU/HDU to consider supportive management whilst awaiting antibiotics to take effect.

[2] The choice of antimicrobial therapy will depend on local resistance patterns and guidelines, in combination with available data on previous susceptibilities. Empiric therapy should be given, and then individualised once more information becomes available. Antimicrobials with good penetration into the urinary system should be used, and specific host characteristics such as renal function and allergies should be taken into account. In a patient who has deteriorated despite standard treatment, drug resistance should be considered and incorporated into antimicrobial therapy decisions. Trimethoprim resistance is reported in around a fifth of *E. coli* isolates causing cystitis. In addition, a number of uropathogenic organisms demonstrate inducible beta-lactamase resistance, including *Serratia*, *Citrobacter* and *Proteus* and if identified as causative organisms, reports of susceptibility to beta-lactamases should be interpreted with caution and specialist advice sought.

[3] The presence of specific urinary tract abnormalities should be considered carefully. For example, the presence of a urethral stent or long-term indwelling catheter may be a factor in recurrence of UTIs, and changing or removal may be indicated, often with urological guidance. If post-void residual urine is present, this should be investigated, with consideration given to urodynamic studies and urological input.

[4] Urological opinion may be considered in the setting of renal stones, or in men with acute prostatitis, as this is considered a complicated UTI.

[5] Delirium is an important condition associated with increased morbidity and mortality, and is more likely to occur in susceptible patients such as the frail elderly. A holistic approach to this patient includes early identification of delirium and use of measures to reduce distress, minimise day–night reversal and facilitate measures to reduce delirium.

[6] It is important to take into account prior patient wishes when initiating treatment. If an Advance Care plan is present, this should be checked to ensure that all aspects of proposed treatment including antimicrobials are consistent with previously documented patient wishes.

[7] Analgesia should be provided, particularly in patients with pyelonephritis, but it is important to take both renal function and susceptibility to opiates into consideration when prescribing. Simple analgesia with paracetamol should be first-line and escalation to other analgesics should be patient-focused and individualised.

[8] Any patient admitted to hospital with an illness that reduces mobility and which increases the risk of VTE should be considered for pharmacological and mechanical prophylaxis.

[9] Infections and hospital admissions, particularly in those complicated by delirium, can impact severely on functional status in the elderly. Assessment by physiotherapists, occupational therapists and dietitian may be useful. In addition, consideration of specific services such as in-reach programmes which allow administration of parenteral antimicrobial therapy in the care home are useful in order to be able to continue appropriate care in a familiar environment, thus reducing the distress and potential for escalating delirium in susceptible patients.

[10] Patients who have recurrent symptomatic UTI should have repeat urine culture performed to identify resistant organisms. Men with recurrent UTIs should undergo urological evaluation to assess for chronic bacterial prostatitis; however, there is limited use for detailed urological investigations for women with recurrent UTIs.

[11] Education should be provided to the patient and if relevant, to carers, on early flagging of symptoms suggestive of cystitis or pyelonephritis. In the care home, acute dysuria is the most specific symptom to suggest symptomatic UTI. There are high rates of asymptomatic bacteriuria in care home residents, and it is important to educate regarding the lack of benefit of screening for and treating based on urinalysis only. It may be useful to consider a plan for patient-

initiated treatment, with antibiotics commenced at symptom onset. This course of action can be considered in women with two or more infections within 6 months, or 3 or more within 12 months. There is evidence to suggest that this approach reduces antibiotic use compared with antibiotic prophylaxis; however, medical review should be sought if symptoms persist despite treatment.

12 Follow-up testing is not generally required, but repeat urine culture should be considered to confirm the resolution of infection for asymptomatic pregnant women and men with prostatitis. In addition, samples with haematuria identified should be considered for repeat urinalysis to ensure resolution of haematuria, and consideration of further investigation with urinalysis to ensure resolution of haematuria, and consideration of further investigation with cytology and urological review if persistent, in case of underlying genitourinary malignancy.

13 Measures to prevent recurrence of urinary tract infections may be considered. Evidence exists to suggest that increased water intake may be useful in premenopausal women, and intravaginal oestrogen therapy may be beneficial due to effects on vaginal flora in postmenopausal women. Other approaches have limited or no evidence, including the use of ascorbic acid, cranberry products and methenamine hippurate. In patients with incontinence, meticulous hygiene measures should be implemented to reduce perineal contamination. Antibiotic prophylaxis may decrease the incidence of urinary tract infections in non-pregnant women, but side-effects include development of drug resistance, candidiasis and long-term effects particularly from nitrofurantoin, including pulmonary, hepatic and peripheral nerve toxicities. Strategies include continuous prophylaxis for 6 months, and intermittent postcoital prophylaxis. With regard to CAUTIs, limiting the use of urinary catheters unless specifically indicated is important, to reduce the infection rates.

CASE 51: Acute inflammatory demyelinating polyradiculoneuropathy

History

- A 34-year-old male taxi driver presents with **progressively worsening lower limb weakness over the last 1 week. The weakness was initially in the toes and ankles but now it has progressed to the level of the knees and hips** [1] . The patient requires the use of crutches to aid his mobility.

- The patient had an **episode of acute diarrhoea** [2] about 2 weeks prior to the current episode of weakness. He needed hospitalisation at the time, and stool MCS and PCR came back with positive result of *Campylobacter jejuni*. He was discharged after the diarrhoea resolved.

- Other than the weakness in the lower limbs, the patient also complains of **pins and needles sensation** [3] in the feet and lower leg bilaterally.

- The patient had no other symptoms and was not reporting any **dyspnoea** [4] .

- There was **no past history of similar episodes** [5] .

- He has **no significant past medical history** [6] . No significant family history was reported. The patient is on no regular medication.

- He **lives with his partner and two children** [7] .

[1] Acute inflammatory demyelinating polyradiculo-neuropathy (AIDP), or Guillain–Barré syndrome – AIDP variant, is an autoimmune process targeting the myelin layer in the peripheral nervous system. The weakness in AIDP is typically ascending motor weakness. The onset is usually acute in terms of time course (as its name suggests, AIDP is usually acute, i.e. <4 weeks). Myelin is the substance that helps with nerve conduction and provides a good living environment for the axon. The destruction of the myelin layer and hence the disruption of this environment results in axonal loss in demyelinating disease. Axonal loss is the core cause of the disabilities in any demyelinating disease.

[2] The development is often associated with preceding respiratory or GI infection. Classically, *Campylobacter jejuni* (shares epitopes with peripheral nerve gangliosides) is the associated organism. Other associated offenders include *Mycoplasma* species, acute viral hepatitis, CMV, EBV and influenza. The associated infective episode can happen in up to 50% of cases about 1–3 weeks before the onset of AIDP.

[3] The patient may complain of paraesthesiae or sensory loss in the limbs affected, although such symptoms are usually minimal. The patient may also experience neuropathic pain due to the destruction of the myelin layer and/or axon.

[4] It is important to explore whether the patient is experiencing any dyspnoea, because acute respiratory failure is one of the most feared complications in AIDP. Any cranial involvement, particularly bulbar lesions (any cranial nerve can be affected except I, II and VIII), should be asked about, as bulbar involvement can be associated with development of respiratory failure. Because autonomic dysfunction can happen in AIDP, it is important to ask whether the patient is experiencing any of postural hypotension, labile blood pressure, arrhythmias or sphincter dysfunction.

[5] The patient should be asked whether they have had any previous episodes of disease. This is because any relapsing course with involvement of sensory symptoms and proximal weakness is suggestive of chronic inflammatory demyelinating polyradiculopathy.

[6] Some precipitating events can contribute to the development of AIDP. Examples include surgical operation, vaccination, malignancy, SLE and HIV infection.

[7] Social history and family support are particularly important to explore, should the patient have any disability resulting from the illness.
Differential diagnoses based on the presenting symptoms are shown in the table below.

Differential diagnoses based on the presenting symptoms

Presenting symptoms	
Ascending muscle weakness	• Relapsed chronic inflammatory demyelinating polyradiculopathy (slower development, less extent, sensory changes including pain) • Acute intermittent porphyria • Diphtheria • Polio • Tick bites • Rhabdomyolysis • Arsenic poisoning • Botulism
Autonomic neuropathy	• Diabetes mellitus • Amyloidosis • Alcoholism • Acute intermittent porphyria

Examination

- A full neurological examination is performed. You noted that there is a pair of **crutches** [1] in the room.
- There is **no obvious muscular atrophy** [2] on inspection. The abnormalities are predominantly found in the bilateral lower limbs with symmetrical distribution.
- The tone is normal bilaterally with **loss of deep tendon reflexes** [3] despite reinforcement manoeuvre.
- The **power** [4] in the lower limbs appeared to be 4/5 in the hip and knee joints but 3/5 in the ankles and feet.
- The **sensation** [5] was intact in all modalities although the patient did occasionally report symptom of paraesthesia during the examination.
- The assessment of the **gait** [6] revealed high stepping gait with appearance of bilateral foot drop.
- The **cranial nervous system** [7] is also examined and there is no evidence of ophthalmoplegia. There is no cerebellar sign identified on examination.
- There is no vascular compromise or **tenderness in the muscles** [8].
- There is no evidence of **postural hypotension** [9] and the patient's cardiovascular examination is unremarkable.
- The **forced expiratory time** [10] is also measured and the patient finished expiration within 4 seconds.

1 Attention should be paid to the presence of walking aids in the room. This may give clinicians an idea of the extent of mobility impairment.

2 Predominantly, AIDP presents with distal muscle weakness without atrophy. If upper limbs are involved, they may be more affected than lower limbs. Any signs of secondary injury such as pressure sores and DVT should be checked in all bed-bound patients.

3 Tendon reflexes are reduced or absent.

4 Ascending muscle weakness in AIDP can be more prominent distally than proximal muscle groups.

5 Sensory loss in AIDP is usually minimal. If it is present, it usually affects the posterior columns (vibration and proprioception).

6 Gait in AIDP can be high stepping, resulting from bilateral foot drop.

7 The cranial nerve system should be examined for the presence of ophthalmoplegia. If ophthalmoplegia is present, it is suggestive of Miller Fisher variant, which typically presents with a triad of ophthalmoplegia, ataxia and areflexia.

8 Muscle tenderness is present in one-third of cases.

9 Autonomic neuropathy can happen in AIDP in the form of postural BP drop and cardiac arrhythmias.

10 Forced expiratory time is a useful clinical utility to assess a patient's respiratory function.

Investigations

- **Nerve conduction and electromyography (EMG)** [1] studies were requested. The nerve conduction study showed conduction in the peripheral nerves in the lower limbs bilaterally. There was no evidence of denervation shown on the EMG.
- The **monospot test and serologies** [2] for mycoplasma, HIV and CMV all came back negative.
- The **antiganglioside antibodies serology** [3] results are still pending.

- An inpatient **pulmonary function test** [4] was requested and it showed normal FEV$_1$ and FVC. The maximum inspiratory and expiratory pressures were also normal.
- The **MRI scan** [5] of the spine was also organised and it did not reveal any abnormality.
- The **ECG** [6] did not show any arrhythmias.
- A **diagnosis of AIDP** [7] is suspected.

[1] Nerve conduction and EMG studies can be used to support the clinical diagnosis of AIDP. Nerve conduction studies typically show slow conduction or conduction block, increased latencies, and F wave latency (can be the only early sign in Guillain–Barré syndrome – AIDP variant). EMG evidence of denervation can take at least 10 days to be evident. The presence of denervation indicates axonal involvement and hence worse prognosis.

[2] Immune stimulus can be tested by using monospot test, cold agglutinins, serologies for CMV, HIV or *Campylobacter* spp.

[3] Antiganglioside antibodies serology can be useful when differentiating variants of AIDP. Anti-GM1 and anti-GD3 are not sensitive. Anti-GM1 and anti-GD1a are associated with axonal variant. Anti-GQ1b Ab is found in 90% of Miller Fisher variant.

[4] Respiratory function tests (FEV$_1$ – forced expiratory volume in 1 second; and FVC – forced vital capacity) are used to assess the progressive involvement of respiratory muscles. Progression to respiratory failure can be rapid (even over hours), requiring intubation.

[5] Neuroimaging of the CNS is mainly used to exclude other possible causes of a patient's symptoms.

[6] ECG can be used to check for arrhythmias resulting from autonomic dysfunction.

[7] It is important to remember that AIDP is a clinical diagnosis. Cerebrospinal fluid examination can be used to look for raised protein level and the relative lack of white blood cells. This is mainly used when the diagnosis is in doubt.

Management

Immediate

The patient was admitted to the neurology ward for further inpatient monitoring of his neurological deficit. Unfortunately, as an inpatient he started to develop acute dyspnoea associated with oxygen desaturation. The patient was on prophylaxis for VTE at the time. An urgent assessment using portable spirometry was performed at the bedside and it showed **FVC of <1 litre** [1] in this patient. Intensive care team was contacted for much-needed critical care support. The patient continued to deteriorate and intubation was required. Permission to use inpatient **intravenous immunoglobulin** [2] was granted and this was administered in the ICU.

Short-term

It took days for the patient to recover from the respiratory paralysis. The patient was extubated before he was transferred back to the neurology ward. The patient's neurological deficits continued to improve while he was on the ward as an inpatient. An early referral to the **physiotherapist** [3] was made and an early physiotherapy programme was initiated. The neurological deficit completely resolved after the patient spent 2 months in a rehabilitation centre.

Prognosis

- Among those diagnosed with AIDP, about 2% die of respiratory failure, PE or arrhythmias. Dysautonomia is observed in two-thirds of cases. About 30% of cases need ventilation.
- 10% have major residual deficit resulting from the illness.

- Poor prognostic factors include rapid onset of symptoms, need of mechanical ventilation, *Campylobacter jejuni* and CMV infection, deficit not starting to improve within 3 weeks, or the presence of autonomic neuropathy.

1 Respiratory support in ICU is needed if FVC is <1 litre.

2 Intravenous immunoglobulin (IVIg) and plasma exchange are both effective treatments. Glucocorticoids are not beneficial in the treatment of AIDP. Oral steroids are contraindicated because they worsen the outcome. Plasma exchange or IVIg shortens time to recovery from respiratory paralysis and hastens the return of mobility. There is no additional benefit to combine plasma exchange with IVIg.

3 Physiotherapy is helpful in preventing contractures. Pressure care and VTE prevention should be considered as a routine practice for a medical inpatient with impaired mobility, if they are not contraindicated. 90% make complete recovery over time, up to a year.

CASE 52: Acute intracerebral haemorrhage

History

- A 22-year-old male university student was brought in by ambulance with altered conscious state at 1900 hours. The patient was intubated on the scene by the paramedics due to a Glasgow Coma Scale (GCS) score of 3. The collateral history was taken from his friend.
- The patient had gone to **play golf** [1] with his friend earlier that afternoon at about 1400 hours.
- He was **hit by a golf ball just behind his right ear** [2]. He was knocked out briefly but later woke up and complained of a mild headache.
- The patient **seemed to be well other than ongoing headache** [3] at the time, according to his friends. They later went to the pub for a drink and

without warning the patient lost consciousness. There was no seizure-like activity such as tonic-clonic movement, tongue biting or incontinence. The ambulance was then called.
- **A traumatic intracranial haemorrhage** [4] **was suspected** [5] **and urgent neuroimaging was requested** [6].
- Meanwhile, the patient was kept intubated due to **the ongoing loss of consciousness** [7] and critical care team consult was requested.
- The patient has **no significant past medical history** [8]. There is no family history of early stroke, intracerebral blood vessel malformation or bleeding diathesis.

[1] Most cases of traumatic intracranial haemorrhage take place during routine activities.

[2] A traumatic aetiology of intracerebral haemorrhage can be diagnosed based on the history of recent trauma and lesions in the location of traumatic injury. Epidural haemorrhage is the bleeding between the dura and the skull. Epidural haemorrhage is uncommon but can be a serious complication of head injury. Again, most cases of epidural haemorrhage are due to head trauma. Epidural haemorrhage is most commonly due to arterial injury. This is different in the case of subdural haemorrhage, where the haemorrhage usually results from venous injury. Non-traumatic acute epidural haemorrhage is rare. Some patients with acute epidural haemorrhage may present with transient loss of consciousness. Characteristically there is a 'lucid interval' with recovery from the initial unconsciousness after the head injury, followed by deterioration over a period of time due to continued arterial bleeding resulting in haematoma expansion.

[3] Intracerebral haemorrhage is the second most common cause of stroke after ischaemic stroke.

[4] There are many ways to categorise the types of intracerebral haemorrhage. Based on mechanism of bleeding, intracerebral haemorrhage is categorised into two types: traumatic and non-traumatic. Based on location of bleeding, it can be categorised into three types: epidural, subdural and subarachnoid.

- Subdural haemorrhage is the bleeding between dura and arachnoid membranes. Head trauma is the most common cause of subdural haemorrhage. The majority of cases result from the rupture of bridging veins between brain surface and the dural sinuses. The bleeding is usually stopped by the increased intracranial pressure and/or direct compression from the clot formed. Arterial bleeding can also happen in 20% of cases. Risk factors for subdural haemorrhage include cerebral atrophy, the elderly, history of chronic alcohol abuse, and previous traumatic brain injury. Although classically described in the epidural haemorrhage, a 'lucid interval' can also happen in about 25% of subdural haemorrhage cases.
- Spontaneous intracerebral haemorrhage is considered non-traumatic. Hypertensive vasculopathy is the most common aetiology of spontaneous intracerebral haemorrhage in general, and cerebral amyloid angiopathy is the most common cause of non-traumatic lobar intracerebral haemorrhage in older adults. Vascular malformations are the most common cause in the paediatric population.
- Subarachnoid haemorrhage is bleeding within the subarachnoid space. In most cases, subarachnoid haemorrhage results from the rupture of an intracranial aneurysm. In contrast to hypertensive intracerebral haemorrhage, where the neurological signs and symptoms are usually gradually increasing, the neurological signs and symptoms in subarachnoid haemorrhage are usually at their maximum from onset. The primary symptom of subarachnoid haemorrhage

is a sudden, severe headache. Patients often describe such headache as the worst headache they've ever had. Nausea or vomiting can also be quite common in subarachnoid haemorrhage. Meningeal irritation may not happen until several hours after the bleed, since it is caused by the breakdown of the blood products leading to aseptic meningitis. Sudden onset headache, regardless of severity or prior history of headache, should always raise clinical suspicion for subarachnoid haemorrhage. The suspicion becomes higher when other features, such as altered consciousness, vomiting and meningismus, are involved.

5 Clinical suspicion for intracerebral haemorrhage should be raised when patients present with acute onset of gradually worsening symptoms, particularly if associated with headache, vomiting, severe hypertension and altered conscious state or coma.

6 A prompt investigation and management plan can be life-saving in the case of intracranial haemorrhage.

7 Symptoms of intracerebral haemorrhage can be highly variable, depending on the location and size of the bleed. Often, patients present with an acute onset of focal neurological deficit that corresponds to the part of the brain affected, and hence neuroanatomy can be quite handy. As the bleed increases in size, the neurological symptoms and signs can increase gradually over time, ranging from minutes to hours. Headache, vomiting and altered conscious state can also develop if the intracerebral haemorrhage is significant in size. Seizure is an important complication of intracerebral haemorrhage and it happens in 15% of patients, more often in those with more superficial bleeds.

8 Major risk factors for spontaneous intracerebral haemorrhage are hypertension, the elderly, the presence of cerebral amyloid angiopathy and the use of anticoagulant therapy.

Examination

- Due to the patient's unconsciousness (GCS of 3 and **intubated** [1]), a neurological examination could not be carried out properly.
- **Patient's pupils were first examined, which revealed bilateral dilated pupils not responsive to light** [2].
- The fundoscopy examination of the fundi revealed **papilloedema of the optic disc** [3] bilaterally.
- The **gag reflex was absent** [4].
- The examination of all four limbs revealed **increased tone and hyperreflexia** [5] in all four limbs, but more prominent in the left upper and lower limbs.
- There was an area of **bruising identified behind the patient's right ear** [6].

1 The examination actually focuses on the assessment of the patient's neurological status, such as the conscious state, as such patients usually present with impaired consciousness or coma. In such situations, it is important to remember that protection of the airway is vital.

2 Full neurological examination is needed provided that the patient is able to participate. However, if patients present with impaired conscious state, the neurological examination would be limited. Pupillary size and response to light can be useful. Pupillary dilation can be an early sign of brain herniation.

3 The papilloedema of optic disc on fundoscopy can also provide vital clues about whether there is an increase in intracranial pressure.

4 Gag reflex can be used to assess cranial nerve IX.

5 Tone and reflexes can be tested in all four limbs. The presence of upper motor neurone signs can be suggestive of CNS damage.

6 Retroauricular or mastoid ecchymosis (Battle sign) and periorbital ecchymosis (raccoon or panda eyes) can be used to diagnose basilar skull fractures. However, it may not appear immediately after the injury and may take 1–3 days to appear. Even if the patient has no evidence of intracranial haemorrhage, those with basilar fracture can have significant risk of future intracranial bleeding. Hence the neurosurgical consultation is needed regardless. It is important to acknowledge that examination plays a limited role in the diagnosis or exclusion of intracerebral haemorrhage and neuroimaging is usually required when intracerebral haemorrhage is suspected.

Investigations

- An **urgent CT brain with no contrast** [1] was carried out.
- While the CT scan did not show any features of cerebral ischaemia, it did reveal a massive **bi-convex** [2] shaped hyperdensity in the right hemisphere region.
- The hyperdensity appears to be **heterogeneous** [3] and sharply demarcated.

- There was also a **marked midline shift** [4] and features suggestive of hydrocephalus in the left lateral ventricle.
- **A fracture in the temporal bone** [5] was also revealed.
- Several adjunct pathology tests were also ordered. **The full blood count, electrolytes, renal function and coagulation profile all came back unremarkable** [6].

[1] Brain haemorrhage and ischaemia cannot be distinguished based on clinical characteristics alone. Neuroimaging with CT brain or MRI is mandatory to confirm the diagnosis of intracerebral haemorrhage. It is also useful in terms of excluding other possible causes, such as ischaemic stroke and stroke mimics. Non-contrast CT brain is more readily available than MRI and is a useful screening test for intracerebral haemorrhage. One downside of this imaging is that it cannot fully exclude subarachnoid haemorrhage when the clinical suspicion is high. In this case, lumbar puncture is usually required. CT angiography or MRI angiography can be useful in terms of identifying aneurysms, vascular malformations and moyamoya disease ('puff of smoke' appearance of collateral vessels on imaging, high risk of rupture). If cerebral venous thrombosis is one of the differential diagnoses, angiography combined with venous phase, i.e. venography, can be used.

Hypertensive haemorrhages tend to occur in the territory of penetrator arteries from the major intracerebral arteries, as they are directly exposed to the pressure of the much larger parent major vessels with no transition of vessel calibre. The locations are usually the same as those affected by hypertensive occlusive disease and diabetic vasculopathy. Common areas affected include pons and midbrain (supplied by penetrators which branch off the basilar artery), thalamus (penetrators branch off the posterior cerebral arteries), and putamen and caudate (penetrators branch off the middle cerebral artery).

In contrast cerebral amyloid angiopathy is an important cause of primary lobar intracerebral haemorrhage. The deposition of congophilic material in small- to medium-sized blood vessels weakens the structure of the vessel walls and makes then structurally prone to bleeding. The location of bleed helps differentiate cerebral amyloid angiopathy-related bleeds from those caused by hypertensive vasculopathy, which is more often seen in putamen, thalamus and pons, as mentioned above.

[2] Because of the presence of firm dural attachment, the collection of haemorrhage usually appears to be bi-convex in the case of epidural haemorrhage. Because subdural haemorrhage can cross sutural margins, it can typically give a crescent-shaped lesion on non-contrast CT brain. In contrast, epidural haemorrhage characteristically gives a lens-shaped appearance (orange) (see *Figure 52.1*).

[3] Heterogeneous appearance of haemorrhagic collection on CT is called swirl sign. This usually indicates active bleed in the intracranial space, with non-clotted fresh blood being less hyperdense than blood clot. This indicates urgent neurosurgical evaluation.

[4] The presence of significant mass effect indicates large haematoma. This is important in making management decisions as the volume of the haematoma correlates with the patient's outcome.

[5] Basilar fracture occurs most frequently through the temporal bone and hence the risk of having epidural haemorrhage is high.

[6] Pathology blood tests are usually supportive but not for diagnostic purposes. Full blood count, electrolyte, renal function and coagulation profile can be helpful when planning management after the diagnosis of intracerebral haemorrhage is made. In addition, those blood tests can provide useful baseline information when the patient is receiving postoperative care. Lumbar puncture is essential if there is a strong suspicion of subarachnoid haemorrhage despite a normal non-contrast CT brain. Elevated opening pressure, elevated red blood cell count, and the presence of xanthochromia can be helpful when performing cerebrospinal fluid analysis for the diagnosis of subarachnoid haemorrhage. A normal non-contrast CT brain and negative lumbar puncture effectively rule out the diagnosis of subarachnoid haemorrhage.

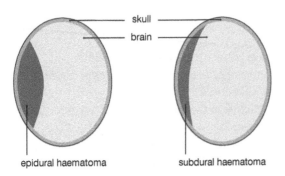

Figure 52.1 *Appearance of epidural haematoma versus subdural haematoma.*

Management

Immediate

The patient was first clinically assessed based on the algorithm of **ABCDE (Airway, Breathing, Circulation, Disability, Exposure/Examination)** [1]. Due to his compromised conscious state (with GCS of 3), the patient was kept intubated while all other investigations were under way. The patient was monitored closely in a **critical care environment with frequent neurological observations** [3] being performed. Once the urgent CT brain came back with the evidence of epidural haemorrhage, the neurosurgical team was contacted for **urgent neurosurgical input** [2]. Since the patient was normally not on any anticoagulant or antiplatelet and there was no evidence suggestive of coagulopathy, **no reversal agent such as vitamin K** [3] was given as part of the management plan.

Short-term

Due to the presence of a heterogeneous collection noted on the neuroimaging, it was highly suggestive that the patient might have ongoing bleed contributing to the **current impaired conscious state** [4]. The decision from the urgent neurosurgical consultation was to perform an **urgent craniotomy with clot evacuation** [5]. The operation itself was uncomplicated and the clot was evacuated successfully and an **external ventricular drain (EVD) was inserted** [6]. There was no bone fragment seen in the intracranial space. The patient was then transferred to the **ICU for further postoperative monitoring** [7]. The patient's conscious state showed improvement when he was monitored in the ICU. He was then extubated on day 3 postoperatively. Unfortunately, he then suffered a generalised tonic-clonic seizure. An urgent CT brain

was performed and it revealed no new collection or bleeding. The CSF from the EVD appears to be clear. He was **afebrile** [8] but biochemistry profile showed **sodium of 114. Hypertonic saline was administered in consultation with the Endocrinology team. Frequent monitoring of the sodium level was in place to avoid overcorrection of the sodium in the setting of severe symptomatic hyponatraemia** [9].

Long-term

Despite the complicated postoperative course, the patient recovered reasonably well. He is now alert and oriented with no cognitive impairment. His repeated sodium is 136 and there was no further seizure episode while he was transferred to normal neurosurgical ward. However, the patient does complain of ongoing left-sided weakness. The weakness was validated on neurological examination and the repeated neuroimaging showed no signs of cerebral ischaemia. **Early physiotherapy** [10] was requested and the patient was transferred to the rehabilitation ward after the recommendation was made by the physiotherapist.

Prognosis

After 1 month spent in the rehabilitation centre, the patient was fully recovered with no residual neurological deficit [11]. Thanks to the prompt treatment and intervention he received, he was then able to return to his university and finish his degree in biomedicine. He is now planning to seek the opportunity to obtain a medical degree and aims to become a neurosurgeon in the future.

1 Close monitoring of regular vital signs such as breathing and neurological observation such as GCS is needed. When the state of consciousness is impaired and a patient has lost their own airway protection, intubation and mechanical ventilation are required for ventilator support. Patients with hypotension need fluid resuscitation to maintain cerebral perfusion. The critical care team should be consulted, although usually this would have already been done in the ED.

2 Intracerebral haemorrhage is a neurological and medical emergency and anyone who is looking after patients with intracerebral haemorrhage should be on high alert. This is mainly because intracerebral haemorrhage is associated with high risk of ongoing bleeding, progressive neurological deterioration, permanent disability and death. Neurosurgical opinion should always be sought upon the diagnosis of intracerebral haemorrhage.

3 If the patient is on anticoagulant, such as warfarin and DOACs, haematology opinion should be sought regarding reversal. Reversal agents for warfarin include vitamin K, prothrombin complex concentrate and frozen fresh plasma. The choice of treatment combination depends on the patient's INR and usually an intensive treatment regime is required as intracerebral haemorrhage can potentially be life-threatening. Dabigatran has its reversal agent, idarucizumab, which is becoming increasingly available. Andexanet alfa is the newly developed antidote for rivaroxaban and apixaban and is not widely available. The treatment options for rivaroxaban and apixaban reversal are very limited. Protamine can be useful in the reversal of heparin. Low molecular weight heparin can only be partially reversed by protamine. Again, Haematology input is important in such situation.

4 Enlargement of haemorrhage is generally associated with neurological deterioration and worse outcomes. Therefore, if there is a deterioration observed on the neurological observation chart, it is vital to repeat neuroimaging and ensure that there is no expansion of the bleeding.

5 Epidural haemorrhage is a neurological emergency that needs prompt stabilisation and interventional treatment to reduce the likelihood of impact from the secondary brain injury from hypoxia, ischaemia and cerebral oedema. The decision of operative vs. conservative management needs to consider multiple factors: GCS, CT brain findings, neurological examination including pupillary signs, clinical stability, acuity of haemorrhage, age and comorbidities. Once the decision is made for surgery, craniotomy and haematoma evacuation are the usual surgical interventions employed for epidural haemorrhage. The elevation of intracranial pressure can be managed with head elevation, hyperventilation (with the aim of $PaCO_2$ 35–40mmHg), and osmotic diuresis using IV mannitol or hypertonic saline. Steroid therapy is not indicated following head injury. Non-operative management is considered for those who are mildly symptomatic, volume of haemorrhage <30cm³ with clot thickness <15mm on CT brain and midline shift <5mm, and no coma with GCS >8 and no focal neurological deficits.

6 An EVD can be inserted for intracranial pressure monitoring and the CSF can be monitored for rebleed or presence of intracranial infection post neurosurgical intervention.

7 The patient is generally transferred to ICU postoperatively for ongoing monitoring for any signs of improvement or deterioration.

8 Any febrile episode with neurological event after any neurosurgical intervention should raise the suspicion of meningitis, encephalitis or intracerebral abscess. CSF analysis and ongoing EVD monitoring can be useful when investigating the cause of a patient's fever.

9 Hyponatraemia after neurosurgery is not uncommon, especially in the presence of traumatic brain injury. Severe, symptomatic acute hyponatraemia requires the administration of hypertonic saline; urgent Endocrinology consultation is also required. However, overly rapid correction of sodium should be avoided, given the risk of osmotic demyelination syndrome, which can carry significant risk of mortality and morbidity.

Acute symptomatic subdural haemorrhage is another neurological emergency that often needs surgical intervention to prevent irreversible brain damage and mortality caused by haematoma expansion, increase in ICP and even brain herniation. Once the decision is made, the neurosurgeons can perform surgical evacuation of symptomatic acute subdural haemorrhage by burr hole trephination, craniotomy or decompressive craniectomy. Small haematoma with thickness <10mm and no clinical or CT signs of brain herniation or elevated ICP may be appropriate for conservative management. Patients who are not surgical candidates due to comorbidities should also be considered for conservative management if the perioperative risk outweighs the benefit.

The management of subarachnoid haemorrhage is a bit different from epidural and subdural haemorrhage. Patients are usually admitted to ICU for ongoing haemodynamic and neurological monitoring. Bed rest, analgesia, VTE prophylaxis using pneumatic compression stockings, and discontinuation of antithrombotics constitute the initial management plan of subarachnoid haemorrhage. After the aneurysm causing subarachnoid haemorrhage is identified, aneurysm repair should be organised as it is the only effective treatment. This should happen within 24–72 hours if possible, because the risk of rebleeding is high. Both coiling and clipping are considered viable treatment options. Hyponatraemia is common and regular monitoring of sodium is required. Fluid status should aim for euvolaemia. Hyperglycaemia is known to be associated with poor outcomes after subarachnoid haemorrhage and hence good glycaemic control is required. Fever is common in subarachnoid haemorrhage and is associated with a poor prognosis. Septic screen is needed before claiming the fever as non-infectious. Symptomatic vasospasm and cerebral infarction are poor prognostic factors. Nimodipine can be used in diffuse vasospasm involving small blood vessels and euvolaemia should be maintained. Hydrocephalus is a common complication of subarachnoid haemorrhage and a ventricular drain is usually inserted to improve the patient's condition. However, ventriculitis is a common complication of external drainage of CSF.

10 Long-term management usually depends on the patient's progress throughout the course of admission. For those with neurological deficits, a period of rehabilitation with MDT input can be helpful. If the patient was previously on anticoagulants or antiplatelets, the benefit of medications and the risk of having bleeding in the future need to be re-addressed.

There is a correlation between aneurysmal subarachnoid haemorrhage and other medical conditions such as autosomal dominant polycystic kidney disease and glucocorticoid-remediable aldosteronism. In such cases, screening for intracranial aneurysm in family members is reasonable.

11 With prompt intervention and appropriate care for postoperative complications, the long-term prognosis is generally pretty good. The patient in this scenario initially had unfavourable prognostic factors, such as impaired conscious state and massive size haematoma with mass effect, but he managed to recover fully with no residual deficit. The hospital journey was, however, quite long. Extension of intracerebral haemorrhage into the intraventricular space can happen and is usually associated with significant complications and worse outcomes. Minimising secondary brain ischaemia and haemorrhage enlargement in the early hours confers better outcome for the patient. As mentioned above, epidural haemorrhage is usually arterial in nature. Unchecked haematoma expansion leads to elevated ICP. Eventually brain herniation and death can occur unless immediate decompression is undertaken. Subarachnoid haemorrhage is associated with a high mortality and survivors of aneurysmal subarachnoid haemorrhage continue to have higher mortality rate when compared with the general population, mainly contributed by cerebrovascular events.

CASE 53: Dementia

History

- An **87-year-old** [1] male retired accountant was brought in by his wife for an outpatient review of his progressive cognitive decline over the last 5 years.
- The wife reports that the patient was noticed to have **significant memory issues** [2].
- While **long-term memory seems to be preserved** [3], short-term memory loss was becoming more prominent over time. He got lost twice over the last 3 months when he went out walking his dog. He also forgot to turn the gas stove off about 3 times over the last 6 months.
- Recently he was also noticed to have issues with **problem solving** [4].
- **His speed of processing information** [5] also seemed to be much slower compared with his baseline cognitive function 5 years ago.

- The patient **denies any issues with his memory** [6].
- He also denies that there was any history of **visual hallucination** [7] and this was confirmed by his wife.
- There is no history of changes in the patient's **social behaviour or personality** [8].
- There is no history of stroke, transient ischaemic attack, frequent falls or head trauma. There is no family history of early onset dementia or Down syndrome. He is an ex-smoker but does not have a history of excessive alcohol consumption. His past medical history includes hypertension, insulin-dependent diabetes mellitus, morbid obesity, hypercholesterolaemia, ischaemic heart disease with previous acute myocardial infarction treated with coronary bypass surgery, and peripheral vascular disease.

[1] Alzheimer's disease is a disease of older age. Its incidence and prevalence increase with age. Early-onset Alzheimer's disease is unusual (it accounts for about 1% of all Alzheimer's disease) and is defined as an onset <65 years of age. It often presents with atypical symptoms and frequently presents in the fifth decade. The patient usually has strong family history, typically in an autosomal dominant pattern. The genes involved are usually the ones that alter beta amyloid protein production and metabolism, such as *APP*, presenilin-1 and presenilin-2. Down syndrome gives additional gene dose of *APP* and hence contributes to the development of Alzheimer's disease. The presenilin-1 mutations have the earliest median age of onset at about the age of 43. Sleep disturbances are common in patients with Alzheimer's disease, with patients often complaining of more fragmented sleep.
Seizures can happen in the late stages of disease. The risk is higher in those with autosomal dominant form of Alzheimer's disease in the early course of disease.

[2] In terms of the clinical presentation, memory impairment is the most common initial symptom of Alzheimer's disease, with declarative episodic memory often profoundly affected. This type of memory depends heavily on the hippocampus. Memory of recent events is prominently impaired early and immediate memory is usually spared early on.

[3] Long-term memory (years ago) is also relatively spared early on.

[4] Executive dysfunction and visuospatial impairment are often present relatively early, usually in the form of difficulties in judgement and problem solving, ranging from subtle to prominent. Patients' procedural and motor learning memories are relatively spared until quite late in the disease. In addition, their memory in vocabulary and concepts often become impaired late in disease. Deficits in language and behavioural symptoms (neuropsychiatric) often manifest late, ranging from apathy to aggression and psychosis.

[5] Vascular disease contributes to 25–50% of all dementias and vascular dementia is the second most common type of dementia in population-based studies. Vascular dementia is often considered as any dementia that is primarily caused by cerebrovascular disease or compromised cerebral blood flow. Because it often coexists with other types of dementia of ageing, such as Alzheimer's disease (the most common coexist pathology), it is challenging to quantify its contribution to patients' cognitive decline in the clinical setting. Vascular dementia is typically recognised in two clinical scenarios. Any cognitive decline after a clinically diagnosed stroke should promote suspicion of vascular dementia. However, patients may present with progressive cognitive decline without any recent stroke and this is usually attributed to patients' 'covert' cerebrovascular disease. The cognitive profile in vascular dementia is characterised by the prominent impairment of executive function, while the episodic memory is often spared. Structural

imaging such as MRI brain should be performed to assess any clinically unrecognised cerebrovascular disease. The identification of history of stroke and/or the presence of 'silent' cerebrovascular disease on neuroimaging is required for the diagnosis of vascular dementia. The management of vascular dementia consists of the secondary prevention of cerebrovascular disease and the use of donepezil and memantine. The optimisation of blood pressure control is highly recommended. Although diabetes and cholesterol control are beneficial in the secondary prevention of stroke, their role in the prevention of vascular dementia is not clearly established. The same principle applies to the use of antiplatelet and homocysteine-lowering therapy. There is no convincing evidence regarding whether the use of donepezil and/or memantine is beneficial. However, given the high incidence of coexisting Alzheimer's disease, their use is reasonable.

6 Reduced insight is common and hence it is important to interview family members to get collateral history.

7 Dementia with Lewy bodies (DLB) is a different entity from Alzheimer's disease. With the onset around age 75, DLB has male predominance and the pathology is associated with cholinergic deficit and presence of Lewy bodies in the brainstem, limbic areas and cortex. Its central feature is the progressive cognitive decline of sufficient magnitude to interfere with normal social or occupational function. Its core clinical features include fluctuating cognition, recurrent visual hallucinations with one or more spontaneous cardinal features of parkinsonism, and rapid eye movement (REM) sleep behaviour disorder. The functions affected typically include attention, executive function, psychomotor speed, constructional praxis and visuo-perceptual functioning. With the presence of fluctuating cognition, recurrent visual hallucination and inattention, DLB can be easily mixed up with delirium. Due to the neuroleptic sensitivity of patients with DLB, the use of antipsychotics needs particular attention from the clinician. This sensitivity can be explained by the cholinergic deficit in DLB and the anticholinergic property of atypical antipsychotics used widely nowadays. While not diagnostic, patients with DLB may present with other supportive clinical features overlapping with Parkinson's disease, such as autonomic features (postural instability, severe autonomic dysfunction), hyposmia, apathy and recurrent falls. Certain psychiatric features may also be present such as hallucinations in other modalities, systematised delusions (a fixed, false system of belief with complex logical structure, constructed in order to protect coherence of a single central delusion) and mood disorders (depression and anxiety). There are now biomarkers available for DLB and they may be used to assist the diagnostic process of DLB or in research. These include low dopamine transporter uptake in basal ganglia demonstrated by SPECT or PET imaging, abnormal MIBG (meta-iodobenzylguanidine) myocardial scintigraphy, and polysomnic confirmation of REM sleep without atonia. Other supportive biomarkers include preserved medial temporal lobe structures on CT/MRI

compared with Alzheimer's disease, generalised low uptake on HMPAO (hexamethylpropyleneamine oxime) SPECT/PET perfusion/metabolism scan with reduced occipital activity with cingulate island sign on FDG (fludeoxyglucose)-PET, and prominent posterior slow wave activity on EEG with periodic fluctuations in the pre-alpha/theta range. The management of DLB can be complex. As in the case of Alzheimer's disease, the screening tests for the reversible causes of a patient's dementia should be carried out. Again, assessing and prioritising issues for patient and carer are important. Review of a patient's medications is a must-do and if appropriate, stepwise removal of deliriogenic, hallucinogenic medications should be planned for (via gradual withdrawal). This is especially true with anticholinergics and dopamine agonists. Pharmacological therapy for cognition may be considered. Donepezil and memantine were originally developed to be used in Alzheimer's disease but they may be considered for use in DLB. However, the evidence for the use of donepezil is limited and for memantine it is mixed. For psychotic symptoms of DLB, cautious use of atypical antipsychotics is advised due to increased sensitivity. Quetiapine can be considered as the first line of antipsychotic therapy and whatever antipsychotics are given, the principle of 'start low and go slow' should always be used in the elderly population. Antidepressants may be used for depressive symptoms; however, tricyclic antidepressants should be avoided at all cost due to their anticholinergic property. Melatonin is considered the first-line therapy for REM sleep behavioural disorders, given its lower risk of side-effects compared with benzodiazepines (e.g. confusion and paradoxical agitation). Treatment of Parkinsonian symptoms in DLB is similar to that for in Parkinson's disease, although patients are usually less responsive.

8 Frontotemporal dementia (FTD) is another mentionable group of neurodegenerative disorders characterised by prominent changes in social behaviour and personality, or aphasia accompanied by degeneration of the frontal and/or temporal lobes. FTD is one of the more common causes of early-onset dementia, with an average age of symptom onset in the sixth decade. Some patients with FTD also develop a concomitant motor syndrome such as parkinsonism or motor neurone disease (MND). There are three distinguishable clinical presentations, including behavioural variant FTD (bvFTD), primary progressive aphasia (PPA) non-fluent variant, and primary progressive aphasia (PPA) semantic variant. Behavioural variant frontotemporal dementia (bvFTD) is the most common clinical subtype. It accounts for about half of all cases of FTD. The hallmark of bvFTD is the progressive change in personality and behaviour. The early behavioural changes usually include disinhibition (may be reported as socially inappropriate behaviours), apathy and loss of empathy (loss of interest and/or motivation for activities and social relationships), hyperorality (altered food preferences, binge eating), and compulsive behaviours (perseverative stereotyped, or compulsive ritualistic behaviours). The patients typically score well on neuropsychological testing in the early stage of the disease, although their executive functions and verbal fluency decline as the disease progresses. In contrast to Alzheimer's disease, the memory and visuospatial functions are usually spared in FTD. MRI brain is often required to exclude structural pathology and may provide supportive findings. The neuroimaging can be normal in the early course of the disease but will show focal frontal or temporal atrophy as the disease progresses. The diagnosis is primarily made by clinical assessment, with any three of the clinical features of disinhibition, apathy or inertia, loss of sympathy and/or empathy, perseverative or compulsive behaviours, hyperorality, and dysexecutive neuropsychological profile. There is no effective treatment available for bvFTD. The aim of currently recommended management strategies is to ameliorate the symptoms, especially the behavioural symptoms of bvFTD. The non-pharmacological therapies include increased supervision, physical therapy, occupational therapy and speech therapy. Other strategies targeting patients' carers include behavioural modification techniques (such as distraction and redirection) and caregiver support and respite. Cholinesterase inhibitors such as donepezil do not have any convincing evidence in the treatment of bvFTD. It should only be considered when the diagnosis of Alzheimer's disease is equally likely as bvFTD. On average, the prognosis of FTD is about 8–10 years. This is shorter in those diagnosed with bvFTD.

Examination

- The patient seemed to be oriented to month, year and person but not to the place or date. He appeared to be calm though not apathetic. He did not seem to be having visual or auditory hallucinations. The conversation did not reveal any delusional thinking. The vital signs were normal and the patient was not febrile.
- A full set of **neurological examinations** [1] was performed. The cranial nerve examination was normal. The examination of all four limbs was also normal.
- There was no expressive or receptive **dysphasia** [2] appreciated in the process of examination. The executive functioning was also preserved on examination, although with slowness.
- A **mini mental state examination** [3] was performed. The patient scored 18 out of 30.
- He lost marks **mainly in the orientation, recall and executive function domains** [4].

[1] Alzheimer's disease typically has normal neurological examination in the early stage of disease. However, pyramidal and extrapyramidal motor signs, myoclonus and seizures occur later in the course of Alzheimer's disease.

[2] Other possible neurological manifestations in Alzheimer's disease include olfactory dysfunction, visual impairment in posterior cortical atrophy, and primary progressive aphasia.

[3] Alzheimer's disease progresses inexorably. The progression of the disease can be monitored with mini mental state examination (MMSE), Montreal Cognitive Assessment and clinical dementia rating scale. Montreal Cognitive Assessment is preferred due to higher sensitivity. The average decline on MMSE is about 3.5 points each year.

[4] MMSE tests a broad range of cognitive functions including orientation, recall, attention, calculation, language manipulation and constructional praxis. A score of <24 points is suggestive of dementia or delirium (sensitivity 87% and specificity 82%). A score <16 in patients with Alzheimer's disease is highly suggestive of impaired capacity in decision-making. However, MMSE is not sensitive for mild dementia and it is also limited by age and education. It is also limited by language, motor and visual impairments. Any change of MMSE score by <2 points is of uncertain clinical significance.

Montreal Cognitive Assessment is more sensitive than MMSE for the detection of mild cognitive impairment. It tests a wider range of cognitive domains including memory, language, attention, visuospatial and executive functions. Its threshold for cognitive impairment is 26, with a sensitivity greater than 94% but with a specificity of only 60%. Its cut-off can be adjusted based on the patient's education level and other appropriate norms.

Clinical dementia rating is mainly used for study and research purposes. It can be used to assess the severity of Alzheimer's disease. It assesses six cognitive domains including memory, orientation, judgement and problem solving, community affairs, home and hobbies, and personal care. Its limitation is time consumption. Though it is mainly used in research settings, it may be useful in following the disease progression over time.

Another cognitive assessment test is the Mini-Cog which is a clock-drawing task and uncued recall of three unrelated words. It is currently under research for its clinical utility. If the patient recalls none of the three unrelated words, a diagnosis of dementia is made. If the patient can recall all three words, the dementia is said to be ruled out. If the patient can only recall 1–2 words, a diagnosis of dementia is made if the clock-drawing test is abnormal, and dementia is ruled out if clock drawing is normal. One advantage of the Mini-Cog test is that it takes much less time to perform.

Investigations

- To rule out other possible causes of the patient's cognitive impairment, an **MRI brain** [1] was performed. The neuroimaging revealed a generalised atrophy which was age appropriate. There was also a notable volume loss of the hippocampus in the bilateral temporal lobe. There were also signs suggestive of chronic small vessel ischaemia.
- The tests for **delirium screening** [2] were also carried out. The laboratory tests returned with unremarkable result and the urine microscopy and culture showed no significant growth.
- The **neuropsychiatric test** [3] was requested and the report revealed moderate cognitive impairment, mainly in the domain of memory and problem solving.
- No **further blood tests or biomarkers** [4] were requested for this patient.

[1] Neuroimaging is often used to rule out other causes. MRI is the preferred modality to document potential alternative or additional diagnoses, and regional brain atrophy suggests other types of neurodegenerative disease. While not widely available, amyloid PET measures amyloid lesion burden. It aids the prognosis and differentiates Alzheimer's disease from other causes of dementia. However, it should not be used to determine dementia severity, nor should it be used in those who meet core clinical criteria for probable Alzheimer's disease and have a typical age of onset.

[2] Delirium screening such as urine microscopy and culturing should be employed to rule out the presence of delirium as a potential cause of functional or cognitive decline.

[3] The neuropsychological testing may provide confirmatory information and aid in the patient's management.

[4] Molecular biomarkers of amyloid beta deposition and tau protein are not recommended for routine diagnostic purposes. To make the diagnosis, the definitive diagnosis of Alzheimer's disease requires histopathological examination, which is rarely done in reality. The laboratory and imaging investigations are mainly to exclude other diagnoses. Probable Alzheimer's disease diagnosis depends on the clinical criteria listed in the following table:

Clinical criteria for probable Alzheimer's disease

Interference with ability to function at work or at usual activities
Cognitive impairment involving >2 of the following domains: ability to acquire and remember new information, language functions, reasoning and handling of complex tasks, ability to make sound judgement, complex attention, visuospatial abilities, and changes in personality, behaviour or comportment
A decline from a previous level of functioning and performance in at least one of the cognitive domains
The cognitive decline cannot be explained by delirium or major psychiatric disorder
Cognitive impairment is established by **history taking** from the patient and a knowledgeable informant; and by **objective bedside** mental status examination or **neuropsychological** testing
Insidious onset of the cognitive impairment
Clear-cut history of worsening of the cognition
Initial and most prominent cognitive deficits include one of the following: • amnestic presentation: impaired learning and recall of recent event • non-amnestic presentation: language with word finding, visuospatial presentation, dysexecutive presentation with judgement
No evidence of substantial concomitant cerebrovascular disease/DLB/FTD/other concurrent conditions or use of medication that could affect cognition substantially

Management

The patient was diagnosed with mixed type dementia with Alzheimer's disease in combination with vascular dementia. **A multidisciplinary meeting** [1] was requested with involvement of physiotherapist, occupational therapist and social worker. The patient was assessed by a physiotherapist and there was no obvious concern of mobility impairment. The **occupational therapist** [2] was called to do a home visit to assess the patient's safety and available facilities at home. The patient was also asked to participate in the driving test organised by the occupational therapist. Several recommendations were made for this patient's care in the community. The gas stove at home was replaced with an electrical cooking unit. A microwave oven was also purchased for heating up prepared meals. The patient also showed safety concerns during the **driving** [3] test and hence he was advised not to drive, and DVLA was informed. The patient's **medication list was also optimised** [4] and the use of psychotropic agents was minimised. **The patient's wife was advised** [5] to place patient's medications in a visible place and a dosette box for patient's medications prepared. The family was also advised to place important reminders in the living place for the patient's memory issues. The social worker was involved in the aged care assessment process. An approval for respite and residential aged care facility was granted, should the need arise. Due to the significant cognitive impairment, the patient and his family were advised to appoint a **substitute decision maker** [6] in case a decision is needed when the patient is incapable of making decisions. **Donepezil** [7] was initiated as part of pharmacological therapy. The patient tolerated the medication quite well and there was a slight improvement of his episodic memory issues. The family decided to keep the patient at home as long as they can, but they do also understand that Alzheimer's disease is a progressive illness of ageing.

Prognosis

- The life expectancy after diagnosis of Alzheimer's disease ranges from 3–11 years.
- The terminal complications are often related to the advanced debilitation such as dehydration, malnutrition and infection.

[1] There is no immediate treatment available for Alzheimer's disease. In the short term, a potential secondary cause of cognitive decline or delirium should be explored. Delirium screening should be carried out and any identified organic cause should be treated promptly. The long-term management of Alzheimer's disease usually involves the assessment and prioritisation of the issues for the patient and their carer. This will often require the involvement of specialists from multiple disciplines, such as physiotherapist, occupational therapist and social worker.

[2] Safety and ease in the home setting should be assessed by the occupational therapist.

[3] Driving can be quite dangerous for those who may get lost while driving. For those with advanced Alzheimer's disease, driving is not recommended.

[4] Medication review should be performed and medication should be optimised for the elderly population, especially with the use of psychotropic medications.

[5] Education for the carer to understand the disease and how to manage a patient's cognitive impairment in the community is paramount. Aged care assessment should be organised early on for potential need of respite or even residential aged care facilities in the future.

[6] Financial planning can be hard for patients with difficulty in making sound judgements. The early appointment of enduring or financial power of attorney should be included as part of the management plan.

[7] There are some pharmacological therapies available for Alzheimer's disease with proven benefit. Donepezil is a cholinesterase inhibitor and is typically used for mild–moderate Alzheimer's disease with MMSE between 10 and 24. However, this drug mainly provides symptomatic improvement. It may also provide non-cognitive improvement such as in apathy and psychosis. It also slows the cognitive decline in moderate–severe Alzheimer's disease group while it also delays entry to nursing home with evidence for up to 3 years. The notable side-effects include GI disturbance, weight loss, muscle cramping, vivid dreams, and less commonly, bradyarrhythmia.
Memantine is another medication available for Alzheimer's disease and is usually used for moderate–severe Alzheimer's disease group with MMSE ranging from 10 to 14. It is an NMDA (N-methyl-D-aspartate) antagonist and can assist with aggression and agitation. Its notable side-effects include constipation, headache and hypertension. There is no evidence of added benefit if combined with donepezil.

CASE 54: Motor neurone disease

History

- A **55-year-old male** [1] carpenter presents with a **4-month history of progressively worsening upper limb weakness** [2].
- **Other than the upper limb weakness, the patient is also complaining of increasing stiffness and difficulty in coordinating movement of his arms and hands** [3].
- There are no complaints of diplopia, dysphagia or dysarthria suggestive of **bulbar palsies** [4].
- There is **no lower limb involvement** [5].
- The weakness **started in the hands and appears to be asymmetrical** [6] at the time of review.

- The **difficulty in coordinating the patient's hands** [7] **and weakness** [8] cause significant stress when the patient is performing at work as a carpenter.
- The patient denies any symptoms suggestive of **cognitive dysfunction, parkinsonism or autonomic dysfunction** [9].
- The patient **denies any sensory changes** [10].
- There was a significant **family history** [11] of amyotrophic lateral sclerosis.

[1] Amyotrophic lateral sclerosis (ALS) is the most common form of motor neurone disease (MND) and is also known as Lou Gehrig's disease, named after the famous baseball player who was diagnosed with the disorder. Although considered as the most common motor neurone disease, ALS is rare, with an annual incidence of about 1 per 100 000 people worldwide. There is no ethnic or racial predisposition to ALS. ALS has an age distribution that peaks between 70 and 80 years old. Prior to age of 65, ALS is more commonly found in men than women, but after 65 the incidence seems to be equal.

[2] MND is a spectrum of progressive neurodegenerative disorder that causes muscle weakness, disability and eventually death.

[3] The hallmark of amyotrophic lateral sclerosis is the combination of upper and lower motor neurone signs and symptoms. The name is derived from the combination of the clinical finding of amyotrophy with the pathological finding of lateral sclerosis. Upper motor neurone findings usually manifest as weakness with slowness, hyperreflexia and spasticity because the upper motor neurones along the corticospinal tract are affected. The lower motor neurone findings usually manifest as weakness associated with atrophy, amyotrophy and fasciculations due to degeneration of lower motor neurones in the brainstem and spinal cord producing muscle denervation.

[4] The spectrum of MND is wide. As mentioned above, ALS is only one (most common) of the multiple degenerative motor neurone diseases that are defined based on the involvement of upper and/or lower motor neurone signs. Other examples include progressive muscular atrophy

(progressive isolated lower motor neurone disorder with slower progression and better survival than ALS), primary lateral sclerosis (progressive isolated upper motor neurone disorder with also slower progression and better survival than ALS), progressive bulbar palsy (progressive upper and lower motor neurone disorder of cranial muscles), flail arm syndrome (progressive lower motor neurone weakness and wasting, predominantly affecting the proximal arm), flail leg syndrome (progressive lower motor neurone weakness and wasting with onset in the distal leg), and amyotrophic lateral sclerosis plus syndrome. The loss of motor neurones in ALS is responsible for the symptoms and signs of ALS. The impairment can affect limb (e.g. difficulty arising from chairs due to proximal leg weakness), bulbar (e.g. dysarthria due to slow and discoordinated tongue movement), axial (e.g. difficulty in maintaining an erect posture due to weakness in truncal extensors) and respiratory (e.g. dyspnoea due to weakness in respiratory muscles) function.

[5] Site of onset, pattern and speed of spread, and the degree of upper and lower motor neurone dysfunction can be significantly variable between individuals.

[6] Initial presentation of ALS can occur in any body segment and may manifest as upper motor neurone or lower motor neurone signs or symptoms. Most ALS cases (80%) initially present with asymmetric limb weakness with upper extremity onset, most often starting in the hands; and lower limb onset, most often starting with foot drop. Rarely, ALS starts with bulbar segment, which most often starts with either dysarthria or dysphagia. Less common onset patterns of ALS are respiratory and axial onset.

7 The loss of upper motor neurones produces slowness of movement, incoordination and stiffness. Upper extremity involvement results in poor dexterity with increasing difficulty in performing activities of daily living. Lower extremity manifestation usually includes spastic gait with poor balance. Dysarthria and dysphagia are the most common bulbar upper motor neurone symptoms. Spastic dysarthria produces slow speech with strained vocal quality. Upper motor neurone dysphagia usually results from slow and discoordinated contraction of the swallowing muscles, which may cause coughing and choking leading to increased risk of aspiration. Laryngospasm can also occur in upper motor neurone bulbar dysfunction. This is a short-lived protective reflex causing closure of the larynx in response to aspiration. The patient typically experiences a squeezing feeling in the throat in this setting. Syndrome of the pseudobulbar affect can also happen in bulbar upper motor neurone dysfunction, leading to inappropriate laughing, crying or yawning. Axial upper motor neurone dysfunction may manifest as stiffness and imbalance.

8 The loss of lower motor neurones produces weakness, usually associated with atrophy and fasciculations. Muscle cramps are common. Instead of losing dexterity from loss of upper motor neurones, upper extremity with lower motor neurone dysfunction often presents with difficulty in performing activities of daily living due to weakness. Distal weakness in lower limbs often results in foot drop and slapping gait. The proximal weakness in the upper limb causes inability to raise the arm above the head and the proximal leg weakness causes difficulty rising from chairs. Dysarthria and dysphagia can also result from weakness produced by lower motor neurone damage. The speech is usually slurred and may have a nasal quality. Hoarseness can occur due to vocal cord weakness. Dysphagia can result from weakness of tongue and swallowing muscles. Dysphagia from lower motor neurone damage can also increase risk of aspiration. Weakness in facial muscles can produce sialorrhoea due to poor mouth sealing and incomplete eye closure. Lower motor neurone weakness in the axial muscle usually manifests as difficulty holding up the head and maintaining an erect posture. Weakness of the diaphragm produces progressive dyspnoea.

9 ALS is generally considered as a pure motor disorder. However, when other regions such as frontal and temporal cortical neurons are involved, other symptoms such as cognitive and autonomic symptoms can develop and the condition is considered as amyotrophic lateral sclerosis plus syndrome, as part of the clinicopathological spectrum of ALS. Those additional features may present like frontotemporal dementia, autonomic insufficiency, parkinsonism and progressive supranuclear palsy. Although patients with MND do not present with overt dementia, cognitive and behavioural dysfunction is present in at least one-third of patients and becomes increasingly common as the disease progresses. The pattern of impairment usually involves issues with executive function, language and letter fluency, with relative sparing of memory and visuospatial function. Such patients can present with apathy, changes in eating behaviours, disinhibition and perseveration. Autonomic symptoms can start as the disease progresses. Constipation occurs frequently, although it is generally considered to be multifactorial. The patient usually complains of early satiety and bloating consistent with delayed gastric emptying. Urinary urgency can also occur without incontinence. Features of parkinsonism may precede or follow motor neurone symptoms. Common presentations include facial masking, tremor, bradykinesia and postural instability.

10 Sensory symptoms are not uncommon in patients with ALS, especially complaints of tingling paraesthesia. However, the objective sensory physical examination is usually normal.

11 ALS is most commonly sporadic, with only 10% of all ALS cases considered genetic or familial. Family history is important as most cases of familial ALS are inherited in an autosomal dominant pattern. While the progression rate of the disease is variable between individuals, the pattern is always progressive over time without intervening remissions or exacerbations. The spread pattern usually involves limb first before moving to bulbar segment. For example, disease that starts in the unilateral arm usually spreads to the contralateral arm, before moving to the ipsilateral leg followed by the contralateral leg, and eventually to the bulbar muscles. Diagnostic criteria of motor neurone disease include:
- evidence of lower motor neurone degeneration by clinical, electrophysiological, or neuropathological examination
- evidence of upper motor neurone degeneration by clinical examination
- progressive spread of symptoms or signs within a region or to other regions, as determined by history or examination.

According to the diagnostic criteria, clinical history taking and examination are important.

Examination

- On **inspection** [1], there was a classic appearance of **'split hand' bilaterally. The muscle atrophy** [2] is significant in the distal upper limbs bilaterally while the proximal muscles were relatively preserved.
- The **tones** [3] in both upper limbs appear to be increased while the tones in the lower limbs were normal and equal.
- There was **hyperreflexia** [4] in both upper limbs with bicep, triceps and brachioradialis reflex response elicited by just flicking the patient's arms.

- The **power** [5] in the finger flexion, extension and abduction appeared to be 3/5 while the power was 4/5 in the wrist flexion and extension. The power was 4/5 in elbow flexion and extension. The power in the shoulder abduction and adduction was 5/5. There was no fasciculation that could be appreciated on close inspection.

- The **Hoffman sign** [6] was positive and the patient had no issues when **standing up from the chair** [7]. The lower limb neurological examination was normal with no evidence of cerebellar lesion.
- The **cranial examination was unremarkable** [8].
- The cardiovascular, **respiratory** [9] and **abdominal examination** [10] were also unremarkable at the time of review.

1 Check posture, looking for stiffness or difficulty maintaining erect posture.

2 Look for 'split hand', a sign due to atrophy in median and ulnar innervated thenar hand intrinsic muscles, with relative sparing of the hypothenar muscles. Also look for muscle atrophy elsewhere in the limbs.

3 Check for tones of limbs. Spasticity is an upper motor neurone sign.

4 Check for reflexes. Hyperreflexia is suggestive of upper motor neurone lesion. Sometimes even a finger flicking can elicit reflex in patients with ALS. Upgoing plantar reflex (Babinski sign) is not present in all ALS patients but it is highly suggestive of upper motor neurone lesion if present.

5 Check for weakness in the limbs, along with any muscle fasciculations. They are lower motor neurone signs.

6 Hoffman sign is checked by flicking the nail of the patient's middle or ring finger. In a patient with positive Hoffman sign the index finger would flex towards the thumb.

7 Ask the patient to rise from their chair. This can be used to assess whether there is any proximal muscle weakness. The same can be tested by asking the patient to squat.

8 Jaw reflex can be prominent due to upper motor neurone lesion. The palmomental reflex is another primitive reflex that can be present in patients with ALS. A twitch of the ipsilateral mentalis muscle is elicited by stroking the thenar eminence of the patient's palm. Tongue fasciculation can be observed as a lower motor neurone lesion if bulbar segment is involved.

9 Listen out for any hoarse voice with reduced vocal volume. This change in speech can be suggestive of respiratory involvement of ALS. One should also look for use of accessory respiratory muscles when assessing the respiratory segment in ALS.

10 The loss of abdominal reflexes is an upper motor neurone sign of axial segment. The lower motor neurone signs include weakness of neck and truncal extension. Look for abdominal protuberance due to abdominal muscle weakness.

Investigations

- EMG was performed and revealed a neuropathic pattern. There were also fibrillations and positive sharp waves on the **electromyography** [1].
- There was no issue identified on the **nerve conduction studies** [2].
- The **repetitive nerve stimulation** [3] yielded unremarkable results.

- The **MRI of brain and spine** [4] was also unremarkable.
- The **creatine kinase** [5] level was mildly elevated.
- The **CSF analysis from lumbar puncture** [6] showed normal cell count and absence of oligoband.

1 Diagnosis of amyotrophic lateral sclerosis does not require electrodiagnostic studies because it is primarily a clinical diagnosis. However, the use of electromyography can be helpful in terms of supporting the diagnosis of ALS. The features of ALS seen on EMG are the combination of acute and chronic denervation and reinnervation. The acute denervation findings include fibrillations and positive sharp waves, whereas chronic denervation and reinnervation findings include large amplitude, long duration, complex motor unit action potentials. The neurogenic recruitment

and a reduced interference pattern are also seen in chronic denervation and reinnervation. Fasciculation potentials may be present in denervated muscles. While those findings can be present in any disease causing chronic denervation, ALS is likely if the abnormalities are observed in widespread muscle groups without the corresponding nerve root compression.

2 Sensory and motor nerve conduction are often normal on nerve conduction studies (NCS). Compound muscle action potential amplitudes may be reduced in atrophic and denervated muscles. The absence of conduction block is part of the electrodiagnostic criteria of ALS. Again, ALS is a motor neurone disease and hence sensory function should be spared and therefore normal on NCS.

3 As myasthenia gravis and Lambert–Eaton myasthenic syndrome can be potential differential diagnoses, repetitive nerve stimulation may be useful.

4 Imaging using MRI is usually used to exclude other possible differential diagnoses. MRI brain should be performed whenever bulbar segment is involved. Cervical and lumbosacral spine MRI is performed to evaluate lower motor neurone disease in the arms and legs. If the patient presents with upper motor neurone disease in legs, the MRI should include brain and whole spine.

5 Other pathology tests are less relevant in terms of diagnosing ALS. Creatine kinase (CK) may be mildly elevated due to denervation. Calcium and parathyroid hormone can be checked, since there is a weak link between primary hyperparathyroidism and ALS. Testing for Lyme disease is reasonable if the patient is from endemic regions. Since HIV can cause ALS-like syndrome, testing for HIV is appropriate in patients from younger and at-risk populations. Serology for the antibodies in myasthenia gravis (anti-AChR and MuSK) and Lambert–Eaton myasthenic syndrome (VGCC) is reasonable if patients present with bulbar dysfunction or ocular motility disturbance.

6 Lumbar puncture and CSF analysis should be performed if Lyme disease or HIV infection are suspected.

Management

While the patient did have neurological deficits at the time of review, there was no immediate threat to his safety. The patient was otherwise well and his vitals were normal. He was sent home from the clinic and was booked for further follow-up appointments in the Neurology clinic.

Immediate and short-term management

There is no crisis or flare known to be associated with MND. A patient may present with acute worsening of respiratory function but it is usually a result of another pathological process, such as chest infection. ALS patients with bulbar involvement are at high risk of having aspiration pneumonia/pneumonitis and hence are prone to chest infections. Those with limb involvement and significantly impaired mobility (e.g. wheelchair-bound) are also at significant risk of having venous thromboembolism. Respiratory failure can be fatal if the acute underlying illness is not recognised and treated early on.

Long-term

The patient was reviewed frequently and the **progression of his MND was monitored** [1]. Unfortunately, the diagnosis of ALS was **overwhelming news to the patient and his family. His independence and ability to work were threatened** [2]. **MDT involvement was requested** [3]. Multiple referrals were made to the psychologist, physiotherapist and social workers. Early referral to the palliative care team was also made for early involvement. Since there was no bulbar or respiratory segment involved in this patient at the time of review, no non-invasive ventilation was organised. However, a referral to a **respiratory physician** [4] was made for serial pulmonary function tests, in case the patient has new development of bulbar or respiratory involvement. General education on the illness was provided. Particular attention was paid to certain symptoms, such as dysphagia, dysarthria and dyspnoea, as they usually indicate notable progression of the disease requiring **specific treatment** [5]. **Riluzole** [6] was also started as it is the only pharmacological medication with good evidence in the management of motor neurone disease.

Prognosis

As ALS progresses, the **final stage of the disease is life-threatening** [7] and it usually involves two aspects: neuromuscular respiratory failure and dysphagia. The most common cause of death in ALS is neuromuscular respiratory failure. Dysphagia increases the risk for aspiration with resultant pneumonia. Dysphagia can lead to reduced oral intake and hence result in malnutrition and dehydration. The median survival of ALS patients from the time of diagnosis is 3–5 years, although a small proportion of ALS patients can live beyond 10 years after diagnosis.

1 Management of ALS consists of two components, symptomatic and disease-modifying. It is always important to keep in mind that ALS is a relentlessly progressive disease and hence disease progress should be monitored, with prompt palliative care involvement as part of the management plan.

2 Breaking bad news can be the first difficult task upon diagnosis. ALS is a progressive disease that can cause significant morbidity and mortality to the patient. Both physical and mental impact on the patient and their family members need to be considered.

3 Because of the complex issues related to ALS, a multidisciplinary approach to the management of ALS should be provided. This usually involves the neurologist, psychologist, physiotherapist, occupational therapist, speech therapist, dietitians, social workers and palliative care team. It does not have to be the end-of-life stage of ALS to have palliative care involvement. It aims to enhance the quality of life in patients and hence is appropriate in all stages of the disease.

4 Respiratory management can be a big issue in the management of ALS. Not only can dyspnoea reduce the quality of life in patients with respiratory involvement, but also the use of non-invasive ventilation appears to provide benefit to patients' mortality. The discussion should ideally happen before the respiratory symptoms occur and the patient and family members should be involved as part of the decision-making process. However, one should remember that the patient always has the right to refuse or withdraw from any treatment. Serial pulmonary function test is an important tool to monitor the progression of respiratory function in ALS. As a general rule, a vital capacity <50% of predicted is enough to cause respiratory symptoms. Non-invasive positive pressure ventilation improves quality of life for patients with respiratory symptoms, if the patient can tolerate it. It is particularly useful for the nocturnal symptoms of respiratory compromise. Immunisation with annual influenza vaccination and pneumococcal vaccine is always recommended.

5 The symptom management includes management of dysphagia, dysarthria, dyspnoea, muscle spasm, sialorrhoea, excessive airway secretion, pressure injury and psychological issues. Dysphagia management should always start with modification of food and fluid consistency. A review by a speech pathologist can be helpful. A percutaneous gastrostomy tube can be used for those with symptoms of dysphagia. For those with no dysphagia but significant weight loss, the use of percutaneous endoscopic gastrostomy (PEG) is also reasonable. Electronic assistive communication device can be helpful in the setting of dysarthria. Dyspnoea in ALS can be multifactorial. General supportive measures for dyspnoea can start with relaxation techniques for components of anxiety. A fan for cool air blowing and chest physiotherapy can also be helpful. Non-invasive ventilation can be helpful in terms of symptom control. The use of opioids such as morphine can be employed to treat breathlessness and can start early on as part of the management. Benzodiazepines can be used as an additional treatment for those with significant anxiety. Muscle spasm can be quite painful and causes discomfort in ALS patients. This can be treated with mexiletine and quinine. Baclofen can be helpful in the management of spasticity. Sialorrhoea and thick mucus production can overlap each other. Atropine and glycopyrrolate are useful in the setting of sialorrhoea, whereas the thick mucus is usually managed with mucolytic acetylcysteine augmented with chest physiotherapy. Pressure care is also important to prevent pressure-induced skin injury and secondary infection.

6 Disease-modifying treatment for ALS is limited. Current evidence suggests only two treatments that can offer mortality benefit. Non-invasive positive pressure ventilation is one of them, as mentioned above. The other is riluzole, a glutamate inhibitor, which is shown to confer mortality benefit and slow the progression of ALS to a modest degree.

7 When the expected prognosis is approaching ≤6 months, a hospice should become involved.

CASE 55: Multiple sclerosis

History

- A **34-year-old female** [1] nurse from New Zealand presented with a 1-week history of **altered sensation** [2] in her right lower leg. The altered sensation was in the form of numbness and is isolated in the right lower leg only. The numbness can also be associated with burning pain.
- She also reported that she had one episode of non-positional vertigo associated with loss of balance about 9 months ago. The previous neurological event **resolved** [3] after 3 weeks without any

treatment and there was no residual deficit after the resolution.
- The symptoms seemed to be worsening while the patient was having a **hot shower** [4]. The symptoms were troublesome to the patient when she was performing day-to-day tasks at work.
- She is a current **smoker and she had Epstein–Barr virus infection** [5] in the past. She has no other significant past medical history.
- There is a **family history** [6] of multiple sclerosis.

[1] Multiple sclerosis (MS) begins in the early stage of adult life. It is more common in females, with a female to male ratio of 2:1. It is also more common in the population living in the regions far from the equator. MS is a chronic autoimmune demyelinating disease. Its pathology happens around the autoimmune process in the central nervous system. In patients with multiple sclerosis, the CNS antigen activates the autoreactive T and B cells, leading to tissue damage in the central nervous system. This in turn results in the further release of autoreactive antigen into the periphery and hence further priming of the autoreactive lymphocytes and continuous cycle. Macrophages and activated microglial cells are the main contributors to damage. The damage to the oligodendrocytes leads to demyelination. Myelin is the substance that helps with nerve conduction and provides a good living environment for the axon. The destruction of the myelin layer and hence the disruption of this environment results in axonal loss in demyelinating disease. Axonal loss is the core cause of the disabilities in MS. Untreated patients have a rate of relapse of about 0.65 attacks a year, though there is high variability between individuals.

[2] There are many other differential diagnoses to consider in patients presenting with acute neurological symptoms. These include paraneoplastic syndrome, CNS neoplasm, vitamin B12 deficiency, vasculitis affecting the CNS, and infective causes such as HIV and syphilis. These potential causes can be explored in the process of investigations. It is also important to know that MS patients do not develop cortical symptoms such as neglect and aphasia in cerebrovascular disease. The presenting symptoms are based on the locations of lesions. Those located in the cerebrum may manifest as cognitive impairment, including executive function and dementia, or upper motor neurone deficit. Any lesion in the optic nerve can present with any

of: unilateral loss of vision, scotoma, reduced visual acuity, colour vision loss or relative afferent pupillary defect. The cerebellum and its pathways can also be affected, with symptoms of tremor or loss of balance. In the brainstem, the presenting symptoms are dependent on the cranial nerve or nerve pathways affected. Symptoms include internuclear ophthalmoplegia, complex ophthalmoplegia, vertigo and trigeminal neuralgia. MS lesions can also cause damage to the spinal cord. The patient may present with upper motor neurone deficit, spasticity, bladder dysfunction, constipation, sensory changes or pain. MS usually starts with an episode of acute neurological disturbance. This is called a clinically isolated syndrome. But a diagnosis of multiple sclerosis requires at least two neurological events separated in time and space within the CNS (McDonald criteria based on radiological findings; see below). The use of MRI brain provides an opportunity for making an early diagnosis of MS, especially if patients present with a single clinical neurological episode and if the MRI brain shows a different area affected suggestive of MS. This would fulfil the McDonald criteria (at least two neurological events) and allow for early treatment for these patients.

[3] In most cases, complete or almost complete resolution of symptoms occurs in this phase of the disease. After 10 years, half of the patients can begin to develop a progressive accumulation of disability. There are different patterns of the disease in MS, illustrated in *Figure 55.1*. The most common pattern of the disease is relapsing–remitting MS, where the patient has relapses with or without complete recovery, but is stable between episodes. Secondary progressive MS happens in about half of the patients with relapsing–remitting multiple sclerosis within 10 years; this shows a relapsing–remitting pattern followed by a gradual progression of the symptoms without distinct episodes. Primary progressive MS

is different. It presents with increasing symptoms without any distinct episodes from the start. It is also considered to be the most aggressive form of MS. The last pattern of multiple sclerosis is progressive relapsing MS, in which there is a gradual worsening of the patient's neurological condition, with episodes of deterioration occurring throughout the course of the illness.

4 Uhthoff's phenomenon refers to any episodes of temporary worsening of the patient's symptoms in the setting of the increase in body temperature resulting from fever, hot weather and exercise. In those who were diagnosed with MS in the past, any episodes of worsening neurological symptoms associated with fever may not be considered as relapses and the possibility of so-called pseudorelapses needs to be considered as well. The risk factors that worsen a patient's neurological symptoms include heat, exercise, fever,

infection and pregnancy (relapse is common postpartum, but there is less activity during pregnancy).

5 Smoking is a major risk factor, while Epstein–Barr virus infection also increases the risk of developing MS.

6 Family history is a risk factor. HLA-DRB1 is the allele with the strongest association. To provide holistic care for the patient, it is important to explore the social impact resulting from the patient's MS. This includes sexual dysfunction, such as erectile dysfunction, depression and euphoria (may create difficulty in the patient's social functioning), cognitive impairment (can be a source of disability and should not be overlooked), seizures and bulbar dysfunction (can create a barrier to employment and can be a source of financial problems).

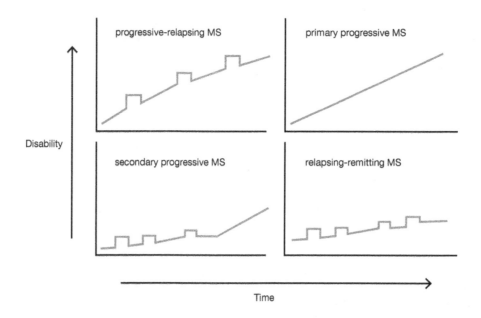

Figure 55.1 *Different patterns of multiple sclerosis.*

Examination

- The patient's vital signs appeared to be normal, with no evidence of fever at the time of examination. A **full neurological examination was performed** [1].
- On examination of the **eyes** [2], visual acuity appears to be normal bilaterally, with normal colour saturation. Fundoscopy did not reveal any abnormality, in particular optic atrophy or swelling. The pupils were also equal bilaterally and both reactive to light. The consensual pupillary response was intact as well. The examination of eye movement did not reveal any features suggestive

of cranial III, IV or VI palsies and there was no pain reported on eye movements.

- There was no **internuclear ophthalmoplegia** [3] appreciated on examination and there was no nystagmus identified. Facial sensation appeared to be intact, with normal corneal reflexes bilaterally. Active facial expression revealed no issues with cranial nerve VII. Testing of hearing did not reveal any sensorineural defect, while the gag reflex was intact bilaterally. There was no tongue or uvula deviation. The function of trapezius and sternocleidomastoid

- muscles were intact on examination, with no features of atrophy.
- The examination of the upper limbs was also unremarkable, with normal tone, reflex and power bilaterally. Sensation was intact in all modalities in both upper limbs. **Lhermitte's sign** [4] was tested by flexing the patient's neck; she reported an electric shock-like sensation from the cervical spine down to the lower limbs bilaterally.

- On examination of the patient's **lower limbs** [5], the tone and reflexes were normal. The power was 5/5 across all joints in the lower limbs. However, there was a loss of fine touch, pinprick and temperature sensations in the right lower leg in the dermatomal distribution of L2–L4. The sensations of vibration and proprioception were intact. There was no cerebellar sign elicited on examination of all four limbs and the patient's gait was not ataxic.

[1] The physical signs in MS can be very variable depending on the locations of the lesions. Examination of the neurological system is a must-do.

[2] The clinician should look for any loss of visual acuity, optic atrophy or swelling. Colour saturation should also be checked and one should look for a relative afferent pupil defect, which can be suggestive of optic neuritis, especially if the patient's visual acuity is reduced. Signs suggestive of neuromyelitis optica (NMO, or Devic's disease) are important to know, as its clinical manifestation may overlap with MS. It usually presents with sudden onset visual loss and pain on eye movements, together with weakness and numbness of the arms or legs. There is usually no cerebellar or cognitive impairment compared with MS, and MRI brain is usually normal. Anti-aquaporin 4 antibodies are present in 70% of patients with NMO and this helps distinguish the condition from MS. The treatment of NMO is different to that for MS and hence it is important to make the right diagnosis.

[3] Internuclear ophthalmoplegia is an important physical sign and it is highly suspicious of MS if such abnormality is seen in a young adult. It is manifested as a weakness of adduction in one eye as a result of damage to the ipsilateral medial longitudinal fasciculus, while there is nystagmus in the abducting eye. In MS, internuclear ophthalmoplegia is often bilateral.

[4] Lhermitte's sign should be tested in any patient with suspected MS, although it may not be positive in every patient. The test is said to be positive if the patient reports an electric shock-like sensation in the limbs or trunk following neck flexion by the clinician. However, it is important to know that Lhermitte's sign can also occur in subacute combined spinal cord degeneration, cervical cord tumour and mantle irradiation.

[5] In the peripheries, the clinician should look out particularly for spastic paraparesis and posterior column sensory loss, as well as cerebellar signs. Because MS is a CNS disease, any motor neurone involvement should manifest as an upper motor neurone lesion.

Investigations

- Since the diagnosis of multiple sclerosis was suspected, an **MRI scan** [1] of the brain and spine with **gadolinium contrast** [2] was organised.
- The T2 images produced from the scan showed multiple enhancing lesions in the periventricular white matter and the spinal cord from the level of L2 extending down to the level of L5, while a **non-enhancing lesion** [3] was identified in the cerebellum at the same time. Lumbar puncture was also performed while the patient was waiting for the MRI scan.

- The **CSF** [4] sample collected was sent for CSF analysis. The test result came back with the presence of oligoclonal bands and lymphocytosis. The CSF microscopy and culture and viral PCR came back with negative results.
- The **anti-aquaporin 4 antibody serology** [5] came back as negative.
- **Septic screening** [6] was conducted to explore possibilities of infections, and the tests came back negative.

1 MRI is the imaging modality of choice and helps to support the clinical diagnosis of multiple sclerosis:

Table 55.1 Sites of demyelinating on MRI scan

Corpus callosum
Periventricular white matter
Optic nerve
Pons, cerebellar peduncles and cerebellum
Juxtacortical white matter
Spinal cord

2 Gadolinium contrast enhancement usually indicates leakage through the blood–brain barrier. This contrast enhancement can last for months after formation of a new lesion. Hence a lesion that was formed a long time ago would be non-enhancing and this will allow the patient to meet the diagnostic criteria early on. A T2-weighted image is usually the MRI image to be used. The extent and number of the lesions on MRI correlates with the clinical severity of the disease, and hence the prognosis. The lesions in the brainstem and spinal cord in particular cause disability to the patient. In contrast, CT scan is not useful in the diagnosis of MS and hence is not used as routine imaging.

3 The radiological version of the McDonald criteria requires dissemination in space on the neuroimaging. The space criterion requires more than one T2 bright lesion in two or more of the typical locations in MS (*Table 55.1*). Please note that the symptomatic lesion in a patient's brainstem and spinal cord does not contribute to the lesion count. As in the clinical version of the McDonald criteria, the radiological version also requires dissemination in time to make the diagnosis of MS. The dissemination in time refers to a new lesion when compared with a previous scan, or asymptomatic enhancing lesion and a non-enhancing T2 bright lesion on any one scan.

4 CSF analysis can be supportive in the diagnosis of multiple sclerosis. Oligoclonal bands are formed from the increased synthesis of immunoglobulin G in the CSF. Its presence supports the diagnosis of MS. However, the presence of an oligoclonal band alone is not enough to make the diagnosis, because it is not specific to MS. Other conditions with oligoclonal bands include bacterial infection, herpes simplex encephalitis, syphilis and sarcoidosis. In patients with MS, the CSF can have pleocytosis with predominance of lymphocytes but again, it is not specific to MS.

5 Anti-aquaporin-4 antibodies can be used to differentiate NMO from multiple sclerosis, although it is unlikely in this case.

6 An exacerbation or recurrence of previously improved symptoms related to an intercurrent infection is usually called pseudorelapse. Management is to treat the underlying infection. Meanwhile, the clinician should also keep in mind that many disorders can also result in multiple lesions in the CNS; examples include CNS SLE, Sjögren's syndrome, Behçet's disease, acute disseminated encephalomyelitis, meningovascular syphilis, sarcoidosis and Lyme disease. It is also important to distinguish MS that predominantly affects the spinal cord from other diseases. Examples include subacute combined degeneration of the cord (can be seen in vitamin B12 deficiency, which usually affects lateral and posterior aspect of spinal cord) and spinal cord compression (can be evident on MRI imaging anyway).

Management

Immediate

Once the diagnosis of MS was made, the patient was started on **steroid pulse therapy** [1] with high dose intravenous methylprednisolone.

Short-term

There was a marked improvement of the patient's neurological deficits. Neither plasma exchange nor intravenous immunoglobulin was needed. **Low dose amitriptyline** [2] was started for neuropathic pain in the lower leg.

Long-term

Long-term use of an **immunomodulator** [3] was planned for the patient after the resolution of her acute exacerbation episode of MS. Based on the information obtained from the history taking, the patient's MS was considered as **relapsing–remitting multiple sclerosis** [4]. After the clearance from multiple pre-immunosuppression screening tests for latent chronic infections, the patient was started on **fingolimod** [5] with 6 hours of close cardiac monitoring after the first dose. Fortunately, the administration of the first dose was uneventful and the patient did not suffer from significant side-effects such as reversible lymphopenia. The patient remained stable with only one episode of exacerbation over 3 years. However, the course of disease turned into an aggressive form after another 3 relapses within 18 months and then transformed into the progressive pattern of MS. The patient's MS was then considered as secondary progressive multiple sclerosis and the medication was switched to **siponimod** [6] after several screening tests proved the patient's eligibility. The patient was also referred to the **clinical trial team for consideration for future treatment** [7]. She was also given the contact details of relevant **support groups and organisations** [8] in the community.

Prognosis

Higher frequency of acute attacks early in the course of the disease predicts more severe disease and poorer outcome overall. The degree of disability correlates with the extent and number of lesions on **MRI imaging** [9]. After the first episode of acute attack, about half of patients will have the second attack within 2 years. At the mark of 15 years after the first episode of acute attack, about 80% of patients have significant symptoms or disabilities that prevent them from working. They often require assistance with normal activities of daily living.

[1] High dose corticosteroid is the mainstay treatment for acute true relapse. An episode of acute 'true' relapse is treated with methylprednisolone 500–1000mg per day for three doses if they are severe. Plasma exchange and intravenous immunoglobulin may be helpful should steroids fail, though they are not needed if steroids prove effective.

[2] Supportive care is important during exacerbations. Severe spasticity can be managed using baclofen, while urinary urgency can be treated with amitriptyline. Low dose amitriptyline can also be used to treat neuropathic pain associated with MS. Trigeminal neuralgia and facial spasm can be helped by using carbamazepine and physiotherapy. The use of propranolol or clonazepam can be considered for intention tremor. The treatment of relapse may hasten recovery but it does not improve the long-term outlook or reduce the risk of further relapses. The long-term benefit is often seen in the use of immunomodulators.

[3] Immunomodulation/immunosuppression provides maintenance treatment for patients with MS. There are multiple immunomodulators available.

[4] The choice of immunomodulatory therapy is largely based on the pattern of the patient's MS.

[5] Fingolimod is an oral agent for MS. It is a lymphocyte sequestrant which acts by keeping lymphocytes in the peripheral lymph nodes and hence limiting the entrance of lymphocytes into the CNS. It is known to be able to cause reversible lymphopenia. Based on research, fingolimod is more effective than interferon. However, it should not be given to patients who had no varicella immunisation or known previous exposure and immunity. One thing to keep in mind is its first dose cardiotoxicity and this should not be missed. The patient needs cardiac monitoring for at least 6 hours post the administration of the first dose.

- Glatiramer acetate is another available treatment for MS. It is slow to act. Its main side-effect is non-cardiac chest pain or dyspnoea and bradycardia.
- Dimethyl fumarate is a well-tolerated MS medication. Rarely it causes lymphopenia. Its main side-effects are flushing and GI upset.

- Natalizumab is a monoclonal antibody targeting alpha 4 integrin which is needed for migration of the autoreactive lymphocytes into the CNS. It is more effective than interferon, according to the research studies, but it is only used in patients with aggressive disease, mainly because of the concerns of progressive multifocal leucoencephalopathy (reactivation of JC virus (John Cunningham virus, also known as human polyomavirus 2) in the CNS, resulting in a fatal disease).
- Alemtuzumab is a monoclonal antibody against CD-52 over the surface of mature lymphocytes. It has high potency and hence limited need for regular dosing. The research shows it has lower sustained accumulation of disability than interferon in the interferon refractory relapsing–remitting MS. However, B-cell mediated autoimmunity can be a problem. Autoimmune thyroid disease, antiglomerular basement membrane glomerulonephritis, and idiopathic thrombocytopenic purpura can happen as complications associated with the use of alemtuzumab.
- Ocrelizumab is an anti CD20 monoclonal antibody (considered as a new humanised version of rituximab). It can be used in relapsing–remitting MS and is the first therapy option available for patients with primary progressive MS. It is a strong immunosuppressant and its side-effect is mainly infection-related.

[6] Siponimod is a newly approved medication that can be used in secondary progressive MS. It is a sphingosine-1-phosphate receptor modulator. It is similar to fingolimod but with higher selectivity. Prior to initiation of the treatment, the patient needs to be screened for CYP2C9 phenotype, as this medication is contraindicated in CYP2C9*3/*3 genotype (poor metaboliser of siponimod resulting in elevated serum siponimod level). Other contraindications include recent myocardial infarction, unstable angina, advanced heart failure, stroke, transient ischaemic attack, and Mobitz type II or higher degree heart block. Interferon beta is a classic treatment for MS. It reduces the frequency of exacerbation by about one-third when it is used at an early stage of the disease, and is also capable of reducing the accumulation of CNS white matter lesions. There is evidence that the use of interferon

improves patients' survival, although the clinician should be aware of its hepatotoxicity and leucopenia. Its psychiatric side-effects should not be overlooked either.

- Mitoxantrone is a chemotherapy agent inhibiting lymphocyte and macrophage proliferation. It can be used in aggressive relapsing–remitting MS, secondary progressive MS and relapsing progressive MS. Its main side-effect is cardiac toxicity and hence it is contraindicated if ejection fraction is <50% or there is a significant drop in ejection fraction during the treatment.

7 Advanced therapy such as stem cell transplantation is presently under research. At the current stage, more long-term data is needed to assess the safety and efficacy of the therapy in the treatment of MS. The availability of such treatment is quite limited.

8 Supportive groups and organisations for patients with MS can be helpful in terms of providing advice to those patients who are distressed. The contact details of such organisations in the community should be offered to all patients.

9 If the initial episode is limited to a single abnormality clinically and the MRI is normal, only 10% of such patients will develop a second episode over the following 10 years. If the MRI is abnormal at the time of the initial attack, up to 80% of the patients will experience further episodes.

CASE 56: Muscular dystrophy

History

- A 21-year-old male presents for the routine review of his Duchenne muscular dystrophy (DMD). His DMD was diagnosed when he was **3 years old with an initial presentation of delayed start of independent standing and walking** [1].
- **His uncle and cousin also suffered from DMD** [2].
- He has been experiencing **progressively worsening weakness in his upper and lower limbs** [3]. The weakness is predominantly proximal.
- As part of the work-up, he was also diagnosed with **dilated cardiomyopathy at the age of 18 years** [4]. He has no previous history of arrhythmias and no permanent pacemakers or automatic defibrillators inserted in the past.
- As the disease progresses, he has an increased requirement for mobility aids, ranging from crutches to walking frame. He became **wheelchair-bound** [5] when he reached the age of 16. Due to the disability, he did not have the opportunity to participate in the same activities as other teenagers.
- He reports symptoms suggestive of **major depressive disorder** [6] and his parents confirm the symptoms reported by the patient. The patient denies any issues with facial expression and the weakness is not predominantly isolated in the upper limbs. However, he does report that he has recently had difficulty in swallowing. Throughout the consultation, the patient was coughing frequently and the cough itself was productive with brownish sputum.

[1] The symptoms of muscle weakness in DMD can start as early as 2 years of age. The proximal muscles are usually affected, followed by the distal muscles, and the lower limbs are affected before the upper limbs. Parents may notice their affected child having difficulty in running, jumping and climbing stairs. The child may find it difficult to sit upright and be unable to keep up with peers. Muscle pain or cramping is not uncommon in the early stage of disease. There are other different types of muscular dystrophy that can cause progressive neuromuscular weakness. Compared with DMD, the age of onset in Becker muscular dystrophy is usually later, varying widely between 5 and 60 years of age. The progression of the disease in Becker muscular dystrophy is also milder. Intellectual disability is not as common or severe when compared with DMD. Unfortunately, although muscle involvement is less prominent in Becker muscular dystrophy, these patients may still find the cardiac involvement to be the major issue in their healthcare. This, in part, may be due to patients with Becker muscular dystrophy having a greater ability to perform strenuous exercise than those with DMD, and thus the associated mechanical stress may further damage the myocardium with abnormal dystrophin.

[2] There are many different types of muscular dystrophies, but the most well-known ones are Duchenne and Becker muscular dystrophy. Because their underlying pathology is caused by the mutations of the dystrophin gene, they are also called dystrophinopathies. The genetic defect happens in the X chromosome and hence dystrophinopathies are inherited in the X-linked recessive pattern. Duchenne muscular dystrophy is resulted from a frame-shifting mutation in the gene encoding dystrophin (causing total absence of dystrophin) and hence has an earlier onset and more aggressive clinical course. In contrast, Becker muscular dystrophy is caused by a non-frame-shifting mutation in the dystrophin gene (which causes reduced dystrophin) and hence has a later onset of symptoms and milder progression. This gives Becker muscular dystrophy a better prognosis in general when compared with DMD. Given the inherited nature of muscular dystrophy, family history is important to obtain. The mutation identified in other affected family members can be helpful in terms of guiding genetic analysis. Female carriers are usually asymptomatic, but a few of them may have variable extent of muscular or cardiac involvement.

[3] Muscular dystrophies are a group of progressive inherited myopathic disorders that result in impairment of muscle function. Muscle weakness is the primary symptom. Weakness of the shoulder and upper arm muscle is characteristic for facioscapulohumeral muscular dystrophy, together with difficulty in facial expression.

- Limb-girdle muscular dystrophy is hard to distinguish from Becker muscular dystrophy and it is phenotypically similar to Becker muscular dystrophy. The calf muscle pseudohypertrophy in limb-girdle muscular dystrophy is not as significant as that in

Becker muscular dystrophy. Family history may help distinguish between these two conditions.

- Spinal muscular atrophy is a disorder caused by degeneration of the anterior horn cells in the spinal cord and motor nuclei in the brainstem, causing progressive muscle weakness and atrophy. The inheritance pattern is autosomal recessive and hence the pedigree would be different. Patients with spinal muscular atrophy may manage to sit with no assistance. However, independent standing and walking is never achieved. Eventually patients' ability to sit independently is lost during the teenage years. Additional features such as tongue atrophy with fasciculations, diffuse areflexia, dysphagia and neuropathic pattern on electromyography are helpful in terms of distinguishing spinal muscular atrophy from DMD.
- Another clinical entity worth mentioning is facio-scapulohumeral muscular dystrophy. The classic form of this disease involves asymmetric involvement of facial, scapular, upper arm, lower leg and abdominal muscles. Unlike DMD, which favours lower extremities more than upper extremities, facioscapulohumeral muscular dystrophy characteristically affects shoulder and upper arm muscles. Scapular winging is a classic physical sign that is hard to miss on inspection.

4 Dilated cardiomyopathy and arrhythmias are not uncommon in patients with DMD because of the involvement of cardiac muscles. The incidence of symptomatic cardiomyopathy in DMD increases with age, particularly during the teenage years. Patients with DMD with significant muscular function impairment are prone to falls. This risk of falls leads to a higher rate of fractures in arms and legs.

5 Duchenne and Becker muscular dystrophies have onset before adulthood. Because of this, when the adult physician sees the patients in their clinic, the patients often already have a few years of progression. Patients with Becker muscular dystrophy may still retain some mobility. Those with DMD, however, may have already become wheelchair-bound due to the aggressive disease progression.

6 When discussing with parents, taking the patient's mental health history is important. Those affected by DMD have a higher risk of autism, attention deficit hyperactivity disorder, obsessive–compulsive disorder and anxiety.

Examination

- On inspection, the patient is sitting in his **wheelchair** [1], with significant muscular atrophy found in all four limbs.
- **Neurological examination** [2] revealed fasciculation in the muscle groups of all four limbs. There was absence of reflexes in all four limbs, despite the use of the reinforcement manoeuvres. The power in all four limbs appeared to be consistently 2/5 in the proximal joints and 3/5 in the distal joints. Since the patient was wheelchair-bound, the gait could not be assessed.
- **There was no positive cerebellar sign appreciated on examination. The sensory examination appeared to be unremarkable** [3].
- There was also evidence of **scoliosis** [4].
- The parents also brought in the patient's **non-invasive ventilation** [5].

- **There was no evidence of scapular winging nor facial muscle atrophy** [6].
- The **cardiovascular** [7] examination revealed a laterally displaced apex beat with a third heart sound. A systolic murmur was best heard at the apex region radiating to the axilla. The audible murmur became louder on expiration and on handgrips. There was no physical sign suggestive of pulmonary hypertension clinically. The respiratory examination, however, revealed an inspiratory coarse crepitation in the posterior lower zone bilaterally and the right middle zone with increased vocal resonance. There was significant peripheral swelling in the patient's lower limbs bilaterally. The vital signs showed decreased saturation of oxygen at the level of 91% on air and the patient was febrile at the time of examination. The patient was haemodynamically stable.

1 Attention should be paid to the presence of walking aids in the room. This may give the clinician an idea of the extent of mobility impairment.

2 Physical examination usually reveals physical signs which may resemble lower motor neurone lesion. However, it is difficult to clinically distinguish myopathy and neuropathy on the basis of physical examination alone. The features in DMD include pseudohypertrophy of the calf, lumbar hyperlordosis, a waddling gait, shortening of Achilles tendons, hypotonia, and hyporeflexia or even areflexia. The patients can have short stature due to growth delay. Proximal muscle weakness can be prominent clinically.

3 The sensory examination and cerebellar examination are usually unremarkable.

4 A scoliosis may be evident on inspection. In combination with progressive weakness, this results in impaired pulmonary function and can contribute to acute respiratory failure.

5 For those with significant respiratory involvement, the patient may need non-invasive ventilation to assist respiratory function.

6 Scapular winging and facial muscular atrophy are typical early features in facioscapulohumeral muscular dystrophy. The respiratory function in facioscapulohumeral muscular

dystrophy is usually spared, while the lower limb muscles can be affected on an individual basis. The distal muscles of the upper limb are typically less affected compared with the proximal muscles.

7 One should never forget to examine the cardiovascular system, which may reveal the physical signs consistent with cardiomyopathy, and a permanent pacemaker may be present. As the disease progresses, significant mitral regurgitation can occur.

Investigations

- By looking at the patient's previous investigations, it was noticeable he did have elevated **creatine kinase** [1] at the time of diagnosis. However, this elevation became less prominent over time and eventually reaches the normal range.
- **Genetic testing** [2] when the patient was a child confirmed the diagnosis of DMD.
- Interestingly, there was a report on the **muscle biopsy** [3] which showed a total absence of dystrophin in the sample collected.
- **Electromyography** [4] was also performed and it was reported with myopathic pattern.
- The nerve conduction study and repetitive stimulation returned as unremarkable. **Electrocardiography** [5] was unremarkable.

- The **transthoracic echocardiogram** [6] performed at the time of diagnosis of dilated cardiomyopathy revealed a dilated left ventricle with markedly reduced left ventricular ejection fraction. Mitral regurgitation was also revealed on the same transthoracic echocardiogram and there was no evidence of pulmonary hypertension at the time.
- The most recent **pulmonary function test** [7] done 6 months ago showed a slightly reduced FEV_1 but markedly reduced FVC, resulting in a normal FEV_1/FVC ratio. The diffusing capacity for carbon monoxide (DLCO) was also normal but reduced total lung capacity and vital capacity. The maximum inspiratory and expiratory pressures were also reduced.

1 Serum creatine kinase levels are usually elevated in DMD in children when the disease is diagnosed. When the patients reach adulthood, creatine kinase levels eventually reach normal ranges in the majority of cases because more muscles are replaced by fat and fibrous tissue over time. Becker muscular dystrophy can also give elevated serum creatine kinase levels. This, however, is at much lesser extent when compared with DMD. An elevated creatine kinase level in a child with muscle weakness should prompt further investigation with genetic analysis. A normal creatine kinase level in a child, however, makes the diagnosis of Duchenne or Becker muscular dystrophy unlikely and the clinician should seek other alternative diagnoses.

2 The diagnosis of Duchenne and Becker muscular dystrophy is confirmed by using genetic testing to find the pathologic mutation in the gene encoding dystrophin.

3 Less often, muscle biopsy is performed to confirm the diagnosis of muscular dystrophy. Dystrophin is totally absent in DMD, whereas it is only reduced in Becker muscular dystrophy.

4 Electromyography may reveal a myopathic pattern and this helps distinguish myopathy from neuropathy as the cause of a patient's muscular weakness. However, it is not specific to Duchenne and Becker muscular dystrophies.

5 Muscular dystrophy causes dilated cardiomyopathy and conduction abnormalities. Because of this, these patients are particularly prone to arrhythmias. Extensive fibrosis can occur in the posterobasal left ventricular wall and can be arrhythmogenic, resulting in characteristic electrocardiographic changes of tall right precordial R waves and deep Q waves in the lateral leads (I, aVL and V5–6).

6 Transthoracic echocardiogram is able to detect structural changes in the myocardium before the onset of symptomatic cardiomyopathy and systolic dysfunction. The cardiac involvement on echocardiography typically shows early right ventricular involvement with later spread of fibrosis to the rest of the heart. Eventually all four chambers of the heart are involved, and the heart failure can be rapidly progressive. For the same reason as in DMD, patients with Becker muscular dystrophy are prone to arrhythmias due to the conduction abnormalities.

7 The pulmonary function test in muscular dystrophies and other types of neuromuscular disorders typically shows restrictive ventilatory defect. This is because the neuromuscular disorders decrease the ability of the patient's respiratory muscles to inflate and deflate the lungs. The gas exchange should be normal, with normal DLCO.

Management

Immediate

The patient appeared to be clinically unwell at the time of the consultation. He was then transferred to the closest ED for an urgent medical review. A diagnosis of **aspiration pneumonia** [1] was suspected. The patient was offered supplemental oxygen to assist his breathing and the saturation of oxygen was corrected to the level of 98% with 2L flow of oxygen. A medical review was performed in the ED and the suspicion of chest infection was validated. A chest X-ray was performed, showing right lower and middle zone opacity and cardiomegaly, together with features suggestive of pulmonary congestion. The patient was then started on IV antibiotics with ceftriaxone and metronidazole as the treatment for aspiration pneumonia given the history of dysphagia. IV diuresis with furosemide was applied to treat the patient's acute infective exacerbation of dilated cardiomyopathy. Since the patient is normally on regular glucocorticoid therapy as the maintenance therapy for DMD, a **doubled dosing of steroids** [2] was given in the form of IV hydrocortisone as stress dosing. The IV steroid was used because the patient was kept nil by mouth to prevent further aspiration until review by the speech pathologist.

Short-term

Although the antibiotics were effective in terms of treating the patient's aspiration pneumonia, and his breathing was improved by the use of diuretics, the assessment by the speech pathologist revealed more concerning issues. The patient's ability to swallow was considered impaired based on assessment with the use of fluoroscopy. His diet was then downgraded to texture C, mainly limited by his ability to keep food down. This in turn is suggestive of disease progression in DMD. The **steroid treatment** [3] was maintained, while no new drugs were added to the patient's medication regimen. Because the patient has been placed on long-term steroids, an assessment of his bone health was carried out. Further investigations with bone mineral density scan and vitamin D level revealed presence of osteoporosis and vitamin D deficiency. Vitamin D replacement was initiated to optimise the patient's bone health and exposure to outdoor sunlight was encouraged. Daily optimal calcium intake was also ensured. A follow-up bone mineral density scan was booked for a few months' time.

Long-term

Because of the complexity of this patient's long-term management, a meeting with the **multidisciplinary** [4] team was called. With the involvement of the **dietitian** [5], the patient's diet and nutritional supplement plan was optimised. The speech pathologist has already provided an opinion regarding the patient's diet texture to avoid further aspiration. However, with the patient's disease progression, it is of concern that the patient may need a feeding tube to be inserted, such as a percutaneous endoscopic gastrostomy tube. **Regular follow-up and serial pulmonary function tests with the respiratory team** [6] were kept as part of the plan, mainly to monitor the progression of the illness from a respiratory perspective. This will also help with the setting of non-invasive ventilation for use at home. A psychology consultation was also organised, given that the patient has disclosed symptoms suggestive of major depressive disorder. A referral to a **psychiatrist** [7] was also made. The patient's **vaccination** [8] schedule was reviewed and updated. Contact details for relevant support groups in the community were provided to the parents in case they need relevant education and advice on the patient's care at home. Referral to the psychological services should also be offered to the parents for their mental wellbeing. The palliative care team was involved early in this patient's care, given the relentlessly progressive nature of DMD and the presence of respiratory issues resulting from the disease. A discussion about the goals of care and **advanced care directive** [9] was carried out with the patient and his parents as part of the process. Pneumococcal and influenza vaccinations were given prior to the patient's discharge from the hospital.

Prognosis

Despite the great effort made by the **multidisciplinary team** [10], the patient continued to deteriorate. Eventually he passed away at the **age of 26 years** [11] from **respiratory failure** [12] despite the use of non-invasive ventilation at home. Thanks to the early involvement of palliative care his suffering at the end stage of his life was minimised.

1 Patients with Duchenne or Becker muscular dystrophy rarely present with a crisis from muscular dystrophy itself. Rather, they usually present with other illness that is precipitated by muscular dystrophy, such as aspiration pneumonia.

2 For those who have been on long-term glucocorticoid therapy and present with acute illness or trauma, a stress dosing of steroid should be employed to avoid acute adrenal insufficiency due to long-term suppression of the adrenal gland by the use of exogenous steroid.

3 Glucocorticoids are the mainstay treatment for DMD and should be started before there is a substantial physical decline. The benefits of steroid have been shown in many aspects of the illness, including improved average muscle strength and timed function testing, improved pulmonary function, reduced mortality related to heart failure, and improved overall survival. However, the use of long-term steroids is associated with many unwanted side-effects, such as weight gain, hirsutism, Cushing's syndrome, growth retardation and osteoporosis. However, if there is no significant obesity or intolerable side-effects, steroid therapy should be continued even for patients who become non-ambulatory, because of the benefits demonstrating delay in development of pulmonary impairment and heart failure. If glucocorticoid therapy is planned to be stopped, a tapering regimen is required to avoid adrenal insufficiency in a patient with a suppressed hypothalamic–pituitary–adrenal axis. In such cases, the tapering should be slow. Again, those who are on a tapering course of steroids and present with acute illness or trauma should still be given stress dose glucocorticoids.

4 Rehabilitation for patients with Duchenne and Becker muscular dystrophy requires involvement of multidisciplinary care because the long-term care needs multiple specialised assessments to improve patients' function and quality of life.

5 Due to the risk of falls, patients with Duchenne and Becker muscular dystrophy are at higher risk of fracture compared with the general population. In addition, the long-term use of steroids results in osteoporosis and further increases the risk of having fractures from injury. Hence, nutrition and bone health are important in fracture prevention. Weight and growth should be monitored and a dietitian should be involved to review patients' nutrition needs. Calcium, vitamin D and sun exposure are helpful in terms of strengthening bone health.

6 Given the cardiac and pulmonary complications resulting from Duchenne and Becker muscular dystrophy, cardiac and pulmonary function monitoring is crucial. Respiratory management is a critical component of DMD care via monitoring the patient's vital capacity annually from the age of 6 years. After the patient becomes non-ambulatory, the monitoring frequency is increased to every 6 months. The baseline assessment of cardiac function should be performed at the time of diagnosis and should be carried out annually.

7 Psychosocial support for patients and their family plays a vital role in the management of the disease. Routine assessment of mental health is a must-do for the patient and sometimes their family members. Referral to a psychiatrist or psychologist should be made if needed.

8 Vaccination is helpful in terms of infection prevention. Annual influenza vaccine and pneumococcal vaccine are recommended.

9 Given that DMD has a poorer prognosis and shorter life expectancy, advanced care planning and palliative care options are usually discussed sensitively with patients and their families early in the course of the disease when compared with Becker muscular dystrophy. For those who need surgery or procedures that require anaesthesia or sedation, a preoperative review by pulmonary, cardiac, and anaesthesia specialists is required due to the higher risk of complications. Succinylcholine is absolutely contraindicated in these patients.

10 Patients with DMD are often wheelchair-bound by the age of 13. The age of mortality is usually between late teens and twenties, from either respiratory failure or cardiomyopathy.

11 Patients with Becker muscular dystrophy may still find themselves able to retain mobility at least until the age of 16 and stay well into adulthood. Some patients may even maintain their ambulation into old age.

12 Marked compromise of respiratory function is the major cause of mortality in patients with muscular dystrophy. In rare cases, heart failure may become the major cause of death, especially in the late stages of the disease.

CASE 57: Myasthenia gravis

History

- A **65-year-old man** [1] with no significant past medical history presents with **drooping eyelids on the right side** [2] **for the last 2 weeks** [3].
- After further history taking, he reports that he has experienced **multiple episodes of similar symptom every few weeks for the last 6 months** [4].
- **Either of his eyes could be affected** [5] **and on one occasion the symptom started in his right eye with later involvement of his left eye** [6].
- He also mentions his current presentation is associated with **weakness in his right leg** [7].
- The right leg weakness **worsens after exercise and at the end of the day** [8].
- The patient **denies any symptoms of dyspnoea, dysarthria or neck weakness** [9].
- He **denies any systemic symptoms** [10] of weight loss, night sweats or fever.
- He does not take any **medications** [11].

[1] The age of onset for myasthenia gravis has a bimodal distribution. Early peak tends to occur in the second and third decades, with female predominance, and late peak tends to occur in the sixth to eighth decades, with male predominance.

[2] 50–85% of patients will present with ocular symptoms. 90% of patients present as diplopia. About half of those who present with ocular symptoms will develop generalised disease within two years. Weakness of the eyelid muscles can result in ptosis. The extraocular muscles are frequently involved in myasthenia gravis as well, leading to binocular diplopia. Some patients may experience both ptosis and diplopia as the ocular presentation.

[3] Early in the course of myasthenia gravis, the symptoms are usually transient and episodic.

[4] Patients may find themselves free of symptoms for hours, days or even weeks. The symptoms of myasthenia gravis may remit spontaneously for weeks.

[5] The ocular symptoms in myasthenia gravis can be unilateral or bilateral.

[6] The ptosis in myasthenia gravis can be characteristically alternating. Patients may find the ptosis starts bilaterally with improvement in one eye, resulting in unilateral ptosis. Alternatively, ptosis can start as unilateral ptosis and later become bilateral. Ptosis in myasthenia gravis may also switch from one eye to the other over time.

[7] As the disease progresses, it is not uncommon for the patient to start experiencing new symptoms in addition to the initial presentation. This development of new symptoms typically happens weeks or months after the initial presentation. The progression of myasthenia gravis usually peaks within a few years from the onset of the disease. More than 80% of patients will experience the maximum extent of the disease within two years. The peripheral muscle weakness in myasthenia gravis is predominantly proximal.

[8] Fatigability is an important character of weakness in myasthenia gravis. Patients may usually find there is a fluctuation in the strength of the affected muscle(s). The weakness of the affected muscle usually gets worse after exercise or use for an extended period of the time. The weakness can also typically get worse at the end of the day. For example, patients may find their ocular symptoms get worse after prolonged periods of reading and weakness in limbs may get worse after activity involving the affected muscle.

[9] 15% of patients may present with bulbar involvement such as dysarthria, dysphagia and fatigability with chewing. Bulbar weakness in myasthenia gravis is usually intermittent, normally with difficulty in swallowing. Isolated neck weakness and isolated respiratory muscle weakness are less common but can result in dyspnoea. Severe respiratory muscle weakness can often lead to myasthenia crisis.

[10] An important differential diagnosis of myasthenia gravis is Lambert–Eaton syndrome. It is a syndrome resulting from presynaptic failure of releasing acetylcholine. This condition can be either paraneoplastic with 50% of cases associated with small cell lung carcinoma, or autoimmune related. The weakness in Lambert–Eaton myasthenia syndrome is more likely to present in the morning and usually improves with exercise. Autonomic dysfunction is another feature in Lambert–Eaton myasthenia syndrome distinguishable from myasthenia gravis.

11 It is important to clarify the list of newly started medication with the patient because some medications can precipitate the symptoms of myasthenia gravis. In particular, the use of certain antibiotics such as aminoglycosides can interfere with neuromuscular transmission.

Examination

- The patient is **not dyspnoeic at rest** [1].
- On cranial nervous examination the patient has **ptosis bilaterally; however, the ptosis is more prominent on the right side** [2].
- It is also noticed that the patient's **right eyebrow is raised, with a wrinkled forehead** [3].
- The ptosis becomes more prominent after the patient was tested by **sustained upward gaze**.
- The ptosis is **partially recovered after resting and the application of an ice pack** [4].
- **Eye movement and the rest of the cranial examination are otherwise normal** [5].
- **No use of accessory respiratory muscles is observed on inspection** [6].
- **The patient is able to lie flat and there is no weakness in their neck flexion** [7].

- **The patient is asked to start counting loudly after maximal inspiration. They can reach 50 in one single breath with no difficulty** [8].
- **No slurred or nasal speech is revealed and the patient's facial expression is otherwise unremarkable** [9].
- On peripheral nervous examination there is **no muscle atrophy on inspection** [10].
- The patient demonstrates weakness in his right hip flexion and knee extension. The **weakness becomes more prominent while the pressure is applied persistently** [11].
- The **reflexes are preserved in all four limbs. There is no sensory change detected on examination** [12].

1 The first thing to check for in myasthenia gravis is whether the patient is in myasthenia crisis. This is characterised by the increasing respiratory muscle and/or bulbar muscle weakness from myasthenia gravis that requires intensive treatment involving intubation.

2 If the ptosis fluctuates throughout the examination, then evidence for fatigability of the levator muscle is present. If fluctuation is not observed during the examination, there are several ways to elicit the fatigability:
- Increase in ptosis either during prolonged upward gaze or upon return to primary gaze suggests fatigability.
- Fast switch from downward gaze to primary gaze triggers the affected eyelid to quickly rise and then fall.
- On passively lifting the more ptotic eyelid above the iris, the contralateral eyelid may become more ptotic by 'curtaining'.
- Look for improvement after the patient is asked to close their eyes and rest for a few minutes.

3 The patient with bilateral ptosis may need to use the frontalis muscle to elevate the eyelids, which gives the forehead a wrinkled appearance.

4 Although it is not used as a diagnostic test, the ice pack test typically gives improvement of ptosis while it is used to raise suspicion of myasthenia gravis. This test has a sensitivity of 80%.

5 Binocular diplopia (diplopia only when both eyes are uncovered) can present in many ocular myasthenia gravis cases. The muscles involved can be individual or bilateral. As with ptosis, ocular motility can demonstrate fatigability. Again, fluctuation in either the degree of diplopia or the direction of gaze that elicits the diplopia during the examination suggests fatigable ocular motor paresis. Prolonged or sustained gaze involving the affected muscle may trigger worsening of ocular motor paresis. Any involvement of trigeminal nerve and/or pupillary abnormality should prompt consideration of an alternative diagnosis such as structural lesion along the brainstem.

6 The use of accessory respiratory muscles is an important indicator of respiratory distress. Usually such effort may not be sustained. However, generalised myasthenia gravis may mask the use of accessory respiratory muscles.

7 Inability to lie supine or speak more than a few words are indicators of diaphragm weakness. Weak neck flexion also correlates with diaphragmatic dysfunction.

8 Single breath count test is a useful bedside tool measuring respiratory function. Ability to reach 50 indicates normal respiratory function and count of less than 15 indicates low forced vital capacity and respiratory muscle weakness.

9 The presence of dysarthria and dysphagia indicates oropharyngeal weakness. When facial muscles are involved, the patient usually appears to be expressionless. Severe slurred speech is also a sign of potential myasthenia gravis crisis.

10 Myasthenia gravis is usually not associated with muscle atrophy. If muscle atrophy is present, the possibility of motor neurone disease can be considered.

11 Fatigability is an important feature of myasthenia gravis. This can be demonstrated by applying persistent pressure while the patient is asked to resist the pressure applied.

12 Myasthenia gravis is a neuromuscular junction disease and hence sensory components should not be involved. Unlike Guillain–Barré syndrome, the reflex in myasthenia gravis is usually preserved. Historically, the Tensilon test can be performed as a diagnostic test for myasthenia gravis. It involves the administration of edrophonium (a short-acting acetylcholinesterase inhibitor). The clinician can then assess the patient for change in signs. Its sensitivity is 60% with low specificity. Atropine should be ready for use at bedside. Amyotrophic lateral sclerosis (ALS) is the most common form of motor neurone disease. While also present with muscle weakness, motor neurone disease is a progressive neurodegenerative disease and is a different entity from myasthenia gravis. ALS can involve the bulbar muscles, resulting in dysarthria, dysphagia and facial weakness. In contrast, ptosis and ocular dysmotility are not typically seen in ALS. Its hallmark is the mix of upper (hyperreflexia and Babinski signs) and lower (atrophy and fasciculations) motor neurone signs.

Investigations

- Serological testing is then ordered. This patient is **anti-acetylcholine receptor antibody positive** [1].
- His **anti-muscle specific kinase antibody is negative** [2]. He then undergoes electrodiagnostic testing to confirm the diagnosis.
- **The repetitive nerve stimulation shows 10% decrement in amplitude after repetitive stimulation and this decrement tends to increase after exercise** [3].
- **Single-fibre electromyography of his ocular muscle shows jittering pattern of the action potentials** [4].
- An MRI is then performed to assess the patient's mediastinum. A thymic mass is revealed with features suggestive of **thymoma** [5].
- **Thyroid function test** [6] and **MRI of the brain** [7] are unremarkable.

1 85% of patients have generalised myasthenia gravis. Of those, 85% are anti-acetylcholine receptor (AChR) antibody positive. 15% of patients have ocular myasthenia gravis and 50% of ocular myasthenia gravis cases have AChR antibody positive.

2 Of those with generalised myasthenia gravis, 6–10% are anti-muscle-specific kinase (MuSK) antibody positive. This proportion is increased to 38% if the patient has negative AChR antibody. MuSK antibody is usually present in non-white young females. It only presents in generalised myasthenia gravis and is not related to thymoma or thymic hyperplasia. Patients with positive MuSK antibody usually have severe disease with respiratory and bulbar involvement. Such patients' response to treatment is generally poor.

3 Repetitive nerve stimulation is widely available and is the most frequently used test for myasthenia gravis. The amplitude of compound muscle action potential (CMAP) is recorded after the electrical stimulation of the nerve. In normal muscles, there is no change in CMAP after stimulation, whereas in myasthenia gravis there may be progressive decrement in CMAP amplitude. 10% decrement in amplitude is diagnostic. This test has sensitivity of 80%.

4 Single fibre electromyography (SFEMG) is less readily available compared with repetitive nerve stimulation. It is able to simultaneously record the action potentials from two muscle fibres that are innervated by the same motor axon. It is best utilised for ocular myasthenia gravis. Jittering is the diagnostic feature of myasthenia gravis. Unfortunately, SFEMG is highly sensitive but not specific. False positives can happen in the case of motor neurone disease, peripheral neuropathy and Lambert–Eaton myasthenic syndrome.

5 Thymoma/thymic hyperplasia is present in 75% of AChR antibody positive myasthenia gravis. Thymic hyperplasia dominates as the most common (85%) thymic abnormality. Thymoma is the predominant tumour form among the thymic tumours identified. MRI is the imaging modality of choice. The presence of thymoma in myasthenia gravis patients indicates the removal of the tumour is possible, because research shows that the thymectomy group has better outcome for those with generalised myasthenia gravis.

6 Graves' disease can mimic ocular myasthenia gravis by producing abnormal eye movement due to constrictive ophthalmopathy. Thyroid function test is a useful screening test that should be performed before instituting treatment for myasthenia gravis.

7 Structural issues in the brainstem can also produce ocular symptoms similar to those in ocular myasthenia gravis. MRI imaging of the brain is essential to exclude any brainstem lesion in unconfirmed cases of ocular myasthenia gravis.

Management

Immediate

For those presenting with myasthenia gravis, **a quick screen for respiratory failure is required** [1]. Monitoring the vitals and ordering investigations should be done early on. Check for the length of sentence the patient is able to speak and perform single breath count test. It is important to identify those with myasthenic crisis because it is a **fatal condition if left untreated** [2]. If there is any sign of respiratory failure, consultation by the **intensive care team is required** [3]. To treat myasthenic crisis, IV **steroid is used as initial therapy. Intravenous immunoglobulin and plasma exchange** [4] can also be used.

Short-term

The use of certain drugs should be **avoided** [5]. Steroids can usually be used in generalised severe cases but paradoxical deterioration should be expected in the **first 1–2 weeks** [6]. For those who are not responding to steroid treatment or are intolerant to steroid, IV immunoglobulin can be used.

Long-term

The use of cholinesterase inhibitors is the **mainstay in mild cases of myasthenia gravis** [7]. However, those patients should be monitored for **cholinergic crisis** [8]. Long-term use of steroid is associated with many unwanted **side-effects** [9] and the benefit of IV immunoglobulin only lasts for a few weeks. In this case, the use of **immunomodulators is reasonable** [10] for the long-term management of myasthenia gravis and for those who do not respond to the use of cholinesterase inhibitor alone. **Thymectomy** [11] is advisable early on for those who present with generalised myasthenia gravis and are positive of anti-AChR antibody. For those who are about to have **surgery** [12] or are **pregnant** [13], plasma exchange can be useful.

---

[1] Clinical tools to monitor myasthenia gravis patients' respiratory function include inspection of accessory muscle use, single breath count test, length of sentence the patient can speak in one breath, and the routine vitals such as respiratory rate and saturation of oxygen. Bedside spirometry can be used as an extra tool if available. The parameters to look out for include maximal inspiratory pressure and tidal volume.

[2] Patients with myasthenic crisis have sudden worsening of symptoms and this can be fatal if respiratory failure develops. The in-hospital mortality rate is about 5%, according to a large cohort study.

[3] Mechanical ventilation may be required in the setting of respiratory failure resulting from myasthenic crisis. Ventilatory support is needed in addition to the use of other immunosuppressive therapies.

[4] IVIg and plasma exchange are the mainstay of treatment but because they take several days to start working and benefit only lasts for a few weeks, IV steroids should also be initiated.

[5] The medications to be avoided include but are not limited to: neuromuscular junction-blocking anaesthetics, streptomycin, aminoglycoside, penicillamine, fluoroquinolones, macrolides, tetracyclines, beta blockers, quinidine, procainamide, hydroxychloroquine, phenytoin and lithium.

[6] 40% of patients with generalised severe disease and treated with steroid therapy can have paradoxical deterioration as aggravation of the disease in the first 7–10 days.

[7] Cholinesterase inhibitors such as pyridostigmine are revolutionary in the management of myasthenia gravis and provide the mainstay of symptom control. However, it is important to watch out for cholinergic crisis.

[8] Cholinergic crisis happens when the use of cholinesterase inhibitor is excessive. The manifestation is usually weakness. Indeed, it is difficult to distinguish weakness from cholinergic crisis and that from the progression of existing myasthenia gravis. Unless the use of cholinesterase inhibitor is truly excessive, one should always expect the weakness is a result of the worsening myasthenia gravis. The treatment of cholinergic crisis is usually the suspension of the cholinesterase and monitoring of the strength of muscles affected.

[9] Steroids are well known for their side-effects resulting from long-term usage. The classical ones include hypertension, adrenal suppression, iatrogenic diabetes, central obesity, immunosuppression, osteoporosis, mood disturbance, proximal muscle weakness and growth retardation in children. The tapering of steroid therapy in myasthenia gravis should be slow and it usually takes months to taper the steroid to the lowest possible dose. *Pneumocystis*

pneumonia prophylaxis should be used for those on high dose prednisolone for a prolonged period of time.

10 For acetylcholine receptor (AChR) antibody-positive or seronegative myasthenia gravis, either azathioprine or mycophenolate mofetil can be used as a first-line steroid-sparing agent. Azathioprine has been shown to be effective at steroid sparing and to reduce relapses. It is also known to prolong remissions. However, azathioprine takes months to start working. In this case, it is not suitable as the initial therapy and hence would require the combination with steroid in the initiation phase. What is also important is the TPMT status of the patient, as TPMT is very important in the metabolism of azathioprine and it has wide variability. The use of FBE and liver function test is also important, to monitor azathioprine's side-effects of bone marrow suppression and liver toxicity. Mycophenolate mofetil is similarly effective but is not safe to be used during pregnancy due to teratogenicity. Bone marrow suppression as a side-effect is another thing to watch out for. If patients do not tolerate azathioprine or mycophenolate mofetil well, then the use of calcineurin inhibitors (tacrolimus and ciclosporin) is the next choice. For anti-MuSK positive myasthenia gravis, rituximab is used as first-line therapy. Those patients usually respond poorly to the use of cholinesterase inhibitors, and the use of azathioprine or mycophenolate mofetil is not enough to spare them from steroid use. If patients with severe myasthenia gravis do not respond to immunomodulators and require particularly high dose of steroid, intravenous immunoglobulin is the next treatment of choice.

11 10% of myasthenia gravis patients have thymoma and another 65% have thymic hyperplasia. After resection, 70% of cases show improvement and among those, 25% undergo remission. For those who do not show response after thymectomy, the reasons of failure include incomplete removal of thymus/thymic tumour, ectopic thymic tissue, and fulminant/widespread thymic disease.

12 Plasma exchange is useful in the perioperative management of patients with myasthenia gravis, especially in the preparation for surgery. With the advances in the management of myasthenia gravis, the prognosis has improved significantly.

13 Management of myasthenia gravis in pregnancy is important. One-third of myasthenia gravis patients have exacerbation, usually during the first trimester or postpartum period. Cholinesterase inhibitor can be used in mild cases. Prednisolone can be used in moderate cases. Azathioprine can be considered for use during pregnancy, especially for those who experience severe disease. In addition, intravenous immunoglobulin and plasma exchange can be used in the management of severe myasthenia gravis during pregnancy. As the mainstay treatment of pre-eclampsia and eclampsia, magnesium sulphate is contraindicated in women with myasthenia gravis due to its ability to precipitate a severe myasthenia crisis. For those with pre-eclampsia and eclampsia, severe hypertension is treated with methyldopa or hydralazine. Seizure prophylaxis usually requires levetiracetam or valproic acid, whereas the use of phenytoin should be avoided. Neonatal myasthenia gravis occurs in 10–20% of infants born to myasthenic mothers, due to transplacental passage of anti-AChR antibodies. Because of this, 48–72 hours of monitoring in special care baby unit or local neonatal unit is required for all infants born to myasthenic mothers. A low to moderate dose of cholinesterase inhibitors can be used during breastfeeding. Steroid is considered safe in lactation. However, azathioprine, mycophenolate and ciclosporin should be avoided as they can cause immunosuppression in infants.

CASE 58 Parkinson's disease

History

- A **73-year-old male** [1] retired teacher presents for review due to concerns of recent increased frequency of falls over the last 2 years. His wife accompanied him at the time of consultation.
- According to the couple, the patient has **been experiencing** [2] falls almost every other day over the first 12 months, and is now experiencing almost daily **falls** [3] over the last 12 months. According to his wife, the patient also has a history of kicking and punching when he was having vivid dreams, months before the onset of his tremors and frequent falls. Constipation has always been an issue for the patient, for which he has been taking laxatives regularly.
- There was also a complaint about ongoing **tremor** [4] at rest which the patient found very bothersome. The tremor disappeared when he was using his hands. The tremor had become more persistent over the last 2 years and has bilateral involvement just prior to his current visit, compared with unilateral tremor at the start.
- On multiple occasions, the wife noticed the patient had an almost **'frozen' posture when he started moving and his movements appeared to be 'shuffling'** [5].
- There is no issue in terms of **maintaining posture** [6] when standing upright. His current list of medications includes aspirin, perindopril, coloxyl and senna, pantoprazole and atorvastatin. His past medical history includes hypertension, hypercholesterolaemia and gastro-oesophageal reflux disease (GORD). He does not have any family history of parkinsonism disorders.

[1] Parkinsonism is a spectrum of movement disorders, with Parkinson's disease (PD) being a progressive neurodegenerative disease with clear aetiology. Other aetiologies of parkinsonism include drug-induced causes, such as phenothiazines and methyldopa and post-encephalitis. Other rare disorders which can also cause parkinsonism include toxins (carbon monoxide, manganese), Wilson's disease, progressive supranuclear palsy, multisystem atrophy, syphilis and malignancy.

[2] Braak staging of Parkinson's disease is used to classify the degree of a patient's PD based on their clinical manifestation. The presymptomatic stage has symptoms of anosmia, constipation, REM sleep behavioural disorder and mood changes. The symptomatic stage is mainly about the motor manifestations of Parkinson's such as tremor, bradykinesia and rigidity. The late stages of PD show manifestation of cognitive impairment and psychiatric symptoms. The late stage can sometimes overlap with the clinical picture of dementia with Lewy bodies.

[3] Cardinal features of Parkinson's disease include tremor, bradykinesia and rigidity. As a result, the patient often finds their mobility greatly impaired and ends up with great risk of falling. There are two broad PD phenotypes, akinetic-rigid and tremor-dominant. Frequent falls are predominantly of the akinetic-rigid subtype, although these two phenotypes can overlap with manifestations of both rigidity and tremor symptoms.

[4] The tremor in PD is typically the pill-rolling type and it is a resting tremor. It differs from action tremors in other conditions such as essential tremor or multiple sclerosis. The tremor itself is most noticeable when the patient is not engaged in purposeful activities. The frequency of the tremor is usually 3–7Hz. The patient often notices the tremor starting intermittently in the early stage of PD. However, this can become more persistent and evident as the disease progresses. Usually it starts unilaterally in the hand and then spreads contralaterally several years after the onset of the symptoms. The starting side tends to be the more affected side throughout the course of the disease. The tremor is not necessarily isolated in the upper limbs solely; it can also happen with the involvement of legs, lips, jaw and tongue.

[5] Another major issue with PD is bradykinesia. The patient often complains of generalised slowness of movement. And as the patient moves, there is a progressive decrement of amplitude and speed. Bradykinesia often presents at the onset of PD and is considered the most common feature of this illness and the major cause of disability in patients diagnosed with PD. Eventually, bradykinesia can be seen in almost all patients as the disease progresses. When the bradykinesia is affecting a patient's arms, they often complain

of decreased manual dexterity of the fingers at the start. When the bradykinesia starts in the legs, the patient is most often found to have issues related to walking. The walking is often in the form of dragging legs, shuffling gait or feeling unsteady on the feet. As the disease progresses, gait freezing and festination may develop (described by James Parkinson as "an irresistible impulse to take much quicker and shorter steps, and thereby to adopt unwillingly a running pace"). Rigidity is the last cardinal feature of PD. It refers to any increased resistance to passive movement about a joint. Like tremor and bradykinesia, rigidity in PD often begins unilaterally, and typically on the same side as the tremor if one is present. Eventually it progresses to the contralateral side and remains asymmetric throughout the disease. Rigidity can affect any part of the body, and may contribute to the complaints of stiffness and pain.

6 Postural instability is another issue with PD. It is defined as an impairment of the patient's postural reflexes. It usually develops in the late stages of PD. If postural instability happens early in the course of the disease, it can be useful to differentiate PD from other Parkinsonian syndromes because early impairment of postural reflex is more often found in other Parkinsonian syndromes such as progressive supranuclear palsy or multisystem atrophy. The patient becomes wheelchair-bound once postural reflexes are lost, because it is the feature least responsive to dopaminergic therapy.

Other motor symptoms in PD are listed in *Table 58.1*.

Table 58.1 Motor symptoms in Parkinson's disease

Category	Notes
Craniofacial	Hypomimia, speech disturbance, hypokinetic dysarthria, hypophonia, dysphagia, sialorrhoea
Musculoskeletal	Micrographia, dystonia, myoclonus, stooped posture
Gait	Shuffling, freezing, festination

Non-motor symptoms in PD are listed in *Table 58.2*.

Table 58.2 Non-motor symptoms in Parkinson's disease

Category	Notes
Autonomic dysfunction	Postural hypotension, constipation, diaphoresis, urinary difficulties and sexual dysfunction
Rapid eye movement sleep behaviour disorder	• Often enact violent dreams during REM sleep • Usually vocalised • Parkinsonism disappears during associated complex behaviours • High frequency in synucleinopathies including PD • A marker of worse outcome for dementia
Cognitive impairment	Dementia (usually late in the course of disease)
Psychiatric	Psychosis and hallucinations, mood disorders
Olfactory dysfunction	

One of the main differentials in patients who present with symptoms suggestive of parkinsonism is multisystem atrophy. It is another alpha synuclein disorder. It typically has onset at a younger age (in the sixth decade) compared with PD. The disease has a triad of autonomic failure (erectile dysfunction, urinary dysfunction, orthostatic hypotension), parkinsonism and cerebellar signs. Its phenotype depends on the predominant symptoms, i.e. autonomic, parkinsonism, cerebellar phenotypes. The mean survival in those diagnosed with multisystem atrophy is about 6–10 years from the onset of the symptoms.

Examination

- Upon inspection, the patient has a **mask-like facial expression** [1].
- Assessment of the patient's **gait** [2] showed that he had difficulty in initiating movements, with a tendency to fall forward, followed by a series of small shuffling steps. The patient also found it hard to stop his movements when he was asked to turn around. There was no ataxia on gait assessment.
- The **'pull' test** [3] was negative, as the patient was able to maintain balance while he was pulled backwards.
- When sitting on the examination table, there was a noticeable **tremor** [4] in both hands with frequency about 4Hz. This appeared to be more prominent in the left hand than the right.

- Finger–nose test was then performed with no past pointing, and the tremor disappeared when the patient was attempting **finger pointing** [5].
- There was **cogwheel rigidity** [6] bilaterally in the patient's upper limbs and this was more prominent on the left side.
- The rigidity persists despite **reinforcement manoeuvre** [7].

- **Rapid hand movement** [8] with repetitive hand gripping movement was tested. The gradual loss of amplitude and speed of hand movement was noticed.
- There was no evidence of **sialorrhoea or hypophonia** [9].
- **Glabellar tap** [10] was performed and it was positive.
- **Eye examination** [11] was unremarkable.

[1] Mask-like facies is often seen in PD, manifested as a lack of facial expression.

[2] Paucity of movement can be prominent. Gait assessment is essential for a patient with suspected PD. The patient is normally asked to walk, turn quickly, stop and then restart walking back to the clinician. The clinician should note difficulty in starting the movement, shuffling gait, freezing and festination. It is important to note that the gait in Parkinson's disease is narrow based and the patient can still move in tandem gait.

[3] The 'pull' test can be used to assess postural instability. The clinician stands behind the patient and pulls the patient's shoulders firmly. The test is negative if the patient is able to maintain balance and step backward (retropulse) by no more than one step. The test is positive if the patient retropulses by more than one step.

[4] After the patient returns to the examination table, the clinician should start looking for resting tremor with the arms relaxed. The tremor in PD can be characteristic as pill-rolling. The pattern can be unilateral or asymmetrical when the tremor is bilateral.

[5] Finger–nose testing can be used to assess cerebellar function. It can also be used to identify any presence of action tremor. The tremor in PD is typically resting tremor type, meaning that the tremor usually diminishes as the patient attempts finger pointing. However, the patient may have action tremor if other pathology is present.

[6] By testing the rigidity, wrist tone is assessed. There are two different types of rigidity: cogwheel and lead pipe rigidity. Cogwheel rigidity is a ratchet pattern of resistance and relaxation as the examiner moves the limb through its full range of motion, whereas lead pipe rigidity is a tonic resistance that is smooth throughout the entire range of passive movement.

[7] Reinforced manoeuvres can be used to confirm the presence of rigidity by asking the patient to perform repetitive movement using the contralateral limbs.

[8] Test for bradykinesia by eliciting rapid alternating movements – ask the patient to perform one of the following movements: finger tapping, hand gripping, pronation–supination hand movements and heel or toe tapping.

[9] Back onto the patient's face, some manifestations may be evident, especially sialorrhoea and hypophonia. The clinician should then start looking for any tremors with the lips, tongue or jaw. This can become prominent with distraction by asking the patient to perform mental calculation. Dribbling of saliva can indicate the presence of sialorrhoea, and this will assist the clinician to formulate the management plan (see below). Speech testing in patients with PD may reveal a monotonous, soft, poorly articulated and faint speech.

[10] Glabellar tap is a primitive reflex that is positive in PD. The clinician taps the patient's forehead while asking them to keep their eyes open. The clinician should keep the finger out of the patient's line of sight. The reflex is positive (Myerson's sign) when the patient's eyes continue to blink after the clinician's middle finger taps several times over the glabella from behind. The test is negative if the patient's eyes are kept open with tapping. Further tests can be useful in revealing additional manifestations of PD: feeling the forehead for greasy or sweaty eyebrows due to autonomic dysfunction, measuring postural blood pressure for postural hypotension and asking the patient to write, for micrographia. Although not routinely performed, the olfactory function can be tested by asking the patient to identify the smell from different scented cards.

[11] Ocular movements should also be checked for supranuclear gaze palsies such as vertical supranuclear gaze palsy in progressive supranuclear palsy, which can also give parkinsonism symptoms.

Investigations

The diagnosis of Parkinson's disease is **mainly clinical** [1]. There are no laboratory or radiological investigations that can be routinely used to diagnose PD.

1 The diagnosis of PD requires both the essential criteria and the presence of supportive features. The essential criteria of PD include bradykinesia plus resting tremor or rigidity. The supportive features of PD include a clear response to dopaminergic treatment, the presence of dopamine-induced dyskinesia, rest tremor of a limb in previous documentation and the presence of either olfactory loss or cardiac sympathetic denervation on metaiodobenzylguanidine scintigraphy.

Management

Non-pharmacological

Based on the information obtained from history taking and clinical examination, a diagnosis of Parkinson's disease was made. It was overwhelming news to the patient himself and his wife. In order to facilitate the management in the future, **a brochure containing information** [1] regarding PD was provided. The contact details of **support groups** [2] in the community were also given to the patient and his wife. As there were no speech or swallow manifestations at the time of the review, no referral to **speech pathology** [3] was made. However, the patient was educated in terms of symptoms suggestive of swallowing or speech disorder and was advised to seek speech pathology opinion should such manifestations occur prior to next review. A referral to the **physiotherapist** [4] was also made for early involvement of regular physical exercise programme. This improves patients' motor functioning, although the patient understands the fact that the motor function may deteriorate as the disease progresses.

Pharmacological therapy

As frequent falls were one of the patient's major concerns, pharmacological therapy **levodopa** [5] was trialled. The medication was started in combination with carbidopa to enhance delivery and to reduce peripheral side-effects. The trial was a success and the patient's motor function greatly improved with almost no further falls for another 2 years. Several attempts were then made to find a **new balance** [6] between the patient's motor manifestations and medication dosing. However, it was becoming increasingly difficult due to more frequent onset of dyskinesia.

As the levodopa in combination with carbidopa is getting increasingly difficult to find the 'on' phase, a decision was made to start other **adjunct therapy** [7] rather than **advanced therapy** [8]. Oral pramipexole was then initiated for added benefit in the patient's control of PD.

Non-motor symptoms [9] can be quite distressing for the patient. This patient had been having issues with **constipation** [10] for a long time while his wife is also complaining of his **enactment of vivid dreams** [11] during the night. **Lifestyle modifications** [12] with high fibre diet and regular exercise were recommended. Melatonin was started to assist the patient's sleep.

Prognosis

The progression of Parkinson's disease is variable and there is no available model to help the clinician to predict the **prognosis** [13] of idiopathic PD. In general, the older the patient and longer the duration of PD, the higher the prevalence of dementia, with the patient's age being the strongest predictor. After 20 years, almost all patients will have developed dementia.

1 Education is essential for the patient and their family to have an understanding and some control over the disorder.

2 Support groups in the community can be a valuable resource.

3 Speech therapy may be helpful in maintaining speech volume and voice quality.

4 Regular physical exercise may offer some benefit for improving patients' functioning.

5 Levodopa is the main precursor in dopamine synthesis. Dopamine can be converted into noradrenaline by dopa decarboxylase in the periphery. Because of this, levodopa is usually combined with dopa decarboxylase inhibitor (e.g. carbidopa) to enhance the delivery of levodopa into the CNS and to reduce the peripheral side-effects of levodopa, such as nausea. Levodopa improves motor function, activities of daily living and quality of life compared with other drug classes. Hence levodopa is the drug of choice as first-line treatment in PD. The benefit is ongoing for many years. Another benefit of levodopa is the decreased chance of requiring add-on therapy compared with other drug classes. However, one downside of levodopa is that it is short-acting and hence requires multiple doses throughout the day. This is particularly burdensome in those already on multiple medications. The side-effects of levodopa include dyskinesia, nausea and vomiting, impulse control disorders if given in high doses (hypersexuality, pathological gambling, excessive shopping, excessive eating), punding (performing repeated pointless actions such as sorting or disassembling objects) and dopamine dysregulation (can lead to dopamine abuse).

6 It is always important to find the balance between patients' symptoms and doses of medication. The phases of motor fluctuation should be noted whenever a dose of dopaminergic medication is changed. The 'on' phase is the honeymoon phase whereas the 'off' phase means the patient is having subtherapeutic effect. The difficulty to find the honeymoon phase is dependent on disease duration but not duration of levodopa therapy. Sometimes the patient is experiencing dose-limiting levodopa-associated dyskinesia as the supratherapeutic effect. As the disease progresses, the patient is more prone to the motor fluctuation and hence more frequent dosing is required. This will in turn lead to more frequent dyskinetic breaches and hence it becomes harder to control the disease. The frequency of dyskinetic breaches is associated with the dosing of levodopa and the disease duration.

7 Dopamine agonists such as oral pramipexole and transdermal rotigotine are the non-ergot dopamine agonists. They directly stimulate postsynaptic dopamine receptors in the striatum and hence provide dopaminergic actions. Though they are dopaminergic medications, they are not as effective as levodopa. However, they are long-acting and hence it is possible for the patient to have single daily dosing. The side-effects of dopamine agonists are mainly dopaminergic: nausea, vomiting, dizziness, hallucinations, orthostatic hypotension, worsening delirium, impulse control disorders and punding. Monoamine oxidase (MAO) B inhibitors such as rasagiline are another adjunct dopaminergic therapy available for those with PD. They are as effective as dopamine agonists and are mainly used in patients with mild/early symptoms or younger age. Their side-effects include hepatic dysfunction. One notable complication from the use of MAOB inhibitor is tyramine hypertensive crisis. Tyramine releases noradrenaline, and ordinarily the MAO system would break down the excessive noradrenaline. In this case, excessive inhibition from MAO inhibitors can block the metabolism of excess noradrenaline and adrenergic crisis can happen. For this reason, the patient needs to be informed to avoid certain types of cheese. Never stop PD medications abruptly as this can lead to a Parkinsonian crisis, which manifests in a similar fashion to neuroleptic malignant syndrome.

8 Deep brain stimulation is one of the advanced therapies available to patients. The device can be used to target different symptoms of PD. To target motor fluctuation, subthalamic nucleus and globus pallidus interna deep brain stimulator should be used. The subthalamic nucleus and thalamic deep brain stimulator is usually used to treat the symptoms of resting tremor, whereas pedunculopontine nucleus deep brain stimulator is used to treat gait freezing

and postural instability in the late stage of PD. The use of deep brain stimulator is indicated if the patient has a low burden of non-motor symptoms, low risk of developing dementia in the next 3–5 years, no non-drug-induced hallucinations and no active or previous recurrent major psychiatric disturbance that could be exacerbated. Its main side-effects include surgical and infective risks, risk of cognitive deficits, risk of psychiatric disturbance, risk of suicide, impulse control disorders, and dopamine dysregulation from subthalamic nucleus stimulation.

9 Drooling can be socially embarrassing for the patient and their family. Topical atropine eye drops can be used in the oral cavity to reduce the production of saliva.

10 Constipation can be a significant issue in patients with Parkinson's disease. High fibre diet and regular exercise can help to reduce constipation associated with Parkinson's disease.

11 REM sleep behaviour disorder can be a significant issue for both the patient and their carer. The treatment is limited. The general strategies include reducing or withdrawing antidepressants, and trial of melatonin and clonazepam. Notably the use of levodopa can sometimes make the symptoms of REM sleep behaviour disorder worse. For patients who are experiencing acute delirium and hallucinations, the first thing to do should be to investigate the cause of delirium (such as infection), followed by treating the cause of delirium accordingly if any source is identified. The dose of non-PD medications should then be reduced, especially those with sedative, anxiolytic and antidepressant properties. If the patient is on any anticholinergic medications, the doses of those medications should also be gradually tapered. Once all those things have been done, the next thing is to strategically withdraw certain anti-PD medications in order. The first one to take off the list should be amantadine, followed by the dopamine agonists. The clinician can finally consider the withdrawal of the MAO inhibitors, followed by levodopa. This order is based on the effectiveness of the medications in the management of PD. If all the above strategies fail to control the patient's hallucination or delirium symptoms, then antipsychotic medications can be considered, including quetiapine, clozapine or pimavanserin. Other neuroleptics should be avoided if possible. If other neuroleptics are needed, they should be used with great caution.

12 Postural hypotension is a major autonomic complication in PD. Non-pharmacological strategies include avoidance of dehydration, high salt diet, domperidone, fludrocortisone, and avoidance of unnecessary antihypertensives.

13 The predictors for nursing home placement include increasing age, dementia and hallucinations. As a general rule, the onset of visual hallucination is always a bad prognostic sign and it usually precedes the patient's death by about 5 years.

CASE 59: Spinal cord injury

History

- A 57-year-old female was complaining of sudden onset of **bilateral lower limb numbness and weakness** [1]. The numbness started from the level of her upper abdomen.
- She was **day 5 post open repair of her abdominal aortic aneurysm** [2].
- Other than the weakness and numbness in her lower limbs, she **denies any presence of pain or pallor in her legs** [3].
- She was unable to stand up from the bed by using her legs alone and requires some assistance with her mobility in the ward. The surgery was performed to repair a pararenal thoracoabdominal aortic aneurysm and the open approach was chosen mainly because of the unfavourable anatomy and patient's relatively young age. The surgery itself was complicated due to the involvement of the renal arteries. Prolonged intraoperative time was required including prolonged aortic cross-clamping and the patient had intraoperative hypotension which required the use of vasopressors. There were no other neurological deficits reported elsewhere.
- The patient's **past medical history** [4] include ex-smoker, hypertension, diabetes mellitus and anxiety.

[1] Spinal cord lesion should always be suspected when there are bilateral motor and sensory symptoms or signs below the level of head. Upper motor neurone signs will dominate the picture, with weakness and long tract signs such as spasticity, hyperreflexia, and upgoing plantar response or Babinski sign.

[2] When talking about injury to the spinal cord, the neuroanatomy of the spinal cord should not be omitted. Our spinal cord consists of 31 segments; each has a pair of nerve roots, ventral (anterior) and dorsal (posterior), on each side of the spinal cord. The nerve roots exit the spinal canal via the neuroforamina of the spine. Longitudinally, the spinal cord is divided into four parts: cervical, thoracic, lumbar and sacral. The spinal cord starts at the base of the skull and ends at the level of L1 vertebral body. Below L1, the nerves from lumbar, sacral and coccygeal nerve roots form a bundle of nerves named the cauda equina. Cross-sectionally, the spinal cord contains the butterfly-shaped central region formed with grey matter, with the surrounding white matter tracts. The neuronal cell bodies in the posterior part of the spinal cord form the dorsal horn, which is responsible for the transmission of sensory information. The neuronal cell bodies in the anterior part of the spinal cord form the anterior horn, which is responsible for mediating information from the descending tracts of the pyramidal and extrapyramidal motor systems (*Figure 59.1*). A single anterior and two posterior spinal arteries form the blood supply system for the spinal cord. The anterior spinal artery supplies the anterior segment of the cord, whereas the posterior spinal arteries primarily supply the dorsal columns. Anterior and posterior spinal arteries originate from the vertebral arteries in the neck and descend from the base of the skull. The anterior spinal artery is the longest artery in the body. Although it is typically continuous, in those with discontinuous course the spinal cord is prone to vascular injury. Along the course of the spinal cord, multiple radicular arteries branch off the thoracic and abdominal aorta to maintain the blood supply to the anterior spinal arteries. The largest and most prominent one is the great ventral radicular artery or the artery of Adamkiewicz, which supplies the anterior spinal artery. This artery enters the spinal cord usually at the level between T9 and T12. Given its location and origin from aorta, the spinal artery at this level is prone to vascular injury after aortic surgeries, particularly after the repair of abdominal aortic aneurysm. The primary watershed area of the spinal cord in most of the population is located in the mid-thoracic region. The posterior spinal arteries, in contrast, run through the length of the spinal cord bilaterally

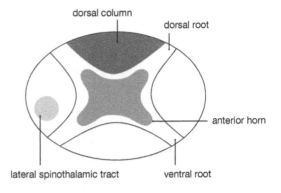

Figure 59.1 *Simplified cross-sectional view of the spinal cord.*

in the posterior lateral sulci. These arteries are supplied by a greater number of radicular arteries than the anterior spinal artery. The posterior spinal arteries often anastomose with each other and supply the dorsal columns and the posterior horns. There are some classic spinal cord syndromes that are worth knowing. They include transection syndrome, dorsal cord syndrome, anterior spinal artery syndrome, Brown-Séquard syndrome, central cord syndrome, pure motor syndrome, conus medullaris syndrome and cauda equina syndrome.

- Anterior spinal artery syndrome results from vascular injury to the anterior part of the spinal cord. The presentation involves the loss of pain and temperature sensation, weakness and bladder dysfunction.
- Central cord syndrome is characterised by segmental loss of pain and temperature. The weakness is often disproportionately more prominent in the upper extremities than the lower extremities. The causes include intramedullary tumour and syringomyelia.
- Dorsal cord syndrome typically involves the dorsal column that is responsible for vibratory and proprioception sensation. Therefore, a patient may present with issues with gait and balance due to difficulty in proprioception.
- Brown-Séquard (hemicord) syndrome can be caused by mechanical insult to the spinal cord. Characteristically the patient can present with ipsilateral weakness and loss of proprioception, and contralateral loss of pain and temperature sensation because the spinothalamic tract crosses just above the level of the nerve root.
- Transection syndrome usually involves the segment that is affected by spinal cord injury. The patient can present with loss of sensation in all modalities, with weakness below the affected level and bladder dysfunction.
- Pure motor syndrome selectively affects the motor function with preserved sensation. It is seen in poliomyelitis, amyotrophic lateral sclerosis and hereditary spastic paraplegia.
- Conus medullaris syndrome is often caused by the lesion at level of L2 and involves bladder and rectal dysfunction and saddle anaesthesia.
- In contrast, cauda equina syndrome often presents with the syndrome of multiradicular pain, leg weakness with sensory loss and sphincter dysfunction. The deficits are usually asymmetric.

3 Surgical repair of thoracic and thoracoabdominal aortic aneurysms is the most common cause of spinal cord infarction. Both open surgery and endovascular repair are associated with spinal cord ischaemia. The clinical picture of spinal cord ischaemia may become apparent immediately after surgery or be delayed for a period up to 27 days after the surgery. Such complication is multifactorial, involving systemic hypotension, aortic cross-clamping causing local arterial hypoperfusion and occlusion of important feeding arteries such as the artery of Adamkiewicz by ligation, resection or embolisation.

4 One of the possible differentials is leg ischaemia post open repair of abdominal aortic aneurysm. Vascular risk factors such as diabetes, smoking and hypertension can contribute to the risk of vascular injury to the spinal cord. Risk factors of vascular injury include age, aortic rupture, history of cerebrovascular or cardiovascular disease, previous aortic surgery, renal impairment, atrial fibrillation, smoking and intraoperative hypotension.

Examination

- On inspection, there was no pallor or cyanosis in the lower limbs suggestive of the presence of ischaemia.
- A full **neurological examination** [1] was performed. There was no muscular atrophy on inspection. The tones and reflexes in the lower limbs were increased bilaterally, while the power in the lower limbs appeared to be 3/5 throughout.
- In terms of sensation, the patient had impaired temperature, pinprick and fine touch sensation in both lower limbs **up to dermatomal level of T9** [2].

- The **sensation modalities** [3] of vibration and proprioception were preserved. The bladder scan showed no urinary retention and the PR exam revealed preserved anal tone. There was no ataxia and there was no cerebellar sign elicited on examination.
- **Lhermitte's sign** [4] was negative and **Romberg's test** [5] was negative.

1 A full neurological examination to all four extremities is essential when assessing a patient's spinal cord. Remembering the neuroanatomy of the spinal cord comes in handy when one is trying to identify the location of the lesion.

2 There will typically be sensory level deficits. Motor-wise, the muscle groups innervated below the affected level will have the upper motor neurone signs and will otherwise be normal above the level involved. A sensory level abnormality is highly suggestive of spinal cord lesion, with normal sensation above, and reduced/absent sensation below the affected level.

3 As mentioned above, identifying the affected level within the spinal cord and the localisation of the lesion is clinically important. Effort should be made to detect the level involved with thorough examination of motor, reflex and sensory functioning. All sensory modalities should be assessed. Sphincter function is important for clinical localisation as well.

4 As in the case of multiple sclerosis, it is worth checking Lhermitte's sign, which presents as an electric shock-like sensation down from the back and legs when the neck is flexed.

5 Romberg's test is not used to test cerebellar function. Rather, it is used to test the functioning of a patient's dorsal columns, particularly proprioception.

Investigations

An **MRI spine** [1] was performed and it showed **hyperintensities** [2] on T2 images from the T8 level extending to the level of L3. The diffusion weighted image also showed restricted diffusion indicative of possible spinal cord ischaemia.

1 Neuroimaging remains the mainstay of the investigation modality for spinal cord lesion. MRI scan of the spinal cord can usually reveal the affected segment and the administration of gadolinium contrast can be helpful. In this case, MRI spine is required in the diagnosis of spinal cord infarction and it may also provide confirmatory information of spinal cord infarction and underlying aetiology. However, it may be deferred if the patient requires urgent surgical intervention due to its limited availability and the emergency nature of spinal cord infarction. A gadolinium-enhanced MRI brain can also be helpful to exclude multiple sclerosis. If other causes of spinal cord infarction are suspected, an aortogram can be carried out to detect aortic dissection. Vascular imaging such as CT angiography can be performed to exclude vertebral artery dissection or vascular malformation. When infection or autoimmune disorders are suspected, lumbar puncture with CSF analysis can also be helpful.

2 Hyperintensities on T2-weighted images often represent the area of spinal cord ischaemia. A finding of restricted diffusion on the diffusion weighted images sequence is more sensitive than standard T2 sequence. The problem is that such appearance, even with restricted diffusion, can be seen in other cases such as transverse myelitis. Infarction in the vertebral body next to the cord signal on MRI makes the finding more specific of infarction, although not commonly seen.

Management

Immediate

Blood pressure augmentation [1] was carried out with filling of volumes. Unfortunately, due to recent vascular surgery and concerns about bleeding complication, the target of blood pressure augmentation is limited. A lumbar drain was inserted and patient's neurological observations were monitored closely. Neurology and neurosurgery consultations were also requested.

Short-term

The patient was **closely monitored in the neurology HDU** [2]. The **haemodynamics** [3] appeared to be stable throughout the course. There was no incident suggestive of **autonomic dysreflexia** [4]. **VTE prophylaxis** [5] and pressure care were performed routinely. Early referral to physiotherapy and occupational therapy was made.

Long-term

Unfortunately, the patient's neurological deficits had never resolved fully despite some improvement with blood pressure augmentation and the use of lumbar drain. The strategies applied for **VTE prophylaxis** [6] and pressure care successfully protected the patient from developing further complication from her impaired mobility as an inpatient. The patient was then transferred to the **rehabilitation ward** [7] for further postoperative rehabilitation. She developed **neuropathic pain** [8] in her lower limbs but it was fully managed by the use of simple analgesia. The newly developed spasticity was treated with baclofen. The sensory changes had never altered but the patient did gain some ground in terms of motor function. She required the use of a single point stick as her walking aid for mobilisation in the community.

She was greatly overwhelmed by the bad news that her **mobility might be permanently impaired** [9] and a referral to the **psychology services** [10] was also made.

Prognosis

Most patients who have spinal cord infarction end up with permanent and disabling neurological deficits depending on the location of the infarction. The severity of the neurological deficits is highly variable and only some of the population manage to make some functional recovery.

[1] Unfortunately, the specific treatment options for spinal cord infarction are very limited. The exception is spinal cord ischaemia resulting from aortic surgery or endovascular repair. There is a specific protocol developed for such situations although the evidence is limited. The treatment usually involves a combination of blood pressure support (to increase mean arterial pressure by 10mmHg every 5 minutes with volume and vasopressor agents until symptoms resolve – but beware of bleeding complications) and reduction of spinal cord canal pressure with lumbar drains (if there is no response to blood pressure augmentation, a lumbar drain should be placed urgently). If there is no response to treatment with blood pressure augmentation and lumbar drain, spinal imaging (either CT or MRI) should be performed to exclude epidural haematoma.

[2] There are some neurological complications post-spinal cord ischaemia that require attention from the clinicians who are looking after the patient. Some of the complications may exacerbate the neurologic injury or even be life-threatening. Moderate to severe deficits resulting from a high thoracic or cervical cord infarct require ICU admission to closely monitor the vital signs and for neurological observation.

[3] Neurogenic shock can be a critical issue. It is the hypotension, accompanied with bradycardia, attributed to interruption of autonomic pathways in the spinal cord resulting in reduced peripheral vascular resistance. Bradycardia often occurs in high spinal cord injury and may require external pacing or the use of atropine.

[4] Autonomic dysreflexia is commonly seen after a traumatic spinal cord injury but can also be seen in spinal cord infarction. It is characterised by paroxysmal hypertension with headache, bradycardia, flushing and sweating. Significant postural hypotension can also happen. When hypertension occurs, it is important to identify the source of insult from the lower part of the body, such as urinary retention, constipation and infections. High spinal cord injury also affects the diaphragm significantly. The weakness of diaphragm and chest wall muscles makes the patient prone to having impaired secretion clearance, ineffective cough, atelectasis and hypoventilation. Signs of respiratory failure should be closely monitored and ventilatory support should be provided if indicated. Chest physiotherapy should be taught and the patient should be encouraged to carry out chest exercises regularly.

[5] Other measures should be taken to avoid VTE, pressure sores, urinary retention and GI stress ulcer. Occupational therapy and physiotherapy should be started as soon as possible and psychological counselling should be offered to the patient and family members.

[6] The prevention of VTE, pressure sores, urinary retention and GI stress ulcer should be ongoing. As mentioned above, possible noxious stimuli such as bladder distension, constipation, pressure sores and infections should be explored in the case of autonomic dysreflexia.

[7] Neurological deficits can be improved by appropriate and early rehabilitation interventions. Early mobilisation and positioning can help prevent contracture and pressure ulcers. If there is a neurological decline, neuroimaging should be organised to exclude syringomyelia or post-traumatic myelomalacic myelopathy.

[8] Neurogenic pain can be treated with simple analgesia and those medications used in neuropathic pain. Chronic use of opioids should be avoided. Spasticity is common post spinal cord injury and the agents available include baclofen, Botox and nerve blocks.

[9] Patients may develop obesity due to impaired mobility, if they become bedbound long-term after a spinal cord injury. This can contribute to the risk of cardiovascular disease in the long run in addition to the cardiac arrhythmias as a result from high spinal cord injury. The impaired mobility also contributes to the development of osteoporosis.

[10] Impairment of patients' functionality presents in many ways post spinal cord injury, including but not limited to impaired mobility and sexual dysfunction. This increases the risk of depression, especially on the background of pre-existing mental illness. Suicidality should be monitored for the long term.

CASE 60: Stroke / transient ischaemic attack

History

- A 75-year-old male retired manager was brought in by ambulance with sudden onset of **dysphasia, right-sided facial droop and right-sided weakness in both upper and lower limbs** [1].
- The **onset of the symptoms** [2] occurred at 18:30. The patient arrived at the ED at 19:00. The patient was known to be right-handed.
- There is no **previous history** [3] of strokes or intracranial haemorrhages. The patient denies any recent history of significant bleeding or recent surgery. There was no history of intracranial

neoplasm, aneurysm or vascular malformation reported. No history of trauma was reported. He was an ex-smoker with a 30 pack year history.
- His **past medical history** [4] includes hypertension, insulin-dependent diabetes mellitus, ischaemic heart disease, hypercholesterolaemia and morbid obesity.
- He **denies any past injuries and does not have any family history** [5] of early onset stroke or vascular malformation in the CNS.
- There was no history of **mechanical heart valve replacement or atrial fibrillation** [6].

[1] 'Cerebrovascular accident' is no longer the term we use. Broadly a stroke can be put into one of two categories: ischaemic or haemorrhagic. However, a stroke can also be categorised based on its aetiology and/or its location. Other types of stroke are mentioned in this section. The symptoms of stroke are highly dependent on the territories affected. In this case the patient has a constellation of symptoms, namely dysphasia (due to the impact to the dominant hemisphere), contralateral hemiparesis and contralateral facial hemiparesis. These are highly suggestive of damage to the left middle cerebral artery territory. Small vessel disease, such as lacunar stroke syndromes, is divided into different subtypes. Pure motor type is the most common lacunar syndrome (up to 50%) and it is usually a result from infarcts in the posterior limb of the internal capsule or the anterior portion of pons (basis pontis). Ataxic hemiparesis type manifests as a combination of cerebellar and motor symptoms. It usually affects the leg more than the arm. It results from infarcts in the posterior limb of the internal capsule, basis pontis or corona radiata. Dysarthria type is usually a result from infarcts in the basis pontis. Pure sensory type is usually a result from thalamic infarcts. Mixed sensorimotor type can also happen and it usually indicates infarct in the thalamus or the posterior limb of internal capsule.

[2] It is important to establish the timing of symptom onset because this will guide the decision making for the management. Once the window of opportunity passes (4.5 hours from time of onset), thrombolysis will no longer provide benefit to the patient's outcome. One different entity to consider is transient ischaemic attack (TIA). Transient ischaemic attack usually manifests as a sudden focal neurological loss that reaches its maximum at the onset

and does not spread or intensify. It is often a result from a focal cerebral ischaemia. By definition, the symptoms must resolve within 24 hours and the imaging should not reveal any permanent cerebral infarct like those in strokes. TIAs that last for more than an hour usually show changes on MRI and hence are not considered a TIA after imaging. 10% of transient ischaemic attack patients have a completed stroke within 90 days and 40% of strokes are preceded by TIAs. Criteria for recommending admission to hospital after a TIA are listed in *Table 60.1*, with a score of ≥3 considered an indication for admission.

Table 60.1 Scoring system ABCD² for admission after a TIA

Age >60	1
BP >140/90mmHg	1
Clinical features	
• focal weakness during episode	2
• impaired speech but no weakness	1
Duration	
• symptoms lasted for >60 minutes	2
• symptoms lasted for >10 minutes but <60 minutes	1
Diabetic patients	1

Amaurosis fugax is a subtype of TIA leading to transient monocular vision loss lasting for seconds to minutes. It is a result of retinal ischaemia with a classic description of a descending curtain of visual loss. Amaurosis fugax can be recurrent. It is generally associated with ipsilateral severe carotid artery stenosis and patients may have retinal emboli. The clinician should also consider giant cell arteritis as a differential diagnosis of the vision loss, especially when the patient is complaining of ipsilateral headache associated with jaw claudication.

3 While the patient is getting work-up for the treatment of stroke, certain questions should be asked to make sure that the treatment, such as thrombolysis, is not contraindicated.

4 It is important to establish the risk factors of stroke. Hypertension is the biggest risk factor for stroke. Other risk factors include diabetes, smoking, dyslipidaemia, alcohol consumption, obesity and sedentary lifestyle.

5 Dissection-related stroke results from a tear in the vessel wall (intima). This then leads to thrombus formation in the wall of artery. If this expands, it can create stenosis or pseudoaneurysm in that artery. Stroke can occur either from thromboembolism or occlusion of the dissected artery. If there is a complete rupture of the artery, subarachnoid haemorrhage can occur. Dissection-related stroke occurs most commonly in the carotid and vertebral arteries. Episodes are usually associated with history of trauma with hyperextension of the neck. Family history of fibromuscular dysplasia and history of connective tissue disorders are additional risk factors. In addition to neurological deficits, the patient may also present with neck pain, headache and partial Horner's syndrome (no anhidrosis as the sudomotor fibres travel adjacent to the external carotid artery and are thus spared).

6 15% of patients have known atrial fibrillation or paroxysmal atrial fibrillation predating the stroke. Previous mechanical heart valves with no appropriate anticoagulation are significant risk factors for strokes.

Examination

- A **full neurological examination** [1] was performed. The patient was alert and oriented. He could follow commands properly. The cranial nerve examination revealed right-sided complete paralysis of the face and there was a right-sided homonymous hemianopia. There was no obvious abnormality in the eye movement. The cranial examination was otherwise normal. Moving on to the peripheries, the patient was found to have complete paralysis of his right upper and lower limbs, while the function of the left side of the body was preserved. The patient denies any sensory changes, although communication was difficult due to the presence of dysphasia and dysarthria. Testing of the higher centres using pre-printed images revealed right-sided visual spatial neglect. A National Institutes of Health Stroke Scale (NIHSS) score of 14 was established. The patient's vital signs showed high blood pressure of 180/90mmHg with heart rate of 80bpm. Other vital signs were normal.

- On **cardiovascular examination** [2], the patient's radial pulse was regular at the time of examination and there was no carotid bruit audible on auscultation. There were no physical signs suggestive of heart failure or previous mechanical valve replacement.

1 A full neurological examination is a must-do and together with knowledge of neuroanatomy it is useful in determining the location and extent of the stroke before proceeding to the imaging investigations. A quick screening based on the National Institutes of Health Stroke Scale should be performed. The determination of deficit also helps establish the baseline of function before the treatment and this will guide future consideration of additional supports for the patient's deficit in performing activities of daily living.

2 A careful cardiovascular examination can usually help determine the aetiology of stroke. The presence of carotid bruits can also be a result from external carotid artery stenosis instead of internal carotid artery stenosis, which is more relevant in the aetiology of stroke. Blood pressure should be measured; it is usually elevated in patients who are having strokes due to a compensatory mechanism to maintain cerebral blood flow. Radial pulse can be palpated for atrial fibrillation. On auscultation of the chest and the praecordium, the clinician should look for the signs suggestive of heart failure or mechanical valve, if there is any. Carotid bruit should be auscultated. However, the absence of carotid bruit does not rule out the presence of carotid artery stenosis.

Investigations

- A stroke code was called after the clinical diagnosis of stroke was made following history taking and physical examination. An urgent CT perfusion mapping was performed following **CT brain** **without contrast** [1]. There was no evidence of intracranial haemorrhage and the CT brain without contrast did not show any evidence of hypodensity suggestive of early stroke.

- The **CT perfusion** [2] mapping revealed a large area of perfusion mismatch in the left MCA territory with a large penumbra (measuring approximately 200ml) surrounding a small infarct core. The angiogram also showed thrombosis in the left internal carotid artery and M1 segment.

- While the patient proceeded to have thrombolysis and clot retrieval, a **cardiac monitoring** [3] **and transthoracic echocardiogram** [4] were organised.
- **Full blood count, coagulation profile** [5] **, fasting lipid profile and HbA1c** [6] level were also ordered.

[1] CT brain without contrast sometimes can show hypodensity that may be suggestive of early stroke. However, it is not sensitive enough in the hyperacute setting.

[2] CT perfusion mapping is more readily available than MRI. It can provide important information of brain perfusion and hence is useful in terms of diagnosing stroke in the acute setting. It can also be used in terms of assessing the size of infarct or penumbra. MRI scan of the brain is a useful modality of imaging to assess the extent of the stroke but its limited availability makes it less ideal in the emergency setting.

[3] ECG and cardiac monitoring is looking for atrial fibrillation. 8% of new diagnosis of AF is made on the first ECG taken; 5% of new diagnosis of AF on inpatient telemetry.

[4] TTE can be used to further illustrate the structure of the heart. Certain features such as ejection fraction, presence of patent foramen ovale or left ventricular thrombosis should be hunted for.

[5] Full blood count and coagulation profile are used to obtain platelet count and coagulation parameters. They provide useful information for the stroke team when they are deciding whether thrombolysis is contraindicated.

[6] Hypercholesterolaemia and diabetes mellitus are two modifiable risk factors of stroke. Diabetes mellitus should always be screened with HbA1c or fasting blood glucose level for those coming in with stroke or TIA.

Management

Hyperacute stroke care

Due to the high NIHSS score and the presence of large penumbra, the patient then proceeded to receive **thrombolysis** [1] with tissue plasminogen activator. The absence of contraindications was again reviewed before the administration of the medication. The patient then underwent **mechanical thrombectomy** [2] for the occlusion in the left ICA and M1 segment. The clot was successfully retrieved and the flow was restored beyond the site of the original occlusion.

Acute stroke care

After the successful clot retrieval, the patient was then transferred to the **stroke care unit** [3] for further management. **Dual antiplatelet therapy** [4] with aspirin and clopidogrel were initiated as an inpatient, with the plan of switching to monotherapy after 3 months. The patient was admitted to the neurology HDU with close monitoring of his **blood pressure** [5].

Long-term

The patient was kept on **dual antiplatelet therapy** [6] for a further 90 days before being switched to monotherapy with clopidogrel. A **carotid Doppler** [7] was performed and revealed a 95% stenosis in the left internal carotid artery. A carotid endarterectomy was planned.

The patient recovered well from the neurological deficits that resulted from the stroke. The carotid endarterectomy was also uncomplicated. The patient's medications for **blood pressure control, diabetes and hypercholesterolaemia** [8] were optimised prior to discharge. New **atrial fibrillation** [9] which was detected at the time of admission is also well controlled. The patient was discharged home after a prolonged period of rehabilitation. However, the family did notice that the patient started having **progressively worsening slowness in problem solving** [10] whereas his memory was largely intact.

1 Thrombolysis uses tissue plasminogen activator pooled data from numerous trials displaying a benefit to the outcome if thrombolysis is provided within 4.5 hours from onset of stroke. Exclusion criteria include stroke or significant head trauma within 3 months, GI or urinary haemorrhage within 3 weeks, major surgery or serious trauma within 2 weeks, arterial puncture at a non-compressible site within 7 days, history of intracranial haemorrhage, intracranial neoplasm/ arteriovenous malformation/aneurysm, symptoms of subarachnoid haemorrhage, active internal bleeding, blood pressure systolic >185 or diastolic >110mmHg, clear and large hypodensity on CT scan indicating old lesion beyond time window and bleeding diathesis. Relative contraindications include minor deficit with NIHSS of ≤5 and not clearly disabling, myocardial infarction in the last 3 months, seizure at presentation and pregnancy (must weigh risks and benefits in the individual circumstances). Risk factors for haemorrhagic transformation include large infarcts, established infarcts, grey matter infarcts, higher NIHSS score, poor collateral history, hyperglycaemia and thrombocytopenia.

2 Thrombolysis does not effectively break down large clots which tend to happen in major blood vessels. This makes thrombolysis less likely to work against large vessel occlusion. In this case, recanalisation with mechanical thrombectomy is needed. However, thrombolysis should be given without delay if it is not contraindicated, even if the mechanical thrombectomy is being considered. Penumbra refers to the area representing potentially salvageable ischaemic tissue around the infarct core on neuroimaging. Though it is supplied by the collateral arteries, it can still turn into infarction if the perfusion is not restored in time. Pooled data demonstrated a strong benefit with mechanical thrombectomy for internal carotid artery- and middle cerebral artery-related strokes. In those patients, early recanalisation is associated with better outcome. Even if the patient was beyond the time window of 4.5 hours, there is still a demonstrable benefit for mechanical thrombectomy performed within 24 hours of onset of symptoms. It can also be performed regardless of whether the patient has received IV alteplase for the same ischaemic stroke event. If mechanical thrombectomy is not contraindicated (see below), it can be performed even when the thrombolysis is contraindicated. Within 6 hours of symptom onset, mechanical thrombectomy is indicated for large penumbra with small infarct core associated with major vessel occlusion and the clinical diagnosis of stroke. Prior to the procedure, brain imaging is needed to rule out intracranial haemorrhage. The NIHSS should be >6. Those patients who present beyond 6 hours but within 24 hours of symptom onset are still eligible for mechanical thrombectomy according to the DAWN trial if thrombolysis failed or was contraindicated, NIHSS score is >10, the patient has no significant pre-stroke disability, the baseline infarct is smaller than one-third of MCA territory on brain imaging, and the intracranial arterial occlusion of the ICA or M1 segment of the MCA is demonstrated on the neuroimaging. There is no proven benefit from mechanical thrombectomy in posterior circulation stroke.

3 The stroke care unit has an MDT which provides assessment and monitoring with stroke protocols. This offers early management including physiological management, early mobilisation and nursing care, and MDT rehabilitation. Mortality and dependency benefits of stroke care unit are proven by research. Hemicraniectomy is usually considered in a younger patient who has extensive MCA territory infarct. Extensive MCA territory infarct can progress into malignant MCA infarct which causes intracranial hypertension resulting from acutely increased swelling. For those <60 years old, hemicraniectomy for infarct involving >50% of MCA territory provides 50% mortality benefit without increased disability. For those >60 years old, there is still survival benefit from hemicraniectomy without increased disability, but the majority of those elderly patients who come in with such significant infarct would usually need assistance with personal ADLs regardless of the surgery. Therapies that do not work include supplemental oxygen (has no role if there is no respiratory issue) and fluoxetine (recent large-scale study showed that it has no benefit in stroke recovery).

4 Antiplatelets are used as part of acute stroke care. They are also useful in terms of secondary prevention of stroke. Short-term (90 days) combined therapy of aspirin and clopidogrel can be used for those who experienced recent large intracranial vessel occlusion, before switching to monotherapy for long-term secondary prevention. For lacunar infarcts, dual antiplatelet with aspirin plus clopidogrel is usually used for 21 days, before switching to monotherapy for long-term secondary prevention.

5 Blood pressure management is vital and complex in post-stroke care. Post stroke, loss of cerebral autoregulation occurs. Because systemic blood pressures directly affect cerebral perfusion pressure, systemic BP needs to be maintained for the improvement of blood flow to the cerebral infarct or penumbra via collateral blood vessels. However, we do not want the BP to go unlimited either. For patients not undergoing thrombolysis, target BP up to 220/120mmHg is reasonable. For patients undergoing thrombolysis, target BP is much lower, with upper limit of 180/105mmHg. If antihypertensive agents are needed, IV labetalol can be used, as well as IV hydralazine. However, this will need to be given in a closely monitored environment.

6 The long-term risk factor control strategy is based on the aetiology of stroke. For those caused by major vessel occlusion, antiplatelet medications (aspirin, clopidogrel and the combination of aspirin–extended-release dipyridamole) are all reasonable options for secondary prevention of recurrent non-cardioembolic ischaemic stroke. Clopidogrel or a combination of aspirin with extended-release dipyridamole are recommended in atherothrombotic strokes, lacunar strokes and cryptogenic strokes. For non-cardioembolic strokes, aspirin and clopidogrel should not be combined as long-term treatment unless otherwise indicated, e.g. recent acute MI requiring placement of stent. For those having carotid endarterectomy, aspirin should be used as indefinite treatment unless contraindicated. Symptomatic carotid stenosis confers an increased risk of stroke compared with asymptomatic stenosis. In the dissection type of stroke there is no evidence that anticoagulation has greater benefit; aspirin is the mainstay of treatment in this type of stroke.

7 Carotid endarterectomy is indicated for patients with non-disabling carotid artery territory stroke or transient ischaemic attack with ipsilateral carotid stenosis measuring 70–99%. Carotid endarterectomy can be considered in selected patients with symptomatic carotid stenosis of 50–69%. In those who had an ischaemic stroke or transient ischaemic attack, carotid endarterectomy should be performed within 2 weeks of stroke. All patients with significant carotid stenosis should be treated with intensive vascular secondary prevention therapy. Carotid stenting is a reasonable choice in selected patients who have unfavourable anatomy for carotid endarterectomy, symptomatic re-stenosis after endarterectomy or stenosis induced by previous radiotherapy.

8 Hypertension is the single most important modifiable risk factor for both ischaemic and haemorrhagic stroke. BP of systolic 120–140mmHg and diastolic 80–90mmHg should be targeted. ACE inhibitor/ARBs and thiazide diuretics have better evidence than other antihypertensives. Control of dyslipidaemia is also important in the primary or secondary prevention of stroke. Atorvastatin and rosuvastatin are considered the most potent statins. Most systematic reviews and meta-analyses have found that treatment with statins does not increase the risk of future intracranial haemorrhage or negatively impact prognosis. Glycaemic control should be optimised in diabetic patients who present with stroke. Once the diagnosis of diabetes is confirmed, diabetes should be treated with medications as per diabetes guidelines. A reasonable goal of therapy is a HbA1C value of not greater than 7% for most patients. The IRIS study showed pioglitazone treatment appears to reduce the risk of recurrent stroke and MI in non-diabetic patients who have insulin resistance, but beware of the side-effects of weight gain, fluid retention and bone fractures.

9 Atrial fibrillation is an important cause of cardioembolic stroke. CHA$_2$DS$_2$VASc score is an important tool for risk stratification (*Table 60.2*). Warfarin is superior to aspirin in terms of prevention of embolic stroke. 150mg dabigatran and 5mg apixaban are superior to warfarin. According to further research, 110mg dabigatran, 20mg rivaroxaban and 2.5mg apixaban are non-inferior to warfarin. In addition to

superiority to warfarin, 5mg apixaban also confers lower rates of all-cause bleeding and lower rates of intracranial haemorrhage. When to start warfarin after stroke depends on the severity of the stroke. Transient ischaemic attack can start from day 0. Minor stroke can start from day 3 and moderate stroke can start from day 6. Severe stroke should start from day 12. As a general principle, novel oral anticoagulation usually have 2 extra days added to the warfarin initiation rule.

Table 60.2 CHA$_2$DS$_2$VASc scoring system

Cardiac failure	1
Hypertension	1
Age >75 years	2
Diabetes	1
Stroke/TIA/thromboembolism	2
Vascular disease (ischaemic heart disease, peripheral vascular disease)	1
Age 65–74 years	1
Sex **c**ategory = female	1

10 Vascular disease contributes to 25–50% of all dementias, and vascular dementia is the second most common type of dementia in population-based studies. Vascular dementia is often considered as any dementia that is primarily caused by cerebrovascular disease or compromised cerebral blood flow. Any cognitive decline after a clinically diagnosed stroke should promote suspicion of vascular dementia. The cognitive profile in vascular dementia is characterised by the prominent impairment of executive function, while the episodic memory is often spared. Structural imaging such as MRI brain should be performed to assess any clinically unrecognised cerebrovascular disease. The management of vascular dementia consists of the use of secondary prevention of cerebrovascular disease and the use of donepezil and memantine. The optimisation of BP control is highly recommended. Although diabetes and cholesterol control are beneficial in the secondary prevention of stroke, their role in the prevention of vascular dementia is not clearly established. The same principle applies to the use of antiplatelet and homocysteine-lowering therapy. There is no convincing evidence regarding whether the use of donepezil and/or memantine is beneficial. However, they are normally used when there is suspicion of coexisting Alzheimer's disease.

CASE 61: Breast carcinoma

History

- A **60-year-old** [1] **woman** [2] presents with **changes in the skin around her left nipple** [3].
- This occurs in the setting of a previous **wide local excision** [4] and course of **radiotherapy** [5] for breast cancer 8 years ago.
- Her breast cancer was previously diagnosed after finding a **breast lump** [6] on **personal examination** [7] and attending a **triple assessment clinic** [8].

- She has been feeling very **lethargic** [9] lately and has also noticed **right-sided abdominal pain** [10] and intermittent **back pain** [11].
- She is also having new issues with **constipation** [12].
- Both her **mother and maternal aunt had breast cancer** [13] in their 40s.
- Other than her previous breast cancer she has no past medical history of note but does drink **2–3 glasses of wine per evening** [14].

[1] Breast cancer incidence is strongly associated with increasing age. The most significant non-modifiable risk factors for breast cancer are female gender, increasing age and genetics.

[2] Breast cancer is the most common cancer in women worldwide. Breast cancer can also occur in men; however, it is much less common, making up <1% of all new male cancer cases.

[3] Nipple changes can include a change in the position of the nipple; for example, it may retract (invert) or turn. Anything that looks or feels different for the patient should alert you to a potential underlying lesion. Malignant nipple discharge is usually from a single duct and may be blood-stained or clear, whereas benign nipple discharge is often multi-ductal which can be creamy/green or brown in colour. Skin changes can include the classic peau d'orange ('orange peel skin') but also eczema on the nipple that does not respond to topical treatment may represent Paget's disease of the breast (a type of breast cancer affecting the nipple or areola region). Breast pain alone is rarely a symptom of breast cancer.

[4] Breast-conserving surgery can be used in patients who have early breast cancer. The surgeon removes the cancer and a margin of normal surrounding tissue. This is called a wide local excision or lumpectomy.

[5] Radiotherapy following breast-conserving surgery is used to reduce the risk of breast cancer recurrence in the breast, chest or lymph nodes. This usually starts 4 weeks post surgery unless chemotherapy is also required. Recurrence rates in breast cancer have significantly improved since the introduction of postoperative radiotherapy, which has reduced the 10-year recurrence rate from around 35% to 19%.

[6] The most common presenting symptom of breast cancer is a breast lump or new changes in the breast. Although the majority of breast lumps are benign (e.g. fibroadenoma, cyst or injury), they should all be investigated with triple assessment in a timely manner. Other signs can include nipple changes or overlying skin changes.

[7] Women should be encouraged to self-examine their breasts regularly and get to know their own breasts so that if any changes do occur, they are more easily detected. However, most breast cancers in developed countries are picked up due to screening programmes. Breast cancer screening is offered in most developed countries for women aged 50–70 inclusive. Those who are at higher risk of breast cancer (e.g. with a strong family history) may be eligible for screening before this time. Current evidence shows that screening does reduce breast cancer mortality; however, as with any screening programme there is a risk of overdiagnosis and treatment.

[8] 'Triple assessment' is the gold standard of investigation for a new breast lump. It combines clinical examination, imaging (either ultrasound or mammogram) and biopsy. Classic mammogram findings in breast cancer are a soft tissue mass and microcalcifications, with the most specific feature being spiculated high density masses. These nearly always represent an invasive cancer.

[9] Lethargy is a non-specific symptom and can be related to many medical problems; however, it can significantly affect a patient's ability to function and their quality of life.

[10] In a patient with previous breast cancer, right-sided abdominal pain should raise concerns regarding liver metastasis, especially if associated with other concerning symptoms.

11 Breast cancer most commonly spreads to the lymph nodes, liver, lungs, bones and brain. Back pain in someone with previous breast cancer and suspected recurrence should alert you to the potential of bone metastases.

12 Constipation can be caused by the treatments and pain relief medications given in breast cancer. However, it can also be caused by hypercalcaemia. Breast cancer is one of the cancers most commonly associated with hypercalcaemia. It can be caused by skeletal metastasis but can also occur in patients in the absence of skeletal metastasis. This can be due to primary hyperparathyroidism from parathyroid adenomas. Symptoms of hypercalcaemia can be very non-specific, such as loss of appetite, nausea, vomiting, constipation and abdominal pain. This can progress to weakness, confusion, headaches, depression and can ultimately lead to death from cardiac arrhythmias.

13 Women with close relatives who have been diagnosed with breast cancer are at higher risk of developing the disease.

Your risk is double that of the general population if you have had one first-degree relative diagnosed with breast cancer (mother, sister, daughter). If two first-degree relatives have been diagnosed, that risk increases to five times the risk of the general population. In some cases, a strong family history of breast cancer has been found to be linked to abnormal genes, the most well-known being *BRCA1* or *BRCA2* (tumour suppressor genes). The checkpoint kinase 2 gene (*CHEK2*) has also been implicated in playing a role in developing breast cancer.

14 Drinking alcohol is a known modifiable risk factor for breast cancer. Other modifiable risk factors include being physically inactive, overweight, taking certain hormones (e.g. HRT) and a woman's reproductive history can play a role as well (such as older age at the time of first pregnancy, not breastfeeding and never having a full-term pregnancy).

Examination

- The patient looks slightly **underweight** [1] and **tired but not unwell** [2]. Her observations are normal.
- She can walk into the room with **no abnormality of gait or shortness of breath** [3].
- Inspection reveals **scleral icterus** [4] and **conjunctival pallor** [5].
- Chest is clear to auscultation and heart sounds are dual with **no added sounds** [6].
- On breast examination her right **nipple is inverted with skin changes** [7] and a further 2–3cm mass is felt in the **right axillary tail** [8], with **swelling felt in the right axilla** [9].

- Her abdominal examination reveals a tender right upper quadrant with a smoothly palpable **liver edge 4cm below the costal margin** [10].
- She complains of **tenderness in her mid-thoracic region** [11], which is reproducible on palpation over T10/11 in the midline.
- There are no overlying skin changes or deformities seen, and **neurological examination is completely normal** [12].

1 Over a third of patients with cancer present with 'unexplained weight loss' at diagnosis. Cachexia (atrophy of adipose tissue and skeletal muscle) may develop, which can affect a patient's quality of life and can worsen prognosis. Although many patients also suffer with anorexia, cachexia is thought to be due to increased energy use and lipolysis by the tumour and/or the body's response.

2 Patients presenting with a new cancer diagnosis may not look particularly unwell. It is important to be able to distinguish between those who are unwell and may need immediate hospital admission for treatment and those who are well enough to remain in the community for investigation and treatment.

3 The ability to walk unaided without becoming significantly short of breath tells us that there is no gross neurological abnormality in the lower limbs, and that their physiological reserve is adequate.

4 As bilirubin levels increase, jaundice may occur in the conjunctiva, known as scleral icterus. This is where the conjunctiva, but not actually the sclera, become stained with bile pigment. Rising bilirubin is a potential sign of liver dysfunction, which may point to liver metastasis in a patient with known breast cancer.

5 Conjunctival pallor is a sign of anaemia. Anaemia is a common problem in patients with breast cancer, either due to the underlying disease itself or as a result of treatment.

6 It is important to carry out a full examination on these patients; even though they may not complain of any chest symptoms, their cancer may still have metastasised to this region. Pericardial and pleural effusions are not uncommon in breast cancer and so it is important to assess for these signs.

7 Nipple and skin changes are common presenting symptoms for patients with breast cancer. Breast examination involves looking at the breasts when in different positions to try to exacerbate any abnormalities that may be seen; a structured breast and surrounding lymph node examination should then follow. Skin changes that indicate a possible breast cancer include a rash, redness, puckering or dimpling of the breast. Some patients present with skin that looks like orange peel, or with a texture that is different to the rest of the breast. A rare cause of skin changes is Paget's disease of the breast. This presents as a scaly, red and sometimes itchy rash that can resemble eczema. These features may represent underlying breast cancer and need further investigation.

8 When performing a breast examination, one needs a systematic approach. This is commonly done by dividing the breast into four quadrants to ensure all areas are covered, including the axillary tail.

9 An important part of the breast examination includes examining for lymph nodes. Swelling around the collarbone (infra- and supraclavicular nodes) or armpit (axillary nodes) could be a sign of breast cancer that has spread to the lymph nodes. These can sometimes be present before there is a palpable breast mass.

10 Breast cancer most commonly spreads to the lymph nodes, liver, lungs, bone and brain. Liver metastases may be asymptomatic initially, but as they grow this can cause the liver to enlarge which can cause pain (liver capsular pain) or obstruct the normal flow of blood and bile (which may cause jaundice, loss of appetite and abdominal swelling).

11 Back pain is a very common symptom for people to present to the doctor with; however, in those with suspected cancer it should raise concerns regarding bone metastasis. It is important to fully examine the spine to assess whether the pain is bony or muscular pain and to see if there are other areas of pain or abnormalities.

12 Patients with back pain should have a thorough neurological assessment to see if there is any evidence of cord compression which would be an oncological emergency, needing immediate investigation and intervention.

Investigations

- **Full blood count** [1] shows a mild anaemia.
- The patient has normal **renal** [2] function but **deranged LFTs with raised transaminases, raised bilirubin and low albumin** [3].
- She had a significantly **raised calcium** [4], and her clotting profile revealed a **raised INR** [5].
- **Mammogram** [6] showed a spiculated soft tissue mass.
- A **chest radiograph** [7] and **thoracolumbar X-ray** [8] showed a T10 compression fracture.
- Given concerns regarding metastatic disease, a **staging** [9] **CT chest/abdomen/pelvis (CT CAP)** [10]

is organised, which unfortunately showed metastatic deposits in the spine and liver.
- A **sentinel node biopsy** [11] was organised to obtain a **histological diagnosis** [12] and to determine nodal involvement.
- Further receptor testing was performed to allow determination of the **hormone profiles** [13] of the breast cancer.
- If there is a concern regarding a strong genetic element to the breast cancer, **genetic testing** [14] for *BRCA* should be considered for family members.

1 Anaemia is common in patients with breast cancer for a variety of reasons, such as the tumour itself (for example blood loss, metastatic deposits with bone marrow infiltration or nutritional deficiencies) or due to the treatments. It is important to identify the likely cause, as it can negatively affect treatment outcomes as well as quality of life and survival outcomes. Patients report that fatigue affects their daily life more than other cancer-associated complications. It is also important to note whether the anaemia is part of a pancytopenia, which may occur as a result of cytotoxic therapy.

2 Renal function may be normal or show an acute kidney injury in patients who have reduced oral intake. Patients may have abnormal renal function at baseline, which can further deteriorate if imaging with contrast is required. For treatment decisions, it is important to have a knowledge of the baseline renal function.

3 LFTs may be deranged in patients with liver metastasis, due to either local invasion or compression of the bile ducts. It is important to assess the synthetic function of the liver by checking for low albumin levels or abnormal clotting profiles. Low albumin may also represent malnutrition.

4 Hypercalcaemia in breast cancer is common. It can be caused either by bone metastasis, or be due to primary hyperparathyroidism. It is important to test for and treat hypercalcaemia if indicated, as it can lead to fatal cardiac arrhythmias if left untreated.

5 Coagulation studies should be sent for all patients with abnormal liver function, as decreased clotting factor synthesis can lead to a coagulopathy. It is also important to assess clotting profiles as most patients will need a biopsy and the presence of a coagulopathy will impact on their risks of bleeding.

6 Imaging is the next consideration. This is to determine the presence of cancer and potential biopsy sites, as well as any potential complications. Mammography is the first line for assessment of breast lumps; however, in those with dense breasts, ultrasounds may be beneficial to assess lumps further, and are useful to distinguish between abnormal tissues and fat lobules or benign cysts.

7 Chest X-rays may show a variety of abnormalities in breast cancer or none at all, depending on whether and where the cancer may have spread to. Some patients develop malignant pleural effusions, or bony metastasis with overlying pathological fractures.

8 Vertebral metastasis and subsequent pathological fractures can cause pain as well as lead to spinal cord or cauda impingement, depending on the level of the lesion. The first-line investigation for concerning symptoms is with plain radiographs if there is no evidence of neurological impairment. Some lesions may require stabilising procedures for symptomatic relief. If there was any evidence of cord compression or impingement, an urgent whole spine MRI should be organised.

9 The tumour, node, metastasis (TNM) staging system is used for breast cancer. The 'T' or tumour describes the size of the tumour and ranges from TX (size can't be assessed), Tis (ductal carcinoma *in situ* – DCIS) and T1–T4 with increasing tumour size. T1 means the tumour is ≤2cm, and T4 means the tumour is large and has spread into surrounding structures or is an inflammatory carcinoma. Node or 'N' reflects whether the cancer has spread to the lymph nodes, with N0 meaning there is no cancer in nearby nodes and N1–3 describing lymph node involvement in progressively distant sites as the number increases. The 'M' or metastasis describes whether the cancer has spread, with M0 showing no spread; cM0(i+) reflects no sign of cancer on exam or imaging but cancer cells have been found via laboratory testing in blood, bone marrow or lymph nodes away from the cancer, and M1 shows that the cancer has metastasised. The most common sites of metastasis for breast cancer are the brain, lung, liver and bone.

This staging system can then be used to categorise cancers into four stages. Stage 1 means the cancer remains within the breast and is small, stage 2 usually means the cancer has not yet started spreading to surrounding tissue but that the tumour is larger. Stage 3 usually means the cancer is larger and has spread to surrounding tissues and lymph nodes. Stage 4 means the cancer has metastasised.

10 Not all patients who present with breast cancer require a CT CAP. Those who just have DCIS or localised disease will not require full body imaging. However, those in whom there is suspicion of metastatic disease will need full body imaging with CT for accurate staging and to allow planning of biopsies and the next steps in treatment.

11 Sentinel node biopsy is a procedure used to determine whether the cancer has spread to the nearby lymph nodes. The 'sentinel nodes' are the first nodes into which the cancer drains. During a sentinel node biopsy, a tracer is injected into the tumour; this allows the surgeon to identify the sentinel nodes which can then be removed and analysed. If the sentinel nodes are cancer-free, then it is unlikely that the cancer has spread.

12 A formal diagnosis is made with a histological sample. Most breast cancers are carcinomas that arise from epithelial cells. However, there are various other histological types of breast cancers, such as sarcomas, to be aware of. The most common epithelial breast carcinomas are:

- infiltrating ductal carcinoma – most common, accounts for 70–80% of invasive lesions
- infiltrating lobular carcinoma comprises ~8%
- mixed ductal/lobular carcinoma, which shows a mixed histological appearance, makes up ~7%
- DCIS is a heterogeneous group of precancerous cells confined to the breast ducts and lobules – it is important to identify these and remove them as they may be a precursor for invasive breast cancer.

Histology also allows a determination of the tumour grade. The grade tells us what the cells look like and gives an idea of how quickly the cancer may grow/spread. In breast cancer there are 3 grades – in grade 1 the cells are usually slow growing; the cancer cells look small and reasonably normal. Grades 2 and 3 represent increasing size and more abnormal-looking cells, which grow faster, the higher the grade.

13 Once breast cancer is identified, hormone receptor status is determined. The newly diagnosed cancers must be tested for oestrogen receptor (ER) and progesterone receptor expression and for overexpression of human epidermal growth factor 2 (HER2) receptors. This information is essential for both prognostic and therapeutic purposes.

14 Those who may have a genetic element to their breast cancer should be advised regarding genetic testing (e.g. *BRCA* gene). They should be referred to a genetics clinic where counselling for them and family members will be provided prior to and following testing.

Management

Immediate

Immediate management should involve **controlling her pain** [1] and treating her hypercalcaemia with **IV fluids and a bisphosphonate** [2] if required. Depending on her INR and whether she has any evidence of bleeding, **vitamin K** [3] may be appropriate. Admission to hospital should be arranged given the clinical picture.

Short-term

A **breast cancer MDT meeting** [4] should be organised to discuss the next steps in management. Initial management is determined by the stage of the cancer. Most patients on initial presentation will not have metastatic disease, and their treatment will involve **primary surgery** [5] of the breast and regional lymph nodes and, depending on the characteristics of the patient's tumour, they may have **neoadjuvant or adjuvant treatment** [6]. This may include **radiotherapy** [7], **chemotherapy** [8], **endocrine therapy and/or biologic therapy** [9].

Long-term

Prognosis in breast cancer [10] depends on the stage at diagnosis. Most breast cancer recurrences occur within 5 years of diagnosis, which is why it is important to ensure patients have **post treatment surveillance** [11] with regular follow-up and annual mammography. Those with metastatic disease at initial presentation will be managed with systemic therapies. The selection of the treatment strategy is dependent on the specifics of the tumour and the patient, usually encompassing chemotherapy, endocrine therapy and/or biologic treatments along with **supportive measures** [12]. The aim of therapy in metastatic breast cancer is to prolong life, alleviate symptoms and maintain or improve quality of life.

[1] Pain management is important when managing patients with cancer and is a key priority for this patient. Bony and liver capsular pain can be significant and difficult to manage. Early involvement of the palliative care and/or pain management teams is often helpful. A multimodal approach using simple analgesia with opiates as well as non-opioid forms of analgesia should be used. Some patients may benefit from specific nerve blocks.

[2] Any life-threatening complications of the primary cancer or metastasis should be managed as an emergency, as with any other patient. Hypercalcaemia can lead to cardiac arrhythmias and death and so should be managed promptly. Initial management includes IV fluids and IV bisphosphonates, if fluids do not reduce the calcium adequately.

[3] Patients with liver dysfunction may develop a coagulopathy due to a variety of factors. This does not necessarily represent an increased bleeding risk; however, many patients with cancer need interventions including biopsies, therefore vitamin K may need to be administered.

[4] Short-term management should focus on symptomatic relief, psychological support and investigations to ensure accurate diagnosis, staging and histopathology are available. Afterwards, discussion at an MDT meeting will occur, during which surgeons/oncologists/pathologists, etc. will make an initial treatment plan for each patient.

[5] Surgery remains the mainstay of early breast cancer treatment. This may consist of an excision of the tumour with surrounding normal breast tissue (breast-conserving surgery) or a mastectomy. Depending on lymph node involvement these will be removed as well.

[6] Non-metastatic breast cancer can be categorised into early stage or locally advanced breast cancer. Following surgery adjuvant therapy may be offered depending on tumour characteristics including size, grade, number of nodes involved and receptor status. Some patients may receive systemic therapy before surgery (neoadjuvant therapy). Those with locally advanced disease will often be offered neoadjuvant therapies to induce tumour response before surgery so breast-conserving surgery may be possible, and this has been shown to improve disease-free survival in these patients. Once a decision has been made to give adjuvant therapy it should be started as soon as clinically possible, and certainly within 31 days of surgery.

[7] Postoperative radiotherapy is for patients who have a high risk of local recurrence, such as those with deep margin involvement or axillary lymph node involvement.

[8] Chemotherapy can be used with both curative and palliative intent. The need for adjuvant or neoadjuvant chemotherapy is determined based on the patient, tumour size, degree of spread, histology and hormone profile of the cancer. It can be used after surgery to reduce risk of recurrence and before surgery to reduce the size of the tumour. Each patient's treatment will be different but in general, chemotherapy will be offered to those with lymph node spread. There are many different chemotherapy

regimens but all node-positive patients considered for chemotherapy will generally be offered a taxane-containing regimen; the most common is 'FEC-T' (fluorouracil, epirubicin, cyclophosphamide and Taxotere (docetaxel)). These chemotherapy agents all have specific side-effects, but the most common are bone marrow suppression, nausea, vomiting and mucositis.

9 Hormone receptor testing is very important, as previously discussed. ER and progesterone receptor are prognostic factors for invasive breast cancer, especially in the first 5 years post diagnosis. Hormone receptor-positive tumours comprise the majority of cases (~80%). Those who have ER-positive cancers will benefit from prolonged anti-oestrogen therapy (tamoxifen +/– aromatase inhibitors). HER2 is overexpressed in ~20% of cancers and treatment with trastuzumab for a year postoperatively has shown good results. However, it is important to assess cardiac function prior to commencing Herceptin as it can cause cardiac damage. If patients are receiving chemotherapy then hormone therapy should be commenced after chemotherapy has finished. It is important to note that hormone therapy does increase the risk of gynaecological cancers, so any vaginal bleeding should be investigated.

10 Prognosis depends on the type of cancer and the degree of spread at presentation.

11 In those who have had treatment for breast cancer, close follow-up involving examinations and annual mammograms is important to ensure any recurrence is detected early. It is also important to recognise any treatment-related complications as well as psychosocial issues that may arise. Treatment for breast cancer can affect many aspects of sexuality and if any concerns are raised, counselling should be organised. As previously mentioned, genetic testing is an important aspect of breast cancer management, especially for men, women under 50 or those with Ashkenazi heritage or a strong family history of breast or ovarian cancer. Before testing it is important that counselling is organised, given the ramifications this can have on not only the patient but also their families.

12 Those with metastatic breast cancer are unlikely to be cured, but with improved therapies prolonged survival has been seen. However, it is important to be open with patients and include them in decision making, as those with advanced disease may choose to have symptomatic management only. Treatment will be tailored to the patient and their cancer, by using a selection of the previously discussed therapies. Symptomatic management includes a range of treatments and depends on what is most distressing to the patient. This can involve just analgesia but may also involve interventions such as pleural or ascitic drainage.

CASE 62: Colorectal carcinoma

History

- A **55-year-old** [1] **man** [2] presents with a **2–3-week history** [3] of a **change in bowel habit** [4], intermittent **abdominal discomfort** [5] and **weight loss** [6].
- He initially went to his GP who diagnosed him with **irritable bowel syndrome (IBS)** [7].
- However, he now presents to hospital 2 weeks later with **severe abdominal pain and distension** [8], nausea and vomiting, and has **not opened his bowels for 3 days** [9].

- He has a past medical history of hypertension but no previous **bowel problems** [10] or **operations** [11]; however, his **father did have bowel cancer** [12] in his 70s.
- He smokes **10–20 cigarettes/day, but does not drink much alcohol** [13].
- He has not yet had his first routine **bowel cancer screening test** [14].

[1] As with many cancers, colorectal cancer is much more common in older ages and most cases are diagnosed in those over the age of 60. Although colorectal cancer mortality is declining, the incidence of colorectal cancers in both men and women under 50 has been steadily increasing over the past few decades, a significant proportion of which are left-sided and rectal cancers.

[2] Colorectal cancer is the third most common cancer in terms of global incidence across both sexes; however, it is the fourth most common cause of cancer death.

[3] In those who present with symptoms, the onset can be gradual as their tumour grows. Concern should be raised in those who are advanced in age with persistent symptoms, and investigations should be promptly organised.

[4] A change in bowel habit is a concerning feature at any stage in life but especially as one gets older. A change in bowel habit can mean a change in frequency, consistency (diarrhoea or constipation), any blood, melaena or mucus in stools. However, many other disease processes can cause similar symptoms, which is why a high level of suspicion is needed.

[5] Abdominal discomfort is a very non-specific symptom and so by itself it is not particularly specific for colorectal cancer, but in the context of other symptoms it should raise concern.

[6] Weight loss in any patient is a concerning feature and should prompt further questioning and/or investigation. Patients unfortunately can be unclear about whether they have experienced weight loss, and whether it is intentional or not. In many bowel pathologies patients lose weight due to GI losses, but it is a red flag.

[7] Irritable bowel syndrome is a group of symptoms including abdominal pain and changes in bowel habit without any clear underlying damage. The pathogenesis of IBS is unclear but is generally a diagnosis of exclusion and concerning signs include onset over 50, blood in a patient's stools or family history of inflammatory bowel disease (IBD).

[8] Severe abdominal pain and distension are concerning symptoms for any patient as they may represent a surgical bowel pathology. An obstructing lesion should be considered, particularly in those with other features suggestive of bowel cancer.

[9] Any patient presenting with nausea, vomiting and constipation should be investigated urgently for bowel obstruction and may need emergency surgery to clear the blockage and prevent bowel perforation.

[10] Non-modifiable risk factors for bowel cancer, apart from age, include a personal history of previous colorectal cancer, colonic polyps, IBD or prolonged inflammation. For this reason, patients with IBD should be screened for colorectal cancer more regularly than the general population.

[11] Taking a thorough history including previous surgical interventions is important, as bowel obstruction can be caused not just by intraluminal lesions such as cancers but by adhesions from previous surgeries.

[12] Patients with inherited syndromes make up ~5% of patients who develop colorectal cancer. These syndromes increase a person's likelihood of developing colorectal cancer due to inherited gene changes. Hereditary non-polyposis colon cancer (HNPCC or Lynch syndrome) is the most common hereditary colorectal cancer syndrome. This syndrome is most commonly caused by defects in genes

responsible for repairing damaged DNA, such as the *MLH1* or *MLH2* genes, but other genes can be involved. The lifetime risk of a person with HNPCC developing colorectal cancer is 80%, and it tends to develop at a young age. There is also an increased risk of endometrial cancer in women, as well as some other cancers.

Familial adenomatous polyposis is another syndrome caused by mutations in the *APC* gene. This leads to the development of hundreds of polyps in the colon and rectum, with cancer developing in at least one polyp by as early as age 20; nearly 100% of patients will develop colorectal cancer by age 40. Patients may have their colon removed to prevent the almost inevitable development of colorectal cancer. They are also at risk of developing other cancers such as stomach, small intestine, pancreatic and liver. Other inherited syndromes that can increase the risk of colorectal cancer include Peutz–Jeghers syndrome and MYH-associated polyposis.

A family history of colorectal cancer or adenomatous polyps is also a risk factor for colorectal cancer. Nearly a third of patients who develop colorectal cancer will have a family member who has also had colorectal cancer. Those with a first-degree relative who has had colorectal cancer are at increased risk, especially those whose relatives developed colorectal cancer below 45 years of age.

13 The modifiable risk factors for colorectal cancer are similar to other cancers. Smoking, significant alcohol intake, minimal physical activity and being overweight all have been shown to increase the risk of both developing and dying from colorectal cancer. A diet that is high in red and processed meats has also been shown to increase the risk of developing colorectal cancer.

14 Bowel cancer screening is usually offered between the ages of 60 and 74 for all men and women every 2 years, and some countries begin screening at the age of 50. The faecal immunochemical test replaced the faecal occult blood test that was previously used. This test detects any occult blood in the stool which may represent a polyp or a cancer. If the screening test returns positive, patients are called in for a colonoscopy. Given that symptoms only develop in colorectal cancer at advanced stages, this screening test allows early detection.

Examination

- The patient looks **unwell** [1] and **is clearly in pain** [2].
- His observations are abnormal, with a **tachycardia (HR 120bpm), hypotension (BP 90/40mmHg), tachypnoea, a temperature of 39°C** [3]; however, oxygen saturation is within normal range.
- He looks **pale** from the end of the bed and has **conjunctival pallor** [4].

- Abdominal examination reveals a **very tender and distended abdomen** [5], worse in the **left iliac fossa** [6] but no **overt masses felt** [7].
- He has **scant tinkling bowel sounds** [8].
- Rectal examination is carried out which finds only an **empty rectum** [9]. There are no abnormalities found on the rest of his examination.

1 On initial assessment it is important to determine whether the patient looks well or unwell. If the patient looks unwell, try to work out what it is about them that is concerning. This will help to focus your examination.

2 Significant pain is a concerning feature for any patient. In those with significant abdominal pain and possible bowel obstruction, a bowel perforation must be considered, which can make patients unwell very quickly.

3 Hypotension, tachycardia and fevers are concerning for septic shock. The source of infection should be determined as quickly as possible. Initial management should also be aimed towards IV fluid resuscitation, blood tests including a lactate and blood cultures, prompt initiation of antibiotics as well as close monitoring of urine output. Early referral to the intensive care and general surgery teams is recommended.

4 Iron-deficiency anaemia is common in colorectal cancers and is caused by a combination of chronic microscopic tumour-induced blood loss and impaired iron homeostasis associated with chronic disease. It is important to be aware of this and ensure appropriate management is put in place for these patients, as their haemoglobin will most likely drop further during treatment.

5 A tender distended abdomen is concerning for an acute abdomen and this patient should be discussed with the surgical team and any relevant imaging performed urgently. This clinical finding is especially concerning for patients with potential bowel cancer as it may indicate an obstructive lesion.

6 In left-sided colorectal cancer, a change in bowel habit and obstructive symptoms are more common than in right-sided disease, whereas PR bleeding and iron-deficiency anaemia are more common in right-sided cancers, especially when the tumour is in the caecum or ascending colon. Rectal cancer can cause the sensation of tenesmus, as well as rectal pain and change in size of stools.

7 Examination can sometimes reveal a palpable mass, as well as an enlarged liver if there has been any metastatic spread to the liver. The liver is the most common site of metastasis for colorectal cancers, but they can spread to the peritoneum, lung, bones and brain. However, distal rectal tumours may metastasise to the lungs first as the inferior rectal vein drains into the inferior vena cava, not into the portal venous system like the rest of the colon.

8 An absence of bowel sounds can indicate either a complete obstruction or an ileus. High-pitched tinkling bowel sounds are concerning for a mechanical bowel obstruction.

9 A digital rectal examination should be carried out on all patients presenting with abdominal symptoms. An empty rectum indicates there is no stool in the rectum, but it also allows assessment for any palpable rectal or prostate (in men) abnormalities such as masses.

Investigations

- **Full blood count** [1] showed the patient was anaemic with a raised WCC.
- **Renal function** [2] showed acute kidney injury; **liver function tests** [3] were normal except for a low albumin.
- A **cross-match** [4] is sent, and **coagulation studies and electrolytes** [5] reveal no abnormalities.
- An urgent **CT of the abdomen and pelvis** [6] revealed a 5cm x 6cm obstructing lesion in the descending colon, with **dilated proximal loops and free fluid** [7] in the abdomen but no clear point of perforation.

- The patient was taken to emergency theatre and the tumour was excised and sent for **histology** [8], including **molecular testing** [9].
- In patients who are stable and do not present with bowel obstruction, a **colonoscopy** [10] is the first-line investigation to get a histological diagnosis, after which a CT CAP is organised for **staging** [11].
- The tumour marker **carcinoembryonic antigen (CEA)** [12] was retrospectively added onto his blood test and found to be very high.

1 As previously mentioned, colorectal cancers can often cause iron-deficiency anaemia through both tumour-induced blood loss and chronic disease affecting iron pathways. In an emergency, if a patient has a haemoglobin of <70g/dl a blood transfusion should be arranged, but if the patient is stable and has proven iron deficiency then iron infusions can be organised. A raised WCC is not abnormal in cancer but if it is significantly raised, an infection should be considered. This patient likely has peritonitis from a perforated bowel.

2 Acute kidney injury (AKI) is a common finding in patients presenting to hospital, and it is important to determine what the cause is (i.e. prerenal, renal or postrenal). In this man, the cause of his AKI is most likely prerenal, given he has been unwell with nausea and vomiting and is likely dehydrated. However, he could potentially have a postrenal obstruction as well as an intrinsic renal cause for his AKI.

3 LFTs may be abnormal in a patient who has liver metastases; however, this may not always be the case. Normal LFTs do not exclude liver metastases.

4 In a patient like this, for whom surgery is probable and who is already anaemic, a cross-match should be organised so that a blood transfusion is ready if needed.

5 Coagulation studies need to be sent to ensure that any coagulopathy can be reversed prior to surgery. It is important to check electrolytes as this patient is at risk of refeeding syndrome postoperatively, given he has not eaten for a while prior to presentation.

6 In the emergency setting, the priority is to investigate the potentially life-threatening abdominal symptoms. CT of the abdomen and pelvis will help to identify any intra-abdominal pathology that needs immediate treatment. If a cancer is revealed, then once the patient is more stable a full screening scan can be organised.

7 This man's CT scan shows an obstructing tumour with free fluid. Although no clear perforation is seen, the suspicion for a perforation must be high in the presence of free fluid. He needs emergency surgery and the general surgeons should be contacted if they have not already been consulted.

8 The majority of colorectal cancers are carcinomas, and of these the majority are adenocarcinomas (90%). Other histological types such as neuroendocrine/lymphomas are much rarer.

9 Molecular testing is involved in guiding treatment for patients with colorectal cancer. *KRAS* mutation testing should be performed to guide decisions about epidermal growth factor receptor inhibitor therapy. *BRAF* mutation testing should be done with deficient mismatch repair and microsatellite instability testing for prognostication and identification of HNPCC.

10 Colonoscopy is the preferred investigation for stable patients following suspicion of colorectal cancer, as it allows for a full assessment of the rectum and large bowel as well as providing histological diagnosis.

11 Colorectal cancers can spread by lymphatic and haematogenous dissemination, as well as contiguous and transperitoneal spread. The most common metastatic sites are lymph nodes, liver and lungs. As with most cancers, the TNM staging system is preferred. The previous Dukes classification is no longer used. The 'T' or tumour is graded from T0 to T4, with T0 representing no evidence of primary, T1 tumours invade the submucosa, T2 invade the muscularis propria, T3 invades through the muscularis propria into the pericolorectal tissues and T4 invades the visceral peritoneum or invades/adheres to adjacent organs or structures. The 'N' or node describes metastasis to regional lymph nodes, ranging from N0 to N2b and describing progressively greater lymph node involvement. The 'M' or metastasis describes whether the cancer has metastasised and by how much, with grades ranging from M0 to M1c, with M0 representing no metastasis and each step representing further metastasis.
The TNM classification can then be used to assign stage grouping for colorectal cancers.

- Stage 0: carcinoma *in situ* – meaning the cancer cells are only in the mucosa.
- Stage I: cancer has grown through the mucosa and has invaded the muscular layer of the colon but has not spread further (T1 or 2 N0 M0).
- Stage II (A–C): cancer has spread through the wall of the colon and may have grown into other structures but has not spread to nodes or elsewhere.
- Stage III (A–C): cancer has spread to regional lymph nodes but no distant metastasis.
- Stage IV (A–C): cancer has spread to a single distant part of the body (A) or it has spread to more than one part of the body (B). C is where the cancer has spread to the peritoneum.

12 Serum CEA levels should ideally be obtained pre-operatively. It has been shown to have prognostic value, and high levels may represent disseminated and more advanced disease.

Management

Immediate

Immediate management of this patient should be focused on stabilising him clinically. Given that he has a bowel obstruction and has likely perforated his bowel, management will involve instructing the patient to be **nil by mouth, having a nasogastric tube inserted**, commencing **IV fluids for his AKI** and **IV antibiotics** [1] to cover for intra-abdominal sepsis. He will need **emergency surgery** [2] to decompress the bowel and remove his cancer.

Short-term

Following surgery, a histological diagnosis will be made. This man should be discussed at the **colorectal multidisciplinary meeting** [3], where next steps in treatment will be discussed and planned. Given he has had a significant operation, he will need adequate **analgesia** [4] and **nutritional review** [5]. Depending on whether he has a **colostomy** [6], support from a stoma nurse is essential.

Long-term

For patients with localised cancer, surgery is the only curative treatment. Some patients may benefit from **neoadjuvant chemoradiotherapy** [7], specifically those with locally advanced rectal cancer. For patients who have undergone potentially curative surgery, they will receive **adjuvant chemotherapy** [8] to eradicate micrometastasis, the **side-effects** [9] of which can be severe. Postoperative radiotherapy is not a routine part of treatment for completely resected colon cancers; however, for patients with rectal cancer **radiotherapy** [10] is used frequently.
For patients who have metastatic disease, surgery for **metastectomy** [11] has shown improved survival outcomes when used in conjunction with chemotherapy, as has the use of **biological therapies** [12]. All patients who have completed treatment for colorectal cancer should have a **surveillance programme** [13] organised for them so that recurrent disease can be detected early.
The most important prognostic indicator following resection of colorectal cancer is **pathological stage at presentation** [14].

1 The most important initial steps are to stabilise the patient with a nasogastric tube to decompress the bowel, commence IV fluids for his AKI and IV antibiotics for likely bowel perforation. Instructing the patient to be nil by mouth is important prior to his emergency surgery.

2 Emergency surgery is needed in this case, given the patient has presented in bowel obstruction. However, surgery is also the only curative treatment available for locally advanced colon cancer (stage I–III) and can also potentially provide a curative option for those with limited metastatic disease (stage IV). The general principle is to remove the tumour with adequate margins. Surgery can range from a hemi-colectomy to total colectomy for excision of the primary tumour. Total colectomy is usually reserved for those with genetic cancer syndromes and a high risk of recurrence due to this. In those with limited metastatic disease, resection of metastases has been shown to improve long-term survival for up to 50% of patients in combination with aggressive medical management.

Surgery is also a palliative option for patients who may gain some symptomatic relief; for example, in those who have bowel obstruction or significant bleeding from the tumour, surgical resection can improve their quality of life.

3 As with all cancers, the multidisciplinary meeting is integral to having a coordinated management approach. All the specialists involved in the patient's treatment can discuss results and next steps together and ensure patients are being followed up appropriately.

4 Pain is a problem that will affect most patients with cancer and ensuring their pain is appropriately controlled using a multimodal approach is integral to their care.

5 Many patients will already be malnourished at presentation, given they have often been unwell for some time. Unfortunately, often the surgery and treatments will cause ongoing difficulty to maintain adequate nutrition, so early involvement of a dietitian can be helpful.

6 Colorectal surgery is a daunting experience, and for many patients having a colostomy or stoma bag is something they never thought they would have to deal with. This can cause a lot of psychological distress and so involvement of the stoma nurse prior to and after surgery is very important.

7 Neoadjuvant chemoradiotherapy is commonly used as initial treatment for patients with locally advanced rectal cancer. It is unclear currently which patients with colon cancer may also benefit from this.

8 All patients who have undergone potentially curative surgery should receive postoperative chemotherapy, the goal of which is to reduce the chance of recurrence by eradicating micrometastasis. The chemotherapy regimens used involve a combination of drugs but the most common are FOLFOX (folinic acid, fluorouracil and oxaliplatin) and CapeOX (capecitabine and oxaliplatin).

9 Chemotherapy can cause significant side-effects, the most common of which include mucositis, nausea, vomiting, diarrhoea, neutropenia, fatigue, hair loss, hand-foot syndrome (pain and peeling of hands and feet) and cardiotoxicity. Most side-effects cease when chemotherapy is stopped, but some can cause long-standing peripheral neuropathy, such as oxaliplatin.

10 Postoperative radiotherapy is used frequently for patients with rectal cancer due to the increased risk of recurrence because of the anatomy and difficulty in getting clear margins. It is used less commonly in colon cancer; however, a selected group of patients with high risk of recurrence may benefit.

11 Approximately 20% of newly diagnosed patients with colon cancer present with metastatic disease, and for these patients a combined approach to treatment is needed. Metastatectomy has been proven to improve outcomes, as has the advent of biologic agents used in conjunction with chemotherapy.

12 Biologic therapies include monoclonal antibodies against vascular endothelial growth factor (e.g. bevacizumab) and epidermal growth factor receptor (EGFR) (e.g. cetuximab). *KRAS* mutations (present in ~40% of colorectal cancers) impact on the efficacy of anti-EGFR treatment, which is why it is important to test this. These treatments have been shown to improve the progression-free survival in patients with metastatic disease.

13 Post treatment surveillance should include annual history and examination with tumour markers, CT scans and colonoscopy to ensure recurrence is picked up as early as possible.

14 The most important prognostic indicator is the pathological stage at presentation for those who present with resectable disease. For those who present with metastatic disease their prognosis is variable and dependent on many factors including patient factors (age, performance status), tumour factors (number of metastases and where they are), molecular factors such as *KRAS*, *BRAF* and DNA mismatch repair/microsatellite instability, and treatment factors (whether they are eligible for surgery, chemotherapy, etc.). However, as with most cancers, the 5-year survival rate is much higher with localised disease (~nearly 90%) than with metastatic disease (<15%).

CASE 63: Head and neck carcinoma

History

- A **56-year-old** [1] **man** [2] presents to the **oncology day unit** [3] for a check-up pre-radiotherapy.
- He is currently at day 10 of his **chemotherapy and radiotherapy regime** [4] for his **head and neck squamous cell carcinoma** [5].
- He is in significant pain with **lesions in his mouth** [6] which have caused him to have a reduced oral intake for the past week.
- He has noticed he has had **darker urine** [7] and has been feeling **hot and feverish** [8] for the last day or so.
- His cancer was detected initially as a **non-healing mouth ulcer** [9] which was found to be a squamous cell carcinoma.
- He has minimal past medical history but is an **ex-smoker** [10], having stopped smoking on diagnosis.

1 The incidence of head and neck cancers increases with age, as with most cancers, with most patients presenting between the ages of 50 and 70 years. However, head and neck cancer can develop at a younger age, especially those cancers that are associated with human papillomavirus (HPV).

2 Head and neck cancer is more common in men, with the highest rates of head and neck cancers being in older males. However, the incidence has been increasing in young non-smokers. This is thought to be due to HPV which is a prominent aetiological factor in development of head and neck cancers.

3 Patients will often present to the oncology day unit to be assessed or to either receive their chemotherapy or wait for their radiotherapy, or both. Often patients are noted to be unwell whilst attending the day unit and will be seen by an oncology or haematology doctor to assess if they need treatment and whether they need to be an inpatient or outpatient.

4 Treatment for these cancers involves surgery and an intensive systemic chemotherapy and concurrent radiotherapy regime. Due to the intensity of these regimes many patients will experience side-effects, some of which will be severe.

5 Head and neck cancers encompass cancers originating in the oral cavity, pharynx, larynx, nasal cavity, paranasal sinuses, thyroid and salivary gland. These cancers include a variety of histopathological tumours; however, the most common is squamous cell carcinoma, making up the majority of these cases.

6 Due to the intensive chemotherapy and radiotherapy treatments required for head and neck cancers patients often develop significant side-effects. One such side-effect is mucositis, which occurs due to acute inflammation of the oral mucosa, tongue and pharynx after radiation exposure and systemic chemotherapy. The grading system developed by the WHO ranges from 0 (none) to IV which is defined as life-threatening mucositis in which oral feeding is impossible. These patients need admission to hospital and parenteral fluids and nutrition to be initiated.

7 Often patients with severe mucositis will be unable to eat or drink properly, and so will have reduced oral intake and become very dehydrated with dark urine. This can lead to acute kidney injury, requiring admission to hospital for IV fluids.

8 Patients with cancer may develop temperatures frequently; however, for those on chemotherapy the concern is that if they are neutropenic, they are unable to fight off even the simplest infections and so may develop neutropenic sepsis. These patients require admission, isolation and treatment with IV antibiotics until their white cell counts have recovered. They may have a reduced chemotherapy dose next cycle to prevent further episodes.

9 Presentation of head and neck cancers varies depending on the site. They may be found incidentally following a dentist appointment or due to patients developing symptoms. Common presenting features by site are listed below:

- Nasopharyngeal carcinoma – neck mass from regional lymph node metastasis. Symptoms from the tumour may include hearing loss, tinnitus, nasal obstruction and pain.
- Oral cavity tumours – often present with non-healing ulcers, mouth pain, dysphagia, odynophagia and/or weight loss. Patients with tongue cancer often have cervical lymph node involvement at presentation; those who present with dysarthria indicate advanced stage, since there is muscle infiltration.

- Oropharyngeal tumours – dysphagia, odynophagia, snoring and bleeding are common presenting complaints. Often, they will present with a neck mass, especially if their cancer is HPV-related.
- Hypopharyngeal tumour – often asymptomatic, thus usually diagnosed at a more advanced stage of disease at presentation. Dysphagia, odynophagia, otalgia, weight loss, haemoptysis and neck masses are some of the presenting symptoms.
- Laryngeal cancer – this depends on the level of the lesion within the larynx. Symptoms can include hoarseness, dysphagia, chronic cough, haemoptysis and stridor.
- Sinus tumours – epistaxis and unilateral nasal obstruction.

10 Smoking is the most important risk factor for head and neck cancers – this includes smokeless tobacco (i.e. chewing, sniffing or placing between gum and cheek). Some people are genetically more affected by the carcinogenic effects of tobacco, and there is evidence that alcohol and smoking synergistically increase head and neck cancer risk. HPV is also a significant risk factor for head and neck cancers. Other risk factors include radiation and other environmental exposures, vitamin deficiencies, immune suppression and betel nut chewing.

Examination

- The patient looks **unwell** [1] from the end of the bed and seems to be in **pain** [2].
- His observations are **abnormal** [3], showing a tachycardia (HR 130bpm), with low blood pressure (85/40mmHg), tachypnoea (25 breaths per minute) and reduced oxygen saturation at 90% on air.
- He is also found to have a **temperature of 38.7°C** [4].
- He has reduced **skin turgor** and his **JVP is not seen** [5].

- He has erythema over his neck, dry chapped lips with **inflamed, erythematous and ulcerated mucous membranes** [6].
- On assessment he is unable to swallow even his **own secretions** [7], which he is spitting into a cup.
- On chest auscultation he has **crepitations at the right base** [8], no added heart sounds and his abdomen is soft and non-tender.

1 Initial assessment includes a decision as to whether the patient is 'well' or 'unwell'. Clinically this can sometimes be difficult with oncology patients as they may look unwell due to their disease process or their cancer treatments, or for another reason such as infections.

2 Pain is a common symptom for patients with cancer. Those undergoing intensive chemoradiotherapy for their head and neck cancers can develop significant side-effects which can be very painful and greatly affect their quality of life. It is important to recognise that a patient is in pain, determine the cause and offer treatment.

3 This patient is in shock. He is most likely in septic shock since he is having chemotherapy and has fevers; however, he may also be hypovolaemic. A patient with these observations should alert you to the fact that they are very unwell, and your next steps need to be quick to prevent further deterioration. Intravenous access is required for blood tests including a blood gas, and then IV fluids and antibiotics can be given. Supplemental oxygen needs to be also commenced promptly. If the patient does not improve with these measures, then early referral to the ICU is recommended.

4 A fever is suggestive of an infection and given that he may have treatment-induced neutropenia, he should be treated as a patient with 'neutropenic sepsis'.

5 Reduced skin turgor and being unable to see this patient's JVP are signs that he is dehydrated and needs fluid resuscitation.

6 Mucositis can occur in patients undergoing both chemotherapy and radiotherapy. In chemotherapy the onset of symptoms is usually 5 days post treatment with a usual peak at around 10 days and gradual improvement over the following weeks. In those receiving radiotherapy it often occurs a couple of weeks after commencing treatment and may last for up to 8 weeks. The mucosal lining of the mouth and oropharynx becomes thinned, sloughs off and then is red, inflamed and ulcerated. This can be extremely painful and often the amount of pain is proportional to the severity of the ulceration. The ulcers can also become infected, which especially in immunosuppressed patients may lead to sepsis.

7 An inability to manage his own secretions tells us that this man has such severe mucositis that he is unable to swallow anything at all. This is potentially life-threatening. He needs immediate management of the ulcer pain (often with mouthwashes) as well as organisation of parenteral hydration and nutrition.

8 This patient may also have a concurrent pneumonia given the crepitations on auscultation of his chest. In all patients, but especially those who are immunocompromised, it is important to be aware that concurrent pathologies can exist and thus a thorough examination is always important.

Investigations

- Initial blood tests reveal a **pancytopenia** [1] on his full blood count, significant **acute kidney injury** [2] and a **low albumin** [3] on his LFTs.
- **Blood, urine and sputum cultures** [4] were sent.
- His venous blood gas shows a **raised lactate and mild metabolic acidosis** [5] with respiratory compensation.
- **Chest radiograph** [6] shows right lower lobe consolidation.
- At initial presentation of his head and neck cancer, **thorough examination** [7] was necessary to identify the lesion followed by examination under anaesthesia with biopsy to obtain a **histological diagnosis** [8].
- Imaging was performed to determine the extent of the primary tumour, and **staging** [9] with CT head and neck as well as chest and abdomen was performed to assess for distant metastasis.
- Close attention is needed to check for **concurrent primary cancers** [10], given these patients often have risk factors for other cancers such as lung cancer.
- **HPV testing** [11] is important for those with newly diagnosed oropharyngeal squamous cell carcinoma.

1 Many chemotherapy agents cause not just neutropenia (neutrophils <1 x10⁹/L) but also anaemia and thrombocytopenia. This is termed pancytopenia. Neutropenia increases the risk of infections, whilst thrombocytopenia increases bleeding risk. In these scenarios, a discussion needs to occur regarding thromboprophylaxis. These patients have an increased risk of thrombosis due to their cancer but increased bleeding risk due to thrombocytopenia. If any procedures are required, platelet transfusions may be necessary.

2 Acute kidney injury is defined as an abrupt decline in renal function. In this patient, his renal impairment is likely due to dehydration (hypovolaemia) because of his poor oral intake in the setting of severe mucositis.

3 Low albumin is a marker of chronic disease and poor nutritional status. Pre-treatment low levels of albumin may be a predictor of poor cancer outcomes.

4 A full septic screen is important in anyone who you are concerned has an infection. Also, in patients with cancer an important source of sepsis is their intravenous lines. Many will have long-term intravenous lines such as PICC lines for delivery of chemotherapy. It is important to look at these lines carefully when assessing patients and take both peripheral and line cultures when doing a septic screen.

5 Venous blood gas sampling allows you to see if a patient is acidotic or alkalotic and whether this is due to respiratory or metabolic causes. A raised lactate is a useful way of determining whether there is tissue hypoperfusion, although it can be caused by other factors. A higher lactate generally means a patient is more unwell and their tissues are not being perfused adequately. The metabolic acidosis in this man is most likely due to a combination of lactate and AKI. His tachypnoea is a compensatory response to the metabolic acidosis and so his carbon dioxide levels will be lower than normal.

6 Chest X-rays should be part of a septic screen to determine if there is any evidence of pneumonia. However, some changes may develop later so a normal chest X-ray does not always mean a patient does not have an early chest infection that may later develop into pneumonia in an immunocompromised patient.

7 In those with head and neck cancers the initial evaluation involves inspection and palpation of lesions and either indirect mirror examination or direct flexible laryngoscopy, depending on where the lesion is. Careful assessment of the nasal and oral cavities is needed, with visualisation and palpation of all mucous membranes. Examination under anaesthesia will often be required to fully assess the tumour and to take biopsies to allow a tissue diagnosis.

8 Most head and neck cancers are squamous cell carcinomas, accounting for 90–95% of these tumours. They are characterised into three groups depending on the percentage of keratinisation seen: well differentiated, moderately differentiated and poorly differentiated. Other histologies include adenocarcinoma, adenoid cystic carcinoma, verrucous carcinoma and mucoepidermoid carcinoma. Squamous cell carcinoma of the head and neck often develops from premalignant cells due to carcinogen exposure. Dysplasia may be found on histopathology and is associated with progression to invasive cancer in around 15–30% of cases.

9 Work-up to assess for metastasis is required for all newly diagnosed patients with head and neck cancers, especially assessing for local lymph node spread. Contrast CT or MRI of the head and neck, as well as chest and abdomen, will determine the extent of tumour infiltration and assess deeper local structures, degree of local infiltration, involvement of lymph nodes and presence of distant metastasis or second primary tumours. The TNM system is used for staging of cancers of the head and neck. The 'T' or tumour indicates the extent of the primary tumour and is site-specific. The 'N' or node indicates the nodal spread and there is significant overlap between different head and neck cancers. The 'M'

or metastasis indicates any evidence of distant spread of the tumour. Distant metastasis at presentation will most often be asymptomatic, the most common sites being the lung, liver and bone.

10 HPV testing via p16 surrogate (increased activity) is incorporated into the staging of oropharyngeal squamous cell carcinomas, given it is a causative agent for these cancers.

11 Head and neck cancers are rare, but frequently aggressive. Patients are often at risk of a second primary, especially in those who continue to smoke and drink alcohol.

Management

Immediate

This patient has neutropenic sepsis which is a medical and oncological emergency. Immediate management should occur promptly, ideally **within one hour, such as IV fluids, broad-spectrum antibiotics** [1] (after blood cultures), urinary catheterisation to monitor urine output and early discussion with **intensive care** [2]. He should be isolated due to his neutropenic sepsis and potentially be started on **granulocyte colony-stimulating factor (GCSF)** [3] to aid improvement in his cell counts. He should be prescribed **mouthwashes** [4] for his mucositis and **analgesia** [5] to improve his pain and prevent further infection.

Short-term

Following treatment of his acute episode his oncology team need to decide when he can restart his treatment and whether a **lower chemoradiotherapy dose is required** [6]. Consideration of his nutrition is important because mucositis can be severe and last a long time, so he may require a **nasogastric tube or a PEG** [7] (percutaneous endoscopic gastrostomy). This may be

discussed at the **MDT meeting** [8], along with all new cases of head and neck cancer. A multidisciplinary approach including surgeons, oncologists (medical and clinical), dentists, dietitians, speech pathologists, rehabilitation teams and prosthodontists is integral to optimal management and decision making.

Long-term

For patients with head and neck cancer, their treatment consists of **surgery** [9], **chemotherapy** [10] and **radiotherapy** [11]. Unfortunately, given the intensity of these treatments patients often experience **toxicities** [12] which can affect their quality of life even after treatment has finished. An important part of their management will involve reconstruction and rehabilitation. Those who present with advanced disease or develop metastatic disease may be managed **palliatively** [13] with surgery, chemotherapy and radiotherapy as indicated. Following successful treatment, **regular follow-up** [14] is essential to monitor for any disease recurrence. The **prognosis** [15] for patients with head and neck squamous cell cancers is dependent on the site and stage at presentation.

1 The recommendation from the Society of Critical Care Medicine and the European Society of Intensive Care Medicine is that within one hour certain tests and therapies should be initiated in patients with septic shock to reduce their morbidity and mortality. In the '1-hour bundle' a lactate measure and blood cultures prior to antibiotics should be taken, and broad-spectrum antibiotics commenced. In those who are hypotensive or with a raised lactate, rapid crystalloid administration (30ml/kg) is recommended and vasopressors should be considered in those who remain hypotensive during or following fluid resuscitation.

2 For patients who remain hypotensive despite adequate fluid resuscitation or are too unwell to be managed on the general wards, early referral to the intensive care unit is recommended to ensure vasopressors can be initiated early.

3 GCSF is a glycoprotein that stimulates the bone marrow to produce granulocytes. This is often used in neutropenic patients to try to improve their neutrophil counts more quickly than they would themselves. Those who have experienced neutropenic sepsis post chemotherapy may be prescribed GCSF prophylactically during their next cycle of chemotherapy to reduce the likelihood of neutropenia occurring.

4 Mouthwashes can provide pain relief and reduce inflammation. Many sites use Difflam or aspirin mouthwashes with morphine.

5 Analgesia for patients with head and neck cancer requires a multimodal approach. For mucositis-related pain, morphine-based or lignocaine mouthwashes may aid in local pain relief.

6 Severe mucositis and neutropenic sepsis are significant complications of chemotherapy and radiotherapy. These complications unfortunately lead to a break in the patient's treatment regimen and potentially this results in dose reductions so that they can continue treatment. It is important to ensure they receive adequate treatment for their cancer, but the treatments and their complications are potentially life-threatening, so there is a fine balance, which is different for each patient.

7 Nutrition for patients with head and neck cancer is often a challenge, as the tumour or the surgery will usually distort the oropharynx and so affect their ability to eat and drink. The treatments can cause significant complications, such as mucositis, which can also affect their nutritional intake. Some patients are unable to continue to eat normally, and require either a nasogastric tube, or in those in whom nutrition will be a long-term problem a PEG can be inserted.

8 As with all cancers the MDT meeting is an integral part of head and neck cancer management, as it brings all different specialists together to determine the best treatment for each patient.

9 The site and stage of a patient's disease will determine the extent of their surgical intervention. The surgical interventions required are varied, given the wide variety of head and neck cancer sites and spread. The surgery will involve removal of the primary tumour, and will often involve neck dissection to remove any spread to the surrounding lymphatics. A large part of head and neck surgery will be reconstruction following initial treatment. The site of head and neck tumours means their treatment can affect not just someone's physical appearances but also their functions, e.g. swallowing and talking. Therefore the goal of surgical intervention in these patients is not just removal of the cancer, but achieving an acceptable reconstruction of the patient's functional status and physical appearance.

10 Chemotherapy is often used as an adjuvant treatment in head and neck cancers, with radiotherapy and surgery being the primary treatments. The stage of the disease will determine whether chemotherapy is required. Studies have shown that chemotherapy improves outcomes when given with radiotherapy instead of separately, and so they will usually be given together. Common chemotherapy agents used in head and neck cancer include cisplatin and cetuximab; however, many other agents may be used.

11 Patients will receive radiation therapy for their cancer, which may be alone if their cancer is localised, or in conjunction with surgery and chemotherapy if it is more advanced. Radiation therapy may also be used for the neck if there is concern the cancer may have spread there. If the tumour is large, radiation therapy may be given to shrink the cancer prior to surgery.

12 Complications of head and neck cancer treatment can be significant. Surgery may alter physical features and function, while the adverse effects of radiotherapy or chemotherapy can be severe, e.g. mucositis, function alteration, dysphagia, fatigue and airway oedema. Delayed toxicity can have an effect on quality of life. Long-term effects of chemoradiation, such as severe dysphagia, osteoradionecrosis, aspiration pneumonia or radiation fibrosis, are related to radiation dose.

13 Palliative management is sometimes the only option for those with advanced disease. This may include surgery, chemotherapy and radiotherapy as well as symptomatic treatments.

14 Surveillance is an essential part of patient care after potentially curative treatment. Patients should have post treatment imaging so that a baseline is available for follow-up. They should be aware of what symptoms to be concerned about (hoarseness, pain, dysphagia, bleeding, lymph nodes) and who to call if these occur. Recurrence is more common in the first 2–4 years following diagnosis, and so follow-up is quite intense initially, involving review every 1–3 months for the first year and decreasing gradually until 5 years after treatment where reviews are often annual.
The important aspects of review are to assess for any late complications (such as hypothyroidism from radiation), any evidence of recurrence or any new cancers. The patient should be encouraged to cease smoking/alcohol consumption if necessary and given any ongoing rehabilitation if needed. Dental complications, dry mouth (xerostomia), osteoradionecrosis, trismus, dysphagia and chronic pain are common long-term complications that need to be followed up and addressed. Specialist follow-up is required in patients who had a laryngectomy or have long-term feeding tubes *in situ*.

15 Prognosis depends on the stage at presentation and the site of the tumour. For those with stage I or II disease, prognosis is excellent, with a 5-year survival of 70–90%; however, for those who present with more advanced disease the prognosis is poorer. Patients with oropharyngeal HPV-associated cancers have a better prognosis than those without; however, their management is currently the same. In those patients with cancers related to tobacco and alcohol use, the risk of a second malignancy is significant, with almost a 20% risk over 5 years.

CASE 64: Hepatocellular carcinoma

History

- A **60-year-old**[1] **man**[2] with a history of **cirrhosis**[3] secondary to **hepatitis B**[4] and excess **alcohol intake**[5], presents feeling generally unwell with **right upper quadrant pain**[6], **weight loss**[7], **diarrhoea**[8] and **increasing ascites**[9].

- He does not attend his routine **follow-up appointments**[10] or take his **regular medications**[11], and unfortunately, he continues to **drink alcohol**[12].
- He has had frequent similar presentations with **decompensated liver disease**[13].

1 Hepatocellular carcinoma (HCC), a primary liver tumour, is more common as people get older, with the peak incidence occurring between ages of 70 and 75 years. However, younger people can also be affected, specifically those with viral hepatitis, who often present with HCC in their 5th and 6th decades. The incidence of HCC in developing countries is also more than double that found in developed countries.

2 HCC is the fourth most common cause of cancer-related deaths in the world. It is much more frequently diagnosed in men than women, possibly due to a combination of increased exposure to environmental toxins, hepatitis carrier states and the potential effects of androgens and oestrogens on cancer cells.

3 Most patients who develop HCC have known chronic liver disease or cirrhosis. There are many risk factors for the development of HCC, most importantly hepatitis B infection, hepatitis C infection, hereditary haemochromatosis and cirrhosis of any cause. This includes patients who develop cirrhosis from non-alcoholic fatty liver disease (NAFLD), which usually develops in the setting of type 2 diabetes, obesity and dyslipidaemia. Given the obesity epidemic in the western world, there is concern that the threat of HCC is going to increase due to an increased incidence of NAFLD and subsequent cirrhosis.

4 Chronic hepatitis B infection is a significant risk factor for developing HCC, with HCC developing even in some patients with chronic hepatitis B infection without cirrhosis. In those with hepatitis B a higher viral load is associated with increased rates of HCC, and although treatment of hepatitis B shows a reduced incidence of HCC, their risk is still higher than that of the general population. Hepatitis C is also a strong risk factor for HCC, accounting for nearly a third of HCC cases, usually in those with advanced fibrosis or cirrhosis. As with hepatitis B, treatment has been shown to reduce the incidence of HCC, but patients remain at higher risk than the general population.

5 Excessive alcohol use is not uncommon in the community, but it is important to realise that alcohol-related liver diseases are not necessarily only present in those considered to be 'alcoholics'. The combination of significant alcohol intake together with hepatitis B infection can significantly increase a patient's chances of developing HCC.

6 Right upper quadrant pain can indicate many different pathologies; however, in a patient with known chronic liver disease or cirrhosis, it raises the possibility of decompensation of their liver disease.

7 Weight loss in any patient is a concerning symptom and can indicate a variety of problems. This can be even more difficult to discern in patients with liver disease as they can frequently be malnourished because of their symptoms and/ or their lifestyles.

8 Patients with HCC may also present with symptoms such as diarrhoea, the mechanism of which is unclear, but potentially due to secretion of peptides such as vasoactive intestinal peptide and gastrin, which can result in significant electrolyte disturbances. Other clinical features associated with HCC include hypoglycaemia (due to tumour metabolic needs, sometimes due to insulin-like growth factor II secretion), erythrocytosis (erythropoietin secretion) and hypercalcaemia (bony metastasis or parathyroid hormone-related protein).

9 Increasing ascites is a sign of decompensated liver disease, which can be caused by a variety of factors such as infections, malignancies and alcohol intake. Ascites should be treated, and patients should undergo investigations to find the underlying cause for the liver decompensation. Especially in those with previously stable cirrhosis, decompensation may be due to extension of the HCC into the liver vasculature.

10 Due to the increased risk of HCC in those with chronic liver disease and cirrhosis, cancer surveillance is recommended for those in high risk groups.

11 Patients with chronic liver disease may be prescribed multiple medications including different diuretics to manage their ascites, such as furosemide and spironolactone. It is important to determine their medication list and their compliance, as this may change their disease management.

12 In those with alcoholic liver disease and/or cirrhosis, continuing to drink alcohol can cause decompensation of their disease. If patients have not yet developed cirrhosis but continue to drink alcohol, this may cause progression to cirrhosis. Often these patients do not have access to the support they need to help them abstain from alcohol, so it is important to find out what is available in your hospital's area and put patients in contact with drug and alcohol teams each time they present to hospital, to help them reduce their intake.

13 Patients with chronic liver disease and/or cirrhosis may present frequently with decompensated disease, especially if they continue to drink alcohol. However, decompensation can also be a sign of HCC. In fact, prior to routine cancer screening of at-risk patients, they would often be diagnosed with HCC at an advanced stage due to presenting with decompensated liver disease, which is often a late sign.

Examination

- He looks unwell; he is **cachectic** [1], **pale** [2] and **jaundiced** [3].
- His observations show a **tachycardia, borderline low blood pressure** [4] with a **low grade fever** [5] and **mildly raised respiratory rate** [6]; saturations are normal.
- **Spider naevi** are noted over his **superior vena cava distribution** [7], he has **asterixis** [8] and is tremulous.
- He has a clearly **distended and tense abdomen** [9] which is tender generally but significantly worse in the **right upper quadrant** [10].
- The **liver is not palpable** [11] and there is evidence of **shifting dullness** [12].
- **Rectal examination** [13] reveals loose stool only, and a normal-feeling prostate. Chest and cardiovascular examinations are normal.

1 Cachexia is the significant loss of weight and muscle that occurs in chronic diseases such as cancer. Patients with liver disease, especially those who consume significant amounts of alcohol, can become very malnourished due to both their poor diet and inability to absorb or utilise nutrients.

2 Anaemia in chronic disease is common; however, in those with significant liver disease a concerning cause of anaemia is GI blood loss. This can be caused by a significant haemorrhage from oesophageal varices, which can be life-threatening.

3 Jaundice is a yellow colouring of the skin and mucous membranes, and reflects raised bilirubin in the bloodstream. It occurs in liver disease when the liver is no longer able to metabolise bilirubin as normal. Bilirubin can be low, normal or raised in patients with cirrhosis.

4 Patients may be seen to have a lower baseline blood pressure than usual; however, a patient who is tachycardic with a low blood pressure should alert you to the fact they may be in shock.

5 A fever can have many different causes, but the underlying cancer and infection are the important ones to consider here. Patients with liver disease are susceptible to infections, and this can cause their liver disease to decompensate. It is important when working these patients up for infection that an ascitic fluid sample is taken and sent for pathogen testing.

6 A raised respiratory rate can indicate many things including pain, fever, infection and compensation mechanisms, and should be investigated further.

7 The terms spider naevi or spider angiomata describe a vascular lesion usually found on the trunk, face and arms that consists of a central arteriole with surrounding smaller vessels that spread out like a spider's web. The cause is not fully understood but is thought to be due to changes in sex hormone metabolism. They can be seen in pregnancy as well as liver disease; however, the number and size of spider naevi are generally proportional to liver disease severity. Potentially those with many large lesions are at an increased risk of variceal bleeds.

8 Asterixis is a flapping of the hands that occurs when the wrists are extended. This can occur in several encephalopathies but most commonly is associated with hepatic encephalopathy. Hepatic encephalopathy occurs because of an increase in nitrogenous waste due to the liver's inability to metabolise it. Specifically, there is a build-up of ammonia which can cross the blood–brain barrier and cause encephalopathy via absorption and metabolism within astrocytes in the brain. Hepatic encephalopathy is graded in severity from 0 (no obvious changes) through to 4 (coma). A tremor is different from asterixis, and many patients may be tremulous without having hepatic encephalopathy. A tremor in a patient who is alcohol-dependent may indicate alcohol withdrawal.

9 A distended abdomen can have many potential causes, but in this patient a distended and tense abdomen most likely indicates significant ascites. However, a mass or bowel obstruction should also be considered.

10 Generalised tenderness in a patient with ascites should make you consider spontaneous bacterial peritonitis, especially if the patient has a fever. The worsening pain in the right upper quadrant is concerning for hepatic pathology such as a mass.

11 In cirrhosis the liver is often small and craggy, and so will commonly not be palpable, especially in a patient with significant ascites. However, a patient's liver may be enlarged in the presence of a mass due to HCC.

12 Shifting dullness is a manoeuvre used to determine the presence of ascites on examination. An air–fluid level is found via percussion and then found to 'shift' when a patient moves, thus indicating the movement of fluid in the abdomen.

13 Rectal examination should be carried out in a patient with liver disease who looks pale and with a change in bowel habit, to ascertain for any evidence of melaena or PR bleeding.

Investigations

- This patient has cirrhosis with decompensated liver disease, so investigations are directed toward finding the **underlying cause for the decompensation** [1].
- A **full blood count** [2] shows a low haemoglobin, borderline low WCC and low platelets.
- Renal function shows an **acute kidney injury** [3] with mild hyponatraemia and hypokalaemia; other electrolytes are normal.
- Liver function shows **raised bilirubin, transaminases and low albumin** [4].
- Coagulation studies show a **raised INR** [5], but **glucose** [6] is normal.
- An **alpha-fetoprotein** [7] level is also raised.
- A full septic screen is sent including urine, stool and ascitic fluid to assess for **spontaneous bacterial peritonitis** [8]. He is not significantly distressed by his ascites and so an ascitic drain is not inserted at this time.
- A **Doppler ultrasound** [9] of his abdomen to assess for the cause of his decompensation shows a **2cm liver lesion** [10].
- For patients who are high risk for developing HCC, diagnosis can be made with dynamic contrast imaging such as **CT or MRI** [11] specific for liver assessment.
- In patients who are not high risk, although the same lesions would be suspicious for HCC, a **biopsy** [12] is required for formal diagnosis and histology.
- Once the diagnosis of HCC is confirmed, **staging** [13] needs to occur to plan appropriate management.

1 There are many causes for decompensated liver disease and each time a patient presents with decompensation, they need to be investigated and a cause found. Common causes can include infections, ongoing alcohol use, variceal bleeding and the development of HCC.

2 A full blood count should be taken in all patients who present unwell to hospital. Patients with liver disease may have a chronic anaemia; however, a low haemoglobin should alert you to potential bleeding, either from varices or other sources. A low WCC may represent infection. Many patients with liver disease have thrombocytopenia (low platelets), and a platelet count of <100 000/μL often corresponds with significant splenomegaly and portal hypertension.

3 Acute kidney injury may be due to dehydration from his diarrhoea. However, given his underlying liver disease and new decompensation, hepatorenal syndrome also needs to be considered. Electrolyte abnormalities are common in these patients; often they are hyponatraemic. This is often multifactorial but in those with cirrhosis and ascites, hyponatraemia can be a marker of advanced disease.

Any patient with significant hyponatraemia should have a formal work-up with paired serum and urine sodium and osmolalities to determine the cause of hyponatraemia and thus appropriate treatment. Hypokalaemia may be a result of diarrhoea, or in some patients this can be a consequence of diuretics (e.g. furosemide). Other electrolytes, such as calcium and phosphate, should also be measured, as some patients with HCC can have hypercalcaemia. Many patients with liver disease are malnourished and so may have a low baseline phosphate level and will be at risk of refeeding syndrome, hence phosphate should be measured frequently whilst in hospital.

4 Elevated liver enzymes reflect liver damage and can be caused by ongoing active hepatitis, alcohol use or other causes. Albumin is synthesised in the liver, and so a low albumin in liver disease represents synthetic dysfunction and is a poor prognostic sign. The Child–Pugh system determines the severity of liver disease using five clinical measures: serum bilirubin, albumin, prothrombin time (or INR) and the presence/absence of ascites and hepatic encephalopathy.

Depending on the severity of the abnormality a score of 1–3 is given for each category, with high scores meaning more severe disease. From this score a Child–Pugh classification is assigned from A–C, from which 1- and 2-year mortality can be predicted. The patient's underlying Child–Pugh score is important as it determines who may be eligible for certain treatments.

5 Patients with liver disease have complex issues with their coagulation, and are both coagulopathic and prothrombotic. A raised INR indicates an inability of the liver to synthesise clotting factors and reflects synthetic dysfunction of the liver. However, unless a patient is actively bleeding or undergoing a large procedure, this coagulopathy often does not need to be reversed.

6 Glucose should be measured for all patients with liver disease because if they are hypoglycaemic it may represent end-stage liver disease (the liver no longer has any glycogen stores), and it can be a clinical feature of HCC, as discussed above.

7 Alpha-fetoprotein (AFP) should be measured at baseline for patients with liver disease and checked frequently (e.g. 6-monthly) according to cancer surveillance guidelines. A level of >400ng/ml is often considered diagnostic of HCC in conjunction with imaging.

8 An ascitic tap or paracentesis is an important aspect of the septic work-up in patients with liver disease. It is important the ascitic tap is carried out prior to antibiotics being commenced. Samples of the ascitic fluid should be sent to microbiology (aerobic and anaerobic cultures, cell count and differential), biochemistry (albumin, protein, glucose, lactate dehydrogenase and amylase) and cytology. A polymorphonuclear cell count of >250cells/mm³, or positive cultures, reflects a positive tap and a diagnosis of spontaneous bacterial peritonitis (SBP) can be made. A serum-ascites albumin gradient can also be calculated and can indirectly measure portal pressures.

9 A Doppler ultrasound of the liver should be organised in all patients who present with decompensated liver disease, to assess for evidence of cirrhosis and lesions such as HCC and to assess blood flow, including any evidence of thrombus.

10 HCC can be identified on ultrasound and generally appear as smooth-edged round lesions with a range of echogenicity. However, for surgical planning and sometimes diagnosis, cross-sectional imaging is required.

11 HCC can be diagnosed with imaging alone in high risk patients, using adequate contrast-enhanced cross-sectional imaging such as triple-phase CT or MRI. To diagnose HCC with imaging alone the Liver Imaging Reporting and Data System (LI-RADS) is used. This is a way of characterising liver lesions in high risk patients (i.e. those with cirrhosis, chronic hepatitis B infection, current or prior HCC diagnosis). The scoring system ranges from LR-1 (benign) to LR-5 (definitely HCC) and LR-M (malignant but not necessarily HCC), LR-NC (unable to characterise) and LR-TIV (tumour in vein). For each category, the next steps are suggested, such as MDT meeting, frequency of surveillance, or biopsy.

12 Some can be diagnosed with HCC using imaging, so an invasive biopsy is not required. However, in non-high risk groups, or in high risk patients in which imaging is not conclusive, a biopsy may be required to determine the diagnosis. Liver biopsy carries significant risks such as spread of the tumour along the needle track, bleeding (which can be significant), hypotension and pneumothorax. These risks should be taken into account when determining the need for a biopsy. The histology of HCC can range from well differentiated to poorly differentiated lesions, with large tumours often having central necrosis.

13 The difficulty in staging for HCC is that the traditional TNM classification takes into account tumour size and spread, but not underlying liver disease, whereas Child–Pugh scores can predict perioperative survival based on the severity of liver disease but the system does not incorporate any information regarding the tumour. The commonly used systems are TNM, the Okuda and Barcelona Clinic Liver Cancer (BCLC) system and the Cancer of the Liver Italian Program (CLIP). A combination of these staging systems may be used. The BCLC system can be useful in deciding potential treatments and incorporates liver function, radiographic findings and performance status in its assessment and classifies patients into four stages (A–D); early, intermediate, advanced and terminal.

Management

Immediate

Immediate management should involve **stabilising the patient** [1] with treatment such as fluids (depending on the cause of hyponatraemia), electrolyte replacement and antibiotics for presumed infection, whilst determining there is no evidence of bleeding. For symptomatic relief of ascites some patients may require an **ascitic drain** [2], as well as analgesia.

Short-term

Prompt investigations as above and discussion at the **MDT meeting** [3] to determine the next steps in management.

Medium- and long-term

The mainstay of treatment for hepatocellular carcinomas are surgical treatments either with **transplantation** [4] or **surgical resection** [5]. Unfortunately, <40% of patients are candidates for surgery due to the extent of the tumour or the severity of their liver disease, and the supply of liver transplants is limited.

Other treatment options include **locoregional therapies** [6] such as embolisation, radiation and ablation, and systemic treatments such as **chemotherapy** [7] and **molecular therapies** [8]. In those who present with **recurrence** [9], treatments will depend

on the same issues as above and will often include the same therapies. High recurrence rates means **surveillance** [10] for these patients is very important. In patients with advanced disease, **palliative care** [11] interventions should be considered. **Prognosis** [12] is dependent on the stage of disease at presentation, with outcomes worsening as the patient progresses from stage A to D of the BCLC staging system.

1 Initial management should involve stabilising the patient and treating any acutely life-threatening conditions whilst investigating the patient for their underlying cancer. In hyponatraemic patients it is important to determine the cause of the hyponatraemia prior to administering fluids, as increased volume can further worsen hyponatraemia, which can be very dangerous.

2 For patients with a significant volume of ascites an ascitic drain can be inserted to drain off fluid to provide short-term symptomatic relief. It is important these drains are inserted by trained staff and that appropriate monitoring and replacement of fluid with albumin is organised.

3 Due to these patients having underlying liver disease and sometimes complex social issues, a multidisciplinary approach is imperative to make the difficult management decisions. This meeting should include hepatologists, hepatobiliary and transplant surgeons, oncologists, interventional radiologists and palliative care teams. This ensures appropriate management is organised in a timely fashion.

4 Liver transplantation is the only curative option for those whose HCC is not resectable. To assess which patients are eligible for liver transplantation the Milan criteria are used. These state that eligible patients will have a solitary HCC ≤5cm or *alternatively* have up to 3 separate lesions, all smaller than 3cm, have no evidence of gross vascular invasion and no regional nodal or distant metastases. Of course, factors such as severity of liver disease or portal hypertension will also affect eligibility for liver transplantation.

5 In those with potentially resectable disease and adequate underlying liver function (Child–Pugh A), a partial hepatectomy can be curative. However, this is only for a small group of patients with solitary lesions, no evidence of invasion and reasonable liver function.

6 Those who are unable to undergo resection or transplantation may benefit from ablation therapies. These can improve mortality, but also may downstage their tumours, thus allowing curative surgical intervention. Common interventions include:
- transcatheter arterial chemoembolisation – this procedure delivers high doses of chemotherapy (e.g.

doxorubicin, cisplatin) to the tumour by cannulating the feeding artery of the tumour. This allows delivery of chemotherapy to the tumour without significant systemic toxicity. This is, however, contraindicated in those with advanced cirrhosis as it can lead to significant decompensation and sometimes death.
- radiofrequency ablation – a needle is inserted into the tumour under ultrasound or CT guidance and a rapidly alternating current is delivered, which generates heat at the tumour site which leads to cell destruction.
- brachytherapy (or radioembolisation) – uses local delivery of radioactive yttrium to the tumour which causes tumour necrosis.

7 For those in whom locoregional therapies have ceased to work, systemic therapy is an option if their performance status and underlying liver disease allow it. However, HCC does not respond well to systemic chemotherapy, with doxorubicin regimes having the best outcomes but still having minimal effect on survival.

8 Molecular targeted therapy has been shown to improve survival rates compared with best supportive care. Some examples include sorafenib and lenvatinib; however, other agents are being assessed and used. Sorafenib is a multi-targeted tyrosine kinase inhibitor that inhibits the vascular endothelial growth factor receptor (VEGFR) and Raf kinase. Lenvatinib is an inhibitor of VEGFR-1, -2 and -3 and fibroblast growth factor receptors (FGFR) 1–4. Side-effects of these agents include hypertension, renal complications, thromboembolism, bleeding and cardiotoxicity.

9 Unfortunately, following liver resection many (up to 75%) patients will develop intrahepatic recurrence by 5 years. Risk factors for recurrence include advanced tumour grade, unclear margins, vascular invasion, the presence of cirrhosis, very high pre-operative AFP and AST levels, hepatitis C and large transfusion requirements intra-operatively. In these patients a personalised treatment plan will be discussed based on both tumour and patient characteristics.

10 Screening high risk patients for the development of HCC should include 6-monthly imaging +/– serum AFP measurements to diagnose HCC early when it is resectable. Post HCC diagnosis and treatment, surveillance is important given the high rates of recurrence. Those who have undergone resection still have a cirrhotic liver and thus are still at significant risk. For the first 2–3 years, 3–6-monthly imaging and AFP measurements are recommended.

11 For those patients in whom resection and transplantation are not possible (Child–Pugh C), many other treatments have the potential to worsen their hepatic decompensation and so treatment focuses on symptomatic management including pain control, management of their oedema and ascites (using spironolactone and furosemide) and their encephalopathy.

12 HCC is an aggressive tumour, and unfortunately is often diagnosed at a late stage. Prognosis is dependent on the stage of the disease and the extent of underlying liver dysfunction. Four important prognostic indicators are: severity of underlying liver disease, size of the tumour, extension of tumour into nearby structures and evidence of metastasis. In those with resectable disease or those who receive a liver transplant, overall survival rates can be excellent (5-year survival >80%); however, in those presenting with advanced disease, treatment options are limited and median survival is less than 4 months.

CASE 65: Melanoma

History

- A **28-year-old** [1] **man** [2] with **fair skin** [3] and a history of **severe sunburn as a child** [4] presents with increasing 'clumsiness' [5] and **new headaches** [6].
- His headaches are **worse in the mornings** and are associated with **nausea and sometimes vomiting** [7]. He has also noticed recently that his headaches are worse on bending down to tie his shoelaces.
- He has no past medical history of note but has always had **many moles** [8].
- His **father** has a past history of **skin cancer** [9], but he is unsure what kind.

[1] Melanoma incidence peaks in the seventh and eighth decades of life, and while the incidence of melanoma is lower in young and middle-aged adults, it is still one of the most diagnosed cancers among young adults.

[2] Men are more likely to be diagnosed with melanoma than women. However, in the <40-year-old age group, melanoma is more commonly diagnosed in women, possibly because of the widespread use of indoor tanning (solariums) by young women. After the age of 40, men are more susceptible to melanoma.

[3] Melanoma is the most serious and fatal form of skin cancer and the annual incidence is rising by around 5% per year, particularly in regions that have fair-skinned populations (e.g. North America, northern Europe, Australia and New Zealand). Melanoma is much more common in people with fair skin, especially those with freckles; however, Asian and dark-skinned people are still at risk.

[4] Ultraviolet (UV) radiation is the most significant risk factor for the development of the majority of melanomas. Both ultraviolet A (UVA) and ultraviolet B (UVB) are implicated, and it is thought to induce melanoma through a combination of free radical production, damage to melanocyte DNA and inhibition of the skin's immune system. However, the amount of sun exposure is not directly related to melanoma development – it is the acute, severe and intermittently blistering sunburns that pose the highest risk factor for melanoma. Parkinson's disease also increases the risk of melanoma four times above that of the general population. There are also other risk factors such as immunosuppression and certain syndromes, e.g. familial atypical mole-melanoma syndrome and xeroderma pigmentosum.

[5] 'Clumsiness' is a non-specific symptom. However, it is concerning for anyone to develop new 'clumsiness', especially young patients, and further exploration during history and examination should help determine the cause.

[6] Headaches are a very common complaint and can be caused by a myriad medical problems ranging from the benign to the very concerning. There are many aspects of the headache history that allow you to try to further determine what the cause of a patient's headache may be, including time of day, frequency, where the headache is, associated symptoms, severity, etc. Sometimes patients may need specialist input at dedicated headache clinics. However, all doctors need to be able to detect concerning features such as those that may indicate raised intracranial pressure (ICP).

[7] Headaches due to raised ICP are classically worse in the mornings, or on bending down/sneezing/coughing (i.e. further increasing your ICP). These headaches can be associated with nausea and vomiting, and sometimes a patient's vision can be blurry. Other symptoms depend on the cause of the raised ICP: too much cerebrospinal fluid, a space-occupying lesion, bleeding or swelling in the brain.

[8] Melanomas can develop either in or near a precursor lesion or in healthy skin (*de novo*). Common precursor lesions include: common acquired naevus, dysplastic naevus, congenital naevus and cellular blue naevus.

[9] A family history of melanoma is a risk factor for melanoma; in fact, ~10% of patients with melanoma have a family history. Those patients with a family history are more likely to develop melanomas at a younger age, and can have multiple primary lesions.

Examination

- On examination the patient looks well but is noted to have an **abnormal gait** [1], and appears unsteady and uncoordinated on walking into the room.
- His observations are within normal limits. Neurological examination reveals **ataxia** [2], particularly on his right side, with **past pointing** [3] and **dysdiadochokinesis** [4].
- Cranial nerve exam shows **papilloedema on fundoscopy** [5] and nystagmus on looking to the right.

- **Skin examination** [6] reveals a lesion on his back that is **very dark, asymmetrical, ~7mm in diameter** [7] and appears to have bled recently.
- A full **lymph node examination** [8] is carried out but no abnormal nodes are identified.
- His cardiovascular, chest and abdominal examination are **normal** [9].

[1] Assessment of gait is useful as it can give you a clue as to the potential pathologies involved in someone's presentation. There are eight basic gait abnormalities that can be attributed to certain neurological conditions: hemiplegic, spastic diplegic, parkinsonian, choreiform, neuropathic, myopathic, sensory and ataxic (cerebellar). The gait described above is a classical description of an ataxic gait.

[2] Ataxia is a lack of voluntary coordination of muscle movements, and is due to damage or dysfunction of parts of the nervous system that coordinate movement – specifically the cerebellum.

[3] Past pointing is a sign that can be elicited in patients who are suffering from dysmetria (the inability to place and position a limb correctly). It is seen during finger–nose testing in which a patient will sequentially touch their nose and then either your finger or a target at arm's length in front of them. This is a cerebellar sign, and most frequently patients with limb dysmetria will have an ipsilateral cerebellar hemisphere lesion.

[4] Dysdiadochokinesis is seen in cerebellar disease and refers to the fragmentation of rapid alternating muscle movements. It is also seen on the ipsilateral side to the lesion. Cerebellar signs include dysdiadochokinesis and dysmetria, ataxia, nystagmus (can be in both directions but usually maximal towards the side of the lesion), intention tremor, slurred speech and hypotonia (useful mnemonic: DANISH).

[5] In anyone whom you are concerned may have raised ICP, a full neurological assessment should be carried out including a cranial nerve exam. Fundoscopy can be difficult to perform but it is important to be able to determine if a patient has papilloedema. Papilloedema is swelling of the optic disc, caused by raised ICP of any cause. It can occur over a period of hours to weeks and is usually bilateral. Findings with an ophthalmoscope include venous engorgement, haemorrhages over/next to the optic disc, blurring of the optic margins and elevation of the optic disc. Patients may have an enlarged blind spot on assessment.

[6] A full body skin examination should be carried out in anyone in whom you are concerned may have melanoma and in those in whom monitoring of lesions is being carried out. A full skin assessment should occur each time and serial photography should be used as an aid. When performing a skin examination the patient should be fully disrobed and a well-lit room should be used.

[7] Abnormal lesions should be assessed using a dermatoscope by those who are trained in its use. Differentiating benign naevi from atypical lesions/melanomas can be difficult. The ABCDE system can be useful:
- **A**symmetry (melanomas are often asymmetrical)
- **B**order irregularity (melanomas usually have irregular borders)
- **C**olour (moles often have uniform colour and are lighter; melanomas are often seen to be black or blue, and sometimes have variations in colour)
- **D**iameter (lesions <6mm in diameter are often benign)
- **E**volution (a change in a lesion or development of a new lesion, especially in those over 40).

[8] A full lymph node examination should be included in the assessment of all patients with melanoma, as it can spread via both lymphatic and haematogenous spread and so both regional and distal nodes can be involved.

[9] A full examination should be carried out, as melanoma can metastasise to the lymph nodes, lungs, liver, bones and brain in particular.

Investigations

- This young man has features concerning for raised ICP and so needs urgent admission to hospital for investigation and management of this.
- **Baseline bloods** [1] (full blood count, renal and liver function) are normal and serum **lactate dehydrogenase level (LDH)** [2] is raised.
- An urgent **CT brain** [3] shows a **right-sided cerebellar lesion** with **surrounding oedema** [4].
- A **chest radiograph** [5] shows no abnormality.
- The lesion on his back is removed with an **excisional biopsy** [6] to assess **histology** [7] and **Breslow thickness** [8].
- In those with advanced melanoma *BRAF* **gene testing** [9] should be carried out. No other lesions are found.

- **Staging** [10] is determined by a combination of the Breslow thickness and evidence of spread using imaging techniques.
- **A sentinel lymph node biopsy** [11] assesses for potential regional lymphatic spread.
- In those presenting with likely distant metastatic disease, a **CT chest and abdomen** [12] should be organised. In those with earlier stage disease this may not be indicated.
- **Positron emission tomography (PET) scans** [13] may be indicated in those with known node involvement, for staging purposes.
- An **MRI brain** [14] should be organised for patients with metastatic disease.

1 Baseline bloods should be performed for all patients who present unwell to hospital. In those with a new melanoma diagnosis, a raised white cell count may indicate an inflammatory response, deranged liver function may indicate liver metastasis and baseline renal function is needed for guiding the next steps in investigation and treatment.

2 Lactate dehydrogenase (LDH) can be elevated in many disease processes. A raised LDH is not specific for melanoma; however, if it is significantly raised on presentation it can indicate metastasis. It can also be useful in monitoring response and follow-up in patients. A raised LDH is now used as part of the staging system for melanoma and is a marker of poor prognosis.

3 An urgent CT brain is indicated for anyone presenting with symptoms of raised intracranial pressure or new neurological signs. A plain CT brain is quick and will show any gross abnormalities; if it is negative and there are still ongoing concerns an MRI can be organised.

4 A space-occupying lesion not only causes raised ICP because of its size but also due to the surrounding oedema. This mass effect can sometimes be improved with the use of steroids in the first instance.

5 A chest X-ray is often organised for all patients presenting with melanoma, although unlikely to have metastases in stage I or II disease. Those with more advanced disease should have a CXR and a CT chest to assess for lung metastases.

6 A complete excisional biopsy should be obtained with a 1–3mm margin of normal skin, and should take in all layers including some subcutaneous fat. If a melanoma is diagnosed re-excision should be performed with specific margins depending on the thickness of the melanoma. Failure to

perform re-excision after biopsy increases the rates of recurrence significantly and so it should always be carried out.

7 The four major subtypes of invasive cutaneous melanoma are: superficial spreading, nodular melanoma, lentigo maligna and acral lentiginous; however, other types are seen such as amelanocytic melanoma. Histopathological diagnosis is based on a combination of features – the presence of atypical melanocytes and architectural disorder are needed for diagnosis. Immunohistochemistry is not needed for diagnosis but is often carried out to ensure complete assessment; S-100 and homatropine methylbromide (HMB45) are positive in melanoma.

8 The Breslow thickness is the thickness in millimetres between the upper layer of the epidermis and the deepest point of the tumour. The thicker the melanoma, the poorer the prognosis.

9 The *BRAF* gene codes for the B-raf protein that is involved with tumour cell growth. Up to 50% of patients with melanoma have a BRAF mutation; knowing the BRAF status allows us to determine which patients will benefit from targeted cancer therapy.

10 Staging for melanoma is performed using the TNM system. In melanoma the tumour 'T' is determined by the thickness of the melanoma and any evidence of ulceration, and ranges from T0 (no evidence of primary tumour) to T4b (>4mm thickness with ulceration). The node 'N' is determined by the presence of nodal disease (including microsatellites, satellites, and in-transit metastases (cutaneous or subcutaneous)) and ranges from N0 (no evidence of nodal disease) to N3c (≥2 clinically occult or detected nodes and/or presence of any matted nodes with presence of in-transit, satellite or microsatellite metastasis). The metastasis 'M' is categorised into M0 (no evidence of distant metastasis) or M1a–d, detailing different sites of distant metastasis, with M1d being distant metastasis to the central nervous system. An elevated LDH level is incorporated into the M scoring system. From the TNM classification patients are divided into different prognostic stage groups:

- Stage I & II include tumours with no nodal or distant metastatic spread.
- Stage III are tumours with nodal but no distant metastatic spread.
- Stage IV are all tumours which have distant metastatic spread.

11 Some patients may have clinically enlarged lymph nodes, and these should undergo a complete lymph node dissection. However, some patients have no clinical evidence of lymphatic spread. To assess for this, a sentinel node biopsy can be performed where the first node into which the tumour's lymphatics drain is assessed for evidence of spread.

12 In all patients with known distal metastasis a CT chest and abdomen should be organised to assess for any evidence of asymptomatic metastasis. The lungs are often the first place to which melanoma metastasises.

13 PET scans are not used in patients with early disease; however, they may be of use in detecting metastatic disease in those with known nodal involvement.

14 An MRI brain should be carried out in those without known metastatic disease and neurological symptoms, but also in all patients with known metastatic disease as it may detect asymptomatic metastatic brain lesions.

Management

Immediate

Immediate management should include investigations as above and management to control the patient's **raised ICP** [1]. Following discussion with the relevant teams, **steroids** [2] may be initiated.

Short-term

Investigations for staging should be organised and a **melanoma MDT meeting** [3] should be held to determine the next appropriate steps for management. Often psychological support will be arranged for patients.

Medium- and long-term

The management of patients with melanoma is based on the stage of their disease. The treatment for those presenting with Stage 0 disease will just involve **excision** [4]. Those with Stage I and II disease will undergo excision plus potentially **lymph node management** [5] which can involve complete lymph node dissection. Patients with Stage III resectable disease will undergo excision, lymph node dissection and if indicated, **adjuvant therapy** [6] such as **immunotherapy** [7]. Those with unresectable Stage III, Stage IV and recurrent melanoma will be treated with a myriad therapies including **surgical metastasectomy** [8], **targeted therapies** [9], **intralesional therapy** [10], **chemotherapy** [11] and **palliative local therapies** [12] (e.g. radiotherapy). **Prognosis** [13], as with all cancers, is dependent on the stage at presentation. However, with the recent discovery of immunotherapies and targeted therapies, outcomes for patients with advanced melanomas have significantly improved.

1 Patients with raised ICP should be investigated and if a lesion is found, it should be discussed with the neurosurgical team as well as oncology teams. In those with acutely symptomatic brain metastases or with a single lesion, neurosurgical management may be used to improve symptoms and control the disease locally.

2 As a short-term measure, steroids can be given to reduce the ICP resulting from space-occupying lesions and surrounding oedema.

3 As with all cancers the MDT is integral to the appropriate and timely management of patients with melanoma.

4 Most cases of malignant melanoma are diagnosed at an early stage, and so surgical excision is curative.

5 For patients in whom a sentinel node biopsy has returned positive, complete lymph node dissection is recommended as it achieves good regional disease control and has been shown to reduce recurrence rates.

6 Adjuvant therapies are therapies used alongside surgery to treat or contain disease. This can include chemotherapies, radiotherapy and immunotherapies.

7 Immunotherapy has significantly improved the outcomes for patients with metastatic melanoma, now allowing them to live for months to years following their diagnosis. Patients may have a delayed response with initial worsening of their disease prior to the treatment working. Checkpoint inhibition with anti-programmed cell death 1 (PD1) antibodies are used (pembrolizumab and nivolumab) and have shown to have better response rates and progression-free survival when used with anti-cytotoxic T-lymphocyte-associated protein 4 (CTLA-4) antibody ipilimumab. Survival data suggests that up to 50% of patients receiving these treatments will be alive three years later. However, as with all treatments these therapies have significant side-effects, including autoimmune adverse effects.

8 Surgical metastasectomy is the surgical excision of metastatic disease. It is used in metastatic melanoma for those with one or a limited number of metastases and has especially shown benefits in those patients with brain metastasis.

9 Almost half of melanomas have a mutation in the *BRAF* gene. This is important because BRAF as well as MEK (downstream) causes tumourgenesis via activating the mitogen-activated protein kinase pathway (MAPK). Thus, inhibition of these can lead to tumour regression; a combination of BRAF inhibitors and MEK inhibitors together have been shown to improve response rates and survival. Examples of BRAF inhibitors include vemurafenib, dabrafenib and encorafenib. The two MEK inhibitors for melanoma are trametinib and binimetinib. Common combinations used are dabrafenib with trametinib and encorafenib with binimetinib.

10 Intralesional therapy is used for melanomas that cannot be removed surgically or have spread to lymph nodes or skin.

It is a form of immunotherapy that is injected directly into the melanoma, called talimogene laherparepvec (T-Vec). This therapy may affect tumours nearby also.

11 Radiotherapy is an important part of metastatic melanoma management, especially in the management of brain metastases, with stereotactic radiosurgery being used for those patients with multiple lesions rather than whole brain radiotherapy. It can reduce symptoms and improve patients' quality of life.

12 Chemotherapy agents used in melanoma (dacarbazine, temozolomide, carboplatin/paclitaxel) have shown very poor response rates, with median responses of 4–6 months only. Thus chemotherapy is only used as a last resort for patients who have progressed through other treatments.

13 Those presenting with localised disease have excellent outcomes (5-year survival ~98%), compared to those with distant disease (5-year survival <25%). Superficial spreading and nodular type melanomas have a worse prognosis than other melanomas. Poor prognostic factors including greater Breslow thickness, mitotic index, the presence of ulceration and bleeding, higher number of affected lymph nodes, evidence of distant metastases and an elevated LDH. However, significant improvements in prognosis for these patients have occurred in the last decade, and research is ongoing.

CASE 66: Pancreatic carcinoma

History

- A **65-year-old** [1] **female** [2] is referred from her GP with **jaundice** [3].
- She complains of **mild epigastric pain** [4] that intermittently **radiates to her back** [5] and has noticed she **feels fuller in her abdomen** [6] in the past few **weeks** [7].

- This has been associated with a **loss of appetite** [8], **weight loss** [9] and **severe itchiness** [10].
- She has a past medical history of **chronic pancreatitis** [11] from alcohol use and was diagnosed with **type 2 diabetes last year** [12].

[1] Increasing age is a non-modifiable risk factor for developing pancreatic cancer. The average age at the time of diagnosis of pancreatic cancer is 71. However, those who have chronic pancreatitis or a family history of pancreatic cancer may develop pancreatic cancer earlier.

[2] The incidence of pancreatic cancer is slightly higher in men than women. Pancreatic cancer is the 12th most common cancer worldwide, but it is the 7th leading cause of cancer death, with the 5-year survival being only 9%. Unfortunately, the incidence rates of pancreatic cancer have been increasing steadily over the last few decades.

[3] 'Painless obstructive jaundice' is the presenting feature most commonly associated with pancreatic cancer. Around two-thirds of pancreatic cancers are localised to the pancreatic head; in these patients jaundice and weight loss are more common. Jaundice in these patients is caused by obstruction of the common bile duct by the pancreatic mass. Unfortunately, initial symptoms are very non-specific, such as fatigue and nausea, which contributes to the difficulty in diagnosing and late presentation of this disease.

[4] Pain is a very common presenting feature of pancreatic cancer and can be seen even with small tumours. Pain often presents in an insidious manner but can become very severe and unrelenting, often found to be worse at night.

[5] Patients will sometimes develop pain that radiates to the back, which is often a bad sign as it may indicate that the tumour is invading the retroperitoneal space and involving the splanchnic nerve plexus.

[6] As pancreatic cancer progresses patients may develop palpable masses from the tumour or metastasis, and also may develop ascites which can cause distension and further discomfort. Pancreatic cancer most commonly metastasises to the liver, peritoneum, lungs and sometimes the bone.

[7] The progression of pancreatic cancer is often insidious, with gradual onset of pain and other symptoms so that by the time a patient presents, the symptoms may have been going on and building for weeks to months.

[8] Weakness, anorexia, weight loss and abdominal pain are the most common presenting symptoms in patients with pancreatic cancer (seen in 80% of patients).

[9] Significant weight loss is a characteristic feature of pancreatic cancer. There are many mechanisms through which this may occur but it is thought to be due to a combination of cancer-associated anorexia and malabsorption plus potential gastric outlet obstruction from the mass in some patients. Due to pancreatic exocrine insufficiency caused by the cancer from pancreatic duct obstruction, patients can develop malabsorption. These patients often have diarrhoea and 'greasy' stools.

[10] Pruritus can often be the most distressing symptom for patients, and is associated with obstructive jaundice, sometimes occurring prior to clinical evidence of jaundice. Depression is also noted to be more common in patients with pancreatic cancer, with a significantly higher rate of suicide being seen in these patients.

[11] Risk factors for pancreatic cancer are tobacco smoking (being linked to 30% of pancreatic cancer cases), diabetes mellitus, pancreatitis, obesity and a family history of pancreatic cancer. Chronic pancreatitis is a significant risk factor in the development of pancreatic cancer, especially in those with hereditary pancreatitis; however, alcohol-induced pancreatitis has also been associated with higher rates and earlier age of diagnosis of pancreatic cancer. Only a small proportion of pancreatic cancers are familial.

12 The relationship between diabetes mellitus and pancreatic cancer is complex and not fully understood. There is an increased risk of pancreatic cancer developing in patients who have had diabetes mellitus for at least 5 years. However, in those patients who develop diabetes mellitus within 2 years of pancreatic cancer diagnosis it is thought that this is caused by the pancreatic cancer. There is difficulty in determining who will benefit from screening following their diabetes diagnosis.

Examination

- On examination the patient is **cachectic** [1] and in **pain** [2] with **jaundice** [3] which is obvious from the end of the bed.
- Her observations show a **mild tachycardia** and **low grade fever** [4]; everything else is within normal limits.
- She has **excoriations** [5] across her skin, and you note a palpable **left clavicular lymph node** [6].
- Abdominal examination finds a **distended abdomen** [7], with a **mass felt in the right upper quadrant** [8].
- You notice a **nodule around her umbilicus** [9].
- Cardiovascular and respiratory examination is normal.

1 Significant weight loss is commonly seen in pancreatic cancer and is caused by a combination of factors, including anorexia and malabsorption, as discussed above.

2 The pain associated with pancreatic cancer can be severe and unrelenting, significantly affecting a patient's quality of life. Almost all patients with pancreatic cancer will experience pain, unfortunately. However, at presentation some may have no pain.

3 Patients who develop painless obstructive jaundice may seek medical attention at an earlier stage. Associated with the jaundice will be dark-coloured urine and light stools, which patients will often notice before the jaundice itself. For jaundice to be clinically noticeable the bilirubin level is usually 2–3 times the upper limit of normal.

4 Tachycardia and low grade fevers can be caused by the underlying disease process in combination with pain, or potentially a superimposed infection which should always be considered.

5 Pruritus can precede clinical jaundice, and can be a very distressing symptom for patients. Palliative care teams have many ways of trying to manage this, including emollients, but often management of the biliary obstruction is the only way in which symptoms will improve.

6 The finding of an enlarged Virchow's node (left supraclavicular lymph nodes) is called Troisier's sign and is an indication of metastatic disease from an abdominal organ. These nodes are the sentinel nodes for many intra-abdominal cancers, as they drain the lymphatics from the abdominal cavity. This is a sign of advanced and thus incurable disease.

7 A distended abdomen in this lady could have multiple causes, including a large mass or development of ascites, both of which are poor prognostic signs. Ascites develops in advanced disease where the cancer has metastasised to the liver.

8 A right upper quadrant mass in those with jaundice may represent a palpable primary tumour or metastasis, or may be evidence of a palpable gall bladder. 'Courvoisier's law' states that a palpable enlarged gall bladder which is non-tender and associated with painless jaundice is *unlikely* to be gallstones, i.e. it should raise suspicion of a malignant cause.

9 'Sister Mary Joseph nodules' are bulging palpable nodules around the umbilicus which are a result of intra-abdominal or pelvic metastasis, with GI malignancies accounting for ~50% of such nodules. These indicate metastatic and advanced disease.

Investigations

- A **full blood count** [1] shows a mild normochromic anaemia and thrombocytosis.
- **Renal function and electrolytes** [2] were normal but **liver function tests** [3] showed a significantly raised bilirubin, ALP and GGT, with mildly raised AST and ALT, as well as a low albumin.
- A **lipase** [4] is sent to assess for acute pancreatitis, and it is raised.
- A **carbohydrate antigen 19-9 (CA19-9)** [5] is also significantly raised.
- An **abdominal ultrasound** [6] shows a dilated biliary tree with a 3cm head of pancreas mass.

- Following this a **CT scan** [7] of the chest, abdomen and pelvis is organised to allow further assessment and **staging** [8]. If the CT provides enough information about the pancreatic cancer and the patient is fit for an operation, biopsy may not be needed prior to surgery.
- If **histology** [9] is required preoperatively, an **endoscopic ultrasound (EUS)-guided or percutaneous biopsy** [10] of the mass can be obtained.
- If there is concern there may be choledocholithiasis, an **ERCP** [11] or **MRCP** [12] may be organised to further assess and/or intervene if indicated.

1 Laboratory findings may be non-specific; the full blood count may be normal or may show a normochromic anaemia of chronic disease. In some cancers a thrombocytosis is seen.

2 Baseline renal function is important to ascertain, as the next steps in investigation and treatment may be affected by this. Many patients with pancreatic cancer will be malnourished, and so it is important to get baseline and repeated electrolytes so that patients can be monitored and treated for refeeding syndrome.

3 Liver function tests in pancreatic cancer will often show an obstructive picture if obstructive jaundice is present (raised bilirubin, ALP and GGT); however, transaminases may be mildly raised also. If a patient has liver metastasis then the transaminases along with the ALP may be more significantly raised. As previously discussed, these patients will often be malnourished, thus a low albumin is common.

4 If there is concern of acute pancreatitis (acute epigastric pain) a lipase and/or amylase should be sent. This can be difficult to interpret in patients with chronic pancreatitis as it may be chronically high or low. Amylase and lipase have also been shown to be raised in some patients with pancreatic cancer. Some patients with pancreatic cancer present with acute pancreatitis, hence in elderly patients with new acute pancreatitis, cancer should be a consideration.

5 CA19-9 is a sialylated oligosaccharide that is normally present within the biliary tract but is found in cancer patients on circulating mucins. It has been shown to be strongly associated with pancreatic cancer and is positive in >80% of pancreatic cancer patients. CA19-9 also appears to be an indicator of cancer stage – those with higher CA19-9 levels often have unresectable and metastatic disease. Hence it can be used as a useful marker to detect response in patients undergoing chemo-/radiotherapies. Carcinoembryonic antigen (CEA) is also raised in ~40% of pancreatic cancer patients, but it is not sensitive or specific for pancreatic cancer.

6 Initial imaging for patients presenting with right upper quadrant pain and jaundice is often an ultrasound. Ultrasound can identify biliary tract dilation and pancreatic masses if they are >3cm in size. Unfortunately, it is not reliable at picking up masses smaller than 3cm, and often the pancreas can be obscured by overlying gas and so may not be reliable.

7 A CT scan allows further assessment of any lesions and assessment of local invasion/metastasis to allow for staging. A triple-phase, helical multi-detector row CT has the highest sensitivity for detecting pancreatic cancer. Typical findings are of an ill-defined hypo-attenuating pancreatic mass. In patients in whom surgical resection is possible, work-up for surgery can commence, instead of obtaining preoperative biopsies.

8 Pancreatic cancers are classified as resectable, unresectable or borderline resectable. Only ~20% of patients have resectable tumours. Accurate preoperative staging is important, as partial resection/non-curative surgeries have not been shown to have any survival benefit.
Pancreatic cancer is staged using the TNM staging system. The 'T' or tumour grade ranges from Tis–T4, with Tis being carcinoma *in situ*, T0 being no evidence of primary tumour, T1/T2 indicating increasing tumour size and T3 indicating extension of the tumour beyond the pancreas. T4 specifies that the tumour involves the coeliac axis or the superior mesenteric arteries. The 'N' or node indicates whether there is any regional lymph node metastasis (N0 or N1) and 'M' or metastasis describes any evidence of distant metastasis (M0 or M1). Patients can then be grouped into stages which allows prediction of prognosis, with stage 0 being carcinoma *in situ* and stage IV representing those with metastatic spread.

9 For a formal diagnosis of pancreatic cancer to be made, a histological diagnosis is required. In patients where resection is possible this may be obtained following removal of the tumour in surgery, whereas in others a biopsy is obtained via endoscopic ultrasound (EUS), percutaneous biopsy or ERCP. A preoperative biopsy is necessary when surgery is not possible and in patients with a diagnosis or suspected diagnosis of chronic or autoimmune pancreatitis. Most pancreatic tumours arise from the exocrine pancreas, with only 5% originating from the endocrine pancreas. Of these the majority are adenocarcinomas (80%) of the ductal epithelium, which generally have a poor prognosis, except colloid carcinomas.

10 A biopsy is generally via fine needle aspiration (FNA) of a lesion using either imaging (CT or US)-guided percutaneous biopsy or with an EUS-guided biopsy. EUS is the best method for obtaining a tissue sample and removes the theoretical risk with percutaneous biopsies that the tumour may seed along the needle path. This involves placing an ultrasound transducer on the end of an endoscope allowing visualisation of the head, body and tail of the pancreas. This allows full assessment of the size and characteristics of a tumour whilst being able to gain tissue samples via FNA.

11 Endoscopic retrograde cholangiopancreatography (ERCP) is used to visualise the biliary tree and pancreatic ducts, and is able to provide intervention at the same time. However, it is not recommended as an initial investigation or for histological diagnosis of pancreatic cancer, as some areas may be missed and it has a lower rate of diagnosis than with EUS. ERCP can be used to provide intervention for those who present with or develop biliary obstruction and require stenting to relieve symptoms. This should be carried out following CT imaging as it can distort the images and make diagnosis more difficult.

12 Magnetic resonance cholangiopancreatography (MRCP) is an alternative to diagnostic ERCP and provides a three-dimensional image of the pancreaticobiliary tree.

Management

Immediate

Immediate management should involve **pain relief** [1] and medication to **alleviate the patient's pruritus** [2] whilst investigations are ongoing. Once imaging has occurred she will likely benefit from **stenting to relieve her biliary obstruction** [3].

Short-term

The above investigations should be completed and a discussion at the **pancreatic multidisciplinary meeting** [4] should be organised. Some patients who have resectable disease on imaging may undergo a **staging laparoscopy** [5].

Medium- and long-term

For those patients with resectable disease, curative **surgery** [6] is the mainstay in management. This may be in addition to **neoadjuvant** [7] **or adjuvant therapies** [8]. Postoperative **surveillance** [9] is essential, as recurrence is common. For those with unresectable or advanced disease, treatment options include **chemotherapy** [10], **local ablation therapies** [11] and early involvement of **palliative care** [12], depending on the stage of their disease. The **prognosis** [13] for pancreatic cancer is very poor, even in those with resectable disease. Research is ongoing to find specific molecular targets that may aid management in the future.

1 Pain is a significant issue in patients with pancreatic cancer, hence initial management should include the use of simple analgesia and opiates if required. Many patients may have significant pain and early involvement of the palliative care team is essential in appropriately managing these patients' pain.

2 Pruritus can be the most significant and distressing symptom for a lot of patients with pancreatic cancer, and can even precede clinical jaundice. It can often be difficult to manage, but emollients, paroxetine and mirtazapine have been shown to help.

3 In certain patients stenting of their biliary obstruction using ERCP may be possible as a palliative measure to help relieve their symptoms. If stenting is not possible some patients may undergo a percutaneous transhepatic cholangiography to allow biliary drainage and decompression. A biliary drain is placed through the site of the malignant biliary obstruction to the duodenum; initially this will have an external drainage component but usually attempts are made to internalise it. This has also been shown to improve patient comfort if ERCP has failed.

4 As with all cancers, an integral part of pancreatic cancer management is the MDT meeting including hepatobiliary surgeons, oncologists and palliative care physicians, to ensure timely diagnosis and management for these patients.

5 Although current imaging techniques allow us to accurately diagnose unresectable disease, because they are unable to detect small volume metastasis they are not always accurate at diagnosing resectable disease. Up to one-third of patients who undergo laparotomy are found to have unresectable disease in the abdomen. To try to avoid this unnecessary surgery some centres and surgeons advocate for staging laparotomies to fully assess the abdomen prior to surgery.

6 Surgical resection is the only cure for pancreatic cancer. Those who are eligible for surgery are those with no metastasis and no evidence of tumour involvement in the mesenteric vasculature. Surgical candidates also need to have few comorbidities and a good performance status preoperatively. A pancreaticoduodenectomy (Whipple procedure) is a well-known surgical procedure for pancreatic cancer; however, many patients will have slightly modified surgeries, depending on their tumour.

7 The role of neoadjuvant therapy is unclear, but it may be beneficial in those with potentially resectable disease. The most common regimen used is FOLFIRINOX (leucovorin/5-fluorouracil plus oxaliplatin plus irinotecan) followed by radiotherapy.

8 All patients should be offered six months of adjuvant chemotherapy which should be started within 8 weeks of surgery. Common regimes include FOLFIRINOX or gemcitabine plus radiotherapy in some centres.

9 Follow-up every 6 months at least for the first 2 years is advised for patients who have undergone potentially curative treatments. Follow-up should include taking a history, performing a clinical examination and serial CA19-9 measurements.

10 The choice of chemotherapy in advanced pancreatic cancers is dependent on their *BRCA* and *PALB2* (partner and localiser of *BRCA2* gene) status, as it has been found that those with these mutations are more sensitive to platinum-based chemotherapy treatments over gemcitabine (e.g.

FOLFIRINOX or FOLFOX regimes). In those without these mutations FOLFIRINOX or gemcitabine-based chemotherapy regimens are offered, based on performance status.

11 In some patients who have unresectable locally advanced pancreatic cancers, local ablative therapies with radiofrequency ablation or other modalities have been shown to provide pain relief and, in some, a small survival improvement.

12 Palliative care is an integral part of pancreatic cancer management. Pain can be a significant issue for patients and management with opiates and sometimes antidepressants can help. In some patients this will not be adequate and other treatments such as neurolysis of the coeliac ganglia and radiation therapy can improve their pain and quality of life.

13 The prognosis for patients with pancreatic cancer is unfortunately very poor, with the median survival being just 4–6 months; the 5-year survival for those with distant disease is just 3%. Even in those able to undergo a successful curative resection, the median survival is still only 12–19 months, with nodal involvement, resection margins and small tumours being the best predictors of long-term survival.

CASE 67: Prostate carcinoma

History

- A **65-year-old** [1] **man** [2] presents to hospital with **progressive bilateral leg weakness** [3], and recent onset of **inability to pass urine** [4] and a single episode of **faecal incontinence** [5].
- This is on the background of progressively **worsening back pain** [6] over the past **2 months** [7].

- Prior to this he has noticed intermittent **difficulty passing urine** and an episode of **haematuria** [8].
- He is otherwise generally well. Past medical history includes T2DM which is controlled by medications.

[1] Incidence of prostate cancer increases with age, being the highest in patients in their late 70s. The majority of prostate cancers are detected at an early stage, although some present with advanced disease. Age is the biggest risk factor for prostate cancer, with genetics seeming to play a role. However, there are no clear links between prostate cancer and any preventable risk factors.

[2] Prostate cancer is the most common cancer in males in the UK and accounts for a quarter of all new cancer diagnoses in men. Although it is the second most common cause of cancer-related death in men, the majority of men diagnosed with prostate cancer are expected to survive 10 years post diagnosis. The clinical behaviour of prostate cancer varies widely, ranging from microscopic well differentiated cancers to very aggressive, invasive cancers that can result in metastasis, morbidity and death.

[3] A serious pathology such as spinal cord compression should be considered in a patient presenting with progressive bilateral leg weakness. A thorough neurological examination, including determination of sensory levels, should be carried out to localise the site of the lesion.

[4] Inability to pass urine may indicate urinary retention, and this needs to be differentiated from oliguria. Whilst acute bladder outlet obstruction may cause suprapubic discomfort and pain, symptoms may be minimal in chronic urinary retention, including those due to neurological dysfunction or spinal cord compression. Bladder scan is a useful bedside tool in diagnosing urinary retention.

[5] The combination of leg weakness, urinary retention and faecal incontinence is concerning for spinal cord or cauda equina compression, which is a medical and surgical emergency and should be investigated and acted on quickly.

[6] 'Red flag symptoms' that can help differentiate benign musculoskeletal causes from more sinister conditions include:
- thoracic back pain
- age <20 or >55 years
- loss of control of bladder or bowel
- weakness or numbness in an arm or a leg
- foot drop/disturbed gait
- fevers
- saddle anaesthesia (numbness of the anus, perineum and genitals)
- history of cancer
- any clear structural abnormality.

[7] In the majority of cases, patients are asymptomatic and the diagnosis of prostate cancer is incidental. Routine screening blood tests are not recommended in asymptomatic patients. However, a subset of patients may often have progression of insidious symptoms over time.

[8] Symptoms of urinary frequency, urgency and haematuria can be caused by prostate cancer but are also commonly caused by benign prostatic hyperplasia (BPH), the incidence of which also increases as men get older. It is important to note that patients can have both BPH and prostate cancer at the same time, which given the similarity of the symptoms can be difficult to delineate.

Examination

- On examination the patient looks reasonably well but appears to be in **pain and is distressed** [1]. His observations are within normal limits.
- There are no obvious abnormalities on inspection of his back, but on palpation he has **significant spinal tenderness around L3** [2].
- Neurological examination of the lower limbs reveals a **lower motor neurone pattern of weakness** [3] with reduced tone and reflexes, bilateral weakness and **downgoing plantars** [4].

- Cranial nerve and upper limb **neurological examination** [5] is normal.
- On **rectal examination** [6] he has **reduced perianal sensation** [7] and **anal tone** [8], and a **large craggy prostate** [9] is felt.
- On abdominal exam he has a **distended and tender abdomen** [10], but it is soft and bowel sounds are present. Cardiovascular and respiratory exams are normal.

1 Metastatic bone pain may be the only presenting symptom in patients with prostate cancer. Vertebral column is the most common site of metastasis for prostate cancer, followed by liver and lung spread.

2 In anyone presenting with back pain, initial assessment should include assessment of gait if possible, inspection of the spine from the side and back and also palpation of each spinous process as well as paraspinally. A tender area over a vertebra is concerning for an underlying pathology such as a fracture.

3 Neurological assessment should ascertain the pattern of weakness, symmetry and associated sensory level to determine the site of lesion.
Upper motor neurone weakness (also known as 'pyramidal' pattern) is indicated by increased tone, weakness of the flexors in the legs and brisk reflexes with upgoing plantars (positive Babinski), and the patient may have a sensory level. This pattern of weakness occurs with spinal cord compression above L1–2 level where the spinal cord terminates (i.e. above the cauda). At or below this level, compression produces lower motor neurone pattern weakness.

4 When compression is below L1–2 level, this results in cauda equina syndrome with lower motor neurone pattern weakness presenting with flaccid tone and weakness in both legs, reduced or absent reflexes and absent plantars.

5 In patients presenting with abnormal neurology in one area of their body, a full neurological examination should be carried out to ensure that there are no other signs that may point to a different problem and potentially aid diagnosis.

6 In any patient presenting with signs concerning for spinal cord or cauda injury a rectal examination should be carried out to assess for perianal sensation as well as anal tone.

7 Perianal sensation is lost in cauda equina syndrome. This can be a difficult symptom for patients to describe – sometimes they may state they cannot feel when wiping after the toilet – but it should be found on examination. In cord compression, often perianal sensation is preserved.

8 Loss of anal sphincter tone is a late sign in cauda equina, but should be assessed with a rectal exam in all patients in whom spinal cord compression is a concern.

9 On rectal examination prostate nodules and asymmetry can be felt; however, only those cancers that are on the posterior and lateral aspects of the prostate gland can be detected via digital rectal examination as this is what is palpable via the rectum. A normal examination does not rule out prostate cancer.

10 There are many causes for a distended abdomen, but in a patient who has not passed urine for some days this may indicate urinary retention.

Investigations

This man has presented with likely cauda equina syndrome or spinal cord compression and needs to be investigated and managed immediately.

- A bladder scan reveals a 1.5L distended bladder. A urinary catheter is inserted and **urine microscopy** [1] is sent.

- Bloods are taken which show a **full blood count** [2] with mildly raised neutrophils.
- **Renal function** [3] is deranged with raised creatinine and urea, and **liver function** [4] shows raised alkaline phosphatase.
- **Electrolytes** [5] show raised calcium and **coagulation profile** [6] is sent.

- An urgent **MRI scan of the whole spine** [7] is organised and shows a **suspicious lesion** at L3 with an **underlying pathological fracture** that is causing **cauda equina compression** [8]. He is discussed urgently with the neurosurgical and the oncology teams.
- A **prostate-specific antigen (PSA)** [9] is added onto his bloods and is found to be significantly raised.

- A **prostate biopsy** [10] is organised to further investigate.
- This is carried out via a transrectal ultrasonography guided biopsy (TRUS). **Transperineal approach** [11] was also considered.
- Further **imaging studies** [12] are discussed to **stage** [13] the cancer.

1 Bladder scan is very useful in those patients who present with 'not passing urine' or 'difficulty passing urine' as it allows us to assess whether any urine is being produced, and also can help us determine if patients have partial outflow obstruction (i.e. with a post void residual). A urine microscopy should be sent for all patients presenting with urinary symptoms to assess for evidence of infection/haematuria, etc.

2 All patients should have a full blood count. A raised neutrophil count could reflect the underlying inflammatory process or potentially a concurrent urinary tract infection which may occur with chronically high residual urine volumes.

3 The most likely cause of acute kidney injury in this man is from post-renal obstruction. Hence with relief of obstruction, the kidney function is expected to improve.

4 LFTs may be abnormal, showing hypoalbuminaemia due to chronic disease, or deranged, due to metastasis. A solitarily raised alkaline phosphatase (ALP) with a raised calcium should alert the possibility of bone metastasis.

5 Electrolytes showing a raised calcium in this clinical picture are concerning for potential bony metastasis.

6 This man has presented with a surgical emergency (spinal cord compression) and may need urgent decompression. Organising appropriate bloods such as group and hold and coagulation profiles early on will help to ensure there are no delays.

7 In any patient with suspected spinal cord compression, a whole spine MRI should be organised, as metastatic disease can involve multiple levels.

8 Metastatic bony lesions can present in many different ways on an MRI scan, resulting in vertebral body destruction or pathological fractures or space-occupying lesions causing impingement of the cord or cauda equina.

9 Routine use of prostate-specific antigen as a screening test is not recommended in the general population level due to limitations with the test. However, in those with prostate cancer a higher PSA is associated with increased risk of more aggressive disease, and is also included in the disease staging system. It is also a useful way of monitoring treatment response and also for recurrence.

10 Adenocarcinoma accounts for the majority (>95%) of prostate malignancies. Other types include transitional cell carcinoma, carcinosarcoma, basal cell carcinomas and lymphomas; these are less common. During a prostate biopsy 10–12 core samples are taken; however, this only samples a small part of the prostate gland and so can miss and/or underestimate cancerous cells. A prostate biopsy allows calculation of Gleason score. The Gleason grade is based on the architectural features of the prostate cancer cells which have been shown to predict clinical behaviour. Based on degree of inflammation and growth pattern, tumours are graded from Grade 1–5, with 5 being the least differentiated (more likely to spread from the prostate). The Gleason score is calculated by adding together the number for the two most prevalent patterns seen in the core biopsies taken. The higher the score, the more likely it is that the tumour will not be confined to the prostate, and also indicates a worse outcome following localised disease treatment.

11 Transrectal ultrasonography (TRUS) is most commonly used to guide the prostate biopsy. However, this can be a very distressing and invasive procedure for men, and often multiple biopsies are required before a diagnosis is confirmed. Because of this a move towards transperineal prostate biopsy has occurred in the last few years. This is due to the advent of the PrecisionPoint Transperineal Access System which has allowed transperineal biopsies to be carried out under local anaesthetic and has shown reduced side-effects.

12 Depending on the initial staging and risk of distant disease some patients will undergo further investigation with imaging studies; this can include radionucleotide bone scans, CT abdo/pelvis or MRI. These imaging modalities are used to assess for any evidence of extraprostatic extension, distant metastasis or nodal spread. These are not recommended for those with very low risk and low risk disease; however, these patients may have an MRI prostate to ensure that higher grade disease is not present. In those with intermediate and high risk disease, bone and pelvic imaging plus sometimes abdominal imaging should be organised.

13 Once a diagnosis of prostate cancer has been made, the extent of staging investigations should be determined by the patient's age and life expectancy, and the clinical stage of the tumour.
The TNM staging system is used for prostate cancer.

Management

Immediate

Immediate management of the patient involves **catheterisation** [1] and urgent discussion with the oncology and **neurosurgical teams** [2]. **Steroids** [3] are initiated and **pain relief** [4] is given whilst a formal plan is made. The patient undergoes an urgent **decompression and fixation** [5] for cauda equina compression with associated pathological fracture. Further **radiotherapy** [6] is arranged to reduce the size of the lesion and provide symptomatic and pain relief.

Short-term

Urgent management as above followed by further investigations to determine the primary lesion and an **MDT discussion** [7] are organised.

Medium- and long-term

Management options for a localised prostate cancer include **active surveillance** [8], definitive local therapy with **radical prostatectomy** [9], **radiation therapy** and **brachytherapy** [10] and **hormone therapy** [11]. For metastatic prostate cancer in this patient, management is focused on **symptomatic relief** with involvement of the **palliative care team** [12] and attempting to **slow progression of the disease** [13]. **Prognosis** [14] and follow-up are further discussed with the patient.

---

[1] Urinary catheterisation relieves symptoms and prevents further obstructive damage to the kidneys.

[2] Any patient with spinal cord or cauda equina compression should be discussed urgently with the neurosurgical team for decompressive surgery to prevent further disability.

[3] Glucocorticoids are part of the initial management of metastatic spinal cord compression (MSCC) as a bridge to either further treatment or palliation. High dose dexamethasone should be given for those patients with neurological deficits or pain caused by MSCC. This can improve symptoms significantly if detected and treated early.

[4] The pain these patients experience can be significant; steroids may improve the pain but this can take time, hence management with opiates is often required.

[5] From clinical and MRI findings the neurosurgical team will be able to determine if the patient has any spinal instability. The patient may require a decompressive surgery for the cord compression and at the same time a surgical fixation to stabilise the spine.

[6] In patients without spinal instability, external beam radiotherapy can treat radiosensitive tumours leading to improvement in pain and symptoms. However, response to radiotherapy can take time and so in those with neurological compromise, surgical decompression should still be considered as a definitive management.

[7] An MDT approach is necessary to determine next steps in investigation and treatment for this patient with metastatic prostate cancer, based on his functional status, comorbidities, cancer stage and personal preferences. A patient-centred approach is discussed.

[8] In those with very low risk disease, active surveillance is often the preferred option.

[9] Radical prostatectomy involves removal of the prostate and the seminal vesicles as well as surrounding lymph nodes, if indicated. Radical prostatectomy is an option for those patients in whom there is localised low risk disease as well as those with locally advanced high risk disease; however, in those with more advanced disease extended lymph node dissection will often be carried out at the same time. Patients may undergo adjuvant or neoadjuvant therapies if they have more advanced disease in conjunction with radical prostatectomy.

[10] There are multiple forms of radiation therapy available. It can potentially cure localised prostate cancer and can be given either as external beam radiation therapy or via the insertion of radioactive seeds into the prostate gland (brachytherapy). Side-effects include proctitis and enteritis, impotence, urinary symptoms and incontinence.

[11] Androgen deprivation therapy (ADT) consists of either surgical castration (bilateral orchidectomy) or medical castration, both of which aim to reduce serum testosterone levels. Gonadotrophin-releasing hormone (GnRH) agonist (egg goserelin, leuprolide) suppresses luteinising hormone-releasing hormone (LHRH) production, and therefore reduces testicular androgen synthesis. However, there can be an initial surge in LHRH levels, hence anti-androgens (e.g. bicalutamide) are often given in conjunction. A GnRH antagonist (degarelix) works by binding to the GnRH receptors in the pituitary

gonadotrophin-producing cells, but does not cause this initial surge in LHRH.

ADT is associated with significant side-effects including loss of libido and erectile dysfunction, hot flushes and gynaecomastia as well as loss of lean body mass, fatigue and osteoporosis.

12 For those with advanced disease, involvement of the palliative care team from early on is beneficial to control symptoms, and if hospice care is needed, this can be organised swiftly.

13 Metastatic prostate cancer may be evidenced by a slowly increasing PSA or with overt metastasis. Treatment options are generally the same for these patients. Men may be offered either ADT alone; in those with high risk disseminated cancer this is often combined with docetaxel (chemotherapy agent) or abiraterone (anti-androgen), as this has been shown to improve survival. Some men may also be offered radiation therapy in conjunction with the systemic therapy outlined above.

14 The overall prognosis for prostate cancer is good, especially in those presenting with early stage disease. The 10-year survival for those diagnosed with prostate cancer is around 85%. The most important indicators for prognosis in prostate cancer are the Gleason grade, the extent of the tumour and evidence of capsular invasion at prostatectomy, with age at diagnosis and PSA levels also contributing. In those who have undergone curative treatment or who are having ongoing hormonal treatments, regular follow-up with PSA levels is important to detect evidence of early recurrence.

CASE 68: Pulmonary carcinoma

History

- A **75-year-old** [1] **man** [2] presents with a **3–4-month history** [3] of gradually worsening **increased shortness of breath** [4] and associated **weight loss** [5].
- He has developed a **change in his cough recently** [6], with some **streaks of blood** [7] in his sputum.
- He has a past medical history of **chronic obstructive pulmonary disease (COPD)** [8].

- He has smoked significantly in the past, with a **30 pack year smoking history** [9], and previously **worked in a shipyard** [10].
- He has noticed a significant **reduction in his exercise tolerance** [11], which has now dropped to only being able to mobilise for 10–15 metres before having to rest.

1 One of the biggest non-modifiable risk factors for lung cancer is age. Lung cancer mainly affects people as they get older, with most people being ~65 years of age or older at diagnosis. However, a very small number of people are diagnosed below the age of 45 years and so consideration must be given to this diagnosis if the history sounds suspicious.

2 Lung cancer (both small cell and non-small cell) is the second most common cancer in both men and women, with prostate cancer being more common in men and breast cancer being more common in women. However, lung cancer is the leading cause of cancer death in both men and women.

3 The presenting history for lung cancer is often insidious, unfortunately with no symptoms until the disease has progressed. Only a small percentage of cases are diagnosed in asymptomatic patients due to incidental findings during work-up for other problems. This unfortunately means that a significant proportion of patients have metastasis at presentation.

4 Shortness of breath along with haemoptysis and cough are the most common presenting symptoms for lung cancers, with shortness of breath being found in up to a quarter of all patients presenting with lung cancer. The signs and symptoms of lung cancer may be due to the primary tumour, local spread and distant metastatic disease or even from paraneoplastic syndromes leading to ectopic hormone spread.

5 Weight loss can be present in many disease processes and is seen in many cancer presentations. It can be due to both the underlying disease processes, or at a later stage due to the treatments we administer. It is felt to be multifactorial, due to a combination of reduced appetite and increased

energy requirements from the malignant process. It is a poor prognostic sign.

6 Cough is the most common presenting symptom of lung cancer, and can be caused by both endobronchial and pleural involvement of the cancer. Unfortunately cough is a very non-specific symptom, and patients with underlying lung disease often have a chronic cough anyway, thus a change in cough pattern must be considered to be suspicious. A new cough or change in a chronic cough that is persistent should raise suspicion of an underlying pathology and prompt referral for a chest radiograph for further investigation.

7 Haemoptysis is another common presenting symptom of lung cancer caused by the primary tumour. It can be a very concerning symptom and leads patients to present more promptly than other common presenting symptoms.

8 Patients with chronic lung pathology such as COPD can have chronic cough and also have weight loss associated with their COPD and so can blur the initial signs of lung cancer. However, in any patients with COPD a high index of suspicion should be had regarding lung cancer, given reported figures of up to 1% of patients with COPD going on to develop lung cancer.

9 Smoking has been shown to be the biggest risk factor for lung cancer. A large proportion of lung cancer cases are due to long-term tobacco smoking, with only 10–15% occurring in those who have never smoked. The majority of lung cancer deaths in both men and women are attributed to smoking. Therefore, lung cancer should always be suspected in a current or former smoker with new onset of cough or haemoptysis.

10 A percentage of lung cancers are, however, not associated with smoking. These are caused by a combination of genetic factors and exposure to different carcinogens or second-hand smoke (radon, air pollution, etc.), with passive smoking leading to an increased risk of lung cancer by 30%. Mesothelioma is a malignant tumour of the mesothelium caused by inhaled asbestos fibres which were used in shipping in the past. Although not technically a lung cancer it often presents in a similar way and in the same demographic of patients and so it is important to be aware of it and its risk factors.

11 Performance status is a way of scoring a patient's functional daily activities, including self-care and physical activity. The initial scoring system, the Karnofsky scale, used a scale from 0–100, with 100 representing normal activity and 0 occurring at death. This score was simplified to the Eastern Cooperative Oncology Group (ECOG) scores of 0–5, with 0 meaning fully active and 5 occurring at death. They are used to make a prognosis in cancer patients as well as to evaluate a patient's functional ability as a result of cancer treatment.

Examination

- The patient is **underweight** [1] and **dyspnoeic at rest** [2], with clear shortness of breath on walking from the waiting room.
- He has **clubbed fingernails** [3]; he is not **cyanosed** [4], but he does look pale and you find **conjunctival pallor** [5].
- You also note he has **drooping of his right eyelid** and on closer inspection he has a **smaller pupil on this side** [6].

- His observations are abnormal – he is **tachycardic at 105bpm, with borderline blood pressure (100/60mmHg), tachypnoeic and hypoxic at 90% with a low grade temperature** [7].
- Chest auscultation reveals a **monophonic wheeze** [8] on the right, with **decreased chest expansion and dull percussion note** [9] to the midzone on this side.
- You also find he has some **left-sided hip tenderness** [10] with reduced range of movement. No other abnormalities are found on examination.

1 Weight loss is a concerning presenting feature of lung cancer and often represents metastatic spread. Its cause is multifactorial but it is a poor prognostic sign.

2 Dyspnoea is one of the most common presenting symptoms in lung cancer. Unfortunately it is very non-specific and can be present in many different pathologies. Initial assessment needs to determine how bad a patient's dyspnoea is, and whether they require acute interventions to manage it.

3 Nail clubbing may occur in many pathologies including lung cancer. It is, however, not seen in COPD and so a patient with COPD and clubbing should be investigated for signs of bronchogenic carcinoma. A specific form of clubbing that is associated with lung cancer is hypertrophic pulmonary osteoarthropathy, which is the combination of clubbing and thickening of the periosteum and synovium, often initially diagnosed as arthritis. Clubbing has five different stages, ranging from no visible clubbing to gross clubbing in which there is thickening of the whole distal part of the finger, often referred to as 'drumstick'. Clubbed nails are mainly associated with non-small cell lung cancer, with <5% of small cell lung cancer patients having clubbed nails.

4 Lung cancer itself, or associated chest infections or pleural effusions, may cause hypoxia and subsequent cyanosis – this is concerning and an indication for admission for investigation, oxygen and treatment.

5 Conjunctival pallor indicates anaemia, which is a common finding in patients with chronic disease and cancers. It is multifactorial but may contribute to a patient's lethargy and fatigue.

6 Horner's syndrome (ipsilateral ptosis, anhidrosis and miosis) should prompt immediate concern regarding a Pancoast tumour. A Pancoast tumour is an apical lung tumour compressing on the sympathetic chain and causing the classical signs listed above. The majority of Pancoast tumours are non-small cell lung cancers.

7 Cardiovascular instability, specifically hypotension with sinus tachycardia, may represent concurrent sepsis; however, one should consider a potential malignant pericardial effusion causing tamponade. If this is a concern, an urgent echo should be arranged and immediate management initiated.

8 Bronchial obstruction may result in a monophonic wheeze due to compression. This can cause lung collapse post the obstruction.

9 Decreased air sounds and dullness to percussion is concerning for pleural effusion, which is most likely malignant in a patient with lung cancer. This should be sampled to determine whether it is a malignant effusion, and can also be used for diagnosis. Depending on the size of the effusion it may need to be drained for symptomatic relief.

10 Findings of bony pain are concerning in a patient with lung cancer as it may represent bony metastasis and should be promptly investigated with radiographs. It can cause significant pain and reduced mobility, which can be distressing to patients.

Investigations

Any patient with concerning clinical examination and observations should have investigations to determine diagnosis and next steps in treatment.

- Initial investigations include blood tests. **Full blood count** [1] shows this patient was anaemic with a raised white cell count.
- **Renal, liver and electrolytes** [2] as well as **coagulation** [3] were within normal range.
- An **arterial blood gas** [4] shows he is hypoxic, and hypocapnic due to tachypnoea.
- A **chest radiograph** [5] shows a right apical opacity 4 x 3cm and a right-sided pleural effusion, and a **left hip radiograph** [6] unfortunately reveals a lytic femoral head lesion.
- His **sputum** [7] is sent for microscopy and culture.
- Given the concerning clinical and radiographic features a **CT chest and upper abdomen** [8] is organised, which shows a large **spiculated right hilar mass** [9] with collapse/consolidation, and a right-sided pleural effusion with perihilar lymph nodes, but no metastatic spread is seen.
- **Pleural aspiration** [10] of the effusion is carried out for diagnostic and symptomatic relief, which reveals an **exudate** [11], but unfortunately is unable to provide cytological diagnosis.
- A **biopsy of the lesion** [12] is organised which shows an adenocarcinoma.
- Depending on the **stage of disease** [13] further imaging may be indicated. In cases where patients may be resection candidates a **PET scan** [14] is performed to determine any evidence of metastasis.
- In some cases, an **MRI of the brain** [15] will be organised if they are symptomatic or have high stage disease.
- If a patient's disease is felt to be resectable, **pulmonary function tests** [16] will be organised to determine their underlying lung function and ability to withstand an operation.

1 Blood tests in lung cancer may show a variety of abnormalities. Commonly, patients will be anaemic due to a variety of factors; this can exacerbate their shortness of breath and so, if indicated, a blood transfusion may be beneficial. Their white cells may be increased or decreased, as in this case – this can be due to either the underlying disease process or a concurrent infection which will need to be treated.

2 Renal and liver function tests should be carried out to assess for any abnormalities as well as for baseline measurements prior to interventions. Abnormal LFTs may reflect liver metastasis, for example, and most of these patients will have a low albumin due to their disease. Many patients as they get older have baseline abnormal renal function, so it is important to compare any results to previous available results. Given their reduced oral intake their renal function may show an acute kidney injury which can be managed with fluids. A lot of these patients are malnourished on presentation and so baseline and recurrent electrolytes are important to replace and monitor for refeeding syndrome.

3 Coagulation should be measured as most of these patients will require some form of intervention to get a diagnosis (pleural aspirate or biopsy of the lesion). Those with abnormal LFTs may have abnormal clotting due to this, so this is important to be aware of and treat if necessary.

4 Arterial blood gas (ABG) is a useful test in patients with respiratory distress, especially those with underlying lung pathology, as it helps us to determine if increased respiratory work is due to primary respiratory or metabolic cause (e.g. respiratory compensation); a patient's level of hypoxia; and whether a patient is a 'carbon dioxide retainer' in whom oxygen therapy should be carefully titrated.

5 A plain chest radiograph is the first-line imaging in any patient who has suspected lung pathology, as it is quick and will show gross abnormalities. It may show lesions in asymptomatic patients and thus bring them to attention. CXR can show where lesions are, and any potential associated collapse, consolidation or effusions. These features should prompt further investigation, e.g. with a CT scan.

6 A plain radiograph of a painful joint/bone is important in lung cancer as this painful joint/bone is concerning for possible metastatic spread +/− pathological fractures. These are important to identify as it changes staging and directs management towards surgical stabilisation of the bone, if indicated. Bony metastatic deposits are not always picked up on X-rays but it is an important starting point. In lung cancer bony mets are more commonly lytic lesions; however, they may be sclerotic, especially in small cell carcinomas.

7 In those with a productive cough, attempts should be made to get a sputum sample, especially if there is concern that the patient has a concurrent chest infection (which is not uncommon in lung cancer). If found or suspected, these patients should be treated for their lung infection.

8 All patients in whom lung cancer is a suspicion should undergo CT scanning of the chest and upper abdomen to assess the extent of the tumour to allow planning for biopsy +/– any metastatic spread, and to provide information for staging. The most common areas of metastasis for lung cancer are to the other lung, adrenal glands, bones, brain and liver.

9 Lesions with spiculated borders are highly suspicious for malignancy (due to malignant cells extending within pulmonary interstitial tissue). However, they are not diagnostic as a similar appearance may also represent being in infectious or inflammatory lesions.

10 A pleural aspirate is important for diagnosis when sent for cytological assessment as well as potentially for symptomatic relief. A diagnosis of lung cancer is made based on either cytological or histopathological (e.g. tissue) specimens.

11 Aspiration of pleural fluid is assessed initially using Light's criteria to determine if it is a transudate or exudate. Pleural fluid associated with lung cancer will show an exudative picture (pleural fluid protein/serum protein >0.5, pleural fluid LDH >⅔ x serum LDH upper limit of normal, pleural fluid LDH/serum LDH >0.6).

12 A biopsy of an appropriate lesion allows histological diagnosis of lung cancer. Non-small cell lung cancer (NSCLC) has four main histological subtypes: adenocarcinoma (most common), squamous carcinoma (~25%), adenosquamous carcinoma and large cell carcinoma (~10%). Although clinical and imaging features may suggest NSCLC rather than small cell lung cancer (SCLC), histological confirmation with a biopsy is required to make this formal distinction, including immunohistochemical staining. Lung cancer has been subclassified into these two major categories due to the difference in clinical features and different approaches to treatment and clinical outcomes. In general, SCLC tends to grow faster with more central/mediastinal growth and earlier metastasis. It has a shorter overall survival time. Based on the way the cancer cells look under a microscope, grading is used; this describes the appearance of the cells and gives an idea of how quickly or slowly the cancer may grow and the likelihood of spread. They are graded on a scale of 1–4, with 1 tending to be slower growing (low grade) and grade 3–4 cells looking very abnormal, with a tendency to grow quickly; they are more likely to spread (poorly differentiated or high grade).

13 The TNM staging system for lung cancer is used internationally to determine extent of disease. It can assist in treatment decisions and is a prognostic indicator. The 'T' is based on the primary tumour characteristics and ranges from T1–T4. It can be subdivided within these categories, from T1 – meaning the cancer is contained within the lung – through to T4 – in which either the tumour is very large (>7cm) or has spread to more than one lobe of the lung or into surrounding structures. The 'N' describes whether the cancer has spread to the lymph nodes and how far, with N0 meaning the lymph nodes do not contain cancer cells and progressive N numbers describing lymph node involvement further from the origin cancer. The 'M' describes whether the cancer has metastasised: M0 means no metastasis while M1 means metastasis and is split into three subtypes, depending on the type of spread.

A 4-stage system is sometimes used which correlates to the TNM classification. In this case, Stage I represents cancer that is only in the lungs and has not spread to any lymph nodes, Stage II is in the lung and nearby lymph nodes, Stage III is described as locally advanced disease and is when cancer has spread to the mediastinal lymph nodes (IIIA or B, whether on the same side as the tumour or opposite) and Stage IV is the most advanced stage, described as advanced disease, i.e. when the cancer has metastasised. Small cell carcinoma is usually staged and managed using a simplified version of clinical limited or clinical extensive disease; however, the TNM classification is useful for prognostication, with worsened survival for more advanced stages.

14 PET scanning is performed in patients who have no evidence of metastasis and so may be resection candidates – to ensure there are no distant metastases.

15 In patients who have symptoms of brain metastasis MRI of the brain with gadolinium will be organised to assess for this. Patients who are asymptomatic but have advanced clinical disease (stage III or IV) may also have this arranged to assess for metastasis.

16 Pulmonary function testing is a useful way of assessing how well a patient's respiratory system is working by assessing airflow, lung volumes and diffusion capacity. Such testing will often be carried out in patients with lung cancer to determine their suitability for treatments. If a patient's disease and their clinical state are felt to be fit for resection of their lung cancer, a work-up for surgery will take place. An important aspect of this is pulmonary function tests, as removal of part of the lung can impact their lung function, and so assessment to ensure their baseline function is good enough to allow for surgery is an important preoperative check.

Management

Immediate

Immediate management of any patient presenting to healthcare should be to stabilise the patient. In this case the patient is given **oxygen therapy** [1] for his hypoxia and commenced on **antibiotics for presumed chest infection** [2]. **Analgesia** [3] is given and initial investigations organised as above. **Discussion** [4] with the patient regarding next steps and concerns from the beginning is very important and allows them to be involved in their management.

Short-term

The above investigations should be organised in a timely manner and referral to the **lung MDT** [5] for discussion and next management steps should be organised. Once the patient has stabilised from their acute illness, treatment for the lung cancer needs to be considered.

Medium- and long-term

For patients with NSCLC initial management is mainly determined by the stage of the disease. **Surgical resection** [6] is the only curative management and is considered for those with early stage disease. Other modalities of treatment include **chemotherapy** [7], **radiotherapy** [8], **targeted therapies such as immunotherapy** [9] and other **non-surgical local therapies** [10]. Unfortunately for those patients presenting with advanced disease there are no curative options and so they are managed **palliatively with either systemic or local palliative treatments** [11]. For patients with SCLC their cancer is almost always disseminated at presentation and so **systemic chemotherapy** [12] is the mainstay of treatment. **Radiation therapy** [13] is often used in combination with chemotherapy to prolong survival.

Side-effects [14] are common with all of the treatments used to treat lung cancer and so it is important to be aware of the types of side-effects experienced and how to manage them.

Prognosis [15] of both NSCLC and SCLC is based on stage at presentation.

---

[1] Initial management should be to stabilise the patient if they have come in unwell or *in extremis*. Oxygen for hypoxia is a simple and important first-line intervention.

[2] As discussed previously, patients often present with concurrent infections, and these need to be treated promptly with antibiotics.

[3] Patients can often present with a significant amount of pain, and as their disease progresses this can intensify. It is important for their pain to be managed effectively from an early stage in their disease and this will involve multimodal approaches and therapies, ranging from simple analgesia to opiates and anaesthetic procedures such as nerve blocks if required.

[4] Open and serious discussions with patients and families from presentation through diagnosis and management are one of the most important interventions we can make. The way we discuss and explain these diagnoses to patients will determine their ongoing trust and interaction with their healthcare, so we must endeavour to be as open and caring as possible so that they can be as involved as they wish to be. This includes having discussions around the seriousness of their diagnosis and prognosis early on so they have time to plan and make decisions regarding end of life if that is the direction of their disease.

[5] MDTs for cancers include all of the healthcare professionals that will be involved in a patient's care, including surgeons, oncologists, pathologists, palliative care team members, clinical nurse specialists and many more. Patients are referred and their imaging/investigations to date are discussed and next steps planned. This may include more investigations or initiation of treatment – patients will be rediscussed each session until a clear plan is in place; they may be referred at any time for further discussion. It not only creates an opportunity for all specialties to get together to organise treatment but also ensures that timelines are being met and if not, a discussion and investigation as to why, so that all patients receive timely care.

[6] For those with early stage NSCLC, surgical resection offers the best opportunity for cure and long-term survival. Patients are assessed for surgical resection by determining the stage of their disease, their performance status and pulmonary function to allow prediction for postoperative function. A patient's cancer may be surgically resectable but if they are not fit enough for the procedure then they are unfortunately not an operable candidate. Patients with stage I or II NSCLC should be treated with complete surgical resection if possible.

7 Adjuvant chemotherapy has been shown to improve survival in patients with stage II disease, and may also have a role in those with stage IB.

8 Radiotherapy also plays an important role in both adjuvant treatment and palliative care.

9 NSCLC subsets for which targeted therapies exist include those with mutations in epidermal growth factor receptor (EGFR) and B-Raf proto-oncogene (*BRAF*), echinoderm microtubule-associated protein-like 4 (*EML4*) anaplastic lymphoma kinase (*ALK*) fusion oncogene and c-ROS oncogene 1 (*ROS1*) fusions. Those without driver mutations may benefit from a combination of chemotherapy and immunotherapy if they express a high level of programmed death ligand 1 (PD-L1), and immunotherapy is in fact available as first-line.

10 Radiofrequency ablation and cryoablation are alternatives to radiation, and photodynamic therapy may also be useful as a primary treatment in patients with superficial airway lesions. This allows for greater monitoring and self-management of their condition, and thus improved outcomes including pain, function and quality of life.

11 Palliative therapies can utilise chemotherapy or radiotherapy or a combination of both to manage symptom control from cancer, although the purpose of these systemic/local therapies is no longer with curative intent.

12 SCLC is a disseminated disease in most patients at presentation and is very responsive to chemotherapy; thus systemic chemotherapy is integral to treatment. Surgery is not used except in rare patients with solitary nodules. For those with extensive stage SCLC, chemotherapy is used as initial therapy with or without immunotherapy. Systemic chemotherapy is the mainstay treatment in SCLC.

13 For patients with limited stage SCLC, thoracic radiation is often used in combination with chemotherapy. Prophylactic cranial irradiation is also used to decrease brain metastasis and therefore prolong survival. Radiation of these areas may also be useful in those SCLC patients with complete or partial response to chemotherapy.

14 Side-effects from both curative and palliative treatments of lung cancer can affect quality of life significantly. Specifically, nausea and vomiting are common with chemotherapy; haematological toxicity (e.g. neutropenia and therefore increased risk of infection), nephrotoxicity (in cisplatin can be severe), neurotoxicity (cisplatin and taxanes), fatigue (from chemotherapy, radiotherapy or the cancer itself) and anorexia and weight loss are very common in lung cancer patients and may be due to either the disease itself or the treatment.

15 The TNM stage at presentation for NSCLC is the factor that has the largest impact on prognosis, with survival decreasing progressively with advancing disease. Poor performance status and weight loss have also been shown to be poor prognostic indicators. Overall the 5-year survival for NSCLC is ~15%; however, the 5-year survival of those who present with stage I resectable disease who undergo surgery is 70%, whereas those with extensive inoperable NSCLC have an average survival of 9 months. In SCLC the most important prognostic factor is the extent of disease at presentation; for those with limited stage disease median survival is 15–20 months, with 5-year survival at 10–13%. This compares with 8–13 months in extensive stage disease and 5-year survival 1–5%. Poor performance status and weight loss in NSCLC are poor prognostic indicators.

CASE 69: Renal cell carcinoma

History

- A **65-year-old** [1] **man** [2] presents with **flank pain** [3] and **haematuria** [4].
- He has noted **frequent headaches** [5] in the past few weeks and has been waking in the **night drenched in sweat** [6].
- He also reports a non-productive **cough** [7] for the same period.
- Recently, he has also noticed **lumps and heaviness in his left testicle** [8].
- He has a medical history of well controlled **hypertension** [9] and is a **current smoker** [10], and has worked in an **office all his life** [11].
- He is otherwise well and has **no personal or family history of cancers** [12].

[1] The incidence of renal cancer increases with age; the diagnosis is most common in those between 60 and 80 years old. The incidence of renal cancer has been seen to increase over the past few decades; however, improved survival rates may be due to lead-time bias from early detection. The 10-year survival for those diagnosed with renal cancer in the UK is 50%.

[2] Renal cell carcinoma (RCC) is nearly 50% more common in men than women, being the 10th most common cancer in women and 7th most common cancer in men in the UK.

[3] The classical triad of flank pain, haematuria and a flank mass is seen only in ~10% patients at presentation, and indicates advanced disease. Flank pain is a common presenting symptom, occurring in nearly half of those presenting with renal cell cancer. Around a third of all patients diagnosed with RCC are asymptomatic at presentation and are diagnosed via incidental findings on imaging studies.

[4] Haematuria is seen in ~40% patients presenting with RCC, and occurs once the tumour has invaded the collecting system. Other causes of haematuria from glomerular origin (e.g. glomerulonephritis) and non-glomerular origin (e.g. cystitis, bladder cancer, transitional cell cancer, renal stones and polycystic kidney disease) need to be considered as differential diagnoses.

[5] In patients with RCC, associated hypertension can cause headaches if untreated.

[6] Fever is seen frequently in patients with renal cell carcinoma, often with night sweats and weight loss. RCC can also cause a variety of other paraneoplastic syndromes via cytokine release or ectopic production of hormones (e.g. erythropoietin, parathyroid hormone-related protein (PTHrP), gonadotrophins, renin, glucagon and insulin). Specific paraneoplastic syndromes include Stauffer syndrome (hepatic dysfunction in the absence of metastasis due to cytokine production in the tumour – often associated with weight loss, fevers and poor prognosis), cachexia, erythrocytosis (erythropoietin), secondary amyloid A (AA) amyloidosis (chronic inflammatory response), thrombocytosis (poor prognosis) and polymyalgia rheumatica. Often with removal of the tumour many of these paraneoplastic syndromes will resolve, and recurrence of the symptoms may indicate recurrence of renal cell cancer.

[7] Around a third of patients with renal cell cancer present with metastatic disease; the most common site is lungs (75%), followed by soft tissues, liver and the brain.

[8] A varicocele is an abnormal enlargement of the veins within the scrotum (pampiniform venous plexus), and represents potential tumour obstruction of the gonadal vein on entering the renal vein. It is sometimes described as looking like a bag of worms. The majority are left-sided, as the right gonadal vein drains directly into inferior vena cava.

[9] Hypertension is a known risk factor for RCC, independent of obesity and use of anti-hypertension medications. Other known risk factors are obesity (having inverse relationship with disease stages), acquired polycystic disease (seen frequently in those undergoing dialysis long-term), prolonged use of analgesics (specifically aspirin and anti-inflammatory drugs), chronic hepatitis C, sickle cell disease, a history of kidney stones and prior use of chemotherapy.

[10] Cigarette smoking is a known risk factor for developing RCC, with heavier smokers often presenting with more advanced disease.

[11] Occupational exposure to certain compounds is also a risk factor for developing RCC; cadmium, asbestos and petroleum by-product exposure have shown increased risk.

[12] There is a potential genetic element in development of RCC; those who have had one RCC are at higher risk of developing a further, and several syndromes are associated with RCCs. In those with relatives who have had a tumour before age 40, genetic component should be suspected.

Renal cell carcinomas caused by hereditary syndromes make up <5% of all RCCs; these syndromes include hereditary papillary cell cancer, tuberous sclerosis, von Hippel–Lindau disease, hereditary leiomyomatosis RCC, Birt–Hogg–Dubé disease and hereditary paraganglionoma and phaeochromocytoma. Polycystic kidney disease is not thought to increase the risk of renal cell carcinoma.

Examination

- On examination the patient looks **pale** [1] with conjunctival pallor and appears **short of breath** [2] .
- Vital signs show **hypertension** [3] (170/90mmHg), but all other observations are within normal range.
- Chest auscultation reveals a few mid-zone **crepitations** [4] , without any pleural effusions.

Cardiovascular examination is normal.
- He has a **palpable left flank mass** [5] on abdominal examination, with an audible **bruit** [6] overlying the paraumbilical region.
- **Scrotal and testicular examination** [7] is carried out which finds a **left-sided varicocele** [8] .

[1] Anaemia is reported in a significant number of patients with renal cell carcinoma and can precede diagnosis by months, and is more often seen in those with advanced disease. In some cases, polycythaemia from excess erythropoietin production may be evident with facial plethora.

[2] Shortness of breath can be exacerbated by anaemia, but in a patient with concerning features for cancer, potential lung metastasis should be considered. Cancer-related chronic venous thromboembolic disease may also present with shortness of breath. Heart failure from underlying anaemia or untreated hypertension may also contribute to symptoms.

[3] Hypertension is both a risk factor for RCC, and can also be seen as a consequence of it, and should be managed appropriately.

[4] Crepitations on this man's chest could be due to changes because of his lifelong smoking; however, any positive finding should be investigated to assess for potential sinister causes such as lung metastasis. Other common sites of metastasis in RCC are bone, liver and brain, and any symptoms or signs within these systems should direct further investigation.

[5] Differentiate between a renal mass and an enlarged spleen on examination – a renal mass should be ballotable and have a palpable upper margin, whereas a spleen will be mobile on inspiration and will move towards the right iliac fossa, and has a palpable notch. A palpable flank mass in renal cell carcinoma is more often felt in those of slim build and is often associated with lower pole tumours – it will often be firm and non-tender.

[6] In renal cell cancers an arteriovenous fistula can form within the tumour and lead to audible renal bruit.

[7] Testicular examination should be carried out in all patients who present with any changes to their scrotum or painful testes.

[8] A varicocele occurs in RCC due to compression of the internal spermatic vein (left testicular vein) by the tumour. Varicoceles are more common on the left, but can in fact also occur on the right.

Investigations

Any patient presenting with haematuria of unknown cause, or with other concerning signs, should be investigated for possible RCC.

- Initial blood tests are organised including **full blood count** [1] which shows a microcytic anaemia.
- **Renal function** [2] and **liver function** [3] are normal.
- **Electrolytes** [4] show hypercalcaemia, and **coagulation profile** [5] is normal.
- **Urinalysis** [6] is sent with urine cytology, which shows evidence of haematuria, and cytology result is pending.
- A plain **chest radiograph** [7] is organised due to his cough and chest signs, which finds multiple 'cannonball' lesions.
- A **CT chest/abdo/pelvis** [8] is organised to allow further assessment and potential **staging** [9] , which shows a left renal mass suspicious for renal cell cancer with multiple cannonball metastasis in the chest.
- **Other imaging** [10] such as ultrasonography and MRI are considered.
- Depending on the patient a **histological sample** [11] is either obtained from a nephrectomy or partial nephrectomy, and less commonly from a **percutaneous biopsy** [12] .

1 Full blood count should be carried out in all patients being worked up for RCC. Anaemia can be severe and can precede other symptoms or RCC diagnosis by months. Anaemia can be normocytic or microcytic, and further iron studies are usually consistent with anaemia of chronic disease.

2 Renal function should be done to detect any new renal impairment, and to get a baseline prior to further investigations and treatments.

3 Given the high rates of paraneoplastic syndromes associated with RCC, investigation and work-up for these patients should include tests to identify any potential paraneoplastic syndromes, including LFTs which may detect Stauffer syndrome.

4 Hypercalcaemia occurs in patients with RCC and can be caused by a variety of mechanisms, including lytic bone lesions, overproduction of PTHrP, or in some due to increased prostaglandin production which can lead to increased bone resorption. Prostaglandin excess may be treated with indomethacin or other NSAIDs.

5 Coagulation profile should be sent, given that this patient will likely need surgery or a biopsy in the near future.

6 Urinalysis should be sent, to assess for any concurrent infection and causes for haematuria. It should specifically be sent for cytology, as in ventral lesions or urothelial carcinomas, a positive cytology can be found from urinalysis.

7 A chest radiograph is a quick and simple investigation for anyone with chest signs. Cannonball metastases are multiple large, well-circumscribed round pulmonary metastases that look like cannonballs on imaging. They are most commonly seen in RCC and choriocarcinoma; however, they have also been seen less frequently in those patients with prostate and endometrial carcinoma, as well as in those with granulomatous polyangiitis.

8 CT, either with or without contrast depending on renal function, is usually the first-line investigation for potential renal cell carcinomas. It allows in-depth assessment of the tumour and can assess for evidence of local invasion as well as being able to evaluate the uninvolved kidney and its vasculature.

9 The TNM staging system is used for renal cell carcinoma. The 'T' describes the primary tumour and ranges from TX (tumour cannot be assessed) to T4. T1 and T2 describe tumours of increasing size that are confined to the kidney. T3 describes tumours that have extended into the major veins, and T4 describes tumours that have invaded beyond Gerota's fascia (and includes extension into the ipsilateral adrenal gland).
The 'N' or node describes the involvement of regional lymph nodes, with NX meaning they are not assessed, N0 indicating no regional nodal involvement and N1 describing metastasis to the regional lymph nodes.
Metastasis or 'M' describes the presence of distant metastasis, with M0 meaning no metastasis and M1 indicating the

presence of distant metastasis.
Using this staging system patients are separated into prognostic stages ranging from I–IV, with I and II indicating tumours with no nodal or metastatic spread, III patients with nodal involvement but no distant metastasis and IV those patients with distant metastasis.
Patients are often separated into localised disease (stage I, II and III) and advanced disease (stage IV) based on this.

10 Other imaging modalities include ultrasound, which may be the initial test for patients presenting with non-specific symptoms. Ultrasound is less sensitive than CT for detecting renal masses but can distinguish between benign cysts and solid masses. In those in whom CT is not possible due to either allergy or renal insufficiency, abdominal MRI can assess the tumour and any evidence of local or venous involvement. In those patients with bone pain or elevated ALP a bone scan may be indicated to assess for bony metastasis. If there is any evidence of brain metastasis from history or examination, MRI of the brain should be organised.

11 Renal cell carcinomas (originating from the renal cortex) are the most common form of renal cancers, accounting for ~80% of cases. Other types of renal cancers include transitional cell carcinoma (~8%) and much rarer causes such as renal sarcomas and oncocytomas.
The most common subtypes of renal carcinoma are clear cell carcinoma (75% of cases), papillary carcinoma, chromophobe and collecting duct carcinomas, as well as rarer subtypes.

12 In patients in whom the diagnosis is felt to not be renal cell carcinoma but potentially a metastatic lesion or lymphoma, or in patients with RCC who are not surgical candidates, a percutaneous biopsy should be organised to determine histology prior to commencing treatment. This is carried out under either CT or US guidance and a core biopsy is taken for assessment.

Management

Immediate

Initial management of the patient should include management of **pain** [1], control of **hypertension** [2] and **fluids +/– bisphosphonate** for **hypercalcaemia** [3]. If **anaemia** is significant he may benefit from a **blood transfusion** [4].

Short-term

Short-term management should involve organising the investigations above and discussion at the **renal cell MDT** [5] meeting to determine next steps.

Medium- and long-term

The approach to renal cell carcinoma management is based on the chance of curative intervention, which can be determined by the stage of disease at presentation. Patients are separated into localised and advanced disease groups; however, management for both involves similar treatments but without curative intent for those with advanced disease.

Treatment approaches for localised disease consist mainly of **surgical** [6] management, with **ablation** [7] in those who are not surgical candidates. In those with **advanced disease** [8], surgery is sometimes a palliative option, but **targeted therapy** [9] and **immunomodulatory agents** [10] are the main treatments offered. **Radiotherapy** [11] is not often used for renal cancers, but can be used in a palliative setting for pain or management of metastasis. In those with advanced disease and who progress through multiple treatments, it is important for **palliative care services** [12] to be involved to aid with symptom control and end of life plans when that time comes.

Prognosis [13] in renal cell carcinoma is dependent on both stage at diagnosis and patient factors such as performance status.

[1] Pain management is an important factor for all cancer patients, and should be managed with both simple analgesics and opiates, with the help of the palliative care team for symptom control if needed.

[2] Hypertension should be treated with oral antihypertensive agents, as prolonged hypertension can cause end-organ damage. As some treatment for RCC may worsen hypertension, it needs to be well-controlled beforehand.

[3] Hypercalcaemia can cause cardiac arrhythmias and death if significant. Ensuring adequate hydration and IV bisphosphonates are the mainstay treatment. Often these paraneoplastic syndromes will cease once the primary tumour is removed; however, hypercalcaemia is often seen in advanced disease.

[4] Anaemia in RCC can often be significant and its effects can impair quality of life, so patients may require blood transfusions until treatment has begun to take effect.

[5] As with all cancers, a multidisciplinary team is essential to ensure timely investigations and management are organised and that all members of the team looking after the patient have an agreed plan of patient-centred care.

[6] Surgery remains the only known curative treatment for RCC, and is also used for palliation in patients with metastatic disease. In those with stage I, II and III disease, it is the preferred treatment.

[7] In those with small tumours who are not surgical candidates, radiofrequency ablation or cryotherapy are potential options.

[8] In advanced renal cell cancers a score called the International Metastatic Renal-cell Carcinoma Database Consortium is used to help prognosticate patients. It is dependent on the following factors and if a patient has none they are considered good risk; if they have one or two they are considered intermediate risk and if they have three or more risk factors they are considered poor risk. Factors include a Karnofsky performance status (KPS) <80, time from diagnosis to treatment <1 year, haemoglobin level < lower limit of normal, serum calcium > upper limit of normal, neutrophil count > upper limit of normal and platelet count > upper limit of normal. Those with advanced but asymptomatic disease and no poor prognostic features may be managed with active surveillance rather than initiation of systemic treatments straight away.

[9] The pathogenesis of renal cell carcinoma has identified the vascular endothelial growth factor (VEGF) pathway and mTOR as targets for intervention in these patients. The VEGF pathway or antiangiogenic treatments include two approaches. One includes the use of small molecule tyrosine kinase inhibitors (TKIs) such as sunitinib, axitinib and sorafenib, to block the intracellular VEGF receptor; the other is with a monoclonal antibody called bevacizumab which binds circulating VEGF and thus prevents it from activating the VEGF receptor. These have shown increased survival for those with advanced renal cell cancers.

The mTOR (mammalian target of rapamycin) pathway has the potential to inhibit tumour progression at multiple points as it is downstream of the phosphoinositide 3-kinase pathway that is regulated by a tumour suppressor gene. However, they are mainly beneficial in those who are refractory to VEGF treatment or with known mutations in the PI3K pathway. Examples include temsirolimus and everolimus.

10 Immunotherapy is an important treatment option for those patients with advanced renal cell carcinoma. Checkpoint inhibitor immunotherapy targets either the programmed cell death receptor 1 (PD-1) pathway (e.g. nivolumab, pembrolizumab), or cytotoxic T lymphocyte-associated antigen 4 (CTLA-4) with ipilimumab. Checkpoint inhibitors used in conjunction with targeted therapies have shown improved outcomes.
Interleukin-2 (IL-2) is an immunotherapy option that activates an immune response against the renal cell cancer and has shown regression of the tumour in some patients.

11 Radiotherapy is not often used in RCC but can be used as a palliative measure either to improve pain and haematuria from the primary tumour, or to treat metastatic disease such as bone or brain metastasis to improve symptoms and thus quality of life.

12 Palliative care involvement for all patients who progress to advanced disease and through treatments is useful, and for those who have symptoms that are difficult to control.

13 Survival rates for renal cell carcinoma are dependent on stage at presentation, worsening as stages get more advanced. Those who have radical nephrectomy for stage I disease have a 95% 5-year survival rate, while those with advanced disease have a 5-year survival of 20%. Poor prognostic features are discussed above, with good prognostic features of metastatic disease being: long disease-free interval between initial treatment and recurrence, good performance status and removal of the primary tumour.

CASE 70: Testicular carcinoma

History

- A **25-year-old** [1] **man** [2] presents with ongoing **discomfort in his left testicle** [3] following an injury **2 weeks ago** [4].
- He feels his testicles are heavier than normal, and sometimes has an associated **ache in his groin and abdomen** [5].
- He is also concerned as he feels he is developing some **fatty areas over his chest** [6].

- He denies any other symptoms such as **cough** or **back pain** [7].
- He has no **past medical history** [8], and no **family history** [9] of note.

[1] Testicular cancer is the most common malignancy in young men aged 15–35 years. Improvements in testicular cancer treatment over the past 40 years have increased the 5-year survival rate from 60% to over 95%. Testicular cancer now accounts for <1% of cancer-related deaths in men.

[2] Although testicular cancer is the most common cancer in younger men, it makes up only 1% of all cancers affecting men of all age groups.

[3] Testicular pain can be caused by many problems ranging from trauma to epididymo-orchitis, and initial concerns in someone presenting with pain following a trauma should be related to potential torsion. However, in some patients, acute pain can be the presenting symptom of testicular cancer.

[4] Ongoing pain in a testicle lasting more than a few days is a concerning feature and should be investigated. Patients often present after either they or their partner notice a nodule or swelling of a testicle.

[5] Nearly a third of patients will notice a dull ache or heaviness in their scrotum, perineum or abdomen.

[6] Gynaecomastia is an endocrine manifestation of testicular cancers that can be very distressing to patients. It is usually associated with human chorionic gonadotrophin (hCG) production; however, this is not always the case. This overproduction of hCG can also lead to hyperthyroidism.

[7] A minority of patients can present with evidence of metastatic disease, and their symptoms can reflect this, e.g. a neck mass from supraclavicular lymph nodes, back pain from bony metastasis, cough or shortness of breath from pulmonary metastasis and neurological symptoms from either a central or peripheral lesion.

[8] Men with a history of cryptorchidism (undescended testes) and prior orchidopexy have a higher risk of developing testicular cancer in both testes, not just the undescended one. Other risk factors include prior testicular cancer and certain genetic syndromes such as Klinefelter syndrome (47XXY), and there also appears to be an increased risk in those patients with male factor infertility.

[9] Those with a first-degree relative with testicular cancer have a higher risk of developing testicular cancer, especially if a brother has been affected.

Examination

- On examination the patient looks **well at rest** [1], with a normal **cardiovascular and respiratory examination** [2], and observations are within normal range.
- However, he has **gynaecomastia** [3] on examination of the chest wall.

- His abdomen is soft with some **mild generalised tenderness** [4].
- **Testicular examination** [5] reveals a **firm, fixed lump in the left testicle** [6].

1 Often patients with testicular cancer are young and appear fit and well, with minimal if any comorbidities. They also often present with early disease, only rarely having metastatic cancer on presentation.

2 It is important to fully examine the patient and assess for any evidence of distant spread such as to the lungs. The most common site of metastasis in testicular cancer is to the retroperitoneal lymph nodes, but it can also metastasise to the lung, liver, bone and brain.

3 Gynaecomastia describes enlargement of breast tissues in men, which presents as a palpable rubbery or firm tissue around the nipples in men. This can be an upsetting symptom for some men and if present, may prompt presentation.

4 Testicular cancers metastasise via lymphatic drainage, and due to the embryology of the testicles the initial drainage for testicles is to the retroperitoneal lymph nodes, which is why it is the most common site of spread. Given this, an abdominal examination is an essential part of the assessment to check for any palpable masses. Abdominal tenderness is a concerning sign for lymphatic spread.

5 Testicular examination should be carried out on any man with testicular pain, swelling or abnormalities. Testicular examination should begin with scrotal content assessment using the bimanual technique, initially assessing the normal testicle. A normal testicle should feel smooth, freely movable and separate from the epididymis.

6 In testicular cancer a firm, hard or fixed lesion may be found which should alert you to something sinister that warrants further investigation.

Investigations

- Any man presenting with a firm mass within the testes has **testicular cancer** [1] until proven otherwise.
- Initial tests include **full blood count** [2], **renal function** [3], **liver function** [4] and **electrolytes** [5], which were all normal.
- **Tumour markers** [6] beta-hCG and LDH were raised, whereas alpha-fetoprotein (AFP) was normal.
- **Testicular ultrasound** [7] shows a well-defined hyperechoic lesion on the left testicle.

- Following this a **CT CAP** [8] is organised to assess for distant disease and to aid in **staging** [9].
- **Testicular biopsy** [10] was not performed due to concerns regarding tumour seeding and hence **histology** [11] was obtained during radical orchidectomy.
- Based on staging and tumour marker levels, patients can then be **risk stratified** [12].
- After discussion about his fertility, he underwent **cryopreservation of sperm** [13] prior to imaging.

1 There is a misconception that testicular cancers cannot present as painful and so are often treated as epididymitis, thus delaying diagnosis, and painless scrotal lesions often do not prompt patients to present early. Differential diagnosis of a testicular mass includes epididymitis, epididymo-orchitis and testicular torsion, with hydroceles, varicoceles, hernias, syphilitic gumma and haematoma being less common.

2 A baseline FBC should be included in the work-up for all patients with testicular cancer, especially because those who present with pain can be misdiagnosed as having epididymitis. A lack of a raised WCC should direct you towards a different diagnosis.

3 Renal function should be assessed to ensure there is no impairment, as this may affect choice of imaging and treatment.

4 Liver function may show abnormalities if there are liver metastases.

5 Electrolytes, especially calcium, are helpful as a patient with back pain and a raised ALP and calcium would be concerning for bony metastasis.

6 Levels of beta-hCG and/or AFP are raised in over 80% of men with non-seminomatous germ cell tumours (NSGCTs); however, these are much less frequently raised in seminomas. Although these tumour markers are useful in initial diagnosis, their main use is in follow-up post treatment. AFP is secreted only in non-seminomas, with concentrations above 10 000ng/ml being seen only in germ cell tumours and hepatocellular carcinoma. Beta-hCG can be secreted by either seminomas or non-seminomas. When the level is very high, sometimes there is nipple tenderness and gynaecomastia. Levels of over 10 000mIU/ml are seen only in germ cell tumours. LDH is seen in both seminomas and non-seminomas and has been found to be an independent prognostic indicator, with higher levels associated with larger tumour burden, increased growth rate and cellular proliferation.

7 Testicular ultrasound can distinguish extrinsic from intrinsic testicular lesions and can significantly aid physical examination. Although many different patterns of lesions are seen on ultrasound, classically seminomas are well-defined and hypoechoic without cystic lesions, compared with NSGCTs which are often ill-defined and inhomogeneous with calcifications and cystic areas. Microlithiasis may be seen on ultrasound, which looks like small echogenic foci. There appears to be a link between microlithiasis and testicular cancer; however, this is unclear and further imaging is not indicated in those with an otherwise normal ultrasound.

8 CT chest, abdomen and pelvis should be organised for all patients with likely testicular cancer to assess for evidence of distant metastasis; however, if sperm preservation is going to be organised every effort should be made for this to occur prior to imaging so that the sperm are exposed to as little radiation as possible.

9 The TNM system is used, combined with tumour marker levels (S) for stages I–III. The tumour or 'T' is classified following radical orchidectomy:

- pTX indicates that the tumour was not assessed, i.e. orchidectomy not performed
- pT1 indicates the tumour is limited to the testes with no local infiltration
- pT2 is when the tumour has extended into the vasculature or lymphatics or through the tunica albuginea
- pT3 indicates the tumour has invaded the spermatic cord
- pT4 is when the tumour has invaded the scrotum.

The node or 'N' is split into N0 which represents no regional nodes, and N1–3, which describe increasingly large lymph nodes, with N3 representing lymph nodes >5cm. The metastasis or 'M' can be either M0 (no metastasis) or M1 (distant metastasis). M1 is divided into M1a (non-regional lymph node or pulmonary metastasis) and M1b (distant metastasis other than that listed in M1a). For testicular cancers the serum tumour marker level (LDH, beta-hCG and AFP) is used in the staging system and is denoted by S, ranging from S1–S3, with rising markers for higher stages. Based on these factors, patients are then grouped into pathological stages ranging from Stage 0 to Stage IIIC. For those with advanced cancer at presentation the International Germ Cell Cancer Collaborative group system is used.

10 Testicular biopsy is not used to get histology for these patients. Almost all patients will undergo a radical orchidectomy and sometimes lymph node dissection, as even those with disseminated disease will need orchidectomy due to the poor penetration of chemotherapy into the testes.

11 Patients with a suspicious testicular mass or concerning ultrasound features should undergo a radical orchidectomy. The vast majority of testicular cancers are germ cell tumours (GCTs), and they can consist of one main histological type or a combination of many. Patients are split into two main groups for treatment purposes: pure seminoma (no non-seminomatous elements present) and all others – non-seminomatous germ cell tumours (NSGCTs). Pure seminomas are much more likely to be localised to the testis at presentation compared with NSGCTs. Less than 50% of germ cell tumours are of a single cell type. The WHO classifies malignant testicular germ cell tumours by histologic type as follows:

1. Intratubular germ cell neoplasia, unclassified
2. Malignant pure germ cell tumours (showing a single cell line) a. seminoma b. embryonal carcinoma c. teratoma d. choriocarcinoma e. yolk sac tumour
3. Malignant mixed germ cell tumour (showing more than one histological pattern) a. embryonal carcinoma and teratoma with or without seminoma b. embryonal carcinoma and yolk scan tumour with or without seminoma c. embryonal carcinoma and seminoma d. yolk sac tumour and teratoma with or without seminoma e. choriocarcinoma and any other element
4. Polyembryoma.

12 Risk stratification is carried out in those with more advanced disease and is based on the characteristics of the tumour and metastasis as well as serum tumour marker levels. Seminomas are classified as good risk (any primary site, no non-pulmonary visceral metastasis, normal AFP, any hCG or LDH) or intermediate risk (any primary site, non-pulmonary visceral metastasis, normal AFP, any hCG or LDH). No seminomas are considered poor prognosis. Non-seminomas are classified as good risk (testicular or retroperitoneal primary tumour, no non-pulmonary visceral metastasis and 'good' markers – i.e. S1 markers), intermediate risk (testicular or retroperitoneal primary tumour, no non-pulmonary visceral metastasis and any intermediate markers – i.e. S2 markers) and poor risk (mediastinal primary, non-pulmonary visceral metastasis and poor markers – i.e. S3 markers).

13 Sperm cryopreservation should be offered to all men diagnosed with testicular cancer, and if possible sperm count and banking should be organised prior to investigations. Many patients with testicular tumours are found to have an element of impaired spermatogenesis for unclear reasons; however, semen quality may further deteriorate following orchidectomy and so early discussions and organisation are essential.

Management

Immediate

Initial management for these patients involves organisation of **sperm preservation** [1] followed by **radical inguinal orchidectomy** [2] to get histological samples and control the tumour. Many of these patients will also undergo a **retroperitoneal lymph node dissection** [3] at the same time.

Short-term

Short-term management involves discussion of the patient at the **germ cell MDT meeting** [4] as well as organising **psychological support** [5] to discuss fertility issues.

Medium- and long-term

Optimal therapy for these patients is dependent on their chance of recurrence, with histology, degree of metastasis and serum tumour markers being used to stratify these patients. For most patients, treatment will involve surgery as discussed above, **chemotherapy** [6] (the length of which depends on the stage of the disease) plus potentially **radiotherapy** [7]. The **prognosis** [8] for testicular carcinoma is excellent, and **follow-up** [9] will be dictated by the histology, stage and risk of recurrence.

1 Sperm preservation is an important management step for these young men undergoing treatment for testicular cancer and it should be discussed as early as possible.

2 Radical inguinal orchidectomy will be performed for almost all patients with testicular cancer. It involves removal of the entire spermatic cord as well as the testicle, via the inguinal approach.

3 Retroperitoneal lymph node dissection is the most reliable method to identify nodal micrometastasis. Unfortunately CT imaging does not provide adequate information. The number and size of affected lymph nodes provides important prognostic information.

4 As with all cancers, discussion of the patient at the relevant MDT meeting is essential for adequate and coordinated care.

5 Psychological support and counselling may be required for some patients facing treatment for testicular cancer, especially regarding fertility issues.

6 Chemotherapy may be given to those with early stage disease for a short course as adjuvant treatment post surgery, or for more extensive disease more prolonged treatment may be required. For those with early stage seminoma, treatment with carboplatin as adjuvant therapy is usually organised, and for those with early stage non-seminoma BEP (bleomycin, etoposide and cisplatin) will be organised. Those with more advanced disease will usually require chemotherapy for a longer period. Side-effects to chemotherapy can be significant, including nausea, weight loss, mucositis, diarrhoea and hair loss. Certain treatments have some specific side-effects: for example, cyclophosphamide can cause haemorrhagic cystitis, and bleomycin can cause pulmonary toxicity.

7 In patients with seminoma that has metastasised to the retroperitoneal lymph nodes, radiotherapy may be organised. Seminomas respond very well to radiotherapy and with a combination of surgery, chemotherapy and radiotherapy most patients have curative treatment. Side-effects of radiotherapy include fatigue, skin damage and diarrhoea.

8 Testicular cancers, including metastatic disease, are generally curable because they are very sensitive to chemotherapy. The cure rate for 'good risk' disease is over 90%. Since the 1970s and the advent of combination chemotherapy, the mortality rates for testicular cancer have decreased by more than 80%. The prognosis does vary based on histologic type of cancer, stage, tumour markers and type of metastasis but the overall prognosis is still excellent, even for those with advanced disease.

9 Most patients relapse within the first one to two years following initial management. Most patients will be followed up for a period with tumour markers and imaging, but the intensity with which this is done depends on their histology and risk of recurrence at initial presentation.

CASE 71: Acute kidney injury

History

- A 79-year-old lady is in the Geriatric unit for inpatient rehabilitation after a fall, fracturing her left hip and requiring a left total hip replacement. Her comorbidities include chronic kidney disease secondary to hypertension, type 2 diabetes on oral antihypoglycaemic agents.
- During her acute inpatient admission, her regular **perindopril** [1] was ceased during the perioperative period, and was restarted two days ago.
- The patient developed a UTI two days ago and was empirically commenced on a three day course of **trimethoprim** [2]. She has received two doses of trimethoprim.

- You are reviewing her routine bloods and noticed that her **eGFR has dropped from 33ml/min/1.73m^2 two days ago to 18 today** [3].
- On review, she denies any **change to her appetite** or **nausea**, **chest pain or discomfort** or **pruritus** [4].
- She also denies any **shortness of breath** [5] but reports mild **thirst** [6].
- However, she also reports that she has been passing **smaller volumes of more concentrated urine** [7] today.

[1] Perindopril is a common cause of acute kidney injury. Perindopril is an ACE inhibitor, which inhibits the function of angiotensin-converting enzyme, which normally converts the inactive angiotensin I to the active angiotensin II (ANGII). ANGII is a very potent vasoconstrictor (hence the name, 'angio' (vascular) + 'tensin' (constriction).

The blood vessels immediately leading to the glomerulus are the afferent arterioles and those immediately downstream of the glomerulus are the efferent arterioles. ANGII leads to the constriction of the afferent and efferent arterioles, but ANGII leads to significantly greater constriction of the efferent arterioles compared to the afferent arterioles.

This effect has discordant effects on the determinants of the glomerular filtration rate (GFR). The determinants of the GFR are renal plasma flow, the difference in hydrostatic pressure between the glomerular capillary and Bowman's capsule, and (to a small extent) the difference in oncotic pressure between the glomerular capillary and Bowman's capsule.

Constriction of the afferent arterioles and efferent arterioles increases the resistance to blood flow across the arterioles, and hence reduces renal blood flow. However, the greater degree of constriction in the efferent arterioles increases the capillary hydrostatic pressure. These two effects have opposing effects on the GFR. However, in usual circumstances, particularly when the pressure head to the kidney is reduced, the net effect generally turns out to be an increase in the GFR.

The commencement of perindopril in this patient would have reduced the production of angiotensin II, and through the mechanisms described above, contributed to a decrease in the GFR.

[2] Trimethoprim has an interesting relationship with the GFR. It is very easy to fall into the trap that trimethoprim is nephrotoxic because it increases the serum creatinine. In fact, trimethoprim does increase the serum creatinine, but it does so by inhibiting creatinine secretion in the tubules, not by inhibiting glomerular filtration.

Plasma creatinine is used as a marker of the glomerular filtration rate. The ideal marker for GFR is a chemical that is cleared exclusively through glomerular filtration (e.g. inulin). In fact, the clearance of inulin is equal to the glomerular filtration rate. Inulin, however, is very expensive. Therefore, we use creatinine instead, which is produced by muscle at a relatively constant rate, and about 90% of creatinine is cleared through glomerular filtration. Most of the remaining creatinine is cleared through secretion through the tubules. In patients with impaired glomerular filtration, a greater proportion of creatinine is cleared through tubular secretion (up to 30% instead of the usual 10%).

Trimethoprim inhibits the tubular secretion of creatinine and therefore causes the serum creatinine to increase. The calculated eGFR, which is dependent on age, sex and serum creatinine, would decrease, and it would appear as though the renal function is worsening. This is a myth, however; the true glomerular filtration rate is actually unchanged.

However, it is very important to know that trimethoprim causes hyperkalaemia, but this is not due to impaired glomerular filtration. Trimethoprim actually also blocks epithelial Na$^+$ channels in the collecting tubule of the kidney (like amiloride, a potassium-sparing diuretic), which inhibits the exchange of Na$^+$ and K$^+$ ions in the collecting tubule and hence inhibits K$^+$ excretion.

Therefore, when looking at changes in serum creatinine in

a patient on trimethoprim, note that at least some of the increase in serum creatinine can be attributed to impaired tubular secretion, rather than worsening glomerular filtration.

3 When the true GFR is decreasing with a concomitant rise in serum creatinine, the eGFR will tend to further overestimate the true GFR.

If a patient's serum creatinine is, for example, 100µmol/L with a calculated eGFR of 50 (ml/min/1.73m^2) and we hypothetically instantaneously halve the GFR, it can take days for the serum creatinine to increase to its new steady state value of 200µmol/L. Therefore, after one day the Cr may be 150µmol/L, and the eGFR reported would be 33ml/min/1.73m^2. However, we know that the patient's glomerular filtration at this point actually corresponds to an eGFR of 25, not 33.

Therefore, if you see a patient with an increasing serum creatinine, note that the new steady state serum creatinine is likely to be significantly higher than the serum creatinine you see as it is approaching its steady state concentration, and the patient's true renal function would be reflective of the steady state concentration, not the concentration at the moment when you are reviewing the patient.

In this patient, the eGFR is 18ml/min/1.73m^2, but the patient's true renal function at that moment is more reflective of an eGFR <18 (if we ignore the competing effect of trimethoprim in this case).

4 Anorexia, nausea, pruritus, and confusion/altered conscious state are the symptoms of uraemia. Uraemia is caused by an accumulation of toxic metabolites from multiple chemical reactions that occur normally throughout the body. These include guanidine-based compounds and phenols. It is important to note that urea accumulates in the body in severe renal failure, but urea is not a primary cause of uraemic symptoms, despite the nomenclature. Rather, a significantly raised urea is an indicator that other toxic metabolites are also not being cleared sufficiently. This is important, because you can have patients with a plasma urea of 20mmol/L with uraemia, but other patients may have a plasma urea of 50mmol/L without uraemia.

Clinically, establishing the presence of uraemia is important because uraemia in acute renal failure is an indication for urgent dialysis.

5 Assessing for shortness of breath is an attempt to screen for pulmonary oedema. In the setting of acute renal failure, pulmonary oedema can be secondary to the volume overload secondary to acute renal failure. This volume overload occurs as impaired glomerular filtration inhibits the ability of the kidney to excrete salt and water from the body, leading to an increased mean systemic filling pressure of the systemic circulation. This can cause increased capillary hydrostatic pressure in the pulmonary circulation (which can be exacerbated by left heart failure), causing transudation of fluid into the pulmonary interstitium.

6 Assessing for thirst is an attempt to assess for hypovolaemia, which can be a cause (rather than a consequence) of acute renal failure. Thirst is stimulated by a number of causes, including hypovolaemia (as sensed by low pressure baroreceptors in the right heart) and angiotensin II (released in hypovolaemia).

7 Oliguria is a complication of acute renal failure, but it is not ubiquitous. This is because, even a patient whose GFR is 5ml/min would be filtering a total of 7L per day. If the patient's kidneys reabsorb 5.5L (which some kidneys do in this setting), the resultant urine output is relatively normal at 1.5L. Oliguria can complicate acute renal failure if there is mechanical obstruction of the tubules (e.g. in acute tubular necrosis where dead and sloughed tubular cells block the tubules, or precipitation of nephrotoxic chemicals inside the tubules), or it can be a clue that hypovolaemia is causing the acute renal failure.

In states of hypovolaemia, aldosterone levels are high (due to the renal hypoperfusion and baroreceptor reflex activating the renin–angiotensin–aldosterone axis) and ADH levels are also higher due to hypovolaemia-induced ADH release by the pituitary. This causes increased retention of salt and water in the kidney, leading to significantly lowered urine output.

Examination

- On examination, the patient looks well, **alert and oriented to time and place** [1].
- There is no evidence of a **uraemic flap** [1].
- BP is 130/75, HR 90, SaO$_2$ 96% on air, RR 21 and temperature is **37.5°C** [2].
- **Peripheries are warm with good capillary refill** [3], and there is no evidence of **excoriations in the limbs** [4].
- **JVP is difficult to visualise** [3].
- There are no **crackles on auscultation of the lungs** [3], and no **pericardial friction rub** [4] on auscultation of the heart.
- Abdomen is soft and non-tender to palpation, with bowel sounds present.
- There is **moderate right flank tenderness to palpation at the right costovertebral angle** [5].
- There is no evidence of **peripheral oedema** [3].

1 Alertness, orientation to time and place and the presence vs. absence of a uraemic flap are indicators of the presence or absence of uraemic encephalopathy. Uraemic toxins are toxic to the brain and cause encephalopathy, which manifests in the same way as encephalopathy due to other causes. This includes altered conscious state including confusion, and the presence of a uraemic flap. In fact, the uraemic flap is actually a manifestation of negative myoclonus at the wrist extensors, where encephalopathy causes a periodic temporary impairment of the neural pathway, leading to wrist extensor contraction and dorsiflexion at the wrist. This periodic impairment causes a 'flap', where the patient's wrist extensors periodically relax, as the patient attempts to maintain a fixed dorsiflexed position at the wrists.

2 In the elderly, the mechanisms that lead to fever are often blunted. Fever is caused by effects of certain signalling molecules on the hypothalamus, causing the hypothalamus to 'reset' its thermostat to a higher temperature. This causes the hypothalamus to activate multiple neuron-mediated mechanisms to increase body temperature, including vasoconstriction to preserve body heat, piloerection and shivering. Such molecules include inflammatory cytokines released during acute inflammation, such as IL-1, IL-6 and TNF-alpha, as well as bacterial endotoxins such as lipopolysaccharide, present in Gram-negative bacteria.

For some reason, in the elderly the production of such inflammatory mediators, and the response of the hypothalamus to these mediators, is diminished. This means that a minor temperature increase to 37.5°C in the elderly can be a sign of serious infection that would cause a fever of up to 38.5°C in a younger person.

3 The mechanism behind similar examination findings is discussed in Case 76: Hyponatraemia.

4 Pericardial friction rub can be a sign for uraemic pericarditis. The uraemic toxins discussed earlier also cause significant levels of pruritus; evidence of scratch marks (excoriations) may be a clue as to whether the patient has uraemia, which would be an indication for dialysis.

5 Flank tenderness is often a sign of renal pathology caused by stretching of the renal capsule (due to a stone, for example), or of inflammation of the kidney and perinephric fat. The kidney is a paired structure derived from intermediate mesoderm, and therefore innervation of nociceptive neurons to each kidney will lead to lateralisation of the pain to the side of the pathology.

In this patient, the flank tenderness is more likely secondary to pyelonephritis.

Investigations

Serum biochemistry results are shown below (all results are in mmol/L unless stated otherwise):

	Two days ago	Today
[Na⁺]	137	135
[K⁺]	4.7	**7.5** [1]
[Cl⁻]	98	**96** [2]
[HCO₃⁻]	24	**15** [2]
Urea	5.5	**16.2** [3]
Creatinine (µmol/L)	140	240
eGFR (ml/min/1.73m²)	33	18

Urine MCS (2 days prior):
Microscopy:
Leucocytes >1000

Erythrocytes >100
Protein +
Bacteria +++
No casts present on microscopy.
No dysmorphic red blood cells [4].
Culture
E. coli >10⁸ [5]
Sensitivities

Amoxycillin	R
Amoxycillin/clavulanate	R
Ceftriaxone	R
Ceftazidime	R
Piperacillin/tazobactam	S
Meropenem	S
Trimethoprim	R

1 Hyperkalaemia is a known and predictable complication of acute renal failure. Remember that the main modality of renal potassium excretion is in the collecting tubule, via the principal cells. The principal cells have epithelial Na⁺ and K⁺ channels on the luminal surface (facing the lumen), whereas the basolateral membrane contains Na/K pumps that maintain the low Na⁺ concentration inside the cell and

high K⁺ concentration inside the cell. Therefore, the presence of the Na⁺ and K⁺ channels in the luminal side favours sodium reabsorption into the cell (from the lumen, which contains a reasonably high Na⁺ concentration) and K⁺ secretion into the tubular lumen.

Now, if there is a high flow rate of tubular fluid through the collecting duct, then any K⁺ excreted into the tubular lumen is quickly swept along the collecting duct. This means that the concentration of K^+ in the luminal fluid is kept low and that of Na^+ is kept reasonably high, and the concentration gradients of Na^+ and K^+ are kept at high levels. This high concentration gradient means the rate of K^+ secretion into the collecting duct remains high.

In renal failure, since there is less fluid filtered at the glomerulus, the flow rate through the collecting duct is quite slow. When this happens, K^+ accumulates in the luminal fluid as the fluid remains in the collecting duct for longer. Additionally, Na^+ concentration in the luminal fluid drops in parallel for similar reasons. This means that the concentration gradient for efflux of K^+ into the tubular lumen is significantly lower, and the rate of K^+ excretion is also significantly lower. Also, the metabolic acidosis induced by acute renal failure worsens the hyperkalaemia. The excess H^+ in the blood and interstitial fluid is exchanged for K^+ inside cells through multiple mechanisms, leading to a shift of K^+ from inside to outside the cells.

In this case, the hyperkalaemia was caused by the acute renal failure with acidosis, with contributions from trimethoprim and perindopril.

2 The low concentration of bicarbonate ions (HCO_3^-) indicates that there is a metabolic acidosis. Renal failure is a cause of metabolic acidosis.

The primary mechanism by which the kidneys excrete acid (H^+ ions) is through Na/H exchangers and H^+ pumps throughout the nephron, with most of the acid being excreted in the proximal tubule.

In renal failure, less fluid is filtered through the nephrons and only a limited amount of acid can be excreted per volume of fluid. This is because if less fluid flows through the nephrons, less sodium can be reabsorbed and hence less H^+ can be excreted through the Na/H exchanger. Additionally, less H^+ can be secreted into the tubule because the fluid pH would drop much more quickly since there are fewer buffering ions such as NH_3 and HPO_4^{2-} ions to resist the drop in pH. This would lead to a significant concentration gradient of H^+ (into the tubular cells), inhibiting the function of the H^+ pump which works against the concentration gradient.

In patients eating western diets, the amount of acid produced in our body through many reactions – the oxidation of sulphur-containing amino acids to produce sulphuric acid, oxidation of phosphorus-containing compounds to produce phosphoric acid, the production of uric acid, oxalic acid, lactic acid and other acids – is greater than the amount of base produced.

Hence, in renal failure, the excess H^+ produced by the body every day would not be excreted completely; this means that H^+ will accumulate in the body. Most of the H^+ produced immediately reacts with the bicarbonate ions in the blood:

$$H^+ + HCO_3^- \rightarrow CO_2 + H_2O$$

with the CO_2 being immediately excreted through the lungs (plasma pCO_2 is kept constant by modulation of minute ventilation in the lungs). The net effect is that $[HCO_3^-]$ decreases significantly, $[H^+]$ increases slightly and pH drops. Notice that in this patient, the $[HCO_3^-]$ is 15mM (in healthy people it is approximately 24mM).

The other important point is that this is a metabolic acidosis with a high anion gap. Remember that the total charge of the cations and the total charge of the anions in the blood and interstitial fluid must be equal. If we consider the main ions in the blood, namely Na^+, K^+, Cl^- and HCO_3^- ions, and consider this sum:

$$[Na^+] + [K^+] - [Cl^-] - [HCO_3^-]$$

this should not be too far away from 0. In fact, this value tends to be approximately 10–15mM, because albumin is present in significant concentrations in the blood, and each albumin molecule has multiple negative charges.

In renal failure, this sum, called the anion gap, increases significantly. This is because the HCO_3^- ions being titrated away by the extra H^+ ions would be replaced by the anionic forms (conjugate bases) of the organic acids that are produced by the body, but not excreted in sufficient quantities. These include sulphate (from sulphuric acid), phosphate, urate, oxalate and other anions.

In this patient, the anion gap is approximately 31mM.

3 Urea is reabsorbed mainly at the proximal tubule (50%) and at the medullary collecting duct. Additionally, urea is recycled from the medullary interstitium into the tubules at the loop of Henle (with most of it being reabsorbed again at the collecting duct).

When urine flow through the tubule is low (in renal failure), there is more time for the urea to be reabsorbed across the concentration gradient to establish equilibrium. This leads to retention of urea.

Also, if poor renal perfusion (e.g. due to hypovolaemia) is the cause of renal failure, then the RAAS system would be upregulated, and ADH would also be secreted in higher amounts. ADH increases the permeability of the medullary collecting ducts to urea as well as water, increasing urea reabsorption further. In these causes of renal failure, you will often see significant rises in urea concentration.

4 Glomerulonephritis (inflammation of the glomeruli) is an important cause of renal failure, with the inflammatory infiltrate causing structural damage to the glomeruli, and sometimes causing mechanical obstruction of the glomeruli (leading to reduced GFR). This structural damage can lead to red blood cells leaking from the blood into Bowman's capsule and trying to pass through the tubules.

The tubules are very tiny passages – the red blood cells passing through them become dysmorphic (look very odd), which can be viewed under a microscope.

The presence of red blood cells which are not dysmorphic suggests they did not have to pass through the renal tubules – and therefore they are more likely to have originated in the ureter or the bladder (or urethra).

5 This patient has a urinary tract infection that is resistant to the trimethoprim she was on. Whilst this may be an isolated finding, it can be a cause of the patient's acute kidney injury, if the infection is causing a septic response.

Sepsis is a condition where a host's immune response to an infection leads to damage of multiple organs, including the kidneys. The mechanism by which AKI occurs in sepsis is complex, but involves a mixture of:

- vasoconstriction of the afferent and efferent arterioles due to high sympathetic tone (in an attempt to maintain an adequate blood pressure); this significantly decreases renal blood flow and can also decrease capillary hydrostatic pressure, leading to a decrease in the GFR

- many other processes that cause mechanical damage to the nephrons, for example thrombosis inside the glomeruli, and apoptosis and necrosis of tubular cells with sloughing into the tubule and causing mechanical obstruction.

Management

Urgently treat hyperkalaemia with calcium gluconate, insulin + dextrose and resonium whilst obtaining urgent cardiac monitoring. This will require a transfer out of the Geriatric ward and into an a cardiac-monitored acute bed.

- **Commence IV fluids** [1] (0.9% NaCl at a rate of 125ml/hour).
- Stop **perindopril** [2] and **trimethoprim** [2].
- Start IV **meropenem** [3].
- **Acute dialysis is not indicated at this stage** [4].

[1] Commencement of IV fluids aims to increase the mean systemic filling pressure of the circulation and hence the preload of the heart. This would increase the ventricular systolic pressure generated in systole and increase arterial blood pressure (transiently). The baroreceptor reflex would downregulate, and any sympathetic vasoconstriction that occurs on the glomerular afferent and efferent arterioles decreases. This increases renal blood flow, and can also increase capillary hydrostatic pressure, leading to an improved GFR.

[2] Cessation of perindopril enables angiotensin II production, allowing adequate constriction of the efferent arteriole and maintenance of an adequate capillary hydrostatic pressure in the glomerulus, improving GFR. Cessation of trimethoprim would not affect GFR, but it would prevent further hyperkalaemia – and it is no longer indicated since the E. coli isolated is resistant.

[3] Treatment with effective antibiotics reduces the systemic inflammatory response to the infection, minimising the damage to the kidney (as described above).

[4] Dialysis involves the filtration of blood across a semipermeable membrane to a dialysate fluid, with water and solutes diffusing out of the blood. These include excess K$^+$ ions, Na$^+$ ions and uraemic toxins (that cause uraemia). The dialysate contains a relatively high concentration of bicarbonate ions; in this case, given the patient has a metabolic acidosis, one would choose a dialysate bicarbonate concentration of about 35mM. This would enable diffusion of bicarbonate into the blood through the dialysate membrane. The addition of extra bicarbonate (as a base) into the blood increases the blood pH and corrects the acidaemia. The extrusion of water and Na$^+$ contracts the extracellular fluid volume, which is essential in patients with volume overload. Urgent dialysis is a risky procedure as it involves having a large intravenous catheter inserted (a 'Vascath') into a large central vein, and the actual dialysis procedure poses the risk of hypotension, infection and other complications. Therefore, urgent dialysis is only indicated in specific settings, including refractory volume overload, severe refractory hyperkalaemia, uraemia, uraemic pericarditis and severe metabolic acidosis. This patient does have severe hyperkalaemia, but it would be reasonable to not proceed with urgent dialysis as we have temporising measures such as insulin/dextrose, as well as causes that we can immediately reverse (cessation of trimethoprim and perindopril, and initiation of IV fluids), that may be able to correct the hyperkalaemia and prevent the need for urgent dialysis.

CASE 72: Chronic kidney disease

History

- A 60-year-old lady (weight **45kg** [1]) is being seen in the Renal Outpatient Clinic for routine review. She is currently living at home with her husband and she has chronic kidney disease secondary to diabetic nephropathy.
- Her baseline serum creatinine is **140μmol/L** [1]
- Her other medical comorbidities include T2DM, hypertension and hypercholesterolaemia. She is on **perindopril 2.5mg daily** [2], **amlodipine 5mg daily** [3], atorvastatin 40mg daily, furosemide 20mg daily, **gliclazide 60mg mane** [4], **linagliptin 5mg bd** [5] and Lantus (insulin glargine) 10 units mane.
- On review, the patient feels generally well. She denies anorexia, nausea, lethargy or **bone pain** [6].
- She makes good volumes of urine and does not have any urinary symptoms. She reports some mild ankle swelling, but no shortness of breath. She is able to manage with her activities of daily living.

[1] The patient's weight is particularly important in the evaluation of the GFR using serum creatinine. Creatinine is the metabolite of creatine, a chemical found in muscle that is used in the ATP-PC muscular energy system (used in short-term intense exercise). The higher the muscle mass, the greater the production of creatinine.

Hence, patients with low muscle mass (e.g. underweight people) will tend to produce less creatinine. Hence, for a given GFR, the steady state serum creatinine would be significantly lower. Thus, in this woman, the relatively benign serum creatinine of 140μmol/L is consistent with an estimated CrCl of 27ml/min (Cockcroft–Gault equation), whereas if the patient were a 40-year-old man weighing 95kg, a serum creatinine of 140μmol/L is consistent with an estimated CrCl of 83ml/min (near normal!).

[2] Perindopril is an ACE inhibitor. It inhibits the production of angiotensin II. Angiotensin II binds to AT_1 receptors in arteriolar smooth muscle, causing smooth muscle contraction and arteriolar vasoconstriction. Hence, perindopril tends to cause arteriolar vasodilation, decreasing the back pressure and lowering arterial blood pressure.

[3] Amlodipine is a dihydropyridine calcium channel blocker. This blocks calcium channels that are found on vascular smooth muscle cells. Preventing entry of calcium into vascular smooth muscle cells weakens the degree of vascular smooth muscle contraction, given Ca^{2+} ions are essential for excitation-contraction coupling.

[4] Pancreatic beta-islet cells contain K^+ channels that close when ATP binds to them. In states of high plasma glucose concentrations, glucose diffuses through GLUT4 channels into the islet cell, and is metabolised with the resultant production of ATP. The higher concentration of ATP leads to a greater closure of K^+ channels, depolarisation of the cell and activation of voltage-dependent Ca^{2+} channels. The Ca^{2+} is a well-known secondary messenger; in this case, it promotes insulin protein production and secretion.

Sulphonylureas (such as gliclazide) bind to these K^+ channels and close them, 'tricking' the pancreas into producing a greater amount of insulin for a given plasma glucose.

[5] GLP-1 is a signalling molecule released by neuroendocrine cells in the small and large bowel in the post-prandial period. It has an anorexic effect, delaying gastric emptying and promoting satiety. GLP-1 also multiplies the effect of glucose-induced insulin release by pancreatic islet cells; however, in the absence of sufficient glucose, GLP-1 has no effect on insulin release by pancreatic islet cells. GLP-1 is antidiabetic and also minimises appetite.

DPP-4 is a proteolytic enzyme found on the surface of vascular endothelial cells, that cleaves GLP-1. Linagliptin is an inhibitor of DPP-4. It is also metabolised through the liver and therefore its levels are not significantly dependent on renal function. Patients with CKD will tend to be on linagliptin (as opposed to other DPP-4 inhibitors such as sitagliptin).

[6] The periosteum is the most densely innervated tissue within bone. Irritation of the periosteum can cause intense bone pain. Renal bone disease causes abnormal bone turnover with abnormally increased osteoclastic activity and bone resorption. This can cause abnormalities in the bony architecture, leading to periosteal irritation and hence bone pain.

Examination

On examination, the patient looks well and there is no **uraemic fetor or uraemic tinge in skin tone** [1]. There is no **uraemic flap** [2].
BP is 139/87mmHg [3], HR 71bpm, RR 16 breaths per minute, SaO_2 97% on air, **temperature is 36.4°C** [4].
Palmar crease and conjunctival pallor [5] are notable. JVP is approximately 4cm vertically from the sternal notch. Chest is clear to auscultation. There is no pericardial friction rub.
Abdomen is soft and non-tender, and there is no evidence of ascites.
There is **mild pitting oedema up to the mid-shin bilaterally** [6].

[1] Patients with chronic kidney disease have a reduced ability to excrete waste, including nitrogenous waste. This results in uraemia which can present as uraemic breath or 'fetor' and uraemic frost on skin. Typically uraemia is a sign of end-stage kidney disease.

[2] The early initiation of dialysis in modern times means that complications secondary to uraemia are not commonly seen. Uraemia is known to result in prolonged bleeding due to impaired platelet function from uraemia, uraemic pericarditis and also uraemic neuropathy.

[3] Hypertension is a common finding in chronic kidney disease. Poorly controlled blood pressure results in worsening kidney function. Thus good BP control is important, as this slows down progression of proteinuric CKD and cardiovascular complications.

[4] Patients with chronic kidney disease are at greater risk of infection and all patients with CKD are advised to be up to date with their vaccinations.

[5] Palmar crease and conjunctival pallor are physical signs of anaemia. Anaemia in CKD is common and is a result of decreased erythropoietin secretion from kidneys. It is important to optimise iron stores before starting erythropoietin therapy in CKD.

[6] JVP, presence of ascites and pedal oedema are physical signs looking for volume overload. In mild–moderate CKD, patients are normally able to maintain relative volume balance, but are less able to respond to rapid intake of sodium, hence are more prone to fluid overload. Fluid overload in these patients is usually responsive to diuretics.

Investigations

Routine blood results are shown below:

Hb (x 10^9/L)	9.4 [1]	Cr (μM)	141
MCV (fl)	85 [1]	eGFR (ml/min/1.73m²)	25
WCC (x 10^9/L)	7.1	Albumin	23
Platelets (x 10^9/L)	215	**Ca^{2+} (mM)**	1.75 [4]
Reticulocyte count	0.9% [1]	**Ca^{2+} corrected (mM)**	2.10 [4]
Na^+ (mM)	138	Mg^{2+} (mM)	1.01
K^+ (mM)	4.6	**Phos (mM)**	2.93 [4]
Cl^- (mM)	101	**PTH (pmol/L)**	31.6 [4]
HCO_3^- (mM)	20 [2]	Transferrin saturation	17%
Ur (mM)	8.6	Ferritin (mg/L)	350
HbA1c	8.1% [3]	**Vitamin D (nmol/L)**	56 [4]

Urinalysis:

Urine protein/creatinine ratio	**1.1g/g** [5]
Urine albumin/creatinine ratio	0.9g/g

1 Erythropoietin (EPO) stimulates red blood cell production. It is produced in the interstitial cells surrounding the peritubular capillaries in the renal cortex.

EPO is a growth factor, a ligand that binds to the EPO receptor on the erythrocyte precursor cell surface. This stimulates a signal transduction pathway mediated by Janus kinase 2 (JAK2), leading to the proliferation and differentiation of these cells into erythrocytes. (Incidentally, a mutation in JAK2 leads to very high Hb levels in a disease known as polycythaemia rubra vera.)

Patients with chronic kidney disease presumably have fewer interstitial cells to produce such EPO, and hence erythropoiesis in the bone marrow is not stimulated as significantly. Given that lack of EPO simply slows down red blood cell production without significant alterations to the red blood cell morphology, the red cell size would be normal, and patients would have a normocytic anaemia, which is what is seen in this patient.

Reticulocytes are immature red blood cells that are released from the bone marrow, which differentiate into erythrocytes in the blood. In patients who are anaemic with a fully functional bone marrow with elevated EPO stimulation, the bone marrow would be producing erythrocytes at a high rate. Many of these would be reticulocytes. This would lead to a greater proportion of the red blood cells being reticulocytes.

No reticulocytosis in the setting of a normocytic anaemia suggests impaired bone marrow function, which could be due to inadequate EPO stimulation.

2 Kidneys excrete excess H^+ through Na/H exchangers, which use the Na^+ concentration gradient to extrude H^+ into the tubular lumen, and H^+ pumps, which use energy to pump H^+ against the concentration gradient into the lumen. H/K pumps are found in the intercalated cells of the collecting tubules and also contribute to acid extrusion.

In severe chronic kidney disease, the flow rate of tubular fluid is low, so there is time for H^+ to increase in the tubular lumen as H^+ gets excreted. This means the concentration gradient is against H^+ secretion to a greater degree. This slows down H^+ extrusion in the kidney.

Additionally, western diets lead to excess H^+ production in the body due to the composition of amino acids consumed. Excess H^+ in the blood and extracellular fluid will titrate the basic HCO_3^- ions to form CO_2 and H_2O, with the CO_2 being excreted in the lungs. This leads to a decrease in the concentration of HCO_3^- ions.

3 HbA1c (%) refers to the percentage of haemoglobin that is present as glycated haemoglobin. Glycated haemoglobin is a form of haemoglobin that is covalently bonded to glucose. This reaction is spontaneous, but slow. However, the higher the concentration of glucose, the faster the reaction.

The usual lifespan of red blood cells is approximately 3 months. Therefore, a HbA1c level gives an index as to the level of glycaemic control over the past 3 months.

4 Vitamin D_3 is involved in calcium balance. There are three forms of vitamin D, only one of which is significantly biologically active. In the skin (at the epidermis) there are ample amounts of a type of cholesterol derivative called 7-dehydrocholesterol. In the presence of UV light, this chemical is converted into an inactive form of vitamin D_3 called cholecalciferol. This is also the form in which vitamin D_3 supplements are given.

The liver converts cholecalciferol to calcidiol by adding a hydroxy (OH) group, a slightly more active form of vitamin D_3, but nonetheless relatively negligible. Calcidiol is known as $25(OH)D_3$, denoting one extra OH group compared to cholecalciferol. When patients' vitamin D levels are checked, it is actually the concentration of calcidiol that is measured. Note that in this patient the calcidiol levels are relatively normal.

The proximal tubular cells in the kidney convert calcidiol to the biologically active calcitriol, by adding yet another hydroxy (OH) group. Note the use of '-diol' and '-triol' as affixes, with the 'ol' denoting the hydroxyl group. Calcitriol is the form of vitamin D_3 that is involved in calcium balance. Vitamin D_3 increases Ca^{2+} absorption in the small bowel and promotes Ca^{2+} reabsorption at the distal tubule in concert with PTH, increasing serum calcium.

The impaired calcitriol production (from calcidiol) in the kidney is what is responsible for the tendency towards hypocalcaemia in patients with CKD.

Additionally, in severe CKD, serum phosphate increases. Most phosphate is absorbed in the proximal tubule, and phosphate reabsorption in the proximal tubule is dependent on a tubular maximum phenomenon. This is where the proximal tubule can reabsorb a maximum of a particular amount of filtered load, and the rest of the phosphate moves past the proximal tubule. This rise in serum phosphate is mitigated by an increase in PTH production (in response to the high phosphate and low calcium), an increase in the tubular maximum mechanism causing a lower fraction of reabsorption of the higher filtered load of phosphate (constant amount of phosphate reabsorbed), and other mechanisms.

The persistent increase in PTH production leads to increased osteoclastic activity in all bones, leading to renal bone disease and higher risk of fractures.

5 At the steady state, the rate of creatinine excretion should be equal to the rate of creatinine production in the body. Between individuals, the rate of creatinine production has relatively minimal variation (although, for example, the amount of creatinine produced by an elderly woman with low muscle mass would be lower than that produced by a young man with high muscle mass).

Importantly, the rate of creatinine excretion should be independent of the rate of urine volume production. We can therefore use the rate of creatinine excretion as an 'index' as to the rate of the excretion of other substances, given that the rate of creatinine excretion has minimal variation between individuals.

Hence, if a substance has a low rate of excretion, its concentration in the urine compared to that of creatinine would be significantly lower, compared to if the substance has a high rate of excretion. In the latter case, the concentration of the substance in the urine would be higher (in comparison to creatinine).

In the example of the rate of protein excretion, we can measure a urinary protein/creatinine ratio. Here, for a sample of urine, we can compare the amount of protein and the amount of creatinine. The higher the rate of protein excretion compared to that of creatinine, the higher the urinary protein/creatinine ratio.

Thus, we can use the urinary protein/creatinine ratio as an approximation to the rate of urinary protein excretion in grams of protein per day.

As it turns out, if the urinary protein creatinine ratio was measured in g/g, and the rate of protein excretion was

measured in g per day, the numerical values of these would be very close to one another.

In this patient, the urinary protein/creatinine ratio is 1.1g/g; this means that in a sample of urine, there is 1.1g of protein for every 1g of creatinine. Hence, a reasonable approximation to the urinary protein excretion rate would be 1.1 g per day. This amounts to significant proteinuria (not necessarily nephrotic-range proteinuria). Proteinuria can be nephrotoxic and therefore should be controlled through medications that can minimise proteinuria, including ACE inhibitors.

Management

Short-term

To treat the renal bone disease, start **calcium carbonate** [1] 600mg tds with meals and a low dose of **calcitriol 0.25mcg daily** [2].

Start darbepoetin alfa (Aranesp) 40mcg weekly subcutaneously for anaemia.

Increase perindopril to 5mg daily and add **metoprolol** [3] 25mg bd.

Instruct GP to increase Lantus if deemed appropriate.

Commence **sodium bicarbonate** [4] 840mg daily.

Long-term

The patient should be reviewed regularly (for example, at 6-monthly intervals).

The following parameters should be monitored:

- Blood pressure: aim for a BP of **125/75mmHg** [5]
- **Postural blood pressure** [6]
- Haemoglobin: aim for **Hb 100–115** [7], but **no higher than 115** [8]
- HbA1c <7%
- Potassium <6mM
- HCO_3^- >22mM
- Calcium, phosphate, PTH within normal limits

A discussion with the patient should be had about the possibility of renal replacement therapy (namely **haemodialysis and peritoneal dialysis** [9]) in the long term, should the need arise.

[1] Calcium carbonate ($CaCO_3$) is an insoluble precipitate that acts as both a source of dietary calcium and as a phosphate binder. The latter is, counterintuitively, the primary function of calcium carbonate.

In the presence of hydrochloric acid, the Ca^{2+} ions from the $CaCO_3$ are liberated into solution; the $CaCO_3$ reacts with H^+ in the stomach acid to form free Ca^{2+} ions and H_2O, with the CO_2 produced likely being burped out, or converted to HCO_3^- ions in the small bowel at the pH ~8 environment.

When dietary phosphate is ingested, it is present primarily as phosphoric acid (H_3PO_4) or superphosphate ($H_2PO_4^-$) ions in the relatively acidic environment of the stomach. Superphosphate can coexist with Ca^{2+} to a great extent in solution.

In the small bowel, however, where the pH increases to approximately 8 owing to the secretion of HCO_3^- ions by the pancreas, the phosphoric acid and superphosphate deprotonate to form predominantly the hydrogen phosphate (HPO_4^{2-}) ion. This ion readily forms a precipitate with Ca^{2+} (unlike superphosphate). Therefore, the HPO_4^{2-} form of the phosphate will readily be bound with Ca^{2+} in a $CaHPO_4$ precipitate and be excreted. Therefore, the amount of free

phosphate ions in the small bowel will be minimised and the amount of phosphate absorbed in the small bowel will be minimised.

The aim is to decrease the serum phosphate in the blood. This will minimise the secretion of PTH from the parathyroid glands and minimise the osteoclastic activity in the bones, minimising the renal bone disease.

The remaining calcium (that does not bind to phosphate) can be part of the dietary calcium intake. Note that only about 30% of calcium gets absorbed in healthy people, and this is modulated to a great extent by calcitriol (activated vitamin D_3). Therefore, serum calcium levels would be optimised by an increase in the blood calcitriol levels.

[2] In most patients, vitamin D is given as cholecalciferol. This is given in patients who have vitamin D deficiency. Cholecalciferol has a half-life of approximately 50 days.

In patients with severe CKD, the kidneys' ability to convert cholecalciferol to the active calcitriol is significantly impaired. Therefore, giving cholecalciferol to increase plasma calcium will likely be ineffective.

Hence, such patients will be given calcitriol instead. It is interesting to note that the effects of calcitriol are likely to be short-lived and dependent on ongoing supplementation; calcitriol has a half-life of approximately 5 hours (compared to 50 days).

The calcitriol here is given to treat the hypocalcaemia.

3 Metoprolol is a beta blocker that has relative selectivity to beta-1 receptors.

Beta-1 receptors are found in the myocardium, the cardiac pacemaker cells and also in the juxtaglomerular cells that produce renin. Beta-1 adrenergic stimulation increases cardiac contractility, increases the heart rate and induces renin production.

Beta blockers will therefore weaken cardiac contractility, slow the heart rate and inhibit the renin–angiotensin–aldosterone axis. All of these mechanisms will serve to lower the arterial blood pressure.

4 A necessary condition for the development of metabolic acidosis in patients with CKD is the consumption of dietary products that will lead to a net production of acid.

Therefore, the oral administration of sodium bicarbonate ($NaHCO_3$) will provide oral HCO_3^- (which is a base), that may minimise the net production of acid and minimise acidaemia. We have to be careful here, though, because the greater the amount of Na^+ ions in the body, the greater the degree of extracellular volume expansion and the propensity towards volume overload. Given that $NaHCO_3$ contains Na^+ ions, this can increase the risk of volume overload.

5 In patients with CKD with proteinuria greater than 1g per day, the BP target is 125/75 (assuming no competing factors such as a high falls risk). Lower systemic blood pressure reduces the degree of proteinuria, likely through decreasing glomerular hydrostatic pressure and hence decreasing convective filtration of protein through the glomerular filtration barrier. A lower systemic blood pressure also decreases the degree of hypertensive renal damage, which can cause further defects in the glomerular filtration barrier, which would worsen the proteinuria.

6 Postural blood pressure is an important parameter to measure, particularly in patients who are approaching old age and are predisposed to falls (due to multiple factors including age-related proprioceptive sensory loss in the lower limbs). This is because postural blood pressure decrease is a well-known cause of presyncope and hence falls.

When a patient assumes an upright position, venous blood redistributes from the large central veins to the lower limbs and splanchnic venous circulation. This occurs because veins are capacitance vessels. Veins have a thin wall, and are usually partially collapsed (with an oval cross-shape). When blood enters a particular segment of vein, the vein can fill and 'open', losing its partially collapsed state and adopting a 'full' state (with a circular cross-shape). Note that the expansion of volume is not associated with wall stretch; incidentally, the actual wall of the vein is an inelastic structure unlike arteries; this is because the vein wall has minimal amounts of the elastic material elastin.

With the redistribution of venous blood away from the central veins and into the splanchnic and lower limb venous circulation, the venous return decreases, which, through the Frank–Starling mechanism, decreases the left ventricular systolic pressure generated and hence decreases the arterial blood pressure. The baroreceptor reflex causes arteriolar vasoconstriction, increased HR and cardiac contractility, and venoconstriction; the latter increases the venous return. The result is that arterial blood pressure reduces only minimally, with a minimal increase in heart rate.

If the patient already has a low volume in the venous circulation (e.g. due to overdiuresis) and/or impaired ability to vasoconstrict (e.g. due to ACEi or other antihypertensives), the decrease in venous return would be so great that even the baroreceptor reflex would not be sufficient to compensate. This would lead to a significant postural BP drop associated with a significant increase in heart rate. However, if the patient has cardiac denervation due to autonomic neuropathy (e.g. from type 2 diabetes, which the patient has), and hence has an impaired baroreceptor reflex, a postural BP drop would occur with minimal changes to heart rate.

7 The aim of keeping Hb high is to maximise oxygen delivery to the tissues. Molecular oxygen is poorly soluble in water, but is highly soluble in blood due to its ability to bind to haemoglobin. The maximum amount of oxygen that can be carried by a particular volume of blood is determined by the haemoglobin concentration.

The equation for the delivery of oxygen is as follows:

$$dO_2 = CO \times [Hb] \times SaO_2 \ (\%) \times 1.39 + CO \times p_aO_2 \times 0.03$$

- CO is the cardiac output (in L/min)
- [Hb] is the concentration of haemoglobin in the blood (in g/dl)
- SaO_2 is the oxygen saturation (from 0 to 100%)
- 1.39 is a correction factor, referring to how much oxygen a particular amount of haemoglobin can carry
- p_aO_2 is the concentration of O_2 dissolved in the plasma (in mmHg)
- 0.03 is a correction factor, referring to how much oxygen a particular volume of plasma can dissolve.

This gives the equivalent volume (in standard laboratory conditions) of O_2 delivered to the tissues per unit time; the unit here is ml/min.

The first term refers to the volume of oxygen bound to haemoglobin that is delivered, whereas the second term refers to the volume of oxygen dissolved in plasma that is delivered. Predictably, the numerical value of the second term is negligible.

The numerical value of [Hb] is highly variable (can vary from 50 in the most severe cases of anaemia to 170+ in those with polycythaemia). The numerical value of SaO_2 would usually vary between 70% and 100%, and the CO would vary between 3–5L/min. Thus, often, the delivery of oxygen can be increased significantly in anaemic patients by correcting the anaemia.

8 Excessively raising the concentration of haemoglobin via increasing the red blood cell count (and haematocrit) causes blood to be more viscous (thicker, having increased intrinsic resistance to flow). This increases the risk of arterial and venous thrombosis through multiple mechanisms.

9 Both haemodialysis and peritoneal dialysis are mechanisms of filtering solutes out of the blood via diffusion across a semipermeable membrane – haemodialysis uses a synthetic membrane in the dialyser, whereas peritoneal dialysis uses the visceral and parietal peritoneum (which, as a serous membrane, forms a semipermeable membrane). Solute filtration is essential for multiple reasons; adequate removal of Na^+ is essential to prevent excessive extracellular volume expansion, adequate removal of K^+ is essential to prevent life-threatening hyperkalaemia, adequate removal of phosphate is essential to prevent secondary hyperparathyroidism, and adequate removal of H_3O^+ ions is essential to prevent acidosis. Additionally, many compounds are produced in multiple biochemical reactions (e.g. guanidine-based compounds, phenols, beta-2 microglobulin) that are normally renally excreted, and are collectively toxic to multiple organs and tissues, including peripheral nerves, the brain and the heart. These are collectively known as uraemic toxins and can be removed through dialysis.

CASE 73: Dialysis-related hypotension

History

- A 65-year-old male has end-stage kidney disease secondary to diabetic nephropathy. He undergoes outpatient haemodialysis on Mondays, Wednesdays and Fridays through a left brachiocephalic arteriovenous fistula. He has residual renal function and is still making urine.
- His comorbidities include hypertension, T2DM on insulin and ischaemic heart disease which is currently medically managed.
- His medications include aspirin 100mg daily, metoprolol 75mg bd, perindopril 5mg daily, **furosemide 80mg daily** [1], lercanidipine 10mg mane, isosorbide mononitrate 30mg daily and nicorandil 5mg daily, as well as a basal-bolus regimen of insulin.
- An hour into one of his dialysis sessions, he becomes light-headed and his BP is measured at 95/40mmHg (baseline BP is 160/80). You are asked to evaluate him.
- On questioning, he reports some **light-headedness** [2] and complains of muscle cramping, but denies chest pain, shortness of breath and palpitations. He also denies any respiratory, GI and urinary symptoms.
- He reports having **taken his antihypertensive medications in the morning** [3].

---

[1] Furosemide is a loop diuretic acting at the Na/K/Cl channel, causing increased excretion of Na^+ ions. Given that the amount, in mol, of Na^+ ions in the body is a major determinant of the extracellular fluid volume, furosemide assists in preventing extracellular volume overload.

The dose of furosemide is high (the standard dose is 40mg). This is because furosemide acts by being filtered at the glomerulus, passing into the tubules, and then blocking the Na/K/Cl channel from the tubular side. In end-stage kidney disease, where there are so few nephrons left, higher doses of furosemide are needed to achieve sufficient Na^+ excretion. A much higher percentage of the existing Na/K/Cl channels needs to be blocked, meaning each nephron needs to secrete high amounts of furosemide into the proximal tubules to be delivered to the loop of Henle. This requires high plasma furosemide concentrations.

[2] The feeling of 'light-headedness' is one of a transiently decreased conscious state, and is due to mildly insufficient cerebral blood flow.

[3] The patient is on multiple medications with an antihypertensive effect, increasing the degree of hypotension. Metoprolol is a beta blocker (selective to the beta-1 receptor). Beta-1 receptors are found in the myocardium, promoting contractility, and are found in the pacemaker cells, promoting a faster heart rate. Hence, metoprolol can lower blood pressure by reducing cardiac contractility.

Perindopril is an ACEi, inhibiting the production of angiotensin II. Angiotensin II binds to its receptors in the arteriolar smooth muscle, causing vasoconstriction and increasing arterial blood pressure. Angiotensin II also stimulates aldosterone production; aldosterone promotes Na^+ retention and hence a high extracellular fluid (ECF) volume. Hence, by lowering the ECF volume (hence lowering venous return) and by preventing vasoconstriction, perindopril lowers blood pressure.

Lercanidipine is a dihydropyridine CCB. This class of drugs is selective to calcium channels found on vascular smooth muscle cells. Smooth muscle cells are largely dependent on calcium influx from the ECF into the cytosol for contraction. Since lercanidipine inhibits entry of calcium via these channels, vascular smooth muscle cells cannot contract as much, arterioles constrict less, leading to a lower blood pressure.

Isosorbide mononitrate and nicorandil are both nitrates. In this patient, they are anti-anginal drugs (that happen to have an antihypertensive effect). These drugs are metabolised in the body via a number of mechanisms to produce nitric oxide (NO) as one of the products. Nitric oxide is a very potent vasodilator and venodilator, crossing cell membranes freely and activating guanylyl cyclase, increasing cyclic GMP production within these cells, leading to vascular smooth muscle cell relaxation. The venodilation reduces the mean systemic filling pressure, preload and hence left ventricular systolic pressure. This, along with the arteriolar vasodilation, significantly reduces blood pressure.

Examination

- On examination, the patient looks well, **alert and oriented to time and place** [1].
- **BP is 95/40mmHg** [2] with **HR 60bpm** [3] and he is afebrile and SaO$_2$ is 96% on air.
- His **'dry weight'** [4] is deemed to be **75.2kg** [4]; prior to dialysis today his weight is **77.1kg** [4].
- He is connected to the dialysis apparatus through two cannulas into his left-sided arteriovenous fistula. His **ultrafiltration rate is 375ml/hour** [5] and the

aim is to have **1.5L of fluid removed** [5] based on the settings of the dialysis machine.
- **Peripheries are warm with good capillary refill** [6].
- **JVP is raised at +5cm** [7] above the sternal notch.
- There are minimal bibasal crackles to auscultation. Heart sounds are dual with nil murmurs, abdomen is soft and non-tender, and there is **minimal peripheral oedema** [8].

---

[1] Alertness and orientation to time and place, in the setting of hypotension, are a sign that the degree of cerebral perfusion is sufficient to maintain conscious state. This is dependent on the cerebral perfusion pressure, which is equal to the difference between mean arterial pressure and the intracranial pressure.

[2] Dialysis causes a potent reduction in blood pressure by introducing a parallel circuit of blood flow; this circuit starts at the AV fistula (where the first cannula introduces blood to the dialyser) and ends at the AV fistula at a site closer to the heart (where the second cannula returns dialysed blood to the body). This parallel circuit reduces total peripheral resistance, just as introduction of a parallel electrical circuit reduces the total resistance of that circuit. A reduction in the total peripheral resistance tends to decrease the arterial blood pressure.

Additionally, dialysis removes fluid from the plasma, decreasing venous return. If the rate of filtration of salt water is high, the plasma volume may contract too quickly before the redistribution of interstitial fluid into the plasma can occur to a significant extent. This potent decrease in venous return causes the left ventricle to contract less vigorously, generating a lower arterial blood pressure.

[3] It is of note that the HR is low–normal, despite the significant drop in BP. One would expect the baroreceptor reflex to be highly active and increase the heart rate. However, in this patient, the heart rate does not increase, for the following reasons:

- the patient is elderly – the SA nodes of the elderly are thought to have a lower responsiveness to beta-1 receptor stimulation, although this notion has been challenged
- the patient is on beta blockers – these drugs inhibit beta-1 receptor stimulation in the SA node
- the patient may have autonomic diabetic neuropathy, hence sympathetic stimulation to the heart may be compromised.

Such patients are highly prone to hypotension.

[4] The density of water is approximately 1.00g/ml. This means that 1L of water weighs approximately 1kg.
Over days, the amount of water in the body can rapidly

fluctuate (given the impaired ability to regulate ECF volume in this patient). In contrast, the mass of fat and muscle changes relatively slowly, with apparent changes to weight being seen over a period of weeks to months, rather than days.
Hence, if a patient's weight decreases from 77 to 76kg within a day, it can be assumed that 1kg of salt water was lost (which has a volume of approximately 1L).
The 'dry weight' is a theoretical weight at which the patient is deemed to be clinically euvolaemic, and this weight is targeted when the patient is on dialysis. The patient is 1.9kg over his dry weight, so it is assumed that the patient has an ECF expansion of approximately 1.9L beyond euvolaemia.

[5] The ultrafiltration rate is the rate at which water is removed from the plasma. As mentioned previously, if this ultrafiltration rate is high, the plasma volume can contract quite precipitously before the interstitial fluid can redistribute into the plasma, causing a decrease in venous return and hypotension.
A removal of 1.5L of isotonic fluid from the ECF should correspond to an approximate decrease of 1.5kg of weight, putting the patient's weight at 75.6kg, just above the 'dry weight'. However, given that this is being removed from the plasma, most of this fluid would be removed from the plasma rather than from the interstitial fluid. Hypothetically, if there were no redistribution of water from the interstitial fluid into the plasma over the 4-hour dialysis session (which is manifestly untrue), then the plasma volume would contract from ~3L (assuming blood volume of 5L and haematocrit of 0.40) to ~1.5L, which is half the plasma volume! This underscores the significance of rapid removal of salt and water from the plasma causing hypotension through decreased venous return.

[6] Warm peripheries indicate that blood flow to the peripheral skin is sufficient to deliver heat (blood is significantly warmer than the outside air, usually). A good capillary refill suggests the same thing.
This indicates that despite the hypotension, there is sufficient blood flow to the extremities (which, in this patient, could be mediated by the lercanidipine!) and reduces the possibility that the patient is in shock.

7 The JVP is a reflection of the right atrial pressure. A high JVP (and right atrial pressure) is consistent with a circulating volume that is high enough to cause a high venous pressure. In this patient, the modestly high JVP of +5cm may be due to a degree of right heart failure (given the history of ischaemic heart disease), and that in this patient, a low plasma volume is associated with a JVP of +5cm, whereas a high plasma volume and mean systemic filling pressure could be associated with a JVP of +10cm.

8 The minimal pedal oedema suggests a normal volume of interstitial extracellular fluid. This provides evidence that the patient could, indeed, be clinically euvolaemic.

Investigations

Serum biochemistry results are shown below (all results are in mmol/L unless stated otherwise):

	2 days ago (post dialysis)	Today (prior to dialysis)
[Na+] [1]	137	132
[K+] [2]	3.9	5.8
[Cl−]	98	94
[HCO3−] [3]	24	22
Urea [4]	24.9	39.1
Creatinine [5] (μmol/L)	630	802
eGFR [6] (ml/min/1.73m²)	8	6

1 Persistent volume overload is a continuous problem for patients with CKD, as sodium retention worsens as kidney function deteriorates. Volume overload can lead to refractory hypertension and recurring hospital admission for congestive heart failure. It is important to use diuretics to correct volume overload in patients with low eGFR.

2 Severe hyperkalaemia is an indication for urgent dialysis (K+ >6.5) or rapidly rising potassium levels + symptoms/ECG changes. Other indications include refractory fluid overload, signs of uraemia, severe metabolic acidosis and certain drug/alcohol intoxications.

3 Severe metabolic acidosis (pH <7.2) is an indication for urgent dialysis, as mentioned before. Dialysis should be considered if a patient still has metabolic acidosis despite optimal medical management, e.g. IV bicarbonate therapy, or if IV sodium bicarbonate cannot be administered due to volume overload.

4 As mentioned previously, uraemia is a strong indication for urgent dialysis and may need to be implemented sooner than usual if a patient presents with clinical symptoms of uraemia. This is less likely, however, if patients are compliant with their treatment.

5 Creatinine is normally elevated in patients with CKD and is a sign of impairment of renal excretion.

6 Dialysis is normally not started on CKD patients unless eGFR is between 5 and 15ml/min/1.73m² + signs/symptoms that could be end-stage kidney disease or eGFR <5ml/min/1.73m². It is advisable to pursue medical therapy if eGFR >15ml/min/1.73m².

Management

Immediate/short-term

Give a bolus of 250ml of IV 0.9% NaCl [1] and reassess blood pressure.

Decrease the ultrafiltration rate and have a lower target for fluid removal, and reassess.

Withhold evening doses of antihypertensive medications.

If the patient's BP does not improve, then consider other diagnoses such as a myocardial infarction or **sepsis** [2] and perform an ECG and take blood cultures accordingly.

Long-term

Minimise salt (Na⁺) intake [3] between dialysis sessions. For future dialysis sessions:

- withhold morning doses of antihypertensive medication on dialysis days
- consider increasing the target 'dry weight'
- instruct the patient to **minimise food intake** [4] during dialysis.

[1] Commencement of isotonic IV fluids (which will remain in the extracellular compartment) aims to increase the mean systemic filling pressure of the circulation and hence the preload of the heart. This would increase the ventricular systolic pressure generated in systole and increase arterial blood pressure (transiently).

However, note that of the 250ml of isotonic fluid reinfused to the patient, only about a quarter of the fluid (~60ml) will remain in the plasma after redistribution.

[2] Sepsis is an inappropriate immune response to infection (bacterial, viral or fungal) that causes impaired function of multiple organs and, at its most severe, multi-organ failure. The vast quantities of inflammatory cytokines produced during the inflammatory response to severe infection can cause this impaired organ function. One effect of these cytokines is vasoplegia (impaired ability of the arterioles to constrict) and increased capillary endothelial permeability. The vasoplegia causes a high capillary hydrostatic pressure and this, along with the increased capillary endothelial permeability, causes increased ultrafiltration of fluid into the interstitium (via convection).

This arteriolar dilation and decreased plasma volume (and hence decreased venous return) can cause profound hypotension.

[3] The amount, in mol, of Na⁺ ions in the body will determine the volume of the extracellular compartment. This is because most of the Na⁺ ions remain in the extracellular compartment due to the ubiquitous Na/K exchanger found in all cells extruding most of the Na⁺ that enters cells. Water will be retained with any excess Na⁺ ions in keeping with osmosis, maintaining an approximate concentration of Na⁺ of ~140mM usually.

In patients with end-stage renal disease (ESRD), the ability to excrete Na⁺ ions is severely reduced (without dialysis). Therefore, to prevent an accumulation of Na⁺ ions and hence an extracellular compartment volume expansion (and its associated pulmonary and peripheral oedema), the intake of Na⁺ ions must remain low.

[4] Oral intake of food, particularly food that is high in carbohydrates, causes significant arteriolar dilation of the splanchnic circulation. This causes a significantly decreased total peripheral resistance and hence hypotension.

During dialysis, the total peripheral resistance is already reduced due to the extracorporeal parallel circuit; splanchnic vasodilation will further decrease the total peripheral resistance, accentuating the dialysis-mediated hypotensive response.

CASE 74:   Hyperkalaemia

History

- A 70-year-old lady with end-stage renal disease (ESRD), on regular haemodialysis, was brought in by ambulance to the ED with severe drowsiness.
- On arrival to ED, she was severely hypotensive and bradycardic with a BP of 85/40mmHg and HR 36bpm.
- She underwent haemodialysis the day prior, but only completed 1 hour of her usual 4-hour session due to being unable to tolerate the **headaches, nausea/vomiting and muscle cramping** [1]; this dialysis session was particularly aggressive, with an attempt to remove large volumes of fluid over a short period of time as she had missed a dialysis session prior to this.
- She is known to have relatively little health literacy and does not adhere to the **low potassium diet** [2] she has been prescribed.
- She has ESRD and is completely dependent on haemodialysis, and does not have any residual urine output. Her medical comorbidities include **type 2 diabetes** [3], hypertension and ischaemic heart disease. She is on metoprolol 75mg bd, moxonidine 400mg mane, Lantus (insulin glargine) and NovoRapid (insulin aspart) tds.

[1] Headaches and nausea/vomiting are non-specific symptoms that are common in dialysis. A possible cause of this, particularly where the dialysis is 'aggressive' and there is rapid small solute removal, is dialysis disequilibrium syndrome.

Cell membranes are generally permeable to urea; however, urea crosses cell membranes rather slowly, and equilibration of urea across cell membranes after dialysis takes hours. If a cell bathed in a high urea concentration solution (with urea equilibrated inside and outside the cell) were removed and hypothetically placed in a low urea concentration solution, a series of events would likely occur:

- the urea inside the cell would remain inside the cell in the immediate term
- water would diffuse by osmosis into the cell from the ECF, expanding the cell volume transiently
- over time, as the urea diffuses slowly out of the cell (over hours), the osmosis of water into the cell would slow, and then reverse direction, until the cell size returns to normal.

An analogous process occurs in the brain, where the blood and ECF are rapidly cleared of urea. This causes a transient cerebral oedema (which can potentially be mild to life-threatening). The mild cerebral oedema can cause headaches, with some nausea and vomiting. However, in severe cases, this can lead to coma and death.

This phenomenon highlights the fact that some solutes can be effective osmoles (cannot permeate cell membranes), ineffective osmoles (can permeate cell membranes immediately), or 'ineffective osmoles' that transiently work as effective osmoles (can permeate cell membranes slowly – during the equilibration period, these osmoles work as effective osmoles). Urea belongs to the latter group.

[2] Some foods are high in potassium ions, including bananas (most famously), some fruits, beans and other legumes. Patients with ESRD can only remove K^+ from the body through dialysis (although a small amount of K^+ can be excreted through the faeces). Therefore, a low potassium diet is important to avoid accumulation of K^+ ions in the body, risking hyperkalaemia.

[3] When K^+ ions are absorbed from the gut into the blood through food, massive hyperkalaemia is avoided due to immediate sequestration of K^+ into the cells via the Na/K pumps present in all cells. This Na/K activity is enhanced by the activity of insulin on skeletal muscle; patients with T2DM and insulin resistance have a greater tendency to develop hyperkalaemia.

Examination

- On examination, the patient is **drowsy, uncooperative and not oriented to time and place** [1].
- Her weight is **82kg** [2], with the weight a week ago being 78kg.
- There is **extensive bruising** [3] of both her arms with **excoriations** [4] visible.
- There is an arteriovenous fistula visible on her left arm, with an **extremely large tortuous vein** [5] visible. This has a palpable thrill that is pulsatile.

- JVP is raised at +10cm vertically from the sternal notch. There are **bibasal crepitations** [6] to auscultation extending up to the mid-zone on chest examination.
- Abdomen is soft and non-tender.
- There is significant **bilateral pitting oedema** [7] up to the knees, with associated **brown-shadowing** [8] of the calves and surrounding erythema.

[1] These symptoms, in this patient, are likely due to decreased cerebral perfusion pressure (CPP). Blood vessels in the brain are able to autoregulate cerebral blood flow relative to demand; however, this mechanism can be overwhelmed in the setting of severely decreased cerebral perfusion pressure.

CPP = mean arterial pressure – intracranial pressure

The intracranial pressure in this patient is very likely to be normal. However, BP is 85/40mmHg (with the mean arterial pressure being approximately 55mmHg, which is very low and unlikely to sustain adequate cerebral perfusion).

[2] Weight changes in the short term will be almost entirely due to changes to the mass of water in the body. This is because changes in body mass due to muscle hypertrophy, or excess fat accumulation, take time to occur.
Hence, short-term weight changes do provide a very useful mechanism of assessing increased water retention.
This patient is likely to have gained an extra 4kg of water, most of it in the ECF. The density of water is approximately 1kg/L (1L of water weighs approximately 1kg). Therefore, 4kg of weight gain is approximately equal to 4L of fluid retained. Patients on dialysis who do not produce urine have very limited means of excreting salt water – they are dependent on adequate dialysis for this purpose.

[3] End-stage renal disease inhibits platelet function (not platelet count) and predisposes patients to abnormal bleeding.

[4] Multiple compounds are produced in the body and are normally excreted renally; however, these compounds accumulate in ESRD. These are known as uraemic toxins. Some of these toxins are highly irritating to the skin and cause pruritus.

[5] The presence of an arteriovenous fistula in the left arm diverts some of the arterial blood directly into a superficial vein. For example, a left brachiocephalic fistula diverts blood from the left brachial artery to the left cephalic vein, a superficial vein on the left arm.
The pressure of blood in the brachial artery, in a normal individual, would range from 80–120mmHg. The blood pressure in the cephalic vein would normally be in the vicinity

of 20mmHg. However, in the presence of a fistula connecting these blood vessels, the pressure in the cephalic vein would increase to the vicinity of 60mmHg.
The vein is a thin structure that is unable to withstand such high pressures. The wall tension generated also causes the cells in the vein wall to further degrade the vein wall, causing further structural damage. The vein is not an elastic structure, and therefore would dilate significantly as the vein wall is chronically stretched. This leads to the cephalic vein becoming very large, tortuous and therefore easy to access using large haemodialysis cannulas.

[6] Pulmonary interstitial oedema causes an increased number of alveoli that collapse on expiration, and that open only on inspiration with adequate 'pulling' of the alveolar wall by the chest wall expanding the lung volume.
On inspiration, as the patient inhales and the lung volume expands, the collapsed alveoli suddenly open, causing sounds known as crepitations.
Distortion of the pulmonary interstitium, including fibrosis, consolidation (due to infection) or fluid, can all cause crepitations to be heard on auscultation.

[7] Fluid retention (given the patient is anuric) leads to an increased venous blood pressure, and hence an increased capillary hydrostatic pressure. This causes increased transudation of fluid (via convection) from the capillaries into the interstitium, causing oedema. This effect is more pronounced in the lower limbs in ambulant patients, due to the effect of gravity.

[8] Sustained high venous pressure causes damage to the vein walls, and this damage allows small amounts of red blood cells to escape into the interstitium. The haemoglobin in the extravasated red blood cells gets converted to the brown pigment called haemosiderin.

Investigations

Urgent blood results show:

Hb (x 10^9/L)	8.9		Cl^- (mM)	98
WCC (x 10^9/L)	7.1		HCO_3^- (mM)	14 [2]
Platelets (x 10^9/L)	210		Ur (mM)	41.0 [3]
Na^+ (mM)	132		Cr (µM)	811 [4]
K^+ (mM)	9.1 [1]		eGFR (ml/min/1.73m²)	5 [5]

The **ECG** [6] is shown below:

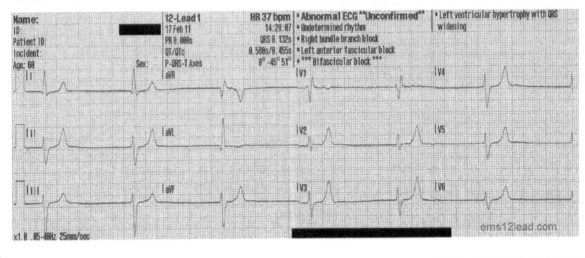

[1] ESRD is invariably associated with hyperkalaemia. Potassium is excreted primarily through the collecting tubules, through epithelial K^+ channels on the principal cells lining the collecting tubules. K^+ flows down its concentration gradient from the principal cell (concentration of K^+ intracellularly is approximately 150mmol/L) to the tubular lumen. Most nephrons are obliterated in ESRD; there are not sufficient nephrons to excrete sufficient amounts of K^+ to offset the amount of K^+ ingested. This invariably leads to hyperkalaemia.

[2] Hyperkalaemia and metabolic acidosis are highly interrelated; the presence of one begets the other. Most cells in the body have a series of ion channels/exchangers/pumps on their cell surface that, in the presence of high extracellular H^+, transfers some of the excess H^+ intracellularly in exchange for extrusion of some of their intracellular K^+ ions. Hence, acidosis can cause hyperkalaemia. Hyperkalaemia can induce acidosis by a similar mechanism, as well as through exchange of H^+ and K^+ in the alpha-intercalated cells of the collecting tubule. Additionally, western diets are generally associated with excess acid production in the metabolism of amino acids compared to base production. Hence, in ESRD, where the capacity to excrete H^+ is impaired, patients are prone to metabolic acidosis.

[3] Urea is a product of the metabolism of amino acids that produce ammonia (NH_3), which is combined with HCO_3^- to produce urea. This process occurs in the liver. The urea is primarily excreted through glomerular filtration, and there is some reabsorption. In ESRD, there is going to be constant urea production due to ongoing protein metabolism, and this urea will accumulate in the body.

[4] Creatinine is a metabolite of creatine, a chemical found in muscle. Creatinine is filtered at the glomerulus, and not reabsorbed (although some creatinine is secreted into the tubules). In patients with ESRD, most of the creatinine that is cleared is through dialysis.

[5] This is a number calculated according to what is called the MDRD formula, based on the patient's age, sex and serum creatinine. In this patient, given that she makes no urine, the true GFR is more likely to be 0. The only reason the serum creatinine is 811 (and not trending upwards indefinitely, assuming 811 is a stable value) is because dialysis can filter out creatinine to some degree. Therefore, the eGFR of 5ml/min/1.73m², in the setting of dialysis, is a meaningless number.

This is important in determining the renal function of patients on dialysis. In these cases, the eGFR is a useless number, because it is based on the serum creatinine, and the formula assumes that glomerular filtration is the only mechanism by which creatinine is removed from the body.

6 Hyperkalaemia causes depolarisation of the cardiac pacemaker cell and cardiac myocyte. This puts the patient at risk of both tachyarrhythmias (e.g. VF) and bradyarrhythmias (e.g. asystole). The depolarisation puts the resting membrane potential closer to the threshold potential for both fast and slow Na^+ channels to open and induce phase 0 depolarisation of the cell, and therefore puts the patient at risk of tachyarrhythmias. The mechanism by which hyperkalaemia can increase the risk of bradyarrhythmias is shown below. When a part of the cardiac myocyte sarcolemma (cell membrane) is depolarised, voltage-gated Na^+ channels open, causing a massive influx of Na^+ into the myocyte. This Na^+ diffuses laterally along the myocyte to the next section of sarcolemma that is undepolarised. The Na^+ (being positively charged) depolarises the negatively charged adjacent sarcolemma, causing Na^+ channels at that part to open, causing a chain reaction. This is how an action potential is propagated along a myocyte. The greater the rate of Na^+ influx, the greater the rate of Na^+ diffusion laterally, and the quicker the rate of propagation of the action potential. After voltage-gated Na^+ channels open, they automatically close after a period of time, and are inactivated (cannot open again) until the cell is sufficiently repolarised. In hyperkalaemia, the resting membrane potential is significantly less negative. At some point, the resting membrane potential is not negative enough to allow the Na^+ channels to become de-inactivated (and be available to open again).

Additionally, a high extracellular fluid $[K^+]$ actually changes the permeability of the K^+ channels to K^+ ions; the K^+ channels become even more permeable to K^+ ions when open. As the hyperkalaemia becomes progressively more severe, increasing amounts of sarcolemma will not have sufficient available Na^+ channels to mount and propagate an action potential. Therefore, propagation of the action potential along cardiac myocytes slows down. The effects this has on the ECG are predictable:

- peaked T waves – given the K^+ channels become extremely permeable to K^+ when open in hyperkalaemia, the repolarisation is associated with a very high rate of influx of K^+, and hence a high voltage and peaking of the T waves
- lengthening of the P wave – reflective of the slowed propagation of the action potential along the atria
- lengthening of the QRS complex – reflective of the slowed propagation of the action potential along the ventricles
- flattening of the P wave – the decreased amplitude reflects the decreased amount of Na^+ current (responsible for the voltage generated in the ECG) due to less Na^+ influx into myocytes due to decreased Na^+ permeability
- junctional or ventricular escape rhythms – reflective of complete atrial 'paralysis' – where action potentials cannot propagate along the atria at all due to a lack of available Na^+ channels
- asystole – complete paralysis of the cardiac myocytes.

In this ECG,
- the P waves are not visible
- the QRS complexes are lengthened
- there is some peaking of the T waves.

Management

Urgent administration of:

- **calcium gluconate IV solution** [1]
- **insulin neutral (ActRapid) 10 units + 50ml of 50% dextrose** [2]; multiple boluses may be required
- **IV isoprenaline infusion** [3]
- **Resonium** [4] orally and/or rectally.

The patient should be monitored overnight with regular K^+ levels and arranged for haemodialysis the next morning with a **low potassium dialysate** [5] (at a slow rate).

Withhold **metoprolol** [6] and all other antihypertensives.

1 IV calcium is known to 'stabilise' the sarcolemma and antagonise the effects of hyperkalaemia.

An increase in the extracellular Ca^{2+} concentration has multiple effects on the electrophysiological properties of the sarcolemma. Through an unclear mechanism, a high extracellular Ca^{2+} increases the threshold voltage required for phase 0 depolarisation, which is protective against tachyarrhythmias. It also, through another unclear mechanism, increases the rate of phase 0 depolarisation, which is the direct opposite effect of hyperkalaemia, where Na^+ influx is paralysed from the hyperkalaemia-induced Na^+

channel inactivation. If the rate of phase 0 depolarisation is increased, the rate of lateral diffusion of the cations across the myocyte increases, and hence, the rate of propagation of the action potential increases.

Finally, Ca^{2+} is a major ion that flows inwards in action potentials that occur in the SA and AV node, noting that the slow Na/Ca channels are the sole channels responsible for phase 0 depolarisation in these cells. A high extracellular Ca^{2+} increases the concentration gradient for Ca^{2+} entry, leading to a higher rate of cation influx and propagation of the action potential.

2 Insulin increases the activity of the Na/K pump in skeletal muscle cells, which cause extrusion of Na$^+$ and sequestration of K$^+$ into cells.

Hence, administration of IV insulin can cause a mass shift of K$^+$ from the extracellular fluid into the intracellular fluid, in exchange for Na$^+$, temporarily reversing the hyperkalaemia. Note that insulin does not remove potassium from the body. The glucose is given with the insulin to prevent hypoglycaemia; insulin binds to insulin receptors at skeletal muscle, liver and adipose tissue. One of its effects is to increase the permeability of these cells to glucose.

3 Isoprenaline is a non-selective beta-agonist (beta-1 and beta-2 receptors). Beta-1 receptors are found in the myocardium and in the pacemaker cells. Beta-1 receptor stimulation causes an increase in the resting membrane potential in pacemaker cells, which is already higher than the threshold potential for phase 0 depolarisation. Hence, with beta-1 stimulation, the rate of phase 4 depolarisation in an attempt to reach the higher value of the membrane resting potential would be increased, and threshold voltage would be reached sooner. This causes an increased heart rate, which makes isoprenaline a positive chronotrope.

Isoprenaline is often used as medical treatment for severe bradyarrhythmias for this reason.

Beta-2 receptors are found in many cell types throughout the body, including skeletal muscle. Like insulin receptor stimulation, beta-2 receptor stimulation causes an increase in the activity of the Na/K pumps in skeletal muscle, causing increased sequestration of K$^+$ into cells in exchange for Na$^+$ ions.

Isoprenaline can also be used here to treat hyperkalaemia. In most patients, we use a beta-2 selective agonist (e.g. salbutamol), but in this patient who is also markedly bradycardic, isoprenaline should be used.

4 Resonium is sodium polystyrene sulfonate. This is taken either orally or rectally, and its purpose is to sequester K$^+$ into the GI tract and facilitate K$^+$ extrusion through the gut. The K$^+$ is exchanged for Na$^+$, which is absorbed from the Resonium into the body.

5 The use of a low potassium dialysate increases the concentration gradient between the blood containing a high K$^+$ concentration, and the dialysate, in the dialysis membrane. This increases the rate of diffusion of K$^+$ across the dialysis membrane, and hence the rate of extrusion of K$^+$.

6 Metoprolol is a beta blocker that is selective to beta-1 receptors. It has the opposite effect of isoprenaline on heart rate and cardiac contractility.

CASE 75: Hypokalaemia

History

- A 65-year-old lady who lives at home alone is admitted under General Medicine for **Clostridioides difficile** [1] infection. She had presented with a 3-day history of severe **diarrhoea** [1], with about 6–8 loose bowel motions per day.
- This is not associated with nausea or vomiting, and occurred in the context of a recent episode of a diabetic foot infection for which she had required broad-spectrum antibiotic therapy.

- She has maintained good urine output and appears haemodynamically stable.
- Her comorbidities include congestive cardiac failure secondary to ischaemic heart disease, T2DM and hypertension.
- Her medications include aspirin 100mg daily, atorvastatin 40mg daily, metoprolol 25mg bd, **perindopril 5mg daily** [2], **hydrochlorothiazide 25mg daily** [3], **furosemide 40mg bd** [3], metformin 1g daily and gliclazide MR 60mg daily.

1 Diarrhoea is associated with increased potassium excretion through the faeces, particularly secretory causes including *Clostridioides difficile* infection. In the gut, potassium is mainly secreted in the colon through epithelial K+ channels. The rate of K+ secretion into the colon is increased (through multiple mechanisms) in illnesses that cause diarrhoea, including *C. difficile* infection.

2 Perindopril would be protective against hypokalaemia, in that it tends to cause retention of potassium. This is because it inhibits the production of angiotensin II (through inhibition of angiotensin-converting enzyme). Angiotensin II causes the adrenal gland to increase its production of aldosterone. Aldosterone stimulates principal cells of the collecting tubule of the kidney to increase its permeability to Na+ and K+, and increase the number of Na/K exchangers in the basolateral membrane of these cells. Aldosterone therefore increases the rate of reabsorption of Na+ and rate of secretion of K+ out of and into the collecting duct. Inhibition of aldosterone, therefore, causes retention of K+.

3 Hydrochlorothiazide is a thiazide diuretic that blocks Na/Cl symporters in the distal convoluted tubule of the nephron and impairs Na+ reabsorption at the distal tubule; this increases the amount of Na+ ions that flow through the collecting duct. Furosemide is a loop diuretic that blocks Na/K/Cl symporters in the thick ascending loop of Henle, and impairs Na+ reabsorption at the thick ascending limb of Henle. This, too, increases the amount of Na+ ions that flow through the collecting duct.

Through multiple mechanisms, this natriuresis leads to an increased rate of flow of fluid through the collecting tubules, and increases the concentration of Na+ in this fluid. This has two main effects on K+ at the collecting duct, where K+ is secreted.

The principal cells of the collecting tubules have epithelial K+ and Na+ channels. The concentration of K+ is high inside the cell compared to the tubular lumen, whereas the concentration of Na+ is high in the tubular lumen compared to inside the cell. Therefore, the K+ channels allow diffusion of K+ into the lumen (and hence, secretion) along the concentration gradient, and the Na+ channels allow diffusion of Na+ out of the lumen (and hence, reabsorption) along the concentration gradient.

Two factors can increase the rate of K+ secretion. One factor is the concentration difference of K+ inside the cell and in the tubular lumen. A high flow rate of fluid through the collecting tubule means that any K+ that is secreted is quickly 'flushed away' with its surrounding tubular fluid. This ensures that the [K+] in the lumen is stationary and the [K+] that the unmoving principal cell is exposed to remains low, maintaining this concentration gradient, and therefore increases the rate of K+ secretion.

Another factor that increases the K+ secretion rate is if the fluid in the collecting tubule has a high [Na+] concentration. This increases the concentration gradient of Na+ across the principal cell membrane (at the apical side), increasing the flux of Na+ into the cell. This creates a relatively negative voltage inside the lumen, because we are removing positive charges from the lumen. This negative voltage tends to attract positive charges into the lumen as much as possible. K+ is also positively charged, and therefore, the rate of K+ secretion into the lumen is also increased.

This is why loop and thiazide diuretics both cause hypokalaemia by increasing the excretion of potassium in the urine.

Examination

- On general inspection, the patient looks well.
- BP is 110/85mmHg, **HR 114bpm** [1], SaO$_2$ 98% on air, afebrile.
- Mucous membranes are dry.

- JVP is **not visible with the patient at 30 degrees, but is visible when the patient is lying flat** [2].
- Chest, abdominal and lower limb examination is unremarkable.

1 Tachycardia (assuming in this case the patient has sinus tachycardia) is consistent with hypovolaemia in this particular case. Hypovolaemia, which is a low volume in the extracellular fluid and hence the circulating volume in the blood, causes a low mean systemic filling pressure and hence low venous return to the right heart, and hence low venous return to the left heart. Through the Frank–Starling law, this lowers the strength of contraction of the left ventricle during systole, and hence would normally lower arterial blood pressure. However, blood pressure is regulated by the baroreceptor reflex, whose sensors on the carotid sinus and aortic arch sense a low blood pressure, and through a neurogenic mechanism increases sympathetic stimulation to the sino-atrial node, through noradrenaline as a neurotransmitter binding to beta-1 receptors. This increases the rate of phase 4 depolarisation and hence the heart rate.

2 The position of the JVP within the neck varies with the angle at which the patient is inclined.
The pressure of venous blood in the right atrium is some non-negative number; part of the source of this is the blood in the SVC and its tributaries pushing 'downwards' on the blood in the right atrium due to gravity. Due to the fact that gravity is a vertical force, irrespective of the incline of the patient, the vertical height of the column of blood in the internal jugular vein leading to the right atrium remains constant, irrespective of the incline of the patient.
A patient whose right atrial pressure is low due to hypovolaemia will have a low JVP. If the patient were upright, or even at an angle of 30 degrees, the height of the column of blood may not even reach superior to the clavicle, and therefore will not be visible to the examiner. However, if the patient were made to lie relatively flat, even a low JVP may be visible at the neck, as movement up the neck would correspond to only minimal movement vertically.

Investigations

Routine blood results are shown below:

Hb (x 10⁹/L)	15.6	Cr (µM)	110
WCC (x 10⁹/L)	9.7	eGFR (ml/min/1.73m²)	46
Platelets (x 10⁹/L)	310	Albumin	27
Na⁺ (mM)	**131** [1]		
K⁺ (mM)	2.4		
Cl⁻ (mM)	96		
Ur (mM)	11.4		
HCO₃⁻ (mM)	23		

ECG shows the following:

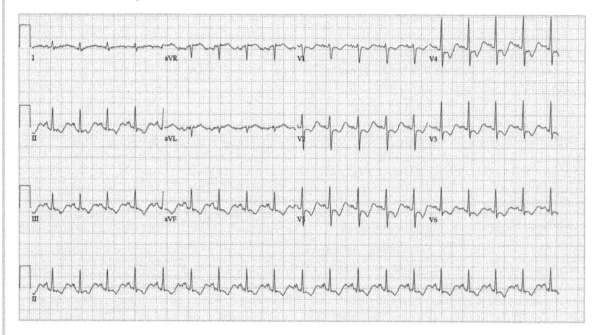

The above ECG shows likely sinus tachycardia (or possible **atrial tachycardia** [2]) with features of hypokalaemia, primarily **T wave inversion with U waves** [3] and **long QT interval** [4] .

However, there is no evidence of **polymorphic ventricular tachyarrhythmias** [2] .

---

1 Hyponatraemia can occur in patients who are hypovolaemic. This is due to the fact that hypovolaemia does cause ADH secretion in the posterior pituitary, irrespective of the plasma osmolality. This causes excessive free water retention at the collecting tubules, causing 'dilution' of the ECF.

The fact the patient is on a thiazide diuretic also predisposes the patient to hyponatraemia.

2 In hypokalaemia low extracellular [K^+] induces arrhythmias by altering the characteristics of the cardiac action potential.

A low extracellular [K^+] causes hyperpolarisation of the cardiac sarcolemma; the sarcolemma is most permeable to K^+ compared to Na^+, Cl^- and other ions. This means that the resting membrane potential will be almost entirely dependent on the relative concentration of [K^+] inside and outside the cardiac myocyte.

However, a low extracellular K^+ paradoxically inhibits the permeability of voltage-gated (not the constitutionally active) potassium channels, through a change in their shape. This means that phase 3 repolarisation is much slower, given the relatively lower capacitance of the cell membrane to potassium at this point. In fact, this repolarisation process can take so long that, by the time the slow voltage-gated Na/Ca channels are de-inactivated, the cell is still not fully repolarised. This increases the risk of these voltage-gated Na/Ca channels activating, causing what is called an early after-depolarisation, with the cell starting to aberrantly depolarise. This can lead to an aberrant action potential, with an ectopic beat. More importantly, it can trigger re-entrant arrhythmias in the atria (e.g. atrial tachycardia) or the ventricles (most notably polymorphic VT).

3 The repolarisation process is delayed in hypokalaemia, but in a heterogeneous manner; different parts of the heart are affected to different extents. This means that the order in which cardiac myocytes repolarise, changes. This leads to characteristic changes in the voltage vector generated from all the individual repolarisation events, which manifests in a change in the direction of the T wave; the T wave initially inverts in many leads, and then becomes normal, forming a U wave.

4 Since the repolarisation process is prolonged, the time between the onset of depolarisation (Q wave) and the end of repolarisation (end of T wave) is prolonged. This leads to a prolonged QT interval.

Management

- Withhold furosemide and hydrochlorothiazide.
- Transfer to a HDU for cardiac monitoring.
- Give a bolus of **250ml of 0.9% NaCl IV** [1], then give a total of 3 bags of **100ml 0.29% NaCl + 10mmol KCl IV** [2] over 3 hours.

- Additional IV K^+ replacement can be given after rechecking plasma K^+; in the interim, a slow infusion of 0.9% NaCl IV can be given.

1 0.9% (w/v) NaCl (normal saline) is approximately isotonic to plasma. Its osmolarity is approximately 30mOsm/L. Administration of 0.9% (w/v) NaCl to a patient would increase the volume of the extracellular fluid without changing the volume of the intracellular fluid.

2 With respect to extracellular fluid volume expansion, administration of 100ml of a mixture of 0.29% (w/v) NaCl + 10mmol KCl is equivalent to giving 100ml of normal saline. These 'minibags' of potassium are also isotonic to plasma. The reason that giving such bags is analogous to giving 100ml of normal saline is because almost all the K^+ ions infused into the ECF would immediately be exchanged for Na^+ ions from inside the cells, owing to the ubiquitous Na/K pumps present in all cells. Hence, the end result is that there is extra water and Na^+ ions in the ECF, amounting to an ECF volume expansion.

However, in most cases, K^+ ions have to be infused slowly to minimise the risk of hyperkalaemia. To illustrate this, the total amount, in millimole, of K^+ ions in the extracellular fluid in this woman (assume she weighs 60kg) is approximately 10L x 2.4mmol/L = 24mmol.

The total amount of K^+ ions in the extracellular fluid is 24mmol, and we are infusing 10mmol extra per hour. Most of this 10mmol will move intracellularly, but if not enough time is provided for that exchange to take place, hyperkalaemia could supervene.

CASE 76: Hyponatraemia

History

- You are an intern in a General Medical unit and are reviewing a 58-year-old man with a Na of **128mmol/L** [1].
- The patient was initially admitted 5 days ago with **community-acquired pneumonia** [2] and had initially been treated with IV benzylpenicillin and oral doxycycline. He is currently on oral amoxycillin and doxycycline and is medically stable.
- He has an active past history of hypertension on **hydrochlorothiazide** [3] and mild gastro-oesophageal reflux disease for which he is on **pantoprazole** [3].

- On review, he denies any **nausea or vomiting, fatigue or confusion** [4].
- His previous plasma sodium levels over the previous few days are as below:
  - 1 day ago   [Na$^+$] = 130
  - 2 days ago   [Na$^+$] = 132
  - 4 days ago   [Na$^+$] = 136

Hyponatraemia is the most common electrolyte disturbance that occurs in hospital inpatients, and it is therefore essential to know how to manage it. Fortunately, the investigation and treatment of hyponatraemia are underpinned by the physiology that you would have learned in your preclinical years.

In simple terms, hyponatraemia is caused by dilution of blood, interstitial fluid and intracellular fluid by excessive water. This can occur due to excessive free water ingestion (e.g. primary polydipsia – where the patient drinks inappropriately excessive amounts of water), or a reduced ability to excrete free water in the kidneys. The main hormone involved is ADH (AVP), also known as antidiuretic hormone (arginine vasopressin). ADH stimulates thirst and causes the cells of the collecting ducts in the kidneys to reabsorb free water (through aquaporin channels), concentrating the urine.

1 In assessing hyponatraemia, make note of the degree of hyponatraemia. A normal plasma [Na$^+$] is in the range 135–145mM. Mild hyponatraemia is 130–134mM, moderate is 120–129mM and severe is <120mM. The patient in this vignette has moderate hyponatraemia.

2 Pneumonias (viral, bacterial or tuberculous) are a known and common mechanism by which non-osmotic ADH secretion occurs. Non-osmotic ADH secretion is the primary mechanism by which hyponatraemia occurs. Commit to memory that lung infections are a cause of SIADH – syndrome of inappropriate ADH secretion.

3 Thiazide diuretics are a common cause of hyponatraemia. I remember seeing a patient who had recently started a thiazide diuretic presenting to hospital with a [Na$^+$] of 114mM! Recall that thiazide diuretics inhibit Na$^+$ reabsorption at the distal tubule (through the Na/Cl channels) and therefore inhibit the osmolality of the urine from decreasing from ~300mOsm/L at the thick ascending limb of the loop of Henle to ~100mOsm/L at the cortical collecting duct from Na$^+$ removal from the tubular fluid (assuming the kidney is not receiving any ADH stimulus). This means that the kidney is not able to dilute the urine sufficiently. Additionally, thiazides can induce some degree of hypovolaemia. Remember that hypovolaemia is also a stimulus for ADH secretion by the posterior pituitary, independent of plasma tonicity. Therefore, we have a combination of urinary dilutional capacity being inhibited by thiazides, and some possible non-osmolar ADH secretion (where ADH secretion increases for a reason other than hypertonicity). Pantoprazole (and other PPIs) are also a known cause of SIADH.

4 Symptomatic hyponatraemia needs urgent treatment. Acute hyponatraemia causes osmosis of water across cell membranes into the intracellular fluid (in osmosis, water diffuses from a hypotonic to a hypertonic solution). This includes intracellular fluid in the neurons in the brain. This causes brain volume expansion, with increasing intracranial pressure (given the brain is encased in a rigid skull). The ICP can progress to the point that the brain is 'squeezed downwards' – the uncus can herniate through the tentorium (flat piece of connective tissue separating the cerebrum from the cerebellum) and press on the midbrain, and the tonsil of the cerebellum can herniate through the foramen magnum and press on the medulla (containing the cardiovascular and respiratory centres), causing cardiorespiratory arrest and death. Symptoms of raised ICP include altered conscious state and nausea/vomiting. Hyponatraemia can also cause seizures.

Examination

- On examination, the patient looks generally well, and is **alert and oriented to time and place** [1].
- His **lying BP is 141/80mmHg and standing BP 135/82, HR 76bpm lying and 80 standing** [2], RR 17 and temperature is 36.5°C, and SaO$_2$ is 97% on air. Pupils are equal and reactive to light.
- He has **warm peripheries and good capillary refill** [3].
- Mucous membranes are moist, and **JVP is visible at 4cm vertically above the sternal notch** [4].
- Chest examination reveals **no bibasal crackles** [5] and heart examination reveals dual heart sounds and nil murmurs.
- The abdomen is soft and non-tender to palpation, and there is **no pedal oedema** [6].

[1] Alertness and orientation are both parameters that assess conscious state. In this setting, decreased conscious state would be due to evolving cerebral oedema that would be minimising cerebral blood flow. Remember the following equation:

CPP = mean arterial pressure – intracranial pressure

This man appears alert and oriented, which suggests that his cerebral perfusion pressure is within normal limits, and therefore the ICP is within normal limits.

[2] Postural blood pressure is a very useful way of determining volume state. Recall that veins are highly collapsible structures and are considered compliant vessels. This is because veins can expand their volume quite significantly, with only a minimal increase in the pressure inside the vein.

When a patient stands up, gravity acts on the venous circulation, causing a downward force on the columns of blood in the veins. This force leads to great venous pressures in the splanchnic and lower limb venous circulations; these veins significantly expand their volume. In this setting, the volume of blood delivered to the right heart significantly drops; in other words, the preload to the right heart drops; the right ventricular output drops, the filling to the left ventricle drops, and hence the left ventricular pressure generated (due to inadequate sarcomere stretching) is lowered. This leads to significantly lowered BP. In patients with an intact baroreceptor reflex and an adequate sympathetic innervation to the heart (which does not apply in patients with severe Parkinson's disease or severe long-standing diabetes mellitus, both of which cause damage to the cardiac sympathetic neurons, among others), the baroreceptor reflex mitigates the significant drop in BP by venoconstriction, arteriolar vasoconstriction and increased cardiac contractility, and causes the heart rate to rise.

In patients who are normovolaemic, the baroreceptor reflex almost completely corrects the drop in blood pressure with only a minimal increase in heart rate. In patients who are significantly hypovolaemic, the initial drop in blood pressure is so great that even the baroreceptor reflex can only partially correct this, and the heart rate is increased significantly. I recall a patient I saw in my internship in the ED who came in with an upper GI bleed, and his lying and standing BP (at 1 minute) was approximately 120/75mmHg and 85/60mmHg, with matched HRs of 100bpm and 150bpm, respectively. He was extremely hypovolaemic and I proceeded to increase his intravascular volume by pumping large volumes of normal saline (and blood).

The patient in this vignette is sufficiently normovolaemic that his postural BP is maintained.

[3] In assessing a patient for hyponatraemia, one thing you want to assess is the patient's volume state. The volume state can give vital clues as to the underlying cause of the patient's hyponatraemia. The patient's 'volume state' is the amount of blood in the systemic circulation. Patients who have a lower volume of blood in their body would have decreased preload to the heart, which requires the baroreceptor reflex to constrict arterioles (as well as increase heart rate and cardiac contractility, and contract great veins). Such vasoconstriction would decrease blood flow to the hands, which would render the hands colder, and slow refilling of the capillary microcirculation after brief occlusion. In the patient in this vignette, it appears that this is not the case.

[4] The JVP is a measure of the pressure of the blood in the right atrium. It uses the concept of a single column of blood starting at the right atrium and moving superiorly up the SVC to the right brachiocephalic vein and to the internal jugular vein. The vertical height correlates with the pressure of the blood in the right atrium. In the right clinical scenario, this is a good measure of the patient's volume state. If the patient is hypovolaemic, you would expect the JVP to not be elevated. The JVP can be relatively normal in hypovolaemia, given that the baroreceptor reflex causes venoconstriction and hence maintains the central venous pressure and right atrial pressure within relatively normal limits. In this patient, the JVP is consistent with a normal volume state.

[5] Bibasal crackles and peripheral oedema can be signs of volume overload. Volume overload is a phrase used to denote either an expansion of the intravascular volume or the interstitial fluid volume. Importantly, these findings reflect an expansion in the volume of the interstitial fluid, which may or may not be associated with an expansion of the intravascular volume. Bibasal crackles can be a sign of pulmonary interstitial oedema. This occurs due to transudation of fluid from the pulmonary capillaries into the pulmonary interstitium, as the pulmonary capillary hydrostatic pressure is

excessively high. This can be due to left heart failure (causing 'back pressure' to the pulmonary capillaries). Peripheral oedema is the equivalent in the lower limbs, where the capillary hydrostatic pressure is excessively high, causing transudation of fluid into the interstitium.

6 Pedal oedema is a sign of peripheral oedema which could be secondary to hyponatraemia in heart failure or

cirrhosis. It is important to take into account the patient's volume status when evaluating hyponatraemia.

Investigations

- UECs reveal a [Na$^+$] of 128mmol/L, a **urea of 6.3mmol/L** [1] and creatinine of 70µmol/L and eGFR >90ml/min/1.73m^2. **Serum glucose is 6.3mmol/L** [1]. **Serum osmolarity was 274mOsm/L** [1]. Serum TSH was normal.

- Paired **urine osmolarity was 200mOsm/L** [2], with urine [Na$^+$] being 30mmol/L and urine [K$^+$] being **20mmol/L** [3].
- Chest X-ray the previous day showed some left lower lobe consolidation, unchanged from the admission CXR, but other lung fields are clear.

1 The serum osmolarity is the sum of the concentrations of all solute particles in the serum. Serum is a mixture of chemicals in a solution of sodium chloride (NaCl). As such, Na$^+$ and Cl$^-$ ions comprise, by far, the major component of the serum osmolarity. Other ions that contribute to a lesser degree are HCO$_3^-$ ions, K$^+$ ions and tiny amounts of other ions such as calcium, magnesium and phosphate. There are also proteins dissolved in serum that contribute to the serum osmolarity, such as albumin, as well as other small uncharged solute particles, such as urea and glucose. Note that these have been highlighted in the vignette above.

Note here that serum osmolarity is not exactly the best concept if you are considering the direction of osmosis of water. This is because serum osmolarity includes solutes that can pass through cell membranes, mainly urea. Urea equilibrates across cell membranes almost instantaneously. Also, glucose has a variable ability to cross cell membranes, depending on the concentration in insulin in the blood (which allows glucose to diffuse into muscle, fat and liver tissue) – although in most people glucose crosses cell membranes reasonably well, albeit slowly. The direction of osmosis of water is dependent only on the concentrations of solutes that cannot pass through cell membranes. A rough estimate of this is the sum of the concentrations of plasma [Na$^+$] and [K$^+$] (multiplied by 2 to include their accompanying anions), plus glucose (given that glucose only diffuses very slowly across cell membranes). Even better, since plasma [K$^+$] can only vary between 3 and 6 (or the patient can become very unwell) and in most healthy people plasma glucose is between 4 and 8, we can use just the plasma [Na$^+$] as an indicator of the tonicity of the plasma. The tonicity of the plasma is the concentration of solutes in the plasma that cannot diffuse across cell membranes. Note that in patients with severe hyperglycaemia (e.g. patients with hyperglycaemic hyperosmolar state (HHS) whose BSLs can be up to 60), the tonicity of the plasma would be much higher than the plasma [Na$^+$] would suggest.

When working up a patient with hyponatraemia, we get

the Pathology lab to measure the serum osmolarity (it is directly measured, not inferred from the concentrations of the chemicals we described above) to ensure that the patient truly has 'dilute' blood, and that there is not some other solute that cannot diffuse across cell membranes that is present at high concentrations (e.g. mannitol from IV infusions to treat cerebral oedema) that could render the plasma hypertonic despite a low [Na$^+$].

2 The urine osmolarity is measured, to assess whether the pituitary is appropriately suppressing ADH production in response to hypotonic plasma. In normal individuals, even a very slight decrease in plasma osmolarity to about 280mOsm/L (assuming normal urea, reflecting a serum sodium of about 135) would cause ADH secretion to be suppressed to practically zero. If there is no ADH action on the collecting ducts of the kidney and hence no water reabsorption in these areas, the urine can get as dilute as 30–50mOsm/L (in the absence of diuretics or severe renal failure). Therefore, if I suddenly infused a patient with high volumes of 5% dextrose (which is practically giving free water without causing haemolysis, given the dextrose would eventually be metabolised by the cells) and cause the plasma [Na$^+$] to drop to about 135mM, the urine should be as dilute as about 50mOsm/L.

The urine osmolarity of the patient in this vignette is 200mOsm/L, which is nowhere near as low as it should be in a patient whose serum osmolality is that low. The urine osmolarity is certainly lower than that of the serum, but this is actually completely irrelevant. I mention this, because this is a common mistake made in interpreting such test results. He clearly has an impaired ability to dilute his urine, and on this occasion this is partly due to diuretics (the hydrochlorothiazide) and inappropriate ADH production by the pituitary, despite the serum osmolality being abnormally low.

3 The most abundant cations in the urine are Na$^+$ and K$^+$. These, along with their corresponding anions, comprise most

of the solute particles that cannot cross cell membranes and, therefore, contribute to the tonicity of the urine. The sum of [Na⁺] and [K⁺] should, therefore, give an index as to the tonicity of the urine. In the patient in this vignette, the sum of the concentrations of these two ions is 50mOsm/L.
A simple rule of thumb is that if the tonicity of the urine is lower than the tonicity of the absorbed solute and water

taken orally or IV, then the tonicity of the plasma should increase. This means that, if the tonicity of the fluids ingested orally or IV is >100mOsm/L (50 x 2), then the tonicity of the plasma should increase and the serum sodium should rise from 128mmol/L.

Management

- **Withhold pantoprazole and hydrochlorothiazide** [1].
- **Commence salt tablets** [2].
- **Commence fluid restriction at 1.5L with no free water** [2].
- **Avoid IV 5% dextrose** [3].
- **Not for 3% saline** [4].
- **Monitor UECs daily** [4].

This would be a standard management plan for such a patient, and as a junior doctor you will be expected to institute such a management plan.

[1] In treating hyponatraemia, a medication review is particularly important. This is because many medications cause SIADH through unclear mechanisms. There are also medications that impair urine dilution (thiazide but NOT loop diuretics) without causing SIADH. If clinically appropriate, these medications should be withheld to improve the ability of the kidneys to dilute the urine appropriately by stopping the pituitary from producing ADH inappropriately, and by preventing excessive salt from being present in the urine through diuretics.

[2] The ultimate aim of these measures is to ensure the fluids ingested are as hypertonic as possible. It is sufficient for the fluids ingested to be more hypertonic than the urine (in this case, equivalent to an NaCl concentration of 50mM). However, as the serum sodium improves and any inappropriate ADH production would be augmented by appropriate ADH production as the blood becomes less hypotonic, during treatment the urine may become even more hypertonic than first measured. Therefore, it is safer for the fluids ingested to be as hypertonic as possible.
The recipe is relatively simple. One thing you can do is minimise the amount of hypotonic fluids ingested. In fact, most fluids you drink have relatively low tonicity. Even orange juice (which is pretty salty) has a total [Na⁺] and [K⁺] concentration of about 50mM, near equivalent to the tonicity of the urine in this patient. Therefore, it is safe to minimise the amounts the patient drinks. Even better, you know that free water has practically no ions and has a tonicity of 0; therefore, ensure the patient drinks no free water during this period. You can also give the patient salt tablets to take with their medication, so as to assist in making the total amount of salt and fluids ingested amount to a more hypertonic fluid.
In this patient, salt tablets are not a bad idea. However, in patients that are volume overloaded due to heart failure or

chronic liver disease, then salt tablets are a terrible idea. This is because the volume of the extracellular fluid is primarily dependent on the total amount, in mol, of Na⁺ ions that are situated in the extracellular fluid; the posterior pituitary (through ADH) ensures that enough water is retained to maintain the ECF [Na⁺] at a relatively steady concentration. Hence, extra Na⁺ ions in the extracellular fluid implies extra water and hence volume in the extracellular fluid.

[3] Patients with hypotonic blood should NEVER be given 5% dextrose as an IV fluid. On face value, 5% dextrose is a relatively isotonic fluid (osmolarity is 278mOsm/L). However, dextrose (glucose) slowly diffuses into cell membranes of all cells, particularly fat, muscle and liver cells, and is either converted to glycogen or carbon dioxide/water, which effectively causes the solute particles (that cannot cross cell membranes) to 'disappear'. Hence, you will have eventually given free water to the patient IV. In fact, 5% dextrose is effectively designed to give 'free water' to the patient without causing massive haemolysis. You cannot inject pure water into a vein because the tonicity of the blood at the site of the vein will drop so significantly that the red blood cells expand and lyse, spilling the haemoglobin into the blood and causing haemoglobinuria and severe acute renal failure.
As explained above, 5% dextrose is effectively free water and, as discussed in *Note 2*, we do not want to give free water to the patient if we want to correct the hyponatraemia.

[4] 3% NaCl solution is very hypertonic (osmolarity 513mOsm/L) and therefore its administration would significantly increase the tonicity of the blood. However, in the patient in this vignette its administration could prove quite dangerous.
In this patient the hyponatraemia took about 4 days to develop. Now, whilst a sudden drop in the plasma tonicity leads to massive osmosis of water into cerebral neurons and causes cerebral oedema and its complications, cerebral neurons have mechanisms (that take about 48 hours to develop) to maintain a relatively constant cell volume in the

face of a change of plasma tonicity. In the face of decreasing plasma tonicity, cerebral neurons will start to extrude extra solute particles from their cytoplasm to reduce their own tonicity, so as to minimise the osmosis of water into the neurons. Importantly, if we reversed the drop in plasma tonicity, the neurons would take a similar amount of time to undo its adaptation, and this is where we can run into trouble. If we increased the plasma Na^+ too quickly (more than about 8mmol/L in a 24-hour period), there would be significant osmosis of water out of the neurons. Since the neurons are still extruding excessive amounts of solute (from the previous adaptation), the osmosis of water out of the neurons can be excessive and render the neurons' cell volume significantly smaller than their usual volume. This can lead to a dangerous, debilitating, disabling and irreversible demyelinating disease called osmotic demyelination syndrome.

CASE 77: Lupus nephritis

History

- A 24-year-old woman is referred to the Renal outpatient clinic by her GP for steadily worsening renal function and a possible diagnosis of lupus nephritis.
- The patient had presented to her GP with a 2–3-month history of generalised tiredness and weight loss, associated with **arthralgias** [1]. She normally works as a hospital nurse and has noticed that she has been having to take multiple days of sick leave because she has been too tired to get up in the morning.
- She also reported left-sided **pleuritic chest pain** [1] that has been long-standing.
- She denied **anorexia, nausea and vomiting** [2], as well as **ankle swelling** [3] and **shortness of breath** [4]. She also denies **frequency** [5], **urgency** [5], **dysuria** [6] or **haematuria** [7].

[1] Arthralgias/arthritis and pleuritic chest pain arise from deposition of immune complexes (a pathogenic hallmark of lupus) in synovial membranes and the parietal pleura. Pleuritic chest pain is worse on inspiration due to the mechanical irritation of the inflamed parietal pleura 'rubbing' against the visceral pleura. The parietal pleura adopts the innervation of the chest wall, where nociceptive fibres project through the intercostal nerves into the spinal cord.

[2] As previously discussed, anorexia, nausea and vomiting are non-specific symptoms of uraemia, the build-up of toxic chemicals that are produced by metabolic reactions in the body.

[3] Ankle swelling is a clinical sign of extracellular volume expansion. This happens for many reasons, and severe renal failure is one of those reasons. In severe renal failure, the kidneys fail to excrete sufficient amounts of Na^+ (and water), leading to fluid retention in the ECF compartment.

[4] Fluid retention in the ECF can involve fluid retention in the pulmonary interstitium. This causes dyspnoea by stimulation of pulmonary C-fibre nerve endings near the gas exchange barrier.

Patients with renal failure can develop pulmonary oedema.

[5] Distension of mechanoreceptors in the bladder wall causes a reflex increasing the tendency of the detrusor muscle to contract; this is how micturition occurs. However, there are also chemoreceptors and nociceptors in the bladder wall which, when stimulated (e.g. by inflammation), also cause the micturition reflex. This leads to frequent micturition, as well as the 'urge' to urinate at inappropriate times.

[6] The flow of urine through an inflamed bladder wall and urethra causes increased nociceptive stimulation (via the inflammation-induced hyperalgesia and allodynia), leading to painful urination or dysuria.

[7] Structural damage to the glomerulus due to acute inflammation can cause defects in the glomerular filtration barrier, leading to red cells being filtered into Bowman's capsule and ending up in the urine. However, in glomerulonephritis, the patient does not usually notice the haematuria, as the number of red cells passing into the urine is too small for the colour of the urine to change significantly.

Examination

- On examination, the patient looks generally well but tired. BP is **150/90mmHg** [1], HR 72bpm.
- Examination of her hands reveals **no boggy swellings of the joints** [2] in the hands and wrists, and there is no evidence of oedema.
- A **malar rash** [3] is notable on the face and shoulders in a **V distribution** [3].
- JVP is 3–4cm vertically from the sternal notch.
- A **pleural friction rub** [4] is evident on auscultation of the left upper zone, and there is **stony dullness to percussion** [2] on the left lower zone, on chest examination. Heart sounds are dual with no murmurs, and there is no pericardial friction rub.
- Abdomen is soft, non-tender and there is no renal angle tenderness, nor are the kidneys ballotable.
- There is no evidence of pedal oedema.

1 Hypertension is a classic feature of the nephritic syndrome. In glomerulonephritis, the kidneys' ability to excrete Na^+ ions (and water) to maintain a normal ECF volume is relatively impaired, through multiple mechanisms. This means that the mean systemic filling pressure increases, as the circulating volume increases; in other words, the preload increases. By the Frank–Starling mechanism, an increased preload to the right heart leads to an increase in the preload to the left heart, increasing left ventricular end-diastolic volume. In systole, the left ventricle contracts harder, generating a higher left ventricular pressure, and hence a higher arterial blood pressure.

2 Boggy swelling of the joints indicates the presence of fluid in the joints. Similarly, stony dullness to percussion of the lung bases indicates the presence of fluid between the percussing finger and the lung, dulling the sound.
Both of these phenomena can occur because of inflammation of the synovial membrane and the pleura due to immune complex deposition from lupus.
Acute inflammation induces an increased permeability of the post-capillary venules to protein by contraction of vascular endothelial cells leaving fenestrations between them. There is a leak of protein into the surrounding tissue; the increased oncotic pressure in the tissue leads to increased fluid filtration from the plasma into this tissue. This fluid leaks out of the tissue into the space that it surrounds; in the lung the space is the pleural space, and in the joint the space is the synovial joint.

3 It is known that UV light damage to the DNA of skin cells causes multiple changes that lead to the exposure of intracellular epitopes on cell surfaces to which autoantibodies are reactive. This leads to localised immune complex formation at sites of skin where there is significant UV light exposure; this includes the cheeks and skin above the V line of clothing at the chest.

4 An inflamed pleural surface is rough in texture; inspiration causes the layers of the pleura to slide past one another. Where the parietal pleura is rough, this rubbing leads to the sound heard on auscultation.

Investigations

Routine blood results are shown below:

Hb (g/dl)	10.1 [1]	Cr (µM)	115
MCV (fl)	83 [1]	eGFR (ml/min/1.73m²)	53
WCC (x 10⁹/L)	2.6	Albumin	26
Platelets (x 10⁹/L)	70 [2]	ANA [3]	+
Na⁺ (mM)	137	anti-dsDNA [3]	+
K⁺ (mM)	3.6	ENA [3]	+
Cl⁻ (mM)	100	C3 [4]	Low
Ur (mM)	11.4	C4 [4]	Low
Serum iron	4 [1]		
Transferrin saturation	10% [1]		
Ferritin	550 [1]		

Urine microscopy:

Protein ++ [5]. Blood ++. **Dysmorphic red cells and red cell casts** [6] present.

24-hour urine collection:

Volume	910ml
Protein concentration (g/L)	**1.54** [5]
Protein excretion (g/day)	1.40
Urine creatinine (mM)	5.17

- Renal biopsy shows diffuse involvement of 16 out of 20 glomeruli, with most glomeruli showing mesangial **matrix accumulation** [7] and **hypercellularity** [8], with a lymphocytic infiltrate.
- There is also evidence of endothelial proliferation on light microscopy. **Crescent formation** [9] is evident.
- Immunofluorescence shows staining of **C1q** [10], **C3** [10], **IgG** [10], **IgA** [10] and **IgM** [10] in the **mesangium** [10] and **glomerular basement membrane** [10].
- Electron microscopy shows **subendothelial** [10], **subepithelial** [10] and **mesangial** [10] electron-dense deposits.
- Chest X-ray reveals a left-sided pleural effusion.

1 The most likely cause of anaemia in this patient is chronic inflammation.

Hepcidin is a signalling molecule released by the liver that modulates iron storage in the body. It inhibits the secretion of iron from the intestinal cells and from the liver into the bloodstream, through inhibition of the ferroportin (FP) channel. This channel is found in hepatocytes and enterocytes. Enterocytes absorb iron from the gut lumen through multiple mechanisms, and secrete this iron into the blood through the FP channel. The liver absorbs iron through transferrin receptors (transferrin is a protein that binds iron in the blood), and secretes iron back into the blood using the FP channel. Hepcidin secretion by the liver is generally dependent on body iron stores; in patients with high systemic iron levels, hepcidin secretion increases.

Hepcidin is also a bactericidal molecule and, therefore, is released in increased quantities in the setting of inflammation, mediated by IL-6. Sustainably high hepcidin levels mean that iron present in the blood can be absorbed by the liver and stored as ferritin, but its release back into the circulation is impaired. This leads to a sequestering of iron out of the blood and into the liver as ferritin. Therefore, there would be less iron available for haematopoiesis, leading to anaemia. Importantly, the serum ferritin (which is a reflection of the amount of ferritin in the liver) would be normal to high, in the setting of a low transferrin saturation rate, indicative of a low circulating amount of iron in the blood.

In addition, other cytokines, including IL-1, cause the bone marrow to be relatively resistant to erythropoietin stimulation of red cell precursor proliferation and differentiation in the bone marrow; it effectively causes bone marrow suppression of red cell production.

The end result is a normocytic anaemia.

2 Severe thrombocytopenia is likely secondary to autoimmune antibody-binding to epitopes on the platelet cell surface, as part of the lupus disease where there is systemic autoimmunity. The platelets, bound to antibody, are phagocytosed by circulating neutrophils, or cells of the reticuloendothelial system in the spleen.

3 A 'positive' antinuclear antibody (ANA) titre carries relatively little meaning; many healthy individuals without lupus will have positive ANA titres. However, it is rare for an individual who has a negative ANA titre to have lupus.

A patient who has a positive ANA titre has serum that contains antibodies to one or more antigens that are found inside cells. The test for ANA is similar to an indirect Coombs test, where the serum of the patient is mixed with a set of human epithelial cells (from another individual) whose cell membranes have been artificially damaged, so as to enable the entry of any autoantibodies into the cytoplasm of these epithelial cells. The cells are washed, and the specimen mixed with a fluorescent-tagged anti-Ig antibody (antibody against antibody). The regions within the cells to which the autoantibodies from the patient bind will fluoresce. A 'positive ANA titre' refers to a specimen where the fluorescence is still present after diluting the plasma above a particular level. Therefore, a positive ANA will confirm the presence of autoantibodies against one or more epitopes usually found

inside cells, but does not tell us which epitopes the patient has autoantibodies against.

In patients with lupus, certain events (e.g. UV damage of skin cells causing expression of normally intracellular epitopes on the cell membrane, which are now accessible to the pre-existing autoantibodies) can cause these autoantibodies to be able to bind to their epitopes, leading to complement fixation and inflammation.

The intracellular epitopes include DNA (for which one can have anti-dsDNA antibodies) and other 'extractable nuclear antigens' or ENAs, such as Ro, La and Smith. Such tests can specify which epitopes the patient has autoantibodies against.

4 In lupus, immune complexes are deposited throughout many different parts of the body; such immune complexes containing IgG will cause complement fixation via the classical pathway. The classical pathway involves the activation of the C1 complex by an antibody–antigen complex, which then activates and cleaves C2 and C4 simultaneously, which then leads to the cleavage of C3. Here, both C3 and C4 are consumed. Since, in lupus, it is likely that this is happening throughout many different parts of the body, enough C3 and C4 would be consumed in the blood to lead to low plasma C3 and C4 levels. Low C3 and C4 levels are suggestive of complement fixation via the classical (antibody) pathway.

5 Glomerular inflammation involves podocyte damage and foot process effacement, which renders the glomerular filtration barrier significantly more permeable to proteins. Podocyte foot processes, as well as the slit diaphragms between them, inhibit the passage of large molecules (including proteins) into the glomerular filtrate.

6 As previously explained, glomerular inflammation also leads to the leakage of red blood cells into the glomerular filtrate. The red blood cells, being large, have to pass through the small tubules. This issue leads to a change to the shapes of the red blood cells; they are termed dysmorphic. Dysmorphic red blood cells on microscopy suggests they originated from the glomerulus.

7 Glomerular inflammation, particularly chronic inflammation, leads to an increase in fibrotic processes; mesangial cells, stimulated by inflammatory cytokines, increase their production of fibrous proteins such as collagen and fibronectin that form the mesangial matrix. This leads to an increase in mesangial area.

8 Glomerular inflammation, similar to acute inflammation of any cause, leads to extravasation of white cells (neutrophils, macrophages and lymphocytes, depending on the chronicity of the inflammation) into interstitial tissues, including the mesangium.

9 Crescents are deposits seen on light microscopy that are found within Bowman's capsule. The presence of crescents indicates destruction and rupture of the glomerular basement membrane due to severe inflammation; this rupture allows plasma proteins that are not normally filtered through the glomerulus to accumulate in Bowman's capsule. One such protein is fibrinogen, which is converted by thrombin (which also leaks) into fibrin. Additionally, significant numbers of white cells infiltrate through the ruptured glomerular filtration barrier into Bowman's capsule and promote inflammation. The end product is a cellular and proteinaceous infiltrate in Bowman's capsule, known as a crescent. The presence of crescents indicates that glomerular damage is extremely severe, and the patient will require intensive immunosuppressive therapy to prevent irreversible renal failure.

10 A major feature of lupus is the presence of many different types of autoantibodies (IgG, IgA and IgM) to many different epitopes, with immune complexes between these formed. Some of these epitopes are 'planted' into the mesangium, or the subendothelial and subepithelial part of the glomerular basement membrane; immune complexes that formed in the blood can filter into these regions too.

Additionally, these immune complexes include IgG1 and IgG3 (and IgM) which can activate complement through the classical pathway. The classical pathway involves activation of C1 (which comprises C1q, C1r and C1s). Activation of the C1 complex leads to the activation/cleavage of C2 and C4, which eventually leads to C3 cleavage. In contrast, the alternative pathway of complement activation involves an upregulation of the pre-existing spontaneous C3 cleavage by bacterial molecules. This pathway does not involve C1, C2 or C4. Therefore, in lupus, you would expect deposits of IgG, IgA and IgM in the glomerulus on immunofluorescence and immunohistochemistry, and you would expect immune complex deposits (which are electron dense) in electron microscopy in the mesangium, and the subendothelial and subepithelial regions of the glomerular basement membrane. Finally, you would see C1q deposition in the glomerulus, due to activation of the classical pathway, and you would see C3 deposition anyhow, due to complement activation.

Management

- The patient is admitted under the Renal unit for intensive immunosuppressive treatment with IV **methylprednisolone** [1], **mycophenolate** [2] and **plasma exchange** [3].

- Once the renal function improves, she is commenced on low dose perindopril, and discharged on oral **prednisolone** [1] and **mycophenolate** [2].

1 Glucocorticoids (e.g. prednisolone, methylprednisolone) have many different effects on various parts of the immune system; all these effects are immunosuppressive. High dose glucocorticoids inhibit the margination of white cells into the interstitium in inflammation, they cause rapid depletion of circulating T cells in high doses, and they invariably inhibit the production of almost all inflammatory cytokines (e.g. IL-1 and TNF-alpha).
Methylprednisolone 1000mg daily IV for 3 days is known as 'pulse steroid' treatment and is an extremely powerful immunosuppressing regimen.
The purpose of glucocorticoids is to disrupt the inflammatory activity occurring in the glomeruli, to prevent further damage.

2 Mycophenolate is a drug that inhibits the enzyme IMDPH, an enzyme that is involved in the *de novo* synthesis of purine nucleotides (adenosine and guanosine phosphates) for production of DNA. Most cells in the body use previously produced free nucleotides or their derivatives to produce purine nucleotides. However, lymphocytes are one of the only cell types that have to synthesise nucleotides *de novo*. Therefore, mycophenolate significantly inhibits lymphocyte production; lymphocytes are ultimately responsible for antibody (and hence immune complex) production, and the production of many pro-inflammatory cytokines.

3 Plasma exchange involves the removal of the patient's plasma, and replacement of that plasma with donor plasma. The idea here is to get rid of immune complexes and autoantibodies that are responsible for precipitating the glomerulonephritis from the blood.

CASE 78: Nephrolithiasis

History

- A 56-year-old male presents to the ED with a 6-hour history of severe **right flank pain that radiates to the right iliac fossa** [1].
- The patient reports haematuria, **mild dysuria and frequency** [2] but denies subjective fevers, sweats and chills. He denies nausea/vomiting or any other GI symptoms.
- He has a long-standing history of **ileocaecal Crohn's disease** [3] that is well controlled on azathioprine.

This section will describe the above symptoms with the assumption that the patient has urolithiasis.

[1] Urolithiasis (ureteric stone) causes flank pain due to urinary obstruction, increased pressure of the urine and interstitial fluid, leading to distension of the renal capsule, which has significant nociceptive innervation.

The kidneys are derived from the intermediate mesoderm and therefore their innervation is lateralised; left-sided kidney capsule distension leads to left-sided pain, and right-sided kidney capsule distension leads to right-sided pain.

This is not the case in, for example, gastritis; the stomach is derived from the endoderm and embryologically was originally a midline structure. Its innervation is not lateralised; gastritis leads to midline epigastric pain, despite the fact that the stomach is primary a left-sided structure.

The left-sided 'loin-to-groin' pain derived from the ureter is likely due to spasm of the ureter (smooth muscle contraction) against an immovable stone. The high pressures generated in the ureteric wall can cause local ischaemia due to blockade of capillary blood supply to the ureter from wall contraction. This local ischaemia can cause intense ureteric pain.

[2] Dysuria and frequency are often associated with urinary tract infections (UTIs). In fact, these two symptoms are simply reflective of urethral and bladder inflammation, which can certainly be caused by UTIs, but can also be caused by vesicoureteric junction stones. Such stones are very close to the bladder, and the resultant local inflammation caused can 'spread' to the bladder and cause symptoms of bladder inflammation.

Frequency occurs in bladder inflammation due to the mechanisms that cause the urge to pass urine. Normally, bladder distension (over 150ml) causes stretch receptors in the bladder to cause an afferent signal to the brain (through pelvic splanchnic nerves) to cause the sensation of the urge to micturate. However, chemoreceptors (that sense chemicals released during inflammation) also produce the same signals to the brain. This is why bladder inflammation leads to the urgency to pass urine, despite minimal bladder volumes.

[3] Ileocaecal Crohn's disease is an important risk factor in the development of oxalate stones. Oxalate ($C_2O_4^{2-}$) ions are ingested in the diet; foods high in oxalate include spinach, nuts and potatoes. It tends to be absorbed in the large bowel, and tends to be excreted renally.

Calcium (Ca^{2+}) and oxalate ($C_2O_4^{2-}$) ions precipitate to form a calcium oxalate precipitate (CaC_2O_4). This can occur in the small and large bowel, as Ca^{2+} and $C_2O_4^{2-}$ ions mix in the chyme and precipitate. The insoluble CaC_2O_4 precipitate cannot be absorbed in the small and large bowel and is excreted. This reduces the absorption of $C_2O_4^{2-}$ ions, while the absorption of Ca^{2+} ions in the bowel is modulated by activated vitamin D (calcitriol). In this vein, Ca^{2+} can be considered an 'oxalate binder', minimising the absorption of oxalate. In fact, a similar principle is used in minimising phosphate absorption in the gut in patients with chronic kidney disease; patients take Ca^{2+} supplements with food to allow precipitation of calcium phosphate in the chyme, reducing phosphate absorption in the gut. Here, Ca^{2+} is considered a phosphate binder.

In patients with ileocaecal disease, the absorption of fatty acids is significantly reduced, and fatty acids remain in high concentrations in the small and large bowel contents. In the high pH environment of the small bowel, the fatty acids exist in their anionic forms, for example stearate ($C_{17}H_{35}COO^-$) ions. These ions also precipitate out Ca^{2+} ions in the same way that hard water (e.g. tap water in the south and east of the UK) containing high calcium concentrations mixes with soap (containing stearate ions) to form soap scum. This phenomenon means that there is less Ca^{2+} to precipitate the oxalate ions in the gut, leading to increased oxalate ion absorption.

With increased oxalate ion absorption comes increased oxalate ion excretion; the higher oxalate ion concentrations in the tubular fluid as the urine becomes more concentrated can lead to calcium oxalate precipitating, leading to urolithiasis.

Examination

- On examination, the patient appears to be in severe pain and is tearful, and **writhing about in the hospital bed** [1]. Routine observations are normal, and **the patient is not febrile** [2], **tachycardic** [2] **or hypotensive** [2].

- General examination is unremarkable. There is moderate left-sided flank tenderness to palpation, but the abdomen is soft and non-tender.

1 'Writhing about' is a classic feature of colicky pain, which may assist in differentiating renal colic from peritonitis due to any cause.

2 A patient with suspected urolithiasis also needs to be assessed for complications such as pyelonephritis and urosepsis. This is important to identify, as such patients can become septic and require urgent fluid resuscitation and antibiotics.

Investigations

Routine blood results are shown below.

Hb (g/dl)	14	Cr (μmol/L)	86
WCC (x 10⁹/L)	9.6	eGFR (ml/min/1.73m²)	>90
Platelets (x 10⁹/L)	215	Corr Ca²⁺ (mmol/L)	2.31
Na⁺ (mmol/L)	139	Mg²⁺ (mmol/L)	0.82
K⁺ (mmol/L)	4.1	Phosphate (mmol/L)	1.04
Cl⁻ (mmol/L)	102	CRP (mg/L)	25
Ur (mmol/L)	9.1		

- CT abdomen/pelvis **without contrast** [1] (CT KUB) shows a 4mm obstructive stone in the left vesicoureteric junction with mild hydronephrosis and hydroureter. **Concurrent abdominal X-ray** [1] corroborated the presence of the same stone. Stone analysis showed a mixture of calcium oxalate (CaC_2O_4) and calcium phosphate as the composition of the stone.
- Urine electrolytes show a **high urine calcium concentration** [2].
- **PTH levels** [3] are normal.

1 CT uses X-rays to differentiate between different types of tissue.

Denser tissue and tissue containing atoms with large nuclei have a greater tendency to absorb/block X-rays, because the X-ray photon 'particles' are more likely to hit particles in denser tissue and bigger nuclei.

For example, contrast contains radioactive iodine usually (an atom with a mass number of 131, much higher than calcium-40 which has a mass number of only 40). Iodine has a really high mass number and therefore tends to block X-rays even better than bone (which is primarily composed of calcium – mass number in the 40s).

In doing a CT KUB, we are trying to find a stone, which is usually made of:

- calcium phosphate or calcium oxalate, which is quite radio-opaque due to the calcium atoms
- uric acid, which is denser than water and will be somewhat radio-opaque.

Therefore, we do not want contrast, because we want to be able to pick out the stone (relatively radio-opaque) from the surrounding tissue. Addition of IV contrast will either make it difficult to differentiate the stone from the surrounding ureteric wall (if the contrast is in the circulation), or from the

surrounding urine (if the contrast is in the ureter, as in a CT intravenous pyelogram).

Radio-opaque stones are potentially likely to be seen on plain abdominal X-ray, but uric acid stones are much less likely to be seen on abdominal X-ray.

2 Each salt has a property called the solubility product (K_{sp}) which is the maximum value of the product of the concentration of each constituent ion in the salt. For example, the K_{sp} of calcium oxalate (CaC_2O_4) is the maximum possible value of $[Ca^{2+}][C_2O_4^{2-}]$.

If the concentration of Ca^{2+} and $C_2O_4^{2-}$ ions in the urine increases sufficiently to increase $[Ca^{2+}][C_2O_4^{2-}]$ beyond the solubility product, Ca^{2+} and $C_2O_4^{2-}$ ions start to precipitate to form solid calcium oxalate. This continues to happen until $[Ca^{2+}][C_2O_4^{2-}]$ decreases sufficiently to reach the value of the solubility product.

A high urinary $[Ca^{2+}]$, which is often idiopathic but can be due to hyperparathyroidism, will therefore increase the risk of developing calcium stones.

3 PTH (parathyroid hormone) increases the mobilisation of Ca^{2+} from bone, promotes the reabsorption of Ca^{2+} in the kidney, and activates vitamin D, which also promotes Ca^{2+} absorption in the kidney and the GI tract.

Primary hyperparathyroidism causes hypercalcaemia and hypercalciuria; presumably, the increased Ca^{2+} load in the glomerular filtrate from the mobilisation of bone Ca^{2+} and increased gut Ca^{2+} absorption dominates the effect of increased Ca^{2+} reabsorption.

As previously discussed, hypercalciuria increases the risk of ureteric stones.

Management

- Acute phase: analgesia with oral oxycodone and PR indomethacin, monitor in the ED short stay unit for stone passage and collect for analysis. **Tamsulosin** [1] not indicated at this stage.

- Post-acute phase:
  - **encourage high volumes of fluid intake** [2]
  - **not for urinary alkalinisers** [3]
  - **encourage oral calcium intake** [4]
  - **low oxalate foods** [5]
  - **thiazide diuretics** [6] .

1 Tamsulosin is an α_1 adrenergic blocker that is selective to the α_{1A} subtype (found in the prostate and distal ureter) compared to the α_{1B} subtype (found in blood vessels). α_{1A} stimulation leads to ureteric smooth muscle contraction. In selected patients with ureteric stones (generally mid-size), tamsulosin can increase the likelihood of spontaneous passage of the stone, by relaxing the ureteric smooth muscle, increasing the lumen width of the ureter, and allowing stone passage.

In the patient in this vignette, the stone is small and is very close to the bladder – the stone is likely to pass spontaneously, with or without tamsulosin.

2 As previously discussed, we need to keep urinary $[Ca^{2+}]$ and $[C_2O_4^{2-}]$ low. One way of doing this is by promoting increased fluid excretion through increased fluid intake. Increased fluid excretion through the tubules means that the Ca^{2+} in the tubular fluid is sufficiently diluted to reduce the risk of precipitation.

3 Urinary alkalinisers can be used to prevent ureteric stones that are composed primarily of uric acid. In this case, since the stones are mainly composed of calcium oxalate and calcium phosphate, urinary alkalinisation (using oral bases such as Ural) is not indicated, and could actually increase the risk of ureteric stones.

4 The pKa of $H_2PO_4^-$ is approximately 7.2. This means that at a urinary pH of 7.2, the concentrations of $H_2PO_4^-$ and HPO_4^- are equal. If the urinary pH is lower, then the phosphate ions would be predominantly $H_2PO_4^-$ and if urine pH is higher, then the phosphate ions would be predominantly HPO_4^{2-}. Calcium superphosphate – $Ca(H_2PO_4)_2$ – is reasonably soluble in water, whereas $CaHPO_4$ is only sparingly soluble in water. Therefore, it stands to reason that increasing the urinary pH in patients who have a predisposition to getting calcium phosphate stones would increase the risk of further calcium phosphate stones, as we get a predominance of the HPO_4^{2-}. ion, which tends to precipitate calcium.

5 Encouragement of calcium intake (with calcium supplementation) is a little counterintuitive here. The aim of maintaining moderate to high calcium ingestion is the use of calcium as an 'oxalate binder' to minimise oxalate absorption in the gut. In patients with Crohn's disease with malabsorption of fatty acids, sufficient calcium ions in the gut may be needed to precipitate the fatty acids and precipitate the oxalate to minimise oxalate absorption in the gut.

In otherwise healthy people, a moderate calcium diet may not necessarily raise calcium absorption, because the permeability of the gut to calcium is dependent on PTH and vitamin D.

6 Thiazide diuretics promote hypocalciuria through multiple mechanisms. One mechanism by which this occurs is by causing a slight hypovolaemia.

This triggers the glomerulotubular balance mechanism. In the face of hypovolaemia and reduced renal blood flow, GFR is maintained by preferential constriction of the efferent arteriole. The blood that passes into the peritubular capillaries will be at a lower pressure (due to efferent arteriolar constriction), and would have a high oncotic pressure due to high protein concentration, since the filtration fraction at the glomerulus is high (normal GFR despite reduced renal blood flow). This promotes reabsorption of fluid from the proximal tubule to the capillaries by convection (rather than diffusion). The convection promotes Ca^{2+} reabsorption in parallel with Na^+ reabsorption at the proximal tubule (where about 65% of Ca^{2+} is reabsorbed and is not subject to hormonal control). This is why patients who are hypovolaemic tend to get mild hypercalcaemia – a situation you will often see in the General Medicine ward.

Thiazide diuretics may be helpful in our patient, given he has a high urinary calcium that is idiopathic.

CASE 79: Nephrotic syndrome

History

- A 55-year-old man has been referred to the Renal outpatients clinic with nephrotic-range proteinuria.
- He reports a 2-week history of **lower limb, upper limb and facial swelling** [1] and **frothy urine** [2]. He otherwise feels well and denies any uraemic symptoms. He also denies fevers, sweats, chills, weight loss, symptoms of GI bleeding or bone pain.
- He has no significant past medical history and is not on any regular medications.

[1] Sodium and water retention (as occurs in nephrotic syndrome) leads to expansion of the extracellular fluid volume. The failure of the kidneys to excrete appropriate amounts of sodium and water leads to an inappropriately high mean systolic filling pressure in the circulation. This high mean systolic filling pressure means a high preload, and hence a greater ventricular systolic pressure and thus arterial blood pressure (prior to the baroreceptor reflex). The baroreceptor reflex would cause, among other things, arteriolar vasodilatation.

This arteriolar vasodilatation means that the drop in pressure across the systemic arterioles is lower; remember that $\Delta P = F \times R$, where ΔP is the change in blood pressure across the arteriole, F is the flow across the arteriole (which can be assumed to be relatively constant) and R is the resistance of the arteriole (which would be lower due to vasodilatation). The lower change in blood pressure across the arteriole means a higher capillary hydrostatic pressure. This leads to increased ultrafiltration/transudation of plasma across the capillary walls into the interstitium. The increase in interstitial volume manifests as swelling in the lower and upper limbs, with facial swelling.

[2] Proteins dissolved in urine reduce the surface tension of the urine. When a liquid has a low surface tension and is agitated (for instance during micturition), it tends to form a foamy mixture with 'bubbles' inside, much like soapy water does. Therefore, significant proteinuria can manifest as bubbly/foamy/frothy urine.

Examination

- On examination, the patient looks well, but grossly oedematous. BP is **160/80mmHg** [1], HR 82bpm, RR 18, SaO_2 98% on air, temperature 36.9°C.
- There is gross **pitting oedema** [2] on the hands and arms, over the orbits and in the lower limbs up to the knees.
- **JVP is visible and elevated** [3].
- There are reduced breath sounds on the right base, with **stony dullness** [4] to percussion on the right base. Abdomen is soft and non-tender.

[1] Whilst hypertension is not a classic feature of the nephrotic syndrome, it can occur. The sodium and water retention that occurs in nephrotic syndrome is postulated to be due to two possible mechanisms. One of these mechanisms is that the proteinuria itself causes the tubular cells in the kidney to inappropriately reabsorb extra Na^+ ions (with extra water being reabsorbed as mediated by ADH to maintain plasma tonicity).

As previously discussed, the extra circulating volume leads to an increase in the mean systemic filling pressure and high preload, and hence a high left ventricular systolic pressure as the left ventricle contracts with greater force, and thus a high arterial blood pressure.

[2] Pitting oedema is a type of oedema where pressing the fingers for a few seconds over the oedema and then letting go leaves a 'dent'. This type of oedema is suggestive of volume overload in the setting of an intact lymphatic system. The extracellular matrix in the dermis and subcutaneous tissue is composed of multiple proteins that form a gel-like structure. This gel-like structure is generally elastic in nature; distension of this matrix and then relieving that distension should cause the matrix to resume its original shape. This is what you see when you press your fingers against the skin of a patient without peripheral oedema. Leakage of extra fluid into this tissue and expansion of its volume would be associated with a significant rise in the extracellular matrix

hydrostatic pressure, limiting further transudation of fluid into the matrix.

However, if sufficient quantities of fluid are infused into the extracellular matrix, and it is distended sufficiently, the matrix becomes plastic in nature; it continues to distend with minimal to no increase in extracellular matrix fluid pressure, and if this distension were to release, the matrix would not resume its original shape. In this setting, when the matrix is compressed by a finger, and the fluid within it dissipates into the surrounding tissues with little to no resistance, upon releasing the finger the fluid is not quickly 'pressed back' into the tissue, as the surrounding tissue is now so much more pliable.

3 As described in *Case 76*, the JVP is a crude estimate of the right atrial pressure, and is a reflection of the central venous pressure. This could be elevated due to excess volume in the extracellular fluid due to 'fluid overload' or due to right heart failure causing back pressure into the central veins.

4 As mentioned earlier, increased ultrafiltration/transudation of plasma across the capillary walls can also leak out into the lungs, resulting in pulmonary oedema. This results in stony dullness upon percussion on physical examination. Patients would generally be short of breath due to reduced lung volume available for gas exchange.

Investigations

Routine blood results are shown below:

Hb (x 10⁹/L)	14.3	Cr (µM)	141
WCC (x 10⁹/L)	8.4	eGFR (ml/min/1.73m²)	54
Platelets (x 10⁹/L)	192	**Albumin**	**17** [1]
Na⁺ (mM)	137	Fasting TAG (mM)	5.6
K⁺ (mM)	3.9	**LDL-C (mM)**	**6.1** [2]
Cl⁻ (mM)	99	**HDL-C (mM)**	**0.6** [2]
Ur (mM)	8.6	ANA, ENA, anti-dsDNA	Neg
		Anti-PLA2 IgG [3]	**+**
		HBsAg	−

Urine microscopy:

Protein +++. Blood +. **Lipid-laden casts and oval fat bodies visible** [4].

24-hour urine collection:

Volume	1429ml
Protein concentration (g/L)	15.2
Protein excretion (g/day)	21.7
Urine creatinine (mM)	4.93

Renal biopsy shows a diffusely **thickened glomerular basement membrane without significant hypercellularity** [6], diffuse IgG and **C3 staining** [6] (granular pattern) but no **C1q staining** [6] on immunohistochemistry and immunofluorescence, and **subepithelial electron-dense deposits** [5] with **podocyte foot process effacement** [7].

Chest X-ray reveals a right-sided pleural effusion.

1 The low plasma albumin is presumably due to the overwhelming proteinuria.

2 Nephrotic syndrome is associated with high LDL, low HDL and high triglycerides. The mechanism by which this occurs is unclear, but it is thought to be due to increased hepatic synthesis of multiple proteins, including ApoB (apolipoprotein B), which is a major constituent of LDL. The mechanism by which low HDL levels and high triglyceride levels occur is unclear at this stage.

3 PLA2 (phospholipase A2) is a protein that is found in the cells of the glomerular basement membrane, closer to the podocyte aspect compared to the vascular endothelial aspect. Autoimmunity to PLA2 leads to the development of IgG antibodies; IgG is produced after a prolonged humoral immune response against an antigen. This leads to a cause of nephrotic syndrome called membranous nephropathy.

4 The presence of lipid-laden casts in the urine and oval fat bodies is strongly suggestive of lipiduria.

Normally, lipoprotein (LDL and HDL) is not filtered significantly at the glomerulus due to its large size. However, in nephrotic syndrome, where there is massive proteinuria, lipoproteins (particularly HDL) are also filtered at the glomerulus. Much of the lipoprotein is reabsorbed at the proximal tubule and the lipid is integrated into the cytosol of the proximal tubular cell. When the proximal tubular cells desquamate and are found in the urinary sediment in microscopy, the lipid inside these cells is referred to as an oval fat body. The unreabsorbed lipoproteins form 'fatty casts'.

5 Subepithelial electron-dense deposits describes matter in the 'subepithelial region' that electrons cannot pass through. An electron microscope operates by shooting electrons rather than photons (light 'particles') at the target of interest, and using electron-sensitive (rather than light-sensitive) lenses to analyse the image.

These electron-dense deposits are generally immune complexes, formed between antigen and antibody. In this patient, the immune complex is likely to involve the PLA2 antigen, which is found in the subepithelial region of the glomerular basement membrane.

6 The location of the immune complexes explains the presence of glomerular basement membrane (GBM) thickening without hypercellularity and the extensive presence of C3 complement protein in the affected GBM. Immune complexes can activate both complement and white cells. However, in this case, the immune complex is located quite 'deep' within the GBM, away from the vascular endothelium and quite close to the podocyte. Even damaged glomerular basement membranes have minimal permeability to white cells, but as a protein, complement would be filtered much more easily. Hence, complement will come into contact with the immune complexes, but not white cells. Hence, the injury the glomerulus is subjected to is almost entirely mediated by complements, not white cells. This explains the lack of hypercellularity.

In primary membranous nephropathy, the antibodies formed against PLA2 are a type of IgG called IgG4 antibodies; these do not activate complement via the classical pathway, but they can do so via the lectin pathway.

The classical pathway involves the following:

- immune complex binds to C1q; C1q is part of a C1 complex protein consisting of C1q, C1r and C1s; C1q is activated; it activates C1r, which then activates C1s; the C1 complex protein is activated
- C1s cleaves C2 and C4 (into C2a + C2b, and C4a + C4b)

- C2b and C4b combine to form a complex protein, known as C3 convertase
- this C3 convertase cleaves C3 into C3a and C3b
- the C3b then triggers a cascade of complement reactions.

Therefore, if the classical pathway were activated, one would expect there to be extensive C1q staining. In primary membranous nephropathy, there is no C1q staining, as the IgG4 against PLA2 cannot bind C1q.

In fact, if there was C1q staining, and therefore the classical pathway was activated, the diagnosis of lupus as a secondary cause of membranous nephropathy should be considered. If complement were activated by any mechanism (classical, alternative, lectin), then C3 staining would be expected; this is because C3 is common to all complement activation pathways.

7 The foot processes of the podocytes, along with the gaps between them (known as filtration slits), bridged by slit diaphragms, provide a major component to the filtration of plasma. Glycoproteins are found on these foot processes, filtration slits and the slit diaphragm; these are negatively charged. Accordingly, they tend to repel negatively charged molecules compared to positively charged molecules. The size of the filtration slits mean that large proteins (particularly negatively charged proteins such as albumin) are filtered only very minimally.

When the foot processes are effaced (obliterated), this barrier is severely impaired, leading to severe proteinuria.

Management

Commence **perindopril 5mg daily** [1] and **furosemide 40mg daily** [2]. Also begin **atorvastatin** **40mg daily** [3] and **prednisolone 60mg daily and cyclophosphamide** [4].

1 Perindopril is an ACE inhibitor that inhibits the production of angiotensin II, and therefore minimises stimulation of AT_1 and AT_2 receptors by angiotensin II. Through a poorly understood mechanism, minimising angiotensin receptor stimulation minimises proteinuria. Theories include that ACE inhibition (or the use of angiotensin receptor blockers) lowers glomerular capillary hydrostatic pressure, which minimises filtration of protein by convection through the glomerular filtration barrier. This is done by lowering systemic blood pressure, and relaxing the efferent arteriole.

It is also known that ACE inhibition causes complex structural changes to the glomerular filtration barrier that renders it more resistant to filtration of protein.

2 Furosemide is a loop diuretic that inhibits the Na/K/Cl symporter at the thick ascending loop of Henle. This leads to increased excretion of Na^+ ions, which, through an osmotic effect and through the attempt by ADH to maintain

a constant plasma tonicity, increases the excretion of water. The ultimate effect is a contraction of the extracellular fluid volume. This would decrease the generalised pitting oedema, as well as the pleural effusion.

3 Atorvastatin inhibits the enzyme HMG coenzyme A reductase. This is an enzyme that catalyses the rate-limiting step of the synthesis of cholesterol in the liver from acetyl coenzyme A. The use of atorvastatin is as an attempt to lower the liver's activity in exporting cholesterol to tissues through LDL and causing atherosclerosis.

4 Prednisolone and cyclophosphamide are both immunosuppressants. Prednisolone suppresses the immune system by many mechanisms, and cyclophosphamide binds to DNA in susceptible cells including white cells. Ultimately, these two drugs impair B cell function in mediating the humoral immune response against PLA2, and hence lowering the burden of immune complexes on the nephrons.

CASE 80: Renal transplant rejection

History

- A 30-year-old man presents to the renal transplant outpatient clinic for routine review for a recent kidney transplant.
- The patient received a live donor single kidney transplant from his wife 6 months ago. He had developed end-stage kidney disease from chronic reflux nephropathy. His immediate postoperative transplant period was uneventful.
- He is currently on **tacrolimus 3mg bd** [1], **mycophenolate 1000mg bd** [2] and **prednisolone 5mg daily** [3].

- He is also on esomeprazole 20mg daily and **magnesium aspartate 1000mg tds** [4]. He has not started any new medications recently.
- On review, he feels generally well. He reports **good urine output** [5] with no symptoms of a urinary tract infection, **no frothy urine** [6] and no haematuria.
- He also denies symptoms of uraemia and reports **normal exercise tolerance** [7].

[1] Tacrolimus is an immunosuppressant drug that inhibits calcineurin. Calcineurin is a secondary messenger protein found in helper T cells. When T-cell receptors (TCR) bind to presented antigen by antigen-presenting cells on their MHC Class II markers, the TCR stimulation leads to a signal transduction pathway involving the activation of calcineurin. The activated calcineurin activates downstream molecules, leading to the expression of genes for multiple cytokines, including IL-2 and IL-4. These cytokines are subsequently secreted into the extracellular fluid.
IL-2 is a cytokine that causes proliferation and differentiation of Th and Tc cells, which promotes cell-mediated immunity. Therefore, tacrolimus primarily inhibits cell-mediated rejection of the renal allograft, which is mediated by T cells.

[2] Mycophenolate is a drug that reversibly and non-competitively inhibits an enzyme involved in the *de novo* synthesis of purine nucleotides. Nucleotides can be synthesised within cells either via *de novo* synthesis or via metabolism of pre-existing nucleotides. B cells and T cells are the only cell types that synthesise nucleotides via *de novo* synthesis. Hence, mycophenolate inhibits DNA nucleotide production in B and T cells selectively.

[3] Prednisolone has many different effects on various parts of the immune system; all these effects are immunosuppressive. Prednisolone inhibits the margination of white cells into the interstitium in inflammation, and invariably inhibits the production of almost all inflammatory cytokines (e.g. IL-1 and TNF-alpha).
Therefore, prednisolone largely inhibits the innate immune response.

[4] Tacrolimus is very well-known (paradoxically) for renal toxicity. One of the effects of tacrolimus is the inhibition of Mg^{2+} reabsorption in the tubules. Patients on tacrolimus can become profoundly hypomagnesaemic; hence, magnesium supplementation is given to balance the profound renal magnesium wasting.

[5] This shows that there is likely sufficient excretion of Na^+ ions and water in the urine to maintain a relatively normal extracellular fluid volume, one of the functions of the kidney.

[6] Proteins such as albumin have a detergent effect on the urine, reducing its surface tension and allowing the formation of bubbles on agitation of the urine (e.g. during micturition). Frothy urine is a sign of severe proteinuria; the absence of this indicates that the glomerular filtration barrier of the graft is sufficiently intact to prevent severe leakage of protein into the urine.

[7] Impaired exercise tolerance may be due to shortness of breath on exertion, which may be due (among other causes) to pulmonary oedema. Any pulmonary oedema, in this case, could be secondary to an extracellular volume expansion causing increased pulmonary capillary hydrostatic pressure and transudation/ultrafiltration of plasma into the pulmonary interstitium.
This pulmonary oedema increases the diffusion distance between the alveolus (at the air–water interface) and the pulmonary capillary containing oxygen, and hence impairs gas exchange. This effect would be heterogeneous in that the oedema would be prominent in the lower lobes of the lung (due to the effect of gravity on pulmonary capillary hydrostatic pressure). The consequent ventilation perfusion mismatch would be partially corrected for by changes to

bronchiolar and pulmonary arteriolar smooth muscle tone throughout the lung.

Exercise increases the pulmonary blood flow and changes the distribution of blood flow as well as distribution of inhaled air throughout the lung which can worsen the ventilation perfusion mismatch, causing exercise-induced hypoxia. Transient hypercapnia can also occur if this distribution change leads to the advent of physiological dead spaces (where regions of lung are being ventilated, but blood flow

to these areas is negligible), worsened by the increased metabolic rate of muscle in exercise producing extra CO_2. This hypoxia and hypercapnia can stimulate chemoreceptors (peripheral and central) and induce severe shortness of breath.

Hence, a good exercise tolerance is a sign that the extracellular fluid volume is sufficiently maintained by adequate renal excretion of Na^+ ions and there is no pulmonary oedema.

Examination

- On examination, the patient looks generally well. BP is **147/89mmHg** [1], HR 64bpm, RR 19, SaO_2 98% on air and afebrile.
- No **coarse tremor** [2] is visible on extension of his arms.
- There is no evidence of **bruising** [3] on his arms.
- JVP is normal, 2cm above the sternal notch vertically.
- Chest was clear to auscultation with normal heart sounds.
- Abdomen was soft to palpation. There is some **mild tenderness over the renal graft site** [4].
- There is no evidence of **peripheral oedema** [5].

1 In patients with a renal transplant, the presence of new hypertension can be secondary to the toxic effects of tacrolimus or due to an extracellular volume expansion from inadequate renal Na^+ ion excretion due to impaired glomerular filtration.

Inadequate Na^+ ion excretion leads to an excess amount of Na^+ ions in the extracellular fluid, leading to a higher volume of ECF (as the osmoreceptors ensure a relatively constant concentration of Na^+ in the ECF by retaining extra free water in the kidney if needed). A higher ECF volume, in this case, is accompanied by a higher volume of venous blood at a higher mean systemic filling pressure; a high mean systemic filling pressure means a high preload, and leads to a high left ventricular systolic pressure and thus a high systemic arterial pressure.

Tacrolimus induces hypertension by itself causing renal Na^+ retention (at the tubules) and renal vasoconstriction. Renal Na^+ retention causes hypertension via the mechanism described previously. Renal vasoconstriction leads to a decreased peritubular capillary hydrostatic pressure. This promotes reabsorption of Na^+ ions and water from the tubular cells back into the peritubular capillaries, which, in turn, promotes reabsorption of Na^+ ions and water from the tubules. This mechanism is referred to as inhibition of pressure diuresis and natriuresis. In addition, renal vasoconstriction leads to an increase in the activity of the renin–angiotensin system in an attempt to maintain normal GFR, with the angiotensin II causing efferent arteriolar constriction, further decreasing the peritubular capillary hydrostatic pressure.

In a well patient with normal kidneys, manually expanding the ECF volume (e.g. by administration of excessive amounts of normal saline) leads to systemic hypertension, followed by an increased peritubular hydrostatic pressure and hence an impairment of reabsorption of Na^+ and water to the peritubular capillaries, increased Na^+ and water reabsorption,

and contraction of the ECF volume. This mechanism is known as pressure diuresis and natriuresis.

2 Tacrolimus is also neurotoxic through unclear mechanisms; a mild manifestation of its neurotoxicity is a coarse postural and action tremor.

3 Via unclear mechanisms, mycophenolate suppresses the production of cells derived from the myeloid lineage in the bone marrow, including red blood cells, neutrophils and monocytes and platelets.

Hence, mycophenolate can induce profound thrombocytopenia; this can impair haemostasis and therefore can lead to easy bruising.

4 Graft tenderness occurs due to a number of causes, including graft pyelonephritis and acute graft rejection. The nerve pathways involved in this are as yet unclear.

5 The lack of peripheral oedema is supportive evidence that the ECF volume is not excessively high; excess extracellular volume is distributed to the interstitium from the blood through high capillary interstitial pressures and ultrafiltration of fluid into the interstitium.

Investigations

Pre-transplant bloods are shown below:

- **HLA typing – 4/6 match between donor and recipient** [1].
- **Donor-specific antibodies** [2] absent.
- **Blood group** [3] – A+ (recipient), O+ (donor).
- **CMV IgG** [4] – negative in both donor and recipient.
- Hepatitis B serology – **core antibodies** [5] negative in donor and recipient, **surface antibodies** [6] positive in both donor and recipient.
- **Hepatitis C IgG** [7] – negative in donor and recipient.
- **EBV IgG** [8] – positive in both donor and recipient.
- **VZV IgG** [9] – positive in both donor and recipient.
- HIV serology – negative in both donor and recipient.

Routine blood results are shown below:

2 weeks prior		Clinic review	
Hb (g/L)	131	Hb (g/L)	126
WCC (x 10^9/L)	5.2	WCC (x 10^9/L)	5.7
Platelets (x 10^9/L)	191	Platelets (x 10^9/L)	210
Na$^+$ (mM)	137	Na$^+$ (mM)	135
K$^+$ (mM)	3.9	K$^+$ (mM)	4.5
Cl$^-$ (mM)	95	Cl$^-$ (mM)	96
Mg^{2+} (mM)	0.82	Mg^{2+} (mM)	0.98
Ur (mM)	5.6	Ur (mM)	6.4
Cr (µM)	98	Cr (µM)	**210** [10]
eGFR (ml/min/1.73m²)	83	eGFR (ml/min/1.73m²)	**34** [10]

Urine MCS performed subsequently showed the following:

- Microscopy:
  - WCC (x 10^9) = 70
  - RCC (x 10^9) = 100
  - protein ++
  - blood ++
  - red cell casts and dysmorphic red cells present.

The results of an urgent renal graft biopsy performed the next morning showed:

- extensive **neutrophilic and monocytic infiltrate** [11] in the mesangium, with evidence of capillaritis and **glomerular basement membrane reduplication** [12], with some evidence of glomerulosclerosis
- extensive monocytic and **T-cell** [13] infiltrate in the interstitium, with evidence of tubulitis
- **C4d staining** [14] on immunofluorescence
- tacrolimus level – 3.5ng/ml (5–15 is therapeutic)
- urine protein–creatinine ratio – **1.3g/g** [15]
- donor-specific antibodies – **positive, MFI** [16] = 4500 (to one donor antigen)

---

1 HLA (human leucocyte antigen) is a set of proteins found on the cell membranes of all cells. These protein molecules present antigens to T cells (self or non-self) by incorporating the antigen onto their extracellular domains. HLA proteins have two categories – MHC class I proteins and MHC class II proteins.

MHC class I proteins are expressed in all nucleated cells, and present antigens to Tc cells. HLA proteins that are in this group are the HLA-A, HLA-B and HLA-C proteins.

MHC class II proteins are expressed in specific white cell types, including B cells, dendritic cells and macrophages (collectively known as antigen-presenting cells). These take up soluble antigens from the extracellular environment and present these antigens on their MHC class II proteins to Th cells. HLA proteins that are in this group are the HLA-DP, HLA-DQ and HLA-DR proteins.

In addition to their antigen-presenting function, HLA proteins are proteins and therefore are themselves antigens. Also, HLA has an additional property that the structure of each HLA protein has extremely high variation between individuals; this is because the genes coding for each individual HLA protein have >3000 alleles for class I proteins and >10 000 alleles for class II proteins. Thus, there is an extremely high number of possible haplotypes (set of alleles at each gene coding for each HLA protein component). This extremely high variation means that HLA proteins themselves are highly prominent antigens in the setting of transplants, and a 'mismatch' of HLA proteins between donor and recipient increases the likelihood of organ rejection.

In HLA typing, the HLA genotype of the donor and recipient at the -A, -B and -DR loci are only determined by molecular testing; each individual has a total of 6 alleles, two alleles at each of the three gene loci. A 'mismatch' occurs if the donor possesses an allele that the recipient does not have a sufficiently similar allele to. For example, suppose the donor had a genotype of HLA-A*2, A*23 (heterozygous for the A*2 and A*23 alleles at the HLA-A gene locus). It is important to note that the A*2 and A*23 'alleles' actually refers to groups of alleles that are similar enough to one another (between A*2 alleles and between A*23 alleles) to render proteins that are structurally sufficiently similar that the risk of rejection is low. Now suppose the recipient had a genotype of HLA-A*2, A*4. The donor and recipient share the HLA-A*2 allele (although they might differ very slightly between the donor and recipient) but they do not share the A*4 or A*23 alleles. This means that when the recipient receives the kidney, the recipient will be exposed to the A*23 allele which will be considered non-self. This constitutes a 1 out of 2 match. Repeating this process for the other four alleles (at the -B and -DR loci), one can determine what the match is, out of 6. The score out of 6 corresponds to the number of donor alleles the recipient will likely recognise as self. In this recipient, the recipient will likely recognise 4 out of the 6 alleles as self. The higher the 'match', the lower the risk of rejection.

2 Donor-specific antibodies (DSAs) are antibodies against non-self HLA proteins. If these are found in the recipient prior to transplant, this means the recipient has already been exposed to these non-self HLA proteins previously, and mounted a humoral immune response against these proteins. This could have occurred in pregnancy (in a female), where the mother may be exposed to foetal HLA proteins (inherited from the father) that are non-self, or in previous transplants. Importantly, if a humoral immune response has already been formed against non-self HLA proteins, this means that memory B cells against these HLA proteins would be present in the donor. Hence, if there are antibodies against non-HLA proteins that coincidentally are also found in the donor kidney, this is a contraindication to transplant. This is because upon exposure to the HLA proteins (for which there are pre-existing antibodies) on transplant, the memory B cells will mount a highly rapid and intense immune response against the graft, leading to hyperacute rejection.

DSAs newly formed after transplant are a sign that a humoral immune response against the graft is occurring with the production of these antibodies.

3 ABO antigens are expressed on red blood cells. They are also expressed on white cells and platelets as well as epithelial and endothelial cells. This means that solid organs, such as kidneys, will have cells (epithelial cells) that express ABO antigens on their cell surfaces. Hence, ABO compatibility with solid organ transplant mirrors that of ABO blood transfusion. The rhesus antigen, however, is not expressed on solid organ cells and therefore is not a consideration in transplant compatibility.

The donor has blood group O, meaning that neither the A or B antigen is expressed on epithelial cells. Hence, the donor kidney will be compatible with respect to the recipient in terms of ABO compatibility. For completeness, the recipient has blood group A, meaning the recipient possesses the A antigen on the relevant cell surfaces, and will have preformed antibodies against the B antigen. The transplant kidney, however, will not express the B antigen.

4 Cytomegalovirus (CMV) is a virus that infects most people during their lifetime; the virulence is low, but CMV is not easily cleared. Hence, in most people, CMV remains

dormant. A humoral immune response is instigated against CMV, leading to the production of IgG. Hence, IgG seropositivity indicates that the individual has been infected with CMV and has mounted a humoral immune response against it.

CMV is relevant as it replicates in immunosuppressed individuals (e.g. those who are on immunosuppressive medications for transplants). Recipients who have been exposed to CMV and mounted an immune response are at intermediate risk of CMV disease after immunosuppression, as CMV remains dormant in previously infected individuals. Recipients who have not been exposed to CMV (and hence are not sensitised to it), and are receiving a kidney from a CMV-exposed donor, are at extremely high risk of CMV infection.

In this case, neither the donor nor recipient has been exposed to CMV, so the risk of CMV disease is very low.

5 The hepatitis B virus has a 'core' antigen on its capsid. When a patient is exposed to hepatitis B virus, a humoral immune response mounts almost immediately against the 'core' antigen, leading to IgM and subsequently IgG production. Lack of core antibodies in both donor and recipient means that neither has been exposed to hepatitis B virus.

6 The hepatitis B virus has a 'surface' antigen on its lipid envelope as well. This surface antigen is also used in hepatitis B vaccines (which are composed of the surface antigen). Patients who have been vaccinated against hepatitis B will therefore have surface antibodies, but NOT core antibodies. Both the donor and recipient have been vaccinated against hepatitis B.

7 Upon exposure to hepatitis C, a humoral immune response mounts, and immunoglobulin is produced, initially IgM and subsequently IgG. Hepatitis C IgM is not tested routinely because it is not considered to have much additional diagnostic power. However, hepatitis C IgG appears at detectable levels in the serum approximately 2 months after initial exposure.

After an individual is infected with hepatitis C, most people are unable to clear the virus and get chronic hepatitis C (unless treated with antiviral therapy which is curative). There is no hepatitis C virus at this stage.

Hence, a positive hepatitis C IgG means the individual has previously been infected with hepatitis C and likely has ongoing hepatitis C infection (unless they have had antiviral treatment).

8 EBV (Epstein–Barr virus) causes glandular fever in adolescents and adults. In infants and toddlers, EBV is relatively asymptomatic or presents as a very mild viral illness. However, new EBV infection in a previously unexposed patient who is immunosuppressed can lead to a potentially fatal lymphoproliferative disorder (known as post-transplant lymphoproliferative disorder).

Most individuals (about 90%) will have previously been exposed to EBV and mounted a humoral immune response. Both the donor and recipient are among these individuals and therefore the risk of the recipient getting post-transplant lymphoproliferative disorder is low.

9 VZV (varicella zoster virus) causes chickenpox on primary infection and shingles on reactivation, for example after immunosuppression. After primary infection with VZV, the virus remains dormant in neuronal ganglia.
Both vaccination and chickenpox infection lead to a humoral immune response with production of anti-VZV IgG. However, vaccination reduces the risk of reactivation of VZV and shingles.

10 Creatinine is a marker of GFR, as its rate of production by muscle is relatively constant, and creatinine is almost entirely cleared through glomerular filtration alone (although there is also some tubular secretion). The serum creatinine is inversely proportional to the glomerular filtration rate assuming it is constant (at the steady state).
The eGFR is a number that is calculated using a mathematical formula, with variables being serum creatinine age, sex and race, and provides a reasonable estimate of the true GFR, assuming the serum creatinine is constant.
However, in this case, the serum creatinine is increasing; it will continue to increase until it reaches its steady state value. This will happen when the concentration of creatinine in the plasma is high enough that the rate of creatinine excretion, in the setting of a low GFR of plasma, is as high as the rate of creatinine production.
Hence, the true GFR will be closer to the eGFR once the serum creatinine increases to its steady state value. Hence, the true GFR is likely to be significantly lower than 34 (unless the serum creatinine value of 210 happens to be the steady state value).

11 During acute inflammation, neutrophils and, later, monocytes, adhere to the vascular endothelium when the endothelial cells express adhesion proteins on their cell surface that binds these two cell types.
Hence, neutrophils and monocytes would be found in the mesangium, as part of an acute inflammatory response.

12 GBM reduplication is where extra extracellular matrix proteins are synthesised in the glomerular basement membrane. Ongoing acute inflammation, mediated by cytokines and signalling molecules released during acute inflammation (e.g. TGF-beta), leads to an upregulation of signalling pathways within mesangial cells to produce

extracellular matrix proteins, which are deposited in the mesangium and the glomerular basement membrane.

13 The presence of T cells in the interstitium indicates the presence of cell-mediated immunity, mediated by Tc (CD8+) cells.

14 C4d staining indicates the presence of antibody-mediated rejection. When a humoral immune response is instigated against antigens (e.g. HLA antigens) of the donor kidney and antibodies against these antigens are produced and bind to these antigens, this leads to the activation of complement, via the classical pathway. The classical pathway involves the activation of the C1 complex, which causes activation of C2 and C4; activation of C4 leads to its cleavage to C4a and C4b. Subsequent cleavage and inactivation of C4b leads to the production of C4d (a fragment). C4d has the property that it can actually covalently bind to molecules on the cell surface of vascular endothelial cells of the kidney. Hence, C4d deposits on the glomeruli, which can be visualised on immunofluorescence.
The alternative pathway does not involve activation of C4.

15 The protein–creatinine ratio is a crude approximation of the rate of protein excretion. As it turns out, the numerical value of the protein–creatinine ratio in g/g is roughly equal to that of the rate of protein excretion in g/day. Hence, the rate of protein excretion is roughly 1g per day, which is excessive. The proteinuria is a sign of a 'leaky' glomerular filtration barrier due to podocyte damage. Podocytes form an integral part of the glomerular filtration barrier and their arrangement, with their foot processes, normally prevents the filtration of significant amounts of protein at the glomerulus.

16 The presence of new DSAs (anti-HLA antibodies against the donor HLA antigens) after transplant is a sign that the recipient is instigating a humoral immune response.
In this test, the recipient serum (containing the DSA) is added onto 'beads' coated with different alleles of different HLA gene loci, and a fluorescent dye binding to recipient antibody that binds to the bead is added. The brighter the bead, the more antibody there is, and the higher the fluorescence, measured by median fluorescence intensity (MFI).
Hence, the MFI is a crude measure of the amount of the specific antibody against a given HLA antigen.

Management

Immediate

Admit the patient under the Renal Unit as an inpatient and collect a urine MCS (shown previously), monitor UECs and strict fluid balance and take a tacrolimus level and perform an urgent renal biopsy.

Given that the renal biopsy showed evidence of both cell-mediated and antibody-mediated rejection, the following treatment regimen is performed:

- **IV methylprednisolone** [1] 500mg for 3 days, then oral prednisolone taper to a final dose of 20mg

- **plasma exchange** [2] on alternate days
- **IVIg** [3] on alternate days
- **rituximab** [4] after completion of plasma exchange and IVIg
- **thymoglobulin** [5] on alternate days.

Tacrolimus and mycophenolate doses should be increased and white cell counts monitored.
The following prophylactic medications should be commenced:

- **trimethoprim/sulfamethoxazole** [6] 160/800mg three times a week
- **valaciclovir** [7].

Short-term

Monitor renal function daily.
Repeat protein–creatinine ratio in 1 week.
Repeat renal biopsy in 1–2 weeks to assess for resolution of acute inflammatory changes and repeat DSAs to assess for depletion of these antibodies.

Long-term

The patient should be maintained on higher doses of prednisolone, tacrolimus and mycophenolate.
Outpatient monitoring should be more frequent, with repeat FBEs, UECs and tacrolimus levels.
Blood pressure and **HbA1c** [8] should be monitored frequently.

1 As previously explained, glucocorticoids are immunosuppressive through many mechanisms, including impairing white cell margination into the interstitium and impairing cytokine production by white cells that mediate acute inflammation.
In very high doses, glucocorticoids cause significant T-cell lymphopenia with sequestration of T cells away from the blood into tissues such as lymph nodes and inhibition of IL-2 production; this effect occurs hours after the initial dose is given. A high dose of prednisolone is >60mg (or 1mg/kg), which is equivalent to a methylprednisolone dose of 48mg. Here, the methylprednisolone dose is 500mg, which is very high.
The purpose of methylprednisolone is to rapidly inhibit the function of T cells and provide rapid immunosuppression.

2 Plasma exchange is where blood is removed from the patient and 'filtered' to remove the plasma, with this plasma being replaced by a fluid such as albumin and fresh frozen plasma. The aim is to remove antibodies against donor antigens from the plasma that are responsible for the acute rejection.

3 IVIg is a mixture of IgG antibodies from pooled plasma donated by multiple individuals. IVIg aims to replace IgG antibodies in the patient that were removed on plasma exchange along with the pathogenic anti-donor tissue antibodies. IVIg also paradoxically has anti-inflammatory and immunosuppressive effects through many different mechanisms.

4 Rituximab is a monoclonal antibody against the CD20 protein. This protein is expressed on most B cells.
Binding of rituximab to the CD20 protein on B cells has multiple effects:
- neutrophils and macrophages bind to the Fc portion of the rituximab, and phagocytose and destroy B cells

- complement is activated by rituximab via the classical pathway, leading to lysis of B cells.
Ultimately, the rituximab causes profound B-cell depletion and hence minimises further plasma cell production (against donor antigens) after the completion of anti-donor tissue antibody removal through plasma exchange and IVIg.

5 Thymoglobulin is a mixture of antibodies against proteins expressed on the surface of thymocytes (lymphocytes residing in the thymus – i.e. T cells). On administration, the antibodies in thymoglobulin bind to Th cells in the bloodstream and, through complement-mediated lysis, cause a massive decrease in the number of circulating Th cells through Th-cell destruction.
Loss of Th cells inhibits both the humoral and cell-mediated immune response, as Th cells are responsible for secreting cytokines that upregulate both responses, and are responsible for direct activation of B cells.

6 *Pneumocystis jirovecii* is an atypical fungus that colonises the alveoli of most individuals in childhood, the proliferation of which is controlled by the immune system. Much of this control is dependent on Th cells and alveolar macrophages. When a patient is immunosuppressed, with loss of number and function of Th cells and alveolar macrophages, *P. jirovecii* can replicate and cause life-threatening pneumonia.
Trimethoprim/sulfamethoxazole (Bactrim) 3 times a week is an antibiotic that also is active against *P. jirovecii*, at a dose that prevents significant replication.

7 Valaciclovir is an antiviral that is particularly effective against herpesviruses, including VZV. It is a nucleoside analogue that binds viral DNA polymerase, inhibiting viral replication intracellularly.
This patient, who has a positive IgG to VZV, may have had chickenpox in the past, and therefore may have VZV virus dormant in neuronal ganglia. T-cell depletion and

immunosuppression can allow VZV to reactivate, replicate, and cause severe shingles (including disseminated shingles). Valaciclovir prevents this VZV replication during the period of intense immunosuppression.

8 Tacrolimus and prednisolone can both cause diabetes. Tacrolimus is toxic to beta-cells of the islet cells in the pancreas that produce insulin, and also directly inhibits insulin secretion. Prednisolone has multiple effects on glucose metabolism, most notably increased gluconeogenesis and increased insulin resistance.

Therefore, HbA1c levels should be measured to assess for the onset of diabetes.

CASE 81: Acute respiratory distress syndrome

History

- A 78-year-old female, who lived at home alone, was admitted into hospital one day ago with **community-acquired pneumonia** [1] after presenting with a **productive cough and fevers** [2].
- She has a **past medical history of hypertension, hypercholesterolaemia and gout** [3]. She has previously had asthma during childhood; however, has no known airways disease in her adult life. She maintained an active and independent lifestyle prior to becoming unwell.
- She has **never smoked** [4]. There was no history of recent travel or trauma. One day prior to presentation, she developed a productive cough without haemoptysis and dyspnoea, mainly on mobilisation.

- There was **no history of orthopnoea, paroxysmal nocturnal dyspnoea or peripheral oedema** [5]. There was also no history of night sweats or loss of weight.
- The patient was commenced on intravenous antibiotics. Despite treatment with appropriate antibiotics, she developed worsening dyspnoea and **required 6L of supplemental oxygen to maintain saturations of 90%** [6].
- The patient was subsequently diagnosed with acute respiratory distress syndrome. **Despite maximal treatment, she passed away during her admission** [7].

[1] Acute respiratory distress syndrome (ARDS) is an acute, inflammatory injury of the lung. ARDS is normally triggered by a precipitating event such as sepsis (most common in hospital cause of ARDS), pneumonia, aspiration pneumonitis and trauma. Other less common causes include massive transfusions, smoke inhalation, transfusion-related lung injury, pancreatitis and drugs. Drug-related ARDS can be caused by chemotherapy agents, amiodarone and radiation. Physiologically, ARDS is due to a diffuse alveolar injury resulting in release of pro-inflammatory cytokines. As a result, there is increased neutrophil infiltration into the lungs, leading to a release of toxic mediations directly causing damage to capillary and alveolar epithelium.

[2] Symptoms initially are related to the underlying aetiology and investigation should be tailored to identify the underlying cause. The specific symptoms of ARDS are dyspnoea, hypoxia and increased oxygenation requirements. Symptoms of ARDS can develop as quickly as 6 hours after onset of the precipitating event; however, late presentations can occur after 72 hours or even up to 1 week after the initial event. In severe cases of ARDS, patients can be confused, cyanotic and diaphoretic.

[3] The diagnosis of ARDS can be difficult to make and can be delayed. A thorough history is required to aid early diagnosis. Past medical history may provide clues for ischaemic heart disease, transfusion requirements, pancreatitis, previous surgeries and possible drug-related causes.

[4] Smoking history is vital to determine in patients who are presenting with dyspnoea.

[5] Paroxysmal nocturnal dyspnoea (PND), orthopnoea and peripheral oedema are all suggestive of an underlying cardiac aetiology. A common differential diagnosis for ARDS is pulmonary oedema. Management and outcomes for these conditions differ greatly.

[6] Patients can improve with treatment of the underlying condition. However, once ARDS develops, patients experience worsening dyspnoea and hypoxia. Oxygen requirements are high and may also warrant consideration of positive end-expiratory pressure.

[7] ARDS is associated with high mortality, estimated to be 40% in hospital. Some poor predictive factors of outcome include increased patient age, severe hypoxia, infection and non-traumatic causes. Patients with fluid overload, packed red blood cell transfusions, and glucocorticoid therapy before onset of ARDS have also been shown to result in high mortality.
Other complications of ARDS include atelectasis, hospital- and intensive care unit-associated complications, multi-organ failure, pulmonary hypertension and pulmonary emboli.

Examination

- On examination, the **patient is confused** [1].
- She is positioned upright in the bed and has an increased work of breathing with **high flow nasal prongs** [2] *in situ*.
- A **CPAP machine** [3] is noted at the bedside.
- She has a **blood pressure of 94/60mmHg** [4], **heart rate of 78bpm (irregular)** [5], oxygen saturations of 90% on FiO_2 40%, and **respiratory rate of 26 breaths per minute** [6].

- She has moist mucous membranes with a **JVP at 2cm** [7]. Her heart sounds are dual with no appreciable murmurs.
- Her **chest examination** [8] reveals reduced chest expansion and bilateral crepitations throughout the lungs.
- The **abdomen is soft and non-tender** [9].
- There is **no evidence of peripheral oedema** [10].
- **No rashes or skin lesions** [11] are seen on examination of the skin.

1 Confusion (delirium) is common in patients who are unwell and require hospitalisation. Confusion is also a feature of severe ARDS and holds a poorer prognosis.

2 General inspection provides an overall assessment of these patients' current clinical state. This patient appears to be in respiratory distress and the need for high flow nasal prongs suggests some positive pressure is required to aid her ventilation.

3 CPAP provides a non-invasive form of ventilation and positive pressure to reduce respiratory effort and aid respiration, which could potentially be a ward-based management or a bridging therapy whilst waiting for intensive care admission. Positive pressure is used to maximise alveolar capacity and improve oxygenation.

4 Hypotension can be a sign of sepsis depending on the rest of the patient's clinical state. Patients can be hypotensive for various reasons, including volaemic state, underlying infection and cardiogenic shock. As part of treatment, maintaining adequate blood pressure will be crucial for organ perfusion.

5 A normal heart rate is 60–100bpm. Patients with severe infection can develop arrhythmias, such as atrial fibrillation.

Treatment of the underlying cause will be a key factor, but further assessment of risks associated with AF will need to be considered, such as anticoagulation to reduce the risk of stroke (CHA_2DS_2-VASc score) and rate control.

6 Despite oxygenation and respiratory support, the patient is saturating at 90%. This is a poor predictor of outcomes.

7 ARDS is diagnosed once acute cardiogenic pulmonary oedema has been ruled out. A JVP of 2cm would not be suggestive of fluid overload. Furthermore, a positive fluid balance is a poor predictor of overall outcomes.

8 Due to their respiratory distress and risk of tiring, patients can have reduced inspiratory effort and hence, reduced chest expansion. Because of the underlying inflammatory changes through the lung fields, bilateral crepitations can be heard.

9 Examination of the abdomen can reveal other causes of ARDS.

10 Peripheral oedema is a sign of fluid overload.

11 In patients with ARDS, skin lesions and rashes can point towards an underlying cause.

Investigations

- There are no direct investigations that confirm the **diagnosis of ARDS** [1].
- A **full blood examination** [2] revealed an elevated WCC and platelet levels.
- There was evidence of **acute kidney injury** [3] with normal sodium and potassium. The liver function tests were normal.
- A **C-reactive protein** [4] was elevated at 208.

- An **arterial blood gas** [5] revealed type 1 respiratory failure.
- A **BNP was <100pg/ml** [6].
- A **CXR** [7] demonstrated bilateral diffuse opacities throughout the lung fields and right basal consolidation.
- An **ECG** [8] showed atrial fibrillation with a rate of 80bpm, without any evidence of acute ischaemia.

1 The diagnosis of ARDS is based on clinical features of dyspnoea and hypoxia with increased oxygen requirements. Chest X-ray findings as described can also be supportive of the diagnosis. Overall, investigations are targeted towards identifying the underlying cause to guide overall treatment.

2 Elevated white cell count on FBC is consistent with infection. Platelets can also be elevated in the setting of an inflammatory response.

3 Acute kidney injury is a common finding in patients admitted to hospital. Causes are broadly defined into pre-renal (dehydration, infection), renal (acute interstitial nephritis, acute tubular necrosis, glomerular nephritis) and post-renal (obstruction).

4 Elevated CRP levels above 100 are suggestive of a bacterial infection.

5 An arterial blood gas (ABG) is particularly important in ARDS to aid diagnosis and also to monitor progress and treatment response. Typically, ABG will reveal hypoxia. A lactate is also measured on ABGs and is useful as a prognostic guide.

6 In ARDS, one of the most important clinical differentials to exclude is acute cardiogenic pulmonary oedema, which can be difficult to tell apart. As such, BNP is a helpful adjunct together with clinical assessment to make that distinction. It is noted that plasma BNP of <100pg/ml may favour ARDS. However, higher levels neither confirm acute cardiogenic pulmonary oedema nor exclude ARDS. Should there still be any confusion between distinguishing the two conditions, a transthoracic echocardiogram can be utilised to look for evidence of cardiac dysfunction.

7 Chest X-ray is helpful to support the diagnosis of ARDS and is useful for evaluating the possible causes for it. Radiological findings are dependent on the severity of ARDS. In the initial phases, chest X-ray would show bilateral diffuse alveolar opacities with dependent atelectasis. Other imaging modalities may help in identifying specific causes for ARDS.

8 As mentioned earlier, acute cardiogenic pulmonary oedema is an important differential to exclude. Should a patient have a myocardial ischaemic event, this could potentially result in acute cardiogenic pulmonary oedema. An ECG would be able to help pick up arrhythmias, right/left ventricular strain or ST segment changes suggestive of myocardial ischaemia.

Management

- There is **no direct treatment** [1] for ARDS.
- Most acute management of ARDS will be focused on improving oxygenation. The main options for management are **ventilation support** [2], **prone positioning** [3] and **conservative fluid management** [4].

1 ARDS has no direct cure. Management is focused on treating the underlying cause and supportive measures whilst alveolar function improves.

2 Ventilation support can be in the form of non-invasive measures (high flow via nasal prongs or a face mask) or invasive measures such as intubation. The majority of patients will require intubation and mechanical ventilation. Oxygenation should be aimed at 95–100%. Other patient factors require consideration prior to intubation, such as patient wishes and baseline level of function.

3 Prone positioning can be considered after 12–24 hours of stable supine ventilation, for up to 36 hours. Prone positioning can be used to help improve oxygenation as it allows more homogeneous ventilation and less overinflation of alveoli due to reduced pressure difference between dorsal and alveoli. This leads to less ventilator-associated lung injury. A prone position also reduces compression of the posterior lung and allows for more even ventilation of the lung parenchyma. Finally, prone positioning improves the ventilation and perfusion match and allows even more blood flow throughout the collapsed lung alveoli. Contraindications to prone ventilation include spinal instability, patients with unstable fractures, anterior chest burns, open wounds and pregnancy.

4 Patients with ARDS require conservative fluid management. This reduces the risk of oedema. More conservative fluid management has been demonstrated to improve oxygenation, reduce long-term lung injury, reduce time on ventilator and shorten an ICU stay.

CASE 82: Asbestosis

History

- A **68-year-old man** [1] who is a **retired electrician** [2] presents with **progressive exertional dyspnoea** [3].
- He reports no cough and is most concerned about a reduction in exercise tolerance to 100m, limited by his breathing. Twelve months ago, he was able to mobilise a kilometre without concern.
- He was a **previous smoker of 20 pack years but ceased 15 years ago** [4].
- He **denies any weight loss, night sweats or fevers** [5].

[1] Asbestosis is a diffuse interstitial lung-fibrosing disease due to exposure to asbestos fibres. There is a spectrum of diseases associated with asbestos exposure. These include asbestosis, benign pleural plaques, lung carcinoma (non-small cell and small cell) and mesothelioma. Males are most likely to have asbestos-related lung disease, mainly due to occupational exposure. There have been reported cases of females with asbestosis, and in the absence of direct exposure through work, many of these have been linked to secondary exposure (e.g. through washing of husband's clothes that have asbestos dust on them).

[2] Asbestos exposure was common in people working in the mining, milling, shipbuilding and construction businesses. Asbestos was found in fire-resistant materials, cement and flooring. Exposure was not only direct but also passive; electricians, painters and plumbers have also been reported to have developed asbestos-related lung diseases. Exposure to asbestos would have been at least a decade prior to symptom development.

[3] The main presenting symptom is insidious exertional dyspnoea. This is due to the fibrotic process occurring within the lung. Other associated symptoms such as cough, sputum and wheeze are not common directly due to asbestos.

[4] Smoking has been found to worsen symptoms of dyspnoea and increase the risk of lung malignancy. Smoking and asbestosis independently are risk factors for lung malignancy, and combined further add risk to development of malignancy.

[5] The presence of such B symptoms would be a red flag for more sinister pathology such as malignancy or mesothelioma. It is important to ask the patient about these key features on initial history. Particularly in mesothelioma, there can be rapid progression and hence deterioration, and early diagnosis would be pivotal.

Examination

- On examination, the patient is a **lean-looking man but does not appear cachectic** [1].
- Examination of his hands revealed **tar staining** [2] and **clubbing of the nails** [3].
- He does not have evidence of **pale conjunctiva** [4] and his **JVP is at 2cm** [5].
- There is **no cervical lymphadenopathy** [6].
- His **trachea is in the midline, without presence of a tug** [7].
- His chest had **reduced chest expansion** [8], although this was noted to be symmetrical.
- There is **no dullness on percussion** [9].
- On auscultation, there were **fine end-inspiratory crackles** [10].
- His cardiovascular examination was normal and there were **no signs of peripheral oedema** [11].

1 General inspection will provide multiple clues as to the patient's clinical state. Cachexia is a prominent feature that is easily identifiable. The presence of cachexia can be an indicator of malignancy or poor nutritional state.

2 Tar staining is a hard sign of the patient's smoking history. The level of staining does not indicate the degree of the patient's smoking history.

3 Clubbing is an important sign, although there are many different causes. These range from cardiovascular (congenital heart disease, infective endocarditis) and respiratory (abscess, bronchiectasis, cystic fibrosis, idiopathic pulmonary fibrosis, malignancy) to GI (ulcerative colitis, biliary cirrhosis).

4 Pale conjunctiva indicates anaemia. If present, it could be a differential cause of the patient's dyspnoea.

5 JVP is a marker of fluid status in the body. A normal JVP is up to 3cm. Elevated JVP indicates fluid overload. Causes of fluid overload would also be important differentials to rule out, as this would greatly alter management for the patient.

6 Cervical lymphadenopathy would be more suggestive of a malignant cause and spread.

7 Tracheal placement is important in a respiratory exam, as displacement can help narrow down potential differentials for the patient's presentation. Displacement towards the side of the lesions may be due to upper lobe fibrosis or collapse. Displacement away from the side of the lung lesion may be suggestive of a tension pneumothorax.

8 Normal chest expansion is 5cm. Due to the fibrotic nature of asbestosis, the lungs as a result become stiff and there is a reduction of chest expansion on examination.

9 Dullness on percussion is an indicator of pleural effusion. Some patients can have asbestos-related pleural effusions. However, this is less common in asbestosis.

10 Fine end-inspiratory crackles are a sign of fibrotic lung disease. At times, these can also be pan-inspiratory. Typically they sound like Velcro being pulled apart.

11 Cor pulmonale or pulmonary hypertension can develop as a result of clinical progression of asbestosis. This can cause peripheral oedema, jugular venous distension, hepatojugular reflux and sometimes a right ventricular heave or gallop.

Investigations

- The initial investigation for the diagnosis of asbestosis is **pulmonary function testing** [1] to assess the severity and character of lung impairment.
- An **initial chest X-ray** [2] can be performed to look for features of asbestosis as well as rule out other contributing factors to the patient's dyspnoea.
- Further imaging can be performed through **high resolution CT (HRCT)** [3] of the chest.
- In certain patients, a **bronchoalveolar lavage (BAL)** [4] may be performed. However, the overall diagnosis of asbestosis can be made through clinical history and HRCT.

1 The initial test is that of pulmonary function which includes spirometry, lung volumes and assessment of the diffusing capacity for carbon monoxide (DLCO). Asbestosis is a restrictive lung disease and spirometry will show a normal forced expiratory volume in 1 second (FEV_1) to forced vital capacity (FVC) ratio. Other expected lung function abnormalities include reduced lung volumes and reduced DLCO.

2 Chest X-ray changes are not always evident in patients with asbestosis. Typical changes are bilateral pleural opacities. There may also be reticular pattern changes, although these are difficult to appreciate on plain X-ray. In asbestosis, changes typically will occur in the lower lobes compared to other pathologies that are more likely associated with upper lobe fibrotic changes. Other differentials for lower lobe fibrosis include rheumatoid arthritis, scleroderma, idiopathic pulmonary fibrosis, drugs (methotrexate, bleomycin, amiodarone) and radiation.

3 HRCT is more sensitive compared to plain chest imaging. Some of the radiological findings include subpleural linear densities, honeycombing and pleural plaques.

4 For patients where clinical history and HRCT combined is not sufficient for diagnosis of asbestosis, and alternative differential diagnoses such as malignancy or infection are yet to be adequately excluded, a BAL can be performed. There may be increased numbers of asbestos bodies found in BAL in patients who have had asbestosis, compared to those who have had previous exposure without development of lung fibrosis.

Management

Unfortunately for patients with asbestosis, there is no specific targeted treatment. **Most management is surrounding primary prevention and supportive treatment of symptoms** [1].

One of the key management strategies is **smoking cessation** [2]. If patients become hypoxic, typically this occurs on mobilisation, but as the disease progresses, this can also occur at rest, then **supplemental oxygen** [3] may be a treatment option.

Patients require **education regarding early recognition of respiratory infections** [4] and early consultation with GPs. Patients should be advised and encouraged to keep up to date with vaccinations including the **annual influenza vaccine and pneumococcal vaccination** [5].

1 Despite there being no specific treatment for asbestosis it is important to engage and provide patients with reassurances of ongoing monitoring and the role of primary prevention.

2 Smoking cessation will not only aid with symptoms of dyspnoea but also reduce the risk of developing lung malignancy. There are multiple strategies available to aid patients with smoking cessation, from the Smokefree National Helpline, to a variety of nicotine replacement therapies (patches, lozenges, inhalers).

3 Supplemental oxygen can be of symptomatic benefit for patients who are hypoxic or subjectively short of breath. There are specific guidelines on eligibility for funded home oxygenation. Contraindications to home oxygen include current smoking.

4 Early recognition of respiratory infections will help reduce the need for hospitalisation in patients with asbestosis and fibrotic lung disease. The presence of a new cough, sputum production and worsening dyspnoea warrants urgent review and consideration of early commencement of antibiotic therapy.

5 Vaccination plays an important role in primary prevention. Annual influenza vaccine and 5-yearly pneumococcal vaccine are recommended.

CASE 83: Asthma

History

- A **16-year-old** [1] boy presents to the ED with acute shortness of breath over the past 5 hours. He also reports chest tightness and wheeziness over the same time period.
- He states that he has had **similar episodes** [2] over the past few weeks after playing soccer with his friends and when **sleeping at night** [3].
- These episodes are associated with a **persistent cough at night** [4].
- He has a **history of eczema** [5] when he was younger, which was managed with corticosteroid cream, and his mum has a history of allergic rhinitis and eczema.

- The boy's mum reports that he had been unwell with a **runny nose and headache** [6] over the past 2 days and has had **friends who were similarly sick** [7] at school.
- The family do not have any **pets** [8] at home and he denies smoking.
- The boy denies a history of trauma or **foreign body inhalation** [9].
- He does not have any other significant past medical history and **has not presented to hospital before with asthma** [10].

[1] Asthma is relatively common in all ages, affecting around 10% of adults and around 15% of children. Most children with asthma tend to improve in adolescence.

[2] The primary symptoms of asthma are episodic shortness of breath and wheezing attacks. These symptoms can be paroxysmal or persistent, especially in poorly controlled asthma.

[3] It is common for asthmatics to wheeze after exercise or inhaling cold dry air. This is secondary to the release of histamine, prostaglandins and leucotrienes from mast cells, and the stimulation of neural reflexes secondary to cooling and drying of the epithelial lining fluid.

[4] Nocturnal cough can sometimes be the predominant symptom in asthma, particularly in children.

[5] Individuals with asthma usually have a family or past history of atopy (asthma, hay fever and eczema). While there is not a single definitive gene for asthma, asthma appears to be associated with a variety of genes connected with the production of cytokines, including IL-3, IL-4, IL-5, IL-9 and IL-13, which are all associated with atopy. Novel genes such as ADAM-33 and DPP-10 have also been identified. However, it is not clear what exact roles those genes play in the pathogenesis of asthma. The form of asthma associated with atopy is also known as 'extrinsic asthma' and the individuals have systemic IgE production with higher levels of circulating IgE. 'Intrinsic' asthma is asthma generally arising in middle age and is less associated with atopy. These individuals usually develop the condition after upper respiratory tract infections. While the mechanism of intrinsic asthma is not

fully understood, it is thought that these individuals have local production of IgE specifically at the bronchial mucosa, as they usually have normal serum concentrations of IgE.

[6] An upper respiratory tract infection is a common potential trigger for an asthma attack. Other potential triggers include allergens (such as dust and mites), cigarette smoke, air pollutants such as sulphur dioxide, ozone and particulate matter, medications such as NSAIDs or beta blockers, anxiety or cold air and exercise, as mentioned above. There are also over 250 recognised workplace materials that can cause asthma, including chemicals such as isocyanates, fungal amylase in wheat flour, and animal allergens in laboratory workers. Occupational asthma can be suspected if the symptoms improve on days off work, such as weekends and holidays, and keeping a symptom diary can assist with diagnosis.

[7] Sick contacts are important to ask in a history, as they can be the source of infection and a potential trigger for exacerbation of asthma.

[8] Animal allergens, including from pets, are another important potential trigger to ask for in the history.

[9] Foreign body inhalation is an important differential for acute shortness of breath. Other important respiratory causes in this age group for acute shortness of breath include pneumothorax, anaphylaxis and pneumonia. Other causes for acute shortness of breath include acute myocardial ischaemia, heart failure, cardiac tamponade or pulmonary embolism.

10 It is important to ask patients with a past history of asthma about any previous ED presentations or hospital admissions, including previous ICU admissions, which can all be indicators of severity of disease.

Examination

- On examination, the patient appears to be **dyspnoeic at rest** and is **struggling to speak in full sentences** [1] secondary to this.
- He is using **accessory muscles of respiration** [2] to assist with his breathing.
- He has a respiratory rate of 32 breaths per minute, a **pulse of 130bpm** [3], a blood pressure of 115/65mmHg, temperature of 36.9°C with an **oxygen saturation of 91% on air** [4].
- He has a **Glasgow Coma Score of 15** [5].

- On examination of his heart, his **heart sounds are dual with no added sounds or murmurs** [6]. His apex beat is not displaced and he does not have an elevated JVP.
- On examination of his respiratory system, his trachea is midline without deviation. He has reduced chest expansion bilaterally. The chest was normal on percussion. On auscultation, there was a **widespread bilateral expiratory wheeze** [7].

1 The patient is currently unable to speak in full sentences. This is one of the signs of an acute severe asthma attack, according to the British Thoracic Society Guidelines. Some of the other signs include tachypnoea (>25 breaths/min), tachycardia >110bpm or reduced peak expiratory flow rate (33–50% of predicted).

2 The use of accessory muscles is another indicator of increased work of breathing and a sign of severity.

3 Tachycardia can be a sign of severity of asthma but it can also be as a result of the side-effect of beta agonist medications such as salbutamol.

4 The patient is currently hypoxic at 91% saturations. Patients are hypoxic in asthma largely secondary to bronchoconstriction, but airway oedema, vascular congestion and luminal congestion may contribute. As this patient is hypoxic, they require supplemental oxygen therapy with usually an aim of oxygen saturations >92% for patients with asthma.

5 Altered mental state is a sign of severity of an asthma attack and is an important part of any examination.

6 It is uncommon for young patients to have heart failure; and if so, it is usually secondary to congenital heart disease or valvular heart disease. The patient does not have any murmurs indicative of valvular heart disease or symptoms of congestive heart failure.

7 An expiratory wheeze is a common sign on examination in asthma. Diffuse wheezing is a sign of airway obstruction. However, wheeze is not necessarily a good marker of severity. For example, a silent chest without a wheeze could indicate imminent respiratory collapse. Wheezing can also be divided into high-pitched polyphonic wheeze (which is caused by disease affecting multiple-sized airways, such as asthma, COPD and heart failure) and low-pitched monophonic wheeze, which is caused by disease affecting a single large airway, such as the trachea or bronchus being blocked by tumour or a foreign body.

Investigations

- The patient has an **ECG** taken which shows **a sinus tachycardia of 130bpm** [1].
- He has a chest X-ray which shows no evidence of consolidation or pneumothorax. He has a **slightly flattened diaphragm with seven ribs visible anteriorly** [2].
- On the full blood examination, the patient has a normal haemoglobin and platelet count. The patient has a **slightly increased white blood cell count** [3]. The patient does not have an elevated CRP.
- The patient has an arterial blood gas taken on air which reveal a pH of 7.49, with a **PaO_2 of 65mmHg** [4] and a $PaCO_2$ of 34mmHg and a bicarbonate of 24mmol/L.

- The patient had a peak expiratory flow rate (PEFR) which was 240L/min, which was **40% of predicted** [5].

He has had recent spirometry testing with the GP, which showed a FEV_1 of 2.9L, which was 80% of predicted, and a FVC of 4.2L which was 110% of predicted. This resulted in a FER (FEV_1/FVC ratio) of 67%. Post bronchodilator therapy, the FEV_1 improved to 3.6L and the FVC improved to 4.5L. The spirometry report concluded that the patient had an **obstructive ventilatory defect with a significant response to inhaled bronchodilators** [6].

1 The ECG helps reassure us that there is no underlying cardiovascular cause of the patient's breathlessness (although unlikely in such a young patient). As mentioned previously, tachycardia can be as a response to the hypoxia and physiological stress of the asthma attack or it may be as a result of administration of beta agonist medications.

2 The flattening of the diaphragm is a sign of hyperinflation. Other signs on chest X-ray include >6 anterior ribs or 10 posterior ribs visible above the diaphragm on the midclavicular line. A chest X-ray also helps exclude other causes of breathlessness, such as a pneumothorax or underlying consolidation.

3 An elevated WCC could be indicative of current or recent infection – potentially related to the upper respiratory symptoms for this patient.

4 The patient has a slightly reduced PaO_2 which is likely secondary to airflow obstruction. However, the patient is not in respiratory failure, which is defined as PaO_2 <60mmHg. The patient's $PaCO_2$ is slightly reduced as a result of increased ventilation to compensate for the hypoxia (also indicated by the increased respiratory rate). The patient has a slightly raised pH indicating respiratory alkalosis.

5 A PEFR of 33–50% of predicted is indicative of acute severe asthma. A PEFR <33% of predicted is a sign of life-threatening asthma. Other signs of life-threatening asthma include any one of silent chest, cyanosis, confusion or coma, bradycardia or hypotension, or feeble respiratory effort or respiratory failure on arterial blood gases.

6 The reduced FVR (FEV_1/FVC) ratio of <70% is indicative of an obstructive defect. The FVC is >80% of the predicted, indicating no presence of restrictive lung disease. The patient had a bronchodilator response >12% and >200ml. Therefore, it can be concluded that there was a significant response to inhaled bronchodilator. These results are consistent with a diagnosis of asthma. However, it is important to note that spirometry results are correct at the time of the test; these can be falsely negative if patients are well at the time of conducting the test. Certain patients may require bronchoprovocation tests such as methacholine challenge test or a mannitol or exercise challenge test to diagnose asthma.

Management

Immediate

The patient is demonstrating signs of a **severe asthma attack** [1]. **Commence supplemental oxygen** [2], aiming for oxygen saturations of 93–95%. Give inhaled bronchodilators, including 12 puffs of **salbutamol** [3] 100mcg and 8 puffs of **ipratropium bromide** [4] 21mcg using a metered dose inhaler **via a spacer** [5]. Continue to **reassess the patient** [6]. If there is limited or no improvement, a further 5mg of nebulised salbutamol and ipratropium 500mcg can be given via a **nebuliser** [7]. If the patient continues to show limited improvement after a further 20 minutes, they can be given further nebulisations of salbutamol and ipratropium. The patient can also be given 10mmol of **IV magnesium sulfate** [8] and commenced on **regular oral prednisolone** [9] for **5 days** [10]. If the patient does not improve, they may require input from the ICU team regarding a potential **ICU admission** [11].

Short-term

The patient is **admitted to hospital** [12] for regular salbutamol and ipratropium nebulisers every 6 hours over the next 24 hours. The patient is also commenced on a regular preventer – containing a combination of an **inhaled glucocorticosteroid and long-acting beta-agonist** [13] to be taken twice a day. In this patient's case, he is commenced on 2 puffs of budesonide 200mcg/formoterol 6mcg twice a day. Once the patient is able to mobilise around the ward without difficulty breathing and is maintaining oxygen saturations with oxygen, they are **suitable for discharge** [14].

The patient should be reviewed by a **respiratory education nurse** [15] prior to discharge. The patient and his family should also be prescribed and educated on a clear **asthma action plan** [16]. He is booked for follow-up with his **GP in 3 days' time** [17].

Long-term

The patient is followed up in the **respiratory clinic in 2 months** [18]. Potential add-on options for therapy if the patient is continuing to have symptoms include adding a **leucotriene receptor antagonist** [19] such as montelukast into the regimen. Another option that could be considered is **theophylline** [20] or to increase the **inhaled glucocorticosteroid dose** [21] and continue to monitor.

Regular oral steroids[22] is another potential management step if the patient continues to have ongoing symptoms. Additionally, new medications available to manage asthma, including **monoclonal** **antibodies**[23] such as omalizumab, mepolizumab and benralizumab, may be indicated. The patient's symptoms should continue to be reviewed in clinic to **titrate therapy**[24].

1 Asthma severity can be determined using the signs discussed previously. In general, a mild–moderate acute asthma attack involves patients who can still speak in whole sentences and are not hypoxic, with oxygen saturations >94%. Severe acute asthma attacks are indicated when they have any of the following: use of accessory muscles or tracheal tug, inability to complete sentences, oxygen saturations 90–94% or signs of obvious respiratory distress. A life-threatening acute asthma attack is indicated by a change in mental state such as drowsiness, cyanosis and oxygen saturations <90%.

2 The recommendation for adults for targeted oxygen therapy between 93% and 95% is to avoid over-oxygenation and the risk of hyperpnoea.

3 Salbutamol, also known as Ventolin, is a short-acting beta-2 adrenergic receptor agonist. Activating of beta-2 receptors leads to smooth muscle relaxation in the lung and bronchodilation. However, the use of beta-2 agonists such as salbutamol is associated with potential side-effects including fine tremor, headache, anxiety and muscle cramps, as well as tachycardia and arrhythmia. Salbutamol also stimulates intracellular shift of potassium, leading to hypokalaemia. Therefore, it can also be used to treat hyperkalaemia.

4 Ipratropium bromide, also known as Atrovent, is a derivative of atropine. It blocks muscarinic acetylcholine receptors, which results in a decreased contractility of smooth muscle in the lungs, inhibiting bronchoconstriction and mucus secretion. While inhaled ipratropium bromide does not generally diffuse into the blood and should not cause systemic anticholinergic effects, some patients have reported dry mouth and sedation as well as urinary retention.

5 The use of a spacer can significantly improve airway deposition of a drug delivered by a pressurised metered dose inhaler (pMDI). It has been shown to be equally effective and safe as nebulised therapy, and is cheaper, portable and convenient.

6 It is important to continually reassess patients with acute asthma, as they can deteriorate quickly and may require further ongoing management.

7 As mentioned, the use of nebulisers and pMDIs with spacers shows a similar level of efficacy. Generally, using a nebuliser is indicated in a life-threatening acute asthma attack or if the patient cannot breathe effectively through the spacer.

8 Magnesium sulfate results in bronchodilation; however, the exact mechanism is unclear. It is thought to potentially be related to the alteration of intracellular calcium concentrations leading to relaxation of bronchial smooth muscles, reducing acetylcholine release at cholinergic nerve endings or increasing the efficacy of beta-2 agonists by increasing receptor affinity.

9 Systemic corticosteroid therapy is ideally indicated within 1 hour of a severe asthma attack. This can be either prednisolone orally or hydrocortisone IV if the patient is too unwell to take oral medications. The primary mechanism by which corticosteroids reduce the severity of asthma is through their anti-inflammatory effects. It is thought that at least half of the patients with asthma have a predominantly eosinophilic-driven inflammation process through IL-4, IL-5 and IL-13. This 'type 2 inflammation' process leads to recruitment of mast cells and eosinophils and release of cytokines. Corticosteroids lead to apoptosis of eosinophils through downregulation of IL-5, as well as inhibiting transcription of IL-4 and IL-5. Corticosteroids also act directly on submucosal glands to prevent increased secretion of mucus.

10 Treatment with a short course of oral steroids for 5–10 days is shown to reduce not only the risks of relapse (probably by reducing the inflammatory process) but also the requirement for further doses of beta-agonists. However, the benefits of steroid therapy are less clear in patients with non-eosinophilic asthma; but it remains standard of care at the moment.

11 Life-threatening asthma patients may require ICU admission for ventilation, either through mechanical ventilation or through non-invasive positive pressure ventilation. Additionally, patients with ongoing life-threatening asthma that has not responded to nebulised salbutamol may receive IV salbutamol in critical care units. These patients require close monitoring of their heart rates, blood electrolytes and acid–base balances due to the systemic effect of the beta-2 agonist.

12 Patients with severe acute asthma who are still requiring regular nebulisers should be admitted to hospital. However, patients who improve after their initial nebulised bronchodilators may be able to be discharged from the ED after monitoring for a few hours, with a clear follow-up plan.

13 The long-term management of chronic asthma involves a stepwise progression of therapy. The first step for patients with intermittent asthma is the PRN use of a short-acting beta agonist such as salbutamol. If patients have regular symptoms or have a severe enough attack requiring hospital admission, they should be commenced on a regular 'preventer' which involves a low dose regular inhaled glucocorticosteroid. This forms step 2 of chronic asthma management. Options for inhaled glucocorticosteroid include budesonide, beclamethasone or fluticasone. This patient has been commenced on step 3 of the asthma therapy – having been commenced on a combination long-acting beta-agonist (LABA) along with an inhaled glucocorticosteroid. Examples of LABAs include formoterol and salmeterol. Long-acting beta-2 agonists have a similar mechanism of action to salbutamol, with the difference being that they remain at the receptor longer and can have a duration of action of up to 15 hours. The benefits for patients of using long-acting beta-2 agonists include improved lung function, significantly reduced symptoms and less requirement of rescue medications. However, there appeared to be a slightly increased risk of asthma-related death in patients using LABA alone (without an inhaled glucocorticosteroid). While the reason behind this is not fully known, it is thought that the use of LABAs may mask symptoms of asthma and delay patients from seeking treatment, leading to an increased risk of a severe asthma attack.

14 Some indicators that an acute asthma patient can be discharged is if they are able to mobilise around the ward without dyspnoea, are not breathless at night and if they are still stable for 24 hours after switching to inhaled bronchodilators.

15 The respiratory education nurse can teach patients to use their inhaler correctly, as this is one of the common reasons for patients to not fully control asthma symptoms with treatment. It is essential that this is regularly reassessed prior to escalating therapy, as an apparent failure of therapy may simply be due to poor inhaler technique. Patients should also be taught to rinse their mouth regularly after using their preventer. One of the side-effects of inhaled glucocorticosteroids is the risk of oral thrush due to the immunosuppressive effects. They should also be made aware that they have to seek medical attention if they have symptoms of oral thrush.

16 Asthma action plans are a set of written instructions for patients, to help them recognise worsening asthma symptoms and know when to seek medical attention. They also outline what regular medications the patient is on and when to take extra doses of medications as required.

17 Early follow-up with the GP to ensure resolution of symptoms is recommended post an acute inpatient admission with acute asthma.

18 Specialty input is not necessarily always required with patients with asthma, as GPs can frequently manage patients and their exacerbations. However, for patients with poorly controlled asthma despite regular preventer therapy, input from a respiratory specialist is suggested.

19 Leucotriene receptor antagonists, such as montelukast, block the activity of leucotriene D4 in the lung, leading to reduced bronchoconstriction. The cysteinyl-leucotrienes are released by eosinophils and bind to receptors in bronchial smooth muscles, leading to bronchoconstriction. The advantage of montelukast is that it is a daily oral tablet which means it can be taken by younger children who may otherwise struggle to comply with adequate inhaler technique. Leucotriene receptor antagonists can be used earlier in the stepwise management of chronic asthma (usually for children) or as an additional aid in adults. Side-effects associated with leucotriene receptor antagonists include diarrhoea and vomiting, insomnia and, rarely, neuropsychiatric changes such as depression, anxiety or changes in behaviour.

20 Theophylline is a xanthine and a competitive phosphodiesterase inhibitor, leading to an increase in cAMP (cyclic adenosine monophosphate) and inhibiting multiple inflammatory pathway mediators, leading to bronchodilation and decreased inflammation. It can also be used in an acute setting intravenously for severe asthma attacks. It has a narrow therapeutic window and is metabolised by the liver cytochrome p450 enzymes, which can be affected by other medications such as sodium valproate, fluoroquinolones and erythromycin. Therefore, plasma levels need to be monitored to avoid toxic adverse effects such as vomiting and diarrhoea, tachyarrhythmias and seizures.

21 Increasing the dose of the inhaled glucocorticosteroid to a regular high dose preventer acts as the next step in the stepwise progressive management of chronic asthma.

22 Regular long-term oral steroids such as prednisolone can be an option in severe chronic asthma and act as a final stepwise increase for asthma management. This is usually only initiated with specialist input in severe refractory asthma. Regular long-term oral steroids are associated with side-effects including growth suppression in children, osteoporosis, cataracts and glaucoma, peptic ulcer disease, hyperglycaemia, weight gain, adrenal suppression and mood/personality changes. Additionally, the systemic immunosuppressive effects increase the risk of infections for these patients.

23 Monoclonal antibody therapy uses monoclonal antibodies that bind specifically to certain proteins to stimulate the patient's immune system to target those cells. Omalizumab binds to circulating IgE in the blood, which prevents cross-linking of IgE receptors on mast cells and reduces allergic activation. Mepolizumab binds to IL-5 and benralizumab binds to the IL-5 receptor. They both block the effect of IL-5 which results in decreased eosinophilic activity. Given these monoclonal antibodies have a very specific target, they are only effective for patients with a particular phenotype of asthma. For example, mepolizumab is specific for eosinophilic asthma as it targets the eosinophilic pathway.

24 It is important to continue to monitor patients with asthma for ongoing symptoms. If they have good control of their asthma for 2–3 months, it may represent an opportunity to step down therapy. Vice versa, if the symptoms continue to worsen, it may mean that the patients should have further escalation of therapy.

CASE 84: Chronic obstructive pulmonary disease

History

- A **70-year-old** [1] woman presents with **increasing shortness of breath** [2] over the **last week** [3].
- She reports having a **runny nose and a sore throat** [4] and has had increasing sputum production over the same time period.
- She reports a **chronic productive cough over the last 4 years with yellow-white sputum** [5].
- She is a current smoker with a **smoking history of 50 pack years** [6].

- She denies any history of **haemoptysis** [7], **night sweats** [8] or **weight loss** [9].
- She is normally able to **walk around 200 metres before having to stop due to dyspnoea, but this has reduced over the past week** [10].
- She has no other past medical history, **particularly no known history of asthma** [11].

[1] Chronic obstructive pulmonary disease (COPD) generally affects middle-aged and older people. Young patients presenting with COPD should be investigated for inherited conditions such as alpha 1-antitrypsin deficiency.

[2] Patients with COPD generally present with dyspnoea, particularly worsening dyspnoea on exertion. The primary pathologic change in COPD is in the airways, where there is chronic inflammation and small airway fibrosis leading to airflow limitation. COPD also affects the lung parenchyma, leading to enlarged air spaces and destruction of airspace walls, known as emphysema. Patients develop dyspnoea in COPD as both the airways and the alveoli play a key role in ensuring oxygenation of blood. Due to the dysfunction with both these processes, patients tend to be hypoxic and feel short of breath.

[3] The onset of dyspnoea can help differentiate between different causes. Acute causes of dyspnoea include cardiac causes (such as acute myocardial infarction), pulmonary causes (such as pneumothorax, pulmonary embolism), upper airway obstruction and psychogenic (such as panic attacks). On the other hand, chronic onset of dyspnoea can indicate chronic inflammatory states such as COPD or asthma, congestive cardiac failure or restrictive lung disease. However, exacerbations of chronic conditions can present acutely, such as in exacerbations of COPD, acute asthma or acute pulmonary oedema.

[4] Coryzal symptoms can indicate an underlying viral illness. Viral infections are common reasons for exacerbation of COPD.

[5] Chronic bronchitis is defined as the presence of a chronic productive cough for at least 3 months in each of the last 2 consecutive years and where other causes of chronic cough have been excluded (such as bronchiectasis). Chronic

inflammation in bronchitis leads to an increase in the number of goblet cells and enlarged submucosal cells. Additionally, the ciliated epithelium is affected, leading to collection of excessive mucus that is produced and increased sputum production. The productive cough is initially present in the mornings but can progress throughout the day. The mucus itself is usually yellowish-white in colour, but in an acute infective setting can turn green due to the presence of a haem pigment in myeloperoxidase expressed by neutrophils.

[6] Cigarette smoking is the most important risk factor for COPD, with significant COPD affecting around 25% of cigarette smokers and 80% of COPD patients having a history of smoking. However, there are other risk factors that can lead to COPD, including passive smoke exposure and the exposure to biomass fuel for cooking and heating. The amount and duration of smoking is associated with disease severity and therefore it is very important to take a detailed smoking history in patients suspected of having COPD.

[7] COPD is not normally associated with haemoptysis. Instead, haemoptysis indicates an underlying more sinister pathology. This can include underlying lung malignancy that can erode pulmonary vessels, or pulmonary embolism. Other common causes of haemoptysis include TB or abscesses, certain forms of vasculitis and coagulopathy.

[8] Night sweats are associated with other conditions such as malignancy, infections such as TB, and certain rheumatic and endocrine disorders. Night sweats are hypothesised to be secondary to raised temperatures due to high levels of released inflammatory markers such as interleukins. As the lowest hypothalamic set point for temperatures is overnight, patients develop excessive diaphoresis to reduce core body temperature. As night sweats are associated with a number of serious conditions, it is important to ask for them on history.

9 Unintentional weight loss is another 'red flag' symptom which is important to ask for on history. Whilst long-standing COPD can cause weight loss, it is more commonly associated with malignancy or other chronic inflammatory conditions. The weight loss also appears to be as a result of increased cytokines, which drives increased catabolism and decreases protein synthesis, leading to cachexia. Additionally, these conditions also appear to increase anorexia, exacerbating the weight loss.

10 Exercise tolerance is an important measure to quantify the severity of dyspnoea. A number of patients with COPD may present with decreasing exercise tolerance as their only primary symptom rather than a productive cough. Additionally, it may be possible to diagnose exacerbation of COPD by a reduction in their exercise tolerance.

11 There is considerable overlap between patients with COPD and those with asthma. Historically, COPD was defined with distinct subtypes, including chronic bronchitis, emphysema and asthma; however, there is no longer any official distinction in the definitions. Rather, patients with asthma whose airflow obstruction does not completely improve with bronchodilators can be considered as having COPD.

Examination

- On general inspection, the patient appears **dyspnoeic at rest** [1] with **use of accessory muscles of respiration** [2], and she is breathing through **pursed lips** [3].
- She is **saturating at 86% on air** [4] with a RR of 26. Her heart rate is 85bpm and regular and her blood pressure is 135/85mmHg.
- On examination of her hands, there is **no evidence of clubbing** [5] but you notice that her fingers are **nicotine-stained** [6].
- There is **no evidence of asterixis** [7] when her hands are outstretched.
- On examination of her face, there is no evidence of Horner's syndrome, **pallor of the conjunctivae** [8] or **central cyanosis** [9].
- Her **trachea is midline** [10] with a **reduced cricoid notch distance** [11].
- On examination of her chest, there is **reduced chest expansion** [12] with **intercostal indrawing during inspiration** [13].
- Chest percussion reveals **symmetrical hyperresonance** [14].
- On auscultation, there is a **widespread bilateral wheeze** [15].
- Her heart sounds are **dual without any added sounds** [16].

1 The pathophysiology behind dyspnoea in COPD patients is multifactorial and complex. Respiratory drive is based upon muscle afferent signals, pulmonary and airway receptors and chemoreceptors that detect CO_2 and O_2 levels. The feeling of shortness of breath is further modulated by the limbic and paralimbic system as a response to the perceived air hunger. In advanced COPD, as there is greater mismatch between the increased neural respiratory drive and restricted ventilatory mechanical response, it leads to an increased feeling of dyspnoea.

2 Chronic dyspnoea along with lung hyperinflation leads to decreased effectiveness of the diaphragm as the primary muscle of respiration. Due to the ongoing increased respiratory drive, accessory muscles of respiration (including sternocleidomastoid, scalene, trapezius, intercostal muscles and pectoralis major and minor) are recruited to help enhance inspiration and expiration.

3 Patients with emphysema usually purse their lips. This narrows the exit of the airways, increasing airway lumen pressure and preventing airways collapse. Therefore, it is easier for these patients to breathe out.

4 Patients with COPD are not able to optimally ventilate themselves due to the loss of alveolar space and gas trapping. Therefore, they have reduced gas exchange, resulting in hypoxaemia. Patients with hypoxaemia require urgent oxygen therapy; however, caution must apply regarding oxygenation aims in patients with COPD (see Management).

5 Finger clubbing is the enlargement of the nailbed and finger tips thought to be secondary to secretion of growth factors in some chronic lung conditions. It is not normally found in COPD, but can be a sign of other comorbid conditions such as bronchogenic carcinoma. Other causes of finger clubbing include interstitial lung disease, TB, cystic fibrosis, bronchiectasis, congenital cyanotic heart disease, endocarditis, Crohn's disease and ulcerative colitis or cirrhosis.

6 Nicotine-stained fingers are a sign of cigarette smoking. Therefore, this has been found to be associated with a number of conditions associated with smoking, including COPD.

7 Asterixis is the involuntary flapping tremor of the hands elicited when the hand is outstretched and bent upwards at the wrist. Normally motor centres in the diencephalon regulate the muscles involved for the hand to maintain position. Hypercapnic respiratory failure affects the function of the diencephalic motor centre, resulting in the flap.

8 Pallor of the conjunctivae is a sign of anaemia. Anaemia is relatively common in elderly patients and these patients can present with dyspnoea. Patients with anaemia should be investigated for sources of bleeding; in particular occult GI blood loss can occur secondary to malignancy. Patients with COPD can actually develop polycythaemia as a result of chronic hypoxaemia.

9 Cyanosis is the bluish discolouration of skin and mucous membranes due to increased concentration of deoxyhaemoglobin in the blood. It is a sign of poor arterial blood oxygenation and can occur secondary to issues with oxygenation in the respiratory system (pneumonia, bronchospasm, pulmonary embolism, COPD, hypoventilation) or due to the cardiovascular system (some congenital heart diseases, heart failure, valvular heart disease) or rarer causes such as methaemoglobinaemia.

10 Tracheal position indicates upper mediastinal position which is determined by intrathoracic pressure. Conditions that change intrathoracic pressure can either push the trachea away (such as the presence of a mass or trapped air) or pull the trachea towards it (in cases of lung collapse or fibrosis). While COPD itself does not cause tracheal deviation, certain complications such as secondary pneumothoraces can deviate the trachea.

11 The distance between the cricoid cartilage and the sternal notch can be used to gauge lung hyperinflation. When examining the patient, you should normally be able to fit 2–3 fingers in this space, with a reduction in distance indicating hyperinflated lung.

12 As a result of gas trapping, patients with COPD have a high functional residual capacity (sign of hyperinflation). This reduces the ability for the chest to expand during deep inspiration, resulting in decreased chest expansion when measured.

13 The paradoxical inward movement of the lower rib cage during inspiration is known as Hoover's sign. As a result of the hyperinflated lungs in COPD, the flattened diaphragm contracts inwards rather than downwards, pulling the inferior chest wall inwards during inspiration.

14 A hyper-resonant sound on percussion over the lung indicates the increased presence of air/hollow structures. This could be secondary to hyperinflation in COPD or a pneumothorax. On the other hand, duller notes during percussion indicate the presence of fluid or a solid mass.

15 A wheeze is a respiratory sound caused by narrowing or obstruction of the airway. Wheezes can be divided into high-pitched polyphonic wheeze or low-pitched monophonic. A polyphonic wheeze indicates obstruction of many different-sized small airways such as in asthma, COPD or cardiac failure (obstruction secondary to oedema). A monophonic wheeze indicates obstruction of a single large airway, such as in tracheal or bronchial obstruction secondary to tumour or foreign body.

16 While COPD does not directly result in a change in heart sounds, chronic severe COPD can lead to pulmonary hypertension. This would lead to a parasternal RV heave and a palpable P2 on examination as well as the development of a tricuspid regurgitation murmur as the right ventricle dilates. As pulmonary hypertension can develop into cor pulmonale and right heart failure, patients can also develop a raised JVP, hepatomegaly, ascites and peripheral oedema.

Investigations

- The patient has an ECG which reveals a **right axis deviation with a dominant R wave in V1 and a dominant S wave in V5 and V6** [1].
- She has a plain chest X-ray which reveals a **flattened diaphragm** [2], **bilateral hyperlucency** [3] and **prominence of hilar vessels** [4].
- There is no evidence of **consolidation** [5] on the chest X-ray.
- She has a set of blood tests including FBE which reveals a **mildly raised haematocrit and white cell count** [6].
- Her UECs reveal a **raised bicarbonate level** [7], but are otherwise normal.

- She has an arterial blood gas which shows a **$PaCO_2$ of 46mmHg and PaO_2 of 67mmHg** [8].
- She has a **sputum MCS** [9] sent which returned as mixed growth.
- She has an **α-1 antitrypsin level** [10] which is normal.
- Her most recent spirometry results showed an FEV_1 of 2.2L which was 60% of predicted, and an FVC of 3.7L which was 90% of predicted. Her **FEV_1/FVC is 60%** [11] with no reversibility with bronchodilators.
- She has a CT scan which shows **centrilobular emphysema** [12].

1 An ECG is an essential investigation in any patients with dyspnoea as it can be used to help rule out urgent cardiac pathology. COPD itself does not cause any ECG changes but patients can develop pulmonary hypertension and right ventricular hypertrophy (RVH) secondary to the increased afterload. RVH can be identified in an ECG as it will result in right axis deviation, a dominant R wave in V1 and a dominant S wave in V5 or V6.

2 A flattened diaphragm is a sign of lung hyperinflation. Other signs of hyperinflation on chest X-ray include >6 anterior ribs or 10 posterior ribs visible above the diaphragm on the midclavicular line. A chest X-ray also helps exclude other causes of breathlessness, such as a pneumothorax.

3 Bilateral hyperlucency occurs in COPD due to the presence of gas trapping within the lung fields. These areas appear dark on the chest X-ray with reduced lung markings peripherally.

4 Prominence of hilar vessels can be seen in a chest X-ray of patients with advanced COPD, leading to pulmonary hypertension and cor pulmonale.

5 Exacerbations of COPD, while often precipitated by infections, may not necessarily lead to consolidation on a chest X-ray. Infective exacerbations of COPD can be due to viruses or bacteria or a combination of both. The most common bacterial pathogens include *Haemophilus influenzae* or *Moraxella catarrhalis*, which do not commonly cause lobar consolidation on chest X-ray. Other common causes of a bacterial infection include *Streptococcus pneumoniae*, which is more commonly associated with lobar consolidation.

6 Patients with COPD can be persistently hypoxic. This can stimulate the release of erythropoietin, leading to increased bone marrow production of red blood cells to help improve oxygen-carrying capacity of blood. Therefore, they can have a raised haematocrit on FBE. COPD is also a chronic inflammatory condition leading to a raised white cell count. Management of COPD also involves the use of corticosteroids, which can also contribute to an increased white cell count.

7 Patients with long-standing COPD are often hypercapnic (see below) and kidneys respond to this chronic respiratory acidosis by retaining bicarbonate ions. This is because the raised arterial $PaCO_2$ increases intracellular $PaCO_2$ in the proximal tubule, leading to increased H^+ secretion into the tubular lumen. This results in increased bicarbonate ion production which enters the circulation (as well as increasing Na^+ reabsorption with H^+ ions, reducing plasma chloride concentrations). The expected chronic compensation is an increase of 4mmol/L of HCO_3 for every 10mmHg in elevation of $PaCO_2$.

8 The patient is hypercapnic (increased $PaCO_2$) and hypoxic. Due to the air trapping and destruction of alveoli in COPD, patients are unable to have adequate gas exchange and therefore, are unable to breathe out carbon dioxide. This patient is close to developing type 2 respiratory failure, which is typically characterised by $PaCO_2$ being >50mmHg and PaO_2 <60mmHg. Patients with type 2 respiratory failure also are usually acidotic due to the increased CO_2.

9 Sputum MCS is not routinely performed for patients with exacerbations of COPD as it does not always affect management. However, for patients who have a history of recurrent infections or previous unusual/resistant microbiology, a sputum MCS can help direct antibiotic treatment choices. Unfortunately, there is significant likelihood that the sputum sample will be contaminated by normal upper respiratory tract flora rather than being a true lower respiratory tract sample. Additionally, many patients with COPD are persistently colonised with bacterial pathogens and a positive culture does not necessarily indicate an acute infection.

10 α-1 antitrypsin is an enzyme produced primarily by the liver that inhibits proteases, including elastase which is released by neutrophils as part of the inflammatory process. Elastase breaks down elastin, which reduces elasticity of the lung and leads to emphysema. α-1 antitrypsin deficiency should be suspected in all patients with COPD, but in particular those who are younger or do not have a history of smoking.

11 A FEV_1/FVC ratio of <70% without bronchodilator reversibility is considered diagnostic for COPD. Other obstructive conditions, such as asthma, also lead to a reduced FEV_1/FVC of <70% but are associated with a significant bronchodilator response (greater than 12% and 200ml).

12 A CT scan is not required for diagnosis of COPD, but rather is used to identify a complication of COPD (pneumonia, bullae, pneumothorax) or for lung cancer screening. However, it is better at detecting emphysema than a chest X-ray. COPD associated with smoking usually leads to centrilobular emphysema, as it generally involves destruction of parenchyma around the terminal bronchiole. On the other hand, emphysema associated with α-1 antitrypsin deficiency is usually panlobular as it affects all areas of the lung. Other findings on CT chest found in COPD include air trapping, bronchial wall thickening and pulmonary artery enlargement once the patients have developed pulmonary hypertension.

Management

Immediate

The patient likely has an acute exacerbation of underlying COPD. Commence **supplemental oxygen** [1] as the patient is hypoxic. Nebulised bronchodilators such as **salbutamol** [2] and **ipratropium** [3] should be given. Patients should be commenced on **systemic corticosteroids** [4]. **Antibiotics** [5] should be considered if there is suspicion of a bacterial infection. **Non-invasive ventilation** [6] should be considered for patients with respiratory failure.

Short-term

Patients should be educated about their condition and prognosis. Discussion about **smoking cessation** [7] should take place. The pharmacologic management should be considered in a stepwise pattern. Patients are usually commenced on short-acting bronchodilators such as ipratropium or salbutamol as necessary. For more symptomatic patients, **long-acting muscarinic antagonists** [8] or a **long-acting beta agonist** [9] can be started. **Inhaled corticosteroids** [10] can be commenced if ongoing symptoms, with usually a **combination inhaler** [11] being used. **Mucolytic agents** [12] can be considered.

Long-term

Patients should be managed by a **multidisciplinary team** [13], ideally coordinated by their GP but including a respiratory physician, physiotherapist and dietitian. They can be referred for **pulmonary rehabilitation** [14]. Patients with severe COPD resulting in significant hypoxaemia will benefit from **continuous home oxygen supplementation** [15]. Patients should have their **influenza and pneumococcal vaccinations** [16]. **Long-term antibiotics** [17] can be considered. Patients can be considered for **surgical intervention** [18] or **lung transplantation** [19]. As their disease progresses, patients should discuss **advanced care planning** [20] and be referred to **palliative care services** [21].

---

[1] Saturation aims for patients with COPD can vary depending on whether patients have a history of CO_2 retention. Patients with chronic COPD with CO_2 retention rely on hypoxia for respiratory drive, and administration of excessive oxygen can reduce the patient's ventilation rate. Therefore, the usual oxygenation saturation aims for these patients are 88–92%. For patients with no history of CO_2 retention, the usual oxygen aims of >94% apply. However, if a patient is acutely unwell, then you commence oxygen at maximal therapy (15L/min via a reservoir/bag-valve mask) and titrate therapy afterwards as appropriate.

[2] Salbutamol, also known as Ventolin, is a short-acting beta-2 adrenergic receptor agonist. It activates beta-2 receptors, leading to smooth muscle relaxation in the lung and bronchodilation. Side-effects of salbutamol include fine tremor, headache, anxiety and muscle cramps, as well as tachycardia and arrhythmia. It also stimulates intracellular shift of potassium, leading to hypokalaemia.

[3] Ipratropium bromide, also known as Atrovent, is a derivative of atropine. It blocks muscarinic acetylcholine receptors, which results in a decreased contractility of smooth muscle in the lungs, inhibiting bronchoconstriction and mucus secretion. Inhaled ipratropium bromide does not usually diffuse into the blood and should not cause systemic anticholinergic effects. However, some patients have reported dry mouth and sedation, as well as urinary retention.

[4] Systemic corticosteroid therapy can be either prednisolone orally or hydrocortisone intravenously if the patient is unable to take oral medications. The duration of a course of corticosteroids can vary but usually 5 days is adequate for most severe exacerbations. Corticosteroids help reduce inflammatory response through a variety of mechanisms, helping with COPD exacerbations.

[5] Antibiotics are not routinely indicated in exacerbations of COPD unless patients have features suggestive of bacterial infection. In most cases, oral antibiotics are adequate to treat most patients, even those in hospital, with amoxicillin or doxycycline being an appropriate choice.

[6] Non-invasive ventilation (NIV) is indicated for patients with type 2 respiratory failure not improving with therapy. NIV has been shown to reduce mortality and usually avoids the need for intubation. Patients on NIV should be closely monitored in a specialist medical ward or in intensive care.

[7] Smoking is the main known cause of COPD in most countries, and smoking cessation is the only intervention that has been shown to improve the long-term prognosis in patients with COPD (apart from oxygen supplementation for those who are severely hypoxaemic). Patients should be counselled regarding reducing smoking; they can be referred to local stop smoking services and assisted with pharmacological agents such as nicotine replacement.

8 Long-acting muscarinic antagonists include aclidinium, tiotropium and umeclidinium. They have similar mechanism of action to ipratropium but with a longer duration of action of 12–24 hours. There have not been many head-to-head studies comparing different LAMAs and it is generally physician/patient preference regarding which to commence.

9 Long-acting beta-2 agonists have a similar mechanism of action to salbutamol, with the difference being that they remain at the receptor longer and can have a duration of action of 14–24 hours. Examples of LABAs include formoterol and salmeterol.

10 Examples of inhaled corticosteroids (ICS) include budesonide, beclamethasone or fluticasone. While the effect of inhaled corticosteroids on mortality in COPD patients is unclear, they are generally used to aim to reduce exacerbation rates.

11 Combination inhalers are available containing both LAMA and LABAs, ICS and LABAs or all three classes of medication. They can make it easier for patients to escalate further therapy for COPD without needing to use a number of different puffers.

12 Mucolytic agents, including *N*-acetylcysteine (NAC), ambroxol, carbocysteine and sobrerol, reduce sputum viscosity and may also have anti-inflammatory or antioxidant effects. There is evidence that suggests the use of mucolytic agents is associated with a slight reduction in risk of exacerbations and potentially hospitalisation. However, it does not appear to have a significant effect on quality of life.

13 The MDT can work together to ensure appropriate puffer technique. Occupational therapists can assess ability to do activities of daily living and physiotherapists can gauge mobility and teach sputum clearance techniques. Dietitians can provide advice regarding appropriate nutritional intake.

14 Pulmonary rehabilitation is usually a 6–8-week programme aimed at patients with chronic lung diseases including COPD. Patients get regular exercise training and are taught energy conservation techniques. Patients are also educated about their condition and provided with psychological support.

15 Long-term continuous oxygen therapy is indicated for patients with COPD and a partial pressure of oxygen (PaO_2) of <55mmHg on an ABG, or those with PaO_2 <60mmHg with cor pulmonale, pulmonary hypertension or polycythaemia. It should ideally be used for 18 hours a day. This has been shown to improve mortality in COPD patients.

16 The influenza and pneumococcal vaccines should be recommended in all elderly patients but even more so in patients with COPD as they have poor underlying respiratory function and significant morbidity and mortality associated with infective exacerbations.

17 Patients with recurrent exacerbations and severe COPD despite maximal therapy may benefit from a long-term low-dose oral macrolide such as azithromycin. However, long-term macrolide use is associated with side-effects including cardiotoxicity, ototoxicity and diarrhoea, and the decision should be made in consultation with specialist respiratory input.

18 Patients with significant emphysema with marked hyperinflation may benefit from lung volume reduction surgery to improve their mechanics associated with ventilation (as it helps reduce inadequate lung emptying). This discussion should ideally happen in tertiary specialist centres.

19 COPD is the most common indication for lung transplantation in adults and is associated with improved survival. However, it is only an option for selected patients and is limited by donor availability. Patients with lung transplants require lifelong immunosuppression and there are significant risks associated with it.

20 Patient wishes regarding end-of-life care, including thoughts on resuscitation and intubation, should be ideally conducted when the patient is stable in an outpatient setting.

21 Palliative care teams can provide strategies to help patients with symptom control at all stages of the disease. An option includes the use of opioids to help with refractory dyspnoea.

CASE 85: Cystic fibrosis

History

- A 30-year-old **Caucasian** [1] **female** [2] with a **history of cystic fibrosis** [3] presents with **increasing cough and daily green sputum production** [4] for 3 weeks associated with some dyspnoea.
- She also reports a chronic **blocked nose** [5].
- She has been commenced on **oral antibiotics** [6] (ciprofloxacin and trimethoprim-sulfamethoxazole) for one week without much improvement.
- She denies any **sick contacts** [7].

- She also has a history of **loose, smelly fatty stools** [8] and is **diabetic** [9], requiring insulin.
- She has already been hospitalised twice in the past 12 months for **intravenous antibiotics** [10].
- She is a **non-smoker** [11].
- She currently works as an architect in an office, where one of her **colleagues also has cystic fibrosis** [12].

---

1 Cystic fibrosis (CF) is more common in people with a European background, as approximately 1 in 25 people of European descent are carriers of a CF mutation.

2 Cystic fibrosis affects both males and females equally. However, historically women have tended to have poorer outcomes (lower life expectancy) with CF, without a clear known reason. In terms of bronchiectasis in the general population, women are more likely to develop bronchiectasis than males.

3 Historically, patients with CF were diagnosed after presenting with symptoms, usually in childhood. However, with the increasing growth of the newborn screening programme, the majority of patients are now diagnosed as a newborn. The screening programme currently involves testing for immunoreactive trypsinogen and cystic fibrosis transmembrane conductance regulator (CFTR) gene mutations with neonates, with two mutations being diagnosed with CF, while those with one mutation have a sweat test to confirm diagnosis.

4 Patients with CF tend to have a persistent, productive cough which can worsen during periods of acute exacerbation. This is due to the effect of the CFTR mutation leading to reduction in ion transport (Na and Cl) of respiratory epithelial cells. As water follows the ion gradient, this leads to reduced volume of airway surface liquid, impairing the function of the cilia and predisposing them to recurrent chest infections. The inflammation associated with recurrent infections leads to epithelial damage and increased luminal debris, resulting in thickened mucus and leading to a cycle of further infections and airway damage.

5 Similar to mucus in the lungs, mucus in the paranasal sinuses is also thick and can block the sinus passage. This can lead to recurrent sinus infections, and the chronic inflammation can lead to development of nasal polyps.

6 Mild exacerbations of CF are often managed with oral antibiotics in the community without requiring hospital admission. The choice of antibiotics is often dependent on previous sputum culture results.

7 Patients with CF are at a higher risk for respiratory infections and have to be careful in maintaining precautions to reduce the risk of acquiring infections. In particular, CF patients who have a history of infections with *Burkholderia cepacia* complex have to ensure that they are segregated from other CF patients.

8 Pancreatic insufficiency is another common feature of cystic fibrosis. Normally, acinar cells in the pancreas release digestive enzymes into the pancreatic duct, where they mix with chloride and bicarbonate ions that are secreted by epithelial cells and travel into the intestines. For patients with cystic fibrosis, CFTR mutation results in decreased secretion of chloride ions into the pancreatic duct, leading to reduced bicarbonate ions (due to reduced HCO_3^-/Cl^- exchange) and water secretion into the pancreatic duct. The thickened pancreatic enzymes do not travel as easily into the intestines and mucus plugs in the pancreatic ducts worsen this process. Over time, the trapped enzymes digest the pancreatic tissue, leading to pancreatic insufficiency.

9 The islets of Langerhans are responsible for the production of insulin. Damage to the pancreas can lead to loss of the islets of Langerhans cells, leading to these patients having diabetes mellitus.

10 Patients with CF may need to come into hospital regularly for 'tune-ups' to manage exacerbations of their disease. These admissions usually involve a course of IV antibiotics and intensive chest physiotherapy. The frequency of these admissions can be used as a sign of the progression of disease.

11 Smoking is associated with worse outcomes for patients with cystic fibrosis. Smoking results in CF patients having more frequent exacerbations, requiring increased IV therapy and with worsening spirometry results.

12 While this may not seem like a key detail, it can be important to clarify the extent of their interactions. Additionally, as mentioned earlier, depending on what pathogens the patient has on their sputum cultures, it can have a large impact on their day-to-day lives as it may limit their ability to go to work.

Examination

- On general inspection, you notice a thin female with an approximate BMI of **19** [1].
- She is alert and responding appropriately, without displaying any **signs of respiratory distress** [2].
- She is currently breathing at a rate of 20 breaths per minute, is **saturating at 96% on air** [3], has a pulse rate of 90bpm and a blood pressure of 115/65mmHg. She is **afebrile** [4].
- On examination of her hands, she has evidence of **finger clubbing** [5].
- Her **heart sounds are dual without any added sounds** [6].
- On auscultation of her chest, she has a moderate **expiratory wheeze** [7] and **bilateral crackles** [8].
- On examination of her abdomen, there is no tenderness and no evidence of **splenomegaly or hepatomegaly** [9].

1 Patients with cystic fibrosis tend to be underweight secondary to pancreatic insufficiency and malabsorption.

2 As patients with CF are well followed-up in the community and commonly present early with their exacerbations, they usually do not present directly with severe respiratory distress. However, in the event of a severe acute infection, they may develop signs of respiratory distress, including tachypnoea, accessory muscle use and nasal flaring.

3 The patient's normal oxygen saturations indicate that she is not in respiratory failure at this stage due to her respiratory disease.

4 Infections are the most common reason for patients with CF to develop worsening pulmonary symptoms. However, given that this patient has already been treated with oral antibiotics and has had symptoms for a few weeks, it is quite likely that she will not present with any fevers.

5 Finger clubbing is the enlargement of the nailbed and fingertips associated with a number of conditions, including CF. While the pathophysiology behind finger clubbing is not fully understood, it is thought to be in relation to secretion of growth factors from the lungs in some chronic lung conditions. Other causes of finger clubbing apart from CF include lung cancer, interstitial lung disease, TB, bronchiectasis, congenital cyanotic heart disease, endocarditis, Crohn's disease and ulcerative colitis or cirrhosis.

6 Patients with long-standing severe CF can develop signs and symptoms of pulmonary hypertension. On examination, these include a loud P2 heart sound with splitting of the second heart sound. With progression of their disease, these patients can develop cor pulmonale, also known as pulmonary heart disease. These patients develop

right ventricular hypertrophy as a response to the increased pulmonary pressures. They could present with signs of right-sided heart failure (shortness of breath, raised JVP, ascites, peripheral oedema) and can have a right parasternal heave.

7 Patients with CF often have an element of airways obstruction that can lead to a wheeze. These patients can improve partially with bronchodilators.

8 Coarse crackles are often a sign of bronchiectasis in patients with CF. In bronchiectasis, they tend to clear with coughing. Other causes of coarse crackles include pneumonia and pulmonary oedema. However, in pulmonary oedema, the crackles do not tend to clear with coughing.

9 Patients with CF can have involvement of the liver as part of their disease process. The CFTR is located in the membrane of the biliary epithelium and similar to its function in the pancreas, secretes chloride and bicarbonate ions, affecting water and solute movement. This results in thickened and slow-moving bile that leads to release of pro-inflammatory factors that increase collagen synthesis within the portal tracts. Eventually, this leads to fibrosis and liver cirrhosis.

Investigations

- The patient has a routine ECG on admission which is **normal** [1].
- Her full blood count reveals a mildly **raised white cell count** along with a **raised C-reactive protein** [2]. Her urea, electrolytes and creatinine are normal.
- She has **mildly elevated liver enzymes** [3].
- Her **albumin is at the lower range of normal** [4].
- Her chest X-ray shows **evidence of hyperinflation** [5] and **prominent bronchovascular markings** [6].
- She had a **spirometry test** [7] recently which shows a reduced FEV_1 (55% of predicted) and reduced FEV_1/FVC ratio (65%).
- She has a high resolution CT (HRCT) of the chest that reveals **mucus plugging, peribronchial thickening, air trapping and airway dilation** [8].
- She also has a **sputum MCS** [9] that grows *Pseudomonas aeruginosa* [10].

[1] ECGs in patients with cystic fibrosis are usually normal. However, with progression of the disease, patients can develop right ventricular hypertrophy. In an ECG, right ventricular hypertrophy is indicated by right axis deviation, a large, dominant R wave in V1 and a dominant S wave in V5 or V6.

[2] A raised white cell count and raised CRP indicate that the patient is currently undergoing an inflammatory process, most likely related to chest.

[3] AST, ALT and GGT can all be elevated in patients with CF and this does not necessarily diagnose patients with CF-related liver disease. However, if patients have any clinical signs of portal hypertension or have ultrasound findings or liver biopsy results that show evidence of cirrhosis, then a diagnosis of CF-related liver disease can be made.

[4] Albumin is a useful marker of both nutrition and synthetic liver function in patients with CF. Patients must have adequate protein intake and absorption to have normal levels of albumin. Additionally, the liver is responsible for synthesising albumin, and patients with CF-related liver disease often have low albumin. Patients with CF bronchiectasis also concurrently have a chronic inflammatory process which can break down proteins including albumin, resulting in a reduced albumin level.

[5] Hyperinflation of the lungs is indicated by a posterior rib count >10 ribs or an anterior rib count >7 ribs. It is one of the earliest changes in patients with CF. While it initially may be reversible, with progression of the disease, the hyperinflation is persistent. As the hyperinflation progresses, it can lead to flattening of the diaphragm and a prominent retrosternal space.

[6] The increased bronchovascular markings are as a result of chronic inflammatory process affecting the airways in CF bronchiectasis. As the pulmonary disease progresses, the dilated and thickened airways appear as parallel lines, also known as 'tram tracks' when seen longitudinally and as ring shadows if seen cross-sectionally. Patients with CF tend to have routine chest X-rays at a minimum of every two years,

even with mild disease, to monitor for pulmonary progression of their disease.

[7] Pulmonary function testing is a reliable way to monitor pulmonary progression of disease in patients with CF. Such patients tend to have normal pulmonary function tests as a neonate (note that this only measures forced expiration and is largely only used for study purposes) but they go on to develop an obstructive pattern over time. In acute exacerbations, FEV_1 may be reduced even further by up to 10–15%, but can improve with treatment. The rate and pattern of decline of pulmonary function tests in patients with CF can vary greatly, depending on their frequency of exacerbations and pathogens involved.

[8] Mucus plugging can frequently occur in patients with CF due to the thickened and excessive mucus production as a result of their disease. This can lead to obstructive respiratory signs and usually requires a strong course of chest physiotherapy to improve it. Post the obstruction, these patients can show evidence of air trapping. Airway dilation is indicated by the 'signet ring' sign which is indicative of bronchiectasis. This relates to the appearance of a large, dilated air-filled bronchus adjacent to a smaller opacity which is a pulmonary artery. The HRCT can also be used to measure pulmonary artery diameter as a surrogate marker for pulmonary hypertension. The utility of regular chest CTs in patients with cystic fibrosis is a contentious issue and needs to take into account the risk associated with repeated radiation exposure versus the benefits of potentially earlier bronchiectasis identification.

[9] A sputum MCS is an essential investigation for patients with CF, as identification and sensitivities of the pathogen will help dictate the management plan. The common bacterial pathogens vary depending on the patient's age, with *Staphylococcus aureus* and *Haemophilus influenzae* being the most common pathogens in childhood, and *Pseudomonas aeruginosa* being more prevalent as they get older. Other common pathogens include *Stenotrophomonas maltophilia* and *Burkholderia cepacia*. Due to the nature of persistent sputum production, most patients with CF are able to

expectorate sputum. Certain patients may require assistance with nebulised sodium chloride. However, some patients may have bronchoalveolar lavage (BAL) cultures to help identify a pathogen.

10 *Pseudomonas aeruginosa* is a Gram-negative rod that frequently colonises the respiratory tract of patients with CF. It is a significant concern due to its high rates of antibiotic resistance and its capacity to develop biofilm, enabling it to survive for long periods of time.

Management

Immediate

As this patient is a chronic CF patient who is currently **haemodynamically stable without any evidence of respiratory compromise** [1], there is no immediate management step required in this situation.

Short-term

The management of an acute exacerbation of CF will commonly require **intravenous antibiotics** [2] for a duration of between **10 days and 3 weeks or more** [3]. While this commonly requires a **hospital admission** [4], some patients may be able to be managed at home. These patients will commonly require a **peripherally inserted central catheter (PICC) line** [5] to administer these antibiotics. The patients will receive **twice-daily chest physiotherapy** [6]. Whilst in hospital, patients would also benefit from a **dietitian review** [7].

Long-term

Once these patients complete their course of IV antibiotics, they are commonly discharged home with a long-term course of **ongoing oral or inhaled antibiotics** [8]. Patients are also commonly commenced on **oral azithromycin** [9]. Other anti-inflammatory treatment such as **inhaled or oral glucocorticosteroids** [10] may also be used. Additionally, patients with evidence of bronchodilator response in spirometry can benefit from **inhaled bronchodilators** [11] such as salbutamol. Patients are also prescribed aerosolised mucolytics such as **dornase alfa** [12] or **nebulised hypertonic saline** [13]. They could benefit from **pulmonary rehabilitation** [14]. In addition to managing the pulmonary component of CF, patients need to be on **pancreatic enzyme supplementation** [15] for their pancreatic insufficiency, along with **insulin and/or oral hypoglycaemics** [16] for their CF-associated diabetes.

Depending on the specific mutation involved in the pathogenesis of CF in patients, drugs targeting the CFTR protein, such as **ivacaftor** [17], may be used.

As the disease progresses, patients can get worsening dyspnoea and hypoxaemia, even at rest. Patients may benefit from home **oxygen supplementation** [18]. Patients may also be considered for **lung transplantation** [19].

1 Cystic fibrosis patients with an element of respiratory compromise or haemodynamic instability will be managed like any other patient, focusing on the DRSABCD algorithm. This is an approach to emergency situations in basic life support: Danger, Respond, Send for help, Airway, Breathing, Circulation/CPR, Defibrillation.

2 The choice of IV antibiotics for exacerbations of cystic fibrosis can vary based upon sputum culture organisms and sensitivities. For patients with *Pseudomonas aeruginosa*, especially as an initial infection, then a protocol aiming for eradication is used. This commonly includes a combination of antipseudomonal penicillin (such as piperacillin/tazobactam) or cephalosporin (such as ceftazidime or cefepime) alongside tobramycin. Tobramycin is an aminoglycoside that is highly effective against certain Gram-negative bacteria including *Pseudomonas* spp. Like other aminoglycosides (such as gentamicin), tobramycin can be ototoxic and nephrotoxic. Therefore, tobramycin needs to be dosed based upon the

patient's body weight, and drug levels need to be monitored. For patients with *Burkholderia cepacia* complex bacteria, there may be limited options as these bacteria are highly resistant to multiple antibiotics. The choice would depend on the sensitivities on sputum culture, but options include ceftazidime or meropenem.

3 There are no set guidelines regarding the duration of antibiotics required during an exacerbation of CF. Generally clinicians use their judgement, taking into account the patient's improvement in symptoms and improvement in FEV_1 to help guide durations. A course of at least 10 days is usually recommended but it can stretch to 3 weeks or more if there is slow, ongoing improvement.

4 While hospital admissions enable closer monitoring of patients and more intensive physiotherapy, some patients may prefer a "Hospital at Home" programme as they can be managed in the comfort of their own house. Provided that patients at home are compliant with their antibiotics and physiotherapy, there is no real significant difference in outcome based upon location of treatment.

5 PICC lines are long catheters usually inserted in a large peripheral vein in the arm (such as the basilic or brachial vein) and advanced towards the heart until the tip sits in the SVC. They are commonly preferred in patients with CF as such patients require a longer course of antibiotics, and a PICC line reduces the necessity of repeat cannulation.

6 Chest physiotherapy is an essential component of the management of pulmonary disease in CF. The aim should be to work on an effective cough which will clear infected bronchial secretions and help relieve airway obstruction. There are a number of different techniques available and the regimen should be tailored to suit the patient, as non-compliance with chest physiotherapy is common.

7 As a result of pancreatic insufficiency, patients with CF are generally recommended to have a high-caloric diet in addition to pancreatic enzyme supplementation, to ensure optimal nutritional status.

8 As with the choice of IV antibiotics, the choice for oral and inhaled antibiotics would depend on the sensitivities of the sputum cultures. Common regimen options for patients with *Pseudomonas aeruginosa* aiming for eradication include oral ciprofloxacin alongside inhaled tobramycin for a minimum of a further 2–3 months. Ciprofloxacin is a fluoroquinolone that inhibits DNA gyrase in bacteria, inhibiting cell division, and is one of the few antipseudomonal antibiotics that has an oral form.

9 Azithromycin is a macrolide antibiotic that is used in treating chronic *Pseudomonas aeruginosa* infection, due to both its antibiotic and anti-inflammatory effects. Azithromycin can penetrate the *Pseudomonas aeruginosa* biofilms and boost neutrophil function. The use of long-term azithromycin has shown to decrease the frequency of CF exacerbations and reduce the progressive decline in lung function.

10 As the progression of pulmonary disease in patients with CF is related to the inflammatory response, treatment with anti-inflammatory medications is used commonly to reduce this progress. Therefore, a significant proportion of patients with cystic fibrosis are prescribed inhaled glucocorticosteroids; however, there is nil clear evidence regarding their benefits. The use of oral glucocorticosteroids is even more controversial due to their systemic effects, including growth suppression in children, osteoporosis, cataracts and glaucoma, peptic ulcer disease, hyperglycaemia, adrenal suppression and mood/personality changes, and is generally not indicated. An exception is in patients with allergic bronchopulmonary aspergillosis, which is a complex hypersensitive immune response to colonisation of airways with the fungus *Aspergillus* in patients with CF or asthma. These patients commonly require treatment with oral glucocorticosteroids in addition to antifungal medications.

11 Short-acting beta-2 adrenergic receptor agonists, such as salbutamol, are commonly used in asthma and COPD. They cause bronchodilation by activating beta-2 receptors in the lungs to stimulate muscle relaxation. While it is likely that inhaled bronchodilators are overprescribed in patients with CF, they can help relieve symptoms in those that have a bronchodilator response.

12 Dornase alfa (also known as Pulmozyme) is a purified solution of recombinant human DNase. Patients with CF have a higher concentration of neutrophil-derived DNA leading to thickened sputum. Dornase alfa hydrolyses this DNA to reduce sputum viscosity and help improve sputum clearance.

13 Nebulised hypertonic saline can help clear mucus through a number of different mechanisms including disrupting the ionic bonds within the mucus, increasing the depth of the liquid layer on the lung epithelial surface and triggering a cough reflex.

14 Pulmonary rehabilitation is a programme aimed at people with chronic lung diseases including CF. It usually involves an MDT including educators about their condition, physiotherapists and exercise physiologists to help improve patients' function, and dietitians regarding ongoing nutritional support. They can also provide counselling or group support for patients to help with anxiety or depression, particularly if associated with their chronic respiratory disease.

15 Pancreatic enzyme supplementation are tablets that contain lipase, amylase and protease which help digest and absorb fats, carbohydrates and proteins. Patients need to take the supplements at the start of meals and dosing can vary between patients (with 40 000 units of lipase per main meal being an approximate starting point for adults). A concern with high doses of pancreatic enzyme supplementation is the risk of fibrosing colonopathy, where there is formation of colonic strictures and increased fibrosis.

16 The management of CF-related diabetes is unlike that of regular diabetes, as patients are encouraged to continue with high calorie diets to ensure adequate nutrition. Depending on the degree of damage to the islets of Langerhans cells, some patients might be able to be managed with oral hypoglycaemics only. However, generally most patients are on at least some insulin supplementation.

17 Ivacaftor is a CFTR potentiator as it binds to the ion channel to increase its likelihood to be open and enabling chloride channels to pass through. Ivacaftor is currently only indicated for patients with a G551D mutation. Ivacaftor is also available as a combination drug with lumacaftor for patients with two copies of F508del mutation. Lumacaftor improves protein folding of the CFTR protein by chaperoning CFTR proteins to the surface.

18 There is no significant evidence regarding oxygen supplementation in patients with CF; however, patients with end-stage lung disease could benefit from oxygen supplementation for comfort. Patients with CF are at high risk for hypercapnic respiratory failure and depending on their blood gas results, could benefit with target oxygen saturations of 88–92%.

19 Lung transplantation in patients with CF would usually involve both lungs, as leaving a native lung involves high risk of infected secretions affecting the transplanted lung. The work-up process and discussions around lung transplantation should occur throughout the disease process, rather than once patients get to end-stage lung disease. Patients with CF who have lung transplants generally have a better prognosis than other indications for transplant, with a median survival of 9.2 years post transplant. Nevertheless, it is still an intensive procedure and many patients opt out of undergoing the transplantation process.

CASE 86: Idiopathic pulmonary hypertension

History

- A 76-year-old female presents to the outpatient clinic with **progressive shortness of breath, mainly on exertion** [1].
- This is associated with **symptoms of fatigue, lethargy** [2] and **intermittent chest pain** [3]. The patient **denies any palpitations** [4].
- Upon further history, she reports having an active and healthy life without any significant past medical conditions. She **denies any previous ischaemic heart disease, connective tissue disease, previous venous thrombotic events, or lung disease** [5].
- There is **no significant family history** [6].
- She occasionally takes **paracetamol for pain but no regular medications** [7].

[1] Exertional dyspnoea is the commonest presentation of idiopathic pulmonary hypertension (IPH). The symptoms developed over a prolonged period and most patients are generally diagnosed in an outpatient setting.

[2] Fatigue and lethargy occur due to reduced cardiac output during exercise.

[3] Chest pain occurs as a symptom of right heart failure, due to increased myocardial demand for oxygen. As pulmonary hypertension progresses, features of right heart failure become more evident. Other symptoms of right heart failure include oedema and weight gain, exertional syncope and abdominal distension.

[4] Palpitations and arrhythmias can also occur in pulmonary hypertension.

[5] There are many causes of pulmonary hypertension. Pulmonary hypertension is classified based on case. Treatment is based largely on the underlying cause. On initial diagnosis of pulmonary hypertension, further investigations for the underlying cause need to be performed. Pulmonary hypertension is classified into five groups:

- Group 1: pulmonary arterial hypertension
  - idiopathic pulmonary hypertension (IPH)
  - hereditary
  - associated with other conditions: connective tissue disease, HIV, portal hypertension, congenital heart disease
- Group 2: left heart failure
- Group 3: lung disease/chronic hypoxia – COPD, obstructive sleep apnoea, interstitial lung disease
- Group 4: chronic thromboembolic pulmonary hypertension
- Group 5: other (sarcoidosis, obstructing tumours, chronic kidney failure on dialysis) or unclear/multifactorial cause

[6] There are some causes of IPH that are heritable forms. These are autosomal dominant with mutations in the transforming growth factor-β (TGF-β) signalling system. Venous thrombotic events can also run through families.

[7] There are some drug causes that can increase the risk of patients having pulmonary hypertension. These include appetite suppressants and tyrosine kinase inhibitors.

Examination

- On examination the patient looks comfortable at rest; however, you noticed she had an **increased work of breathing on mobilising into the outpatient clinic room** [1].
- She has **no signs of arthritic joint disease** [2] on examination of her hands.
- She has moist mucous membranes, with a **JVP at 5cm with the presence of A waves** [3].
- On examination of the cardiovascular system there is a **left parasternal heave** [4] and **auscultation reveals an S3** [5] and **wide splitting of the S2** [6].
- A **pansystolic murmur can be heard over the left parasternal edge over the tricuspid region, which was louder on inspiration** [7]. Examination of the lungs was clear.
- A **pulsatile liver** [8] was palpated on examination of the abdomen.
- There were **no signs of peripheral oedema** [9].

1 Increased work of breathing on mobilisation is consistent with the patient's presenting complaint of exertional dyspnoea. During times of rest and reduced cardiac requirements, the patient can be reasonably symptom-free.

2 An attempt should be made on initial examination to determine the causes of pulmonary hypertension, as outlined above. Close examination of the hands may reveal any underlying connective tissue diseases that may be present. Aside from Group 1 pulmonary hypertension, all treatment is of the underlying causes.

3 An elevated JVP with prominent A waves is suggestive of tricuspid regurgitation, which is a sign of right-sided heart failure.

4 Left parasternal heave is a sign suggestive of right-sided heart failure. Left parasternal heave is due to right ventricular hypertrophy.

5 S3, the third heart sound, is also called a 'gallop'. The third heart sound occurs at the beginning of diastole after the second heart sound. (It is best heard with the bell.)

The potential causes of an S3 include volume overload (congestive cardiac failure), physiological (young, athletes, pregnancy).

6 On very close auscultation, splitting of the second heart sound can be normal. However, wide splitting of S2 occurs when there is delayed right ventricular emptying, such as in RBBB and right heart failure.

7 A pansystolic murmur in the setting of A waves in the JVP is indicative of tricuspid regurgitation. Other causes of a pansystolic murmur include mitral regurgitation and ventral septal defects. Right-sided murmurs will be louder on inspiration, compared to those that are left-sided (i.e. mitral regurgitation), which will become louder in expiration.

8 Pulsatile liver is a sign of right heart failure due to backward pressure onto the liver. This can also cause congestion of the liver and subsequently result in hepatomegaly.

9 Peripheral oedema is typically a late sign of right heart failure.

Investigations

- All patients with IPH should undergo investigation with **baseline blood tests** [1], **electrocardiogram** [2], **chest X-ray** [3] and **transthoracic echocardiogram (TTE)** [4].
- Confirmation of idiopathic pulmonary hypertension should be made with a **right heart catheter study** [5].
- Once the diagnosis of pulmonary hypertension has

been confirmed, further investigation is required to rule out other causes of pulmonary hypertension. These include **left heart catheterisation** [6], **CT chest** [7], **pulmonary function test** [7], **ventilation-perfusion (V/Q) scan** [8], **HIV serology** [9], **liver function test** [10] and **autoantibody titres** [11].

- An **arterial blood gas** [12] may also need to be performed for management.

1 Baseline blood tests would include full blood count to rule out any contributing infection and anaemia as the cause of shortness of breath and fatigue. Urea, electrolytes and creatinine will assess any renal dysfunction that may also be contributing to dyspnoea. There are no specific pathology blood tests that will diagnose IPH.

2 ECG can be normal. Patients with IPH who have right ventricular hypertrophy or strain can have right axis deviation and RBBB. ECG changes are not an indicator of severity.

3 Chest X-ray can be normal. It may reveal right ventricular enlargement, right atrial dilation and enlargement of the central pulmonary arteries. In some cases, it may provide additional information regarding other potential causes of pulmonary hypertension.

4 TTE is the initial test of choice that will aid the diagnosis of pulmonary hypertension. TTE uses the tricuspid regurgitant jet velocity (TRV) to estimate the pulmonary artery systolic pressure (ePASP). Using a combination of TRV and ePASP, the likelihood of IPH can be determined and guide

further investigation. TTE will also be able to assess right ventricular size, wall thickness and function.

5 Not all patients with pulmonary hypertension need to undergo right heart catheterisation as it is an invasive procedure with associated risks. However, if all causes have been ruled out then right heart catheterisation will be required to confirm the diagnosis of IPH. Pulmonary hypertension is defined as a resting mean pulmonary artery pressure of ≥25mmHg.

6 Investigations for left heart disease (Group 2) include TTE and can be further investigated with left heart catheterisation. However, this diagnosis is largely made on risk stratification, clinical history, examination and TTE findings.

7 Investigation for chronic lung disease and hypoxia (Group 3) is required through HRCT of the chest, pulmonary function testing and 6-minute walk tests. Patient may also be required to undergo overnight oxygen monitoring or overnight sleep study.

8 To further investigate for chronic thromboembolism pulmonary hypertension, a V/Q scan or CT of the pulmonary arteries can be performed. Patients with underlying airways disease such as COPD will have mismatch on their V/Q scan and results cannot be accurately interpreted. For these patients CTPA is required to confirm chronic pulmonary artery obstruction.

9 HIV is an associated condition for Group 1 pulmonary hypertension.

10 LFTs can provide information regarding presence of portal hypertension.

11 Autoantibodies are used to diagnose any underlying connective tissue disease.

12 Arterial blood gas is reserved for patients who remain hypoxic. Chronic hypoxia proven on an ABG will be important for patients who may qualify for home oxygen.

Management

IPH needs to be managed in a **specialised pulmonary hypertension centre** [1]. IPH has no current treatments for primary prevention. **Calcium channel blockers** [2] have been used in patients who have proven response to therapy. Other **drug classes specific** [3] for IPH are **endothelin receptor antagonists** [4], **PDE-5 inhibitors** [5], **prostacyclins** [6] and soluble guanylate cyclase stimulators.

Other considerations in treatment of IPH include **hypoxia and eligibility for home oxygenation** [7]. There are no specific diet and exercise regimes recommended directly for the treatment of IPH. Patients should be advised to maintain physical activity as much as possible, understanding that there are limitations due to their symptoms, particularly dyspnoea.

Close monitoring is required through review of symptoms, repeat TTEs and regular medication reviews.

1 IPH is a rare condition and requires specialty input from pulmonary hypertension specialists who are typically cardiologists or respiratory physicians. Treatment will depend on symptomatology and WHO functional class.

2 CCBs are trialled in patients who demonstrate vasodilator response of decrease in mean pulmonary artery pressure of ≥10mmHg. CCBs work as vasodilators and lower the pulmonary artery pressure. Of patients who are proven responders to CCBs, 50% will see benefit to treatment and have an improved quality of life. The response, however, is short-lived and eventually they will require alternative or additional treatment. Common CCBs used are nifedipine sustained-release or diltiazem. The most common side-effects of CCBs are hypotension and peripheral oedema.

3 Pulmonary hypertension-specific therapy has been shown to improve symptoms and the 6-minute walk test distance, and reduce WHO functional class.

4 Endothelin receptor antagonists (ERAs) such as ambrisentan, bosentan and macitentan act to block endothelin-1, a vasoconstrictor. By blocking endothelin receptor A and B, there is a resultant vasodilator effect. Ambrisentan is a selective endothelin receptor A blocker, whilst bosentan and macitentan are non-selective blockers. The main side-effects of ERAs are hepatotoxicity and peripheral oedema.

5 Phosphodiesterase-5 inhibitors (PDE-5Is) such as sildenafil and tadalafil work to promote the action of nitric oxide, which has vasodilator effects. The most adverse effects are headache, flushing, myalgias and arthralgias.

6 Prostacyclin receptor agonists such as selexipag are non-prostanoid prostacycline receptors. Activation results in vasodilation. Typically, these medications are used after trial of ERAs and PDE-5Is.

7 Patients who are persistently hypoxic, confirmed on ABG, may be eligible for home oxygenation. The main contraindications to home oxygen include current smoker, or family member in the same household who smokes.

CASE 87: Interstitial lung disease

History

- A **67-year-old** [1] male presents to his local doctor with worsening **shortness of breath** [2] on exertion and a **non-productive cough** [3] over the last **12 months** [4].
- He denies any **chest pain** [5].
- He denies any **orthopnoea or any swollen ankles** [6].
- He denies any **joint pain** [7].

- He has no previous significant past history and **no family history** [8] of respiratory conditions.
- He does not take any **regular medications and has not had radiotherapy** [9].
- He is an **ex-smoker** [10], having smoked for 40 pack years before quitting 10 years ago.
- He **worked** [11] as a teacher, before retiring 3 years ago.

1 The presentation of patients with interstitial lung disease (ILD) varies depending on their underlying pathology. Patients with idiopathic pulmonary fibrosis (IPF) generally tend to present over the age of 60. On the other hand, patients with connective tissue disease-associated ILD, sarcoidosis, pulmonary Langerhans cell histiocytosis or some inherited forms of IPF present between 20 and 40 years of age.

2 Dyspnoea is one of the most common presenting symptoms for patients with interstitial lung disease. However, it is not uncommon for patients to attribute the gradual progression of exertional dyspnoea to ageing or deconditioning. Some patients may subconsciously limit their activity and therefore, deny the presence of any dyspnoea. Other causes of dyspnoea in the elderly to consider include other respiratory causes such as COPD and bronchiectasis, cardiac causes such as congestive cardiac failure and angina, or anaemia.

3 A dry cough is common in most patients with interstitial lung disease but it is unusual for ILD patients to have a productive cough. Rather, a productive cough would indicate an acute infection or another underlying lung pathology such as bronchiectasis.

4 The length of time between onset of interstitial lung disease and diagnosis can vary depending on the cause. Acute idiopathic interstitial pneumonia, eosinophilic pneumonia or hypersensitivity pneumonitis are relatively acute, presenting over days to weeks, while IPF and sarcoidosis present over months to years.

5 Most patients with interstitial lung disease do not have chest pain. However, certain causes of ILD such as rheumatoid arthritis (RA), SLE or mixed connective tissue disease can present with pleuritic chest pain.

6 Orthopnoea, paroxysmal nocturnal dyspnoea and swelling of the ankles indicate a fluid component as a cause of the dyspnoea and will indicate congestive cardiac failure as a likely diagnosis.

7 One of the group of conditions that cause ILD is connective tissue and autoimmune diseases including RA, SLE, systemic sclerosis, polymyositis and dermatomyositis. These patients can present with joint pain, weakness, photosensitivity, dry eyes and mouth. However, in rare cases, the pulmonary manifestation of ILD can occur prior to the development of other systemic symptoms of the inflammatory conditions.

8 While the specific genetic factors involved in idiopathic pulmonary fibrosis are not known, there does appear to be a genetic predisposition, with several cases of IPF occurring within families with potential autosomal dominant inheritance.

9 A thorough medication history is essential in cases of suspected interstitial lung disease, as a number of medications are known to cause ILD. These include amiodarone, chemotherapeutic agents such as bleomycin or methotrexate, certain antimicrobials such as nitrofurantoin or new biologic agents such as rituximab. Radiotherapy is also known to cause lung disease and is related to cumulative dose of radiation. Acute radiation pneumonitis can occur within 1–2 months of radiation, while fibrotic radiation pneumonitis develops after 6–12 months.

10 Smoking has a known strong association with a number of causes of ILD including idiopathic pulmonary fibrosis. However, smoking is also strongly associated with other causes of dyspnoea in adults such as ischaemic heart disease or COPD.

11 An occupational history is another important component of the history for patients with suspected interstitial lung disease, as a number of occupational exposures are associated with ILD. These include inhaled silica, asbestos, coal dust, metals such as tin, animal proteins and fungi and certain fumes.

Examination

- On general inspection, the patient appears to be slightly short of breath as he moves to the examination bed. His pulse is 70bpm and regular and is normotensive with a blood pressure of 118/65mmHg. His respiratory rate is 20 breaths per minute and he is **saturating at 95% on air at rest, but desaturates to 88% with slight mobilisation** [1]. He is afebrile.
- On examination of his hands, there is evidence of **finger clubbing** [2]. There is no evidence of joint inflammation, **finger deformity** [3], **sclerodactyly** [4] or **Gottron's papules** [5].
- The **JVP is not elevated** and he had **no evidence of peripheral oedema** [6].
- On examination of his heart, the **heart sounds were dual with no added sounds or murmurs** [7].
- On examination of his chest, his trachea was midline without any deviation. Chest expansion was equal. On auscultation of the chest, there were bilateral **basal fine end-inspiratory crepitations** [8].

1 The patient is not significantly hypoxic at rest. Patients with early-stage ILD have normal oxygen saturations at rest but as the disease progresses, they can become hypoxic even at rest. Oxygen desaturation is common with exertion in ILD and is generally associated with poorer outcomes.

2 The enlargement of the nailbed and fingertips, known as clubbing, is associated with a number of conditions, including some causes of ILD. It is common in advanced idiopathic pulmonary fibrosis and asbestosis; however, it is rare in sarcoidosis and hypersensitivity pneumonitis. Other causes of finger clubbing include lung cancer, TB, bronchiectasis, congenital cyanotic heart disease, endocarditis, Crohn's disease and ulcerative colitis or cirrhosis.

3 Rheumatoid arthritis is a possible cause for interstitial lung disease and can present with swan neck deformity (where there is flexion of the distal interphalangeal joint (DIPJ) and hyperextension of the proximal interphalangeal joint (PIPJ)), boutonnière deformity (where there is flexion of the PIPJ and extension of the DIPJ) or a Z deformity of the thumb (with flexion at the metacarpophalangeal joint (MCPJ) and hyperextension of the interphalangeal joint).

4 Sclerodactyly is the thickening of skin around the fingers and toes and is associated with scleroderma and other mixed connective tissue disorders.

5 Gottron's papules are purple plaques found on bony prominences such as knuckles and are pathognomonic for dermatomyositis. Dermatomyositis generally presents with a heliotropic skin rash and muscle weakness, but can also affect the lungs.

6 An elevated JVP and peripheral oedema would be signs of fluid overload and indicate that the cause of the patient's dyspnoea is likely secondary to congestive cardiac failure or renal failure.

7 The cardiac examination is usually normal in patients with ILD. However, pulmonary hypertension and cor pulmonale may develop in advanced pulmonary fibrosis or may be a primary presentation of some connective tissue disorders associated with ILD, such as systemic sclerosis. The main examination findings in cor pulmonale would be loud P2, right-sided gallop, right ventricular heave and evidence of signs of right heart failure such as peripheral oedema.

8 Crackles can originate from either the alveoli or the airways; when from the airway secretions they are described as coarser and lower pitch, while those originating in the interstitium or alveoli are described as fine. As the crepitations are bilateral and basal, either oedema or pulmonary fibrosis are potential causes for them. However, the patient does not appear fluid-overloaded, making it more likely that pulmonary fibrosis is the cause of the crepitations. The crackles from idiopathic pulmonary fibrosis are typically described as being soft and high-pitched and like the sound of opening a Velcro fastener.

Investigations

- The patient had a set of blood tests including FBE, UEC and LFTs which was unremarkable and revealed a **normal haemoglobin level** [1].
- He had **tests looking for systemic autoimmune diseases** [2], including an antinuclear antibody, rheumatoid factor, anti-extractable nuclear antigen, myositis-associated antibodies, anti-neutrophil cytoplasmic antibody and anti-double-stranded DNA antibodies, which are all unremarkable.
- He has an ECG which is **normal** [3].
- He has a chest X-ray which reveals **non-specific reticular infiltrates** [4].
- The patient goes on to have an HRCT scan of his chest which revealed **peripheral opacities associated with honeycombing and traction bronchiectasis** [5] predominantly in **the lower zones** [6].

- The patient also had pulmonary function tests which revealed a **significantly reduced FEV$_1$ and significantly reduced FVC with a normal FVR (FEV$_1$/FVC ratio) with no bronchodilator response**. He also had reduced **lung volumes** and **reduced DLCO** [7].
- The patient also had a 6-minute walk test which found a **reduced walk distance with oxygen desaturation** [8].
- The patient's case was discussed at a respiratory MDT meeting. Given the clinical and radiological findings, it was decided that the patient did not require a **bronchoalveolar lavage** [9].
- It was also decided that he did not warrant a **lung biopsy** [10].

[1] Anaemia is a another relatively common cause for dyspnoea in the elderly and it is easy to rule out on the full blood count. Additionally, some of the causes of ILD, such as rheumatoid arthritis, can also cause anaemia of chronic disease.

[2] An autoimmune screen should ideally be conducted based upon findings on clinical history and examination and pleural disease on imaging. A reasonable starting point would be to order antinuclear antibodies (ANA) and rheumatoid factor (RF) as a screening tool, ordering further tests only if they are positive. ANA is a sensitive test for SLE, systemic sclerosis and mixed connective disease and can also return positive results for polymyositis/dermatomyositis, RA and Sjögren's syndrome, but it is not a specific test. A positive ANA should warrant further investigations such as anti-extractable nuclear antigen (ENA) which includes anti-Ro and anti-La (specific for SLE/Sjögren's), anti-Scl70 (specific for scleroderma) and anti-Jo (specific for dermatomyositis). Further tests for SLE include anti-double-stranded DNA and anticardiolipin antibodies. Rheumatoid factor is a reasonable screening test for rheumatoid arthritis but can also flag positive in most other autoimmune diseases. Anticyclic citrullinated peptide antibodies (anti-CCP) would be a more specific test for rheumatoid arthritis if the RF is positive. A positive anti-neutrophil cytoplasmic antibody (ANCA) would indicate a diagnosis of vasculitis. Other specific blood tests that are not commonly ordered include a serum angiotensin-converting enzyme (ACE) that tests for sarcoidosis, and an ESR, which is a marker of inflammation. However, a serum ACE level has low specificity and sensitivity for sarcoidosis and is therefore not routinely performed. Similarly, an ESR is very non-specific and can be elevated even in IPF.

[3] An ECG can help rule out some cardiac causes of dyspnoea/pulmonary oedema. For patients with early-stage IPF, the ECG would normally be normal. However, as the disease progresses it can lead to pulmonary hypertension and right ventricular hypertrophy. This can be identified on ECG as it will result in right axis deviation, a dominant R wave in V1 and a dominant S wave in V5 or V6.

[4] Reticular infiltrates are a 'net-like' shadowing, seen on chest X-ray as multiple fine white lines crossing over each other. The lines represent thickened interstitium secondary to IPF. However, this is a non-specific finding and may also be seen in cardiac failure and other causes of interstitial lung disease.

[5] All patients suspected of interstitial lung disease should have an HRCT. HRCT involves using a narrow beam collimation to take thin-section slices, which provides higher definition images of lung parenchyma. Idiopathic pulmonary fibrosis characteristically has 'honeycombing' which refers to clusters of cystic air spaces (usually 3–10mm in diameter) which normally have a subpleural location. Traction bronchiectasis involves the dilation of bronchi secondary to areas of pulmonary fibrosis. However, other types of interstitial lung disease would have different findings on HRCT. For example, patients with sarcoidosis generally have bilateral hilar adenopathy and upper lobe reticular changes. Pleural plaques with basilar reticular changes suggest asbestosis. Centrilobular nodules are associated with Langerhans cell histiocytosis and hypersensitivity pneumonitis.

[6] Different causes of pulmonary fibrosis predominantly tend to affect different lobes of the lung. Upper lobe

causes of fibrosis include silicosis, sarcoidosis, coal miner's lung, ankylosing spondylitis, allergic bronchopulmonary aspergillosis, radiation and TB. Causes of predominant lower lobe fibrosis include idiopathic pulmonary fibrosis, asbestosis, RA, scleroderma and medication-associated fibrosis.

7 The spirometry findings of reduced FEV_1 and FVC, but normal FVR, indicate a predominant restrictive lung disease with a reduced DLCO. This is the usual finding in idiopathic pulmonary fibrosis, as alveoli expansion is restricted and some alveoli are replaced by the fibrosis. This means that total lung volume and lung expansion is limited, but as the airways themselves are relatively unharmed, there is no evidence of airway obstruction. The DLCO is reduced as there is reduced surface area for gas exchange due to the loss of alveoli.

8 While patients with early interstitial lung disease may have normal oxygenation at rest, as the demand for oxygen increases with exercise, patients with ILD may desaturate and have a significant increase in respiratory rate. Regardless, not all patients with ILD will require a structured 6-minute walk test but it can be especially useful in patients with unclear significance of symptoms or imaging findings, as a normal 6-minute walk test practically excludes significant ILD.

9 Bronchoalveolar lavage (BAL) is a procedure that can be performed as part of a bronchoscopy, where a camera is inserted through either the mouth or nose to visualise the airways. As part of the lavage, some fluid is squirted onto areas of the lung and then recollected to analyse. A BAL is only indicated if the clinical suspicion is high for infection or for hypersensitivity pneumonitis (when BAL lymphocyte counts are >40%). Other potential indications for BAL

include the presence of haemoptysis or acute-onset, rapidly progressing ILD. Given that our patient has typical features of idiopathic pulmonary fibrosis on imaging and has clinical findings consistent with IPF, there is no strong indication for a BAL.

10 The decision whether or not a patient with suspected interstitial lung disease warrants a biopsy is usually made at a multidisciplinary meeting with respiratory physicians and radiologists on a case-by-case basis. It will take into account the patient's other comorbidities, the risks of the procedure itself and whether a biopsy is likely to have significant diagnostic yield. There are a few different methods that can be utilised for lung biopsies. One option is for an open thoracotomy biopsy, which involves a surgical incision into the chest wall with a sample of lung taken. While it leads to good diagnostic yield, it is associated with the highest mortality of biopsy procedures. A more common approach recently is performing a VATS (video-assisted thoracic surgery) biopsy, where an endoscope is inserted through small keyholes in the chest wall and lung samples are taken; this is associated with lower mortality. Transbronchial lung biopsy can be done in conjunction with a BAL and involves inserting forceps through a bronchoscope to take a sample of the airway wall and lung tissue. It is generally the preferred procedure when likely diagnosis is sarcoidosis, hypersensitivity pneumonitis or an infective (such as TB) or malignant cause (such as lymphangitis carcinomatosa) is suspected. While a transbronchial biopsy is the safest option, it has much lower diagnostic yield for most other types of ILD than open or VATS biopsies due to the small size of samples.

Management

Immediate

Given the history, examination and imaging findings, it is likely that the patient has **idiopathic pulmonary fibrosis** [1]. As this is a gradual progressive disease, this patient does not require any immediate treatment.

Short-term

The patient requires an urgent referral to a **respiratory physician** [2] who can organise further investigations (such as a biopsy) as required and discuss the patient in a multidisciplinary meeting. Once the diagnosis is confirmed, the physician should have a **clear discussion with the patient regarding prognosis and aims of management** [3].

Long-term

Patients should be referred for **pulmonary rehabilitation** [4]. As their condition progresses, they will likely require **supplemental oxygen** [5]. Patients should have their **influenza and pneumococcal vaccinations** [6].

Patients may also benefit with **treatment for gastro-oesophageal reflux** [7]. Previously, patients have been managed with **glucocorticosteroids and azathioprine** [8]. Recently, **nintedanib** [9] and **pirfenidone** [10] have been approved for management of IPF. Patients with idiopathic pulmonary fibrosis may be considered for **lung transplantation** [11]. As the disease progresses, patients should also be referred to **palliative care services** [12] for symptom control and support for end-of-life care.

1 The diagnosis of idiopathic pulmonary fibrosis requires other causes of interstitial lung disease to be excluded and features of IPF to be found on HRCT and/or lung biopsy. There are conflicting views regarding the necessity of lung biopsies to make the diagnosis, but if the clinical presentation and HRCT findings are typical of IPF and an MDT is confident of the diagnosis, then a lung biopsy is not required. If patients do have a lung biopsy, then the biopsy results must be correlated with HRCT before making the diagnosis.

2 The initial diagnosis and management of idiopathic pulmonary fibrosis normally requires specialist respiratory input, given the wide range of potential causes for interstitial lung disease with similar presentations. Respiratory physicians usually also have access to multidisciplinary meetings in hospitals involving pathologists and radiologists, which is essential to coming to a diagnosis.

3 The natural progression of idiopathic pulmonary fibrosis is variable; however, most patients experience ongoing, gradual worsening of lung function. The average survival time is a maximum of 3–5 years after diagnosis. The potential symptomatic care options must be discussed and whether they would wish to have a lung transplant. There should also be a discussion about end-of-life choices and the formation of an advanced care directive.

4 Pulmonary rehabilitation is usually a 6–8-week programme aimed at patients with chronic lung diseases, including IPF. Patients receive regular exercise training as well as energy conservation techniques. Patients are also educated about their condition and provided with psychological support.

5 Almost all patients with IPF will eventually require supplemental oxygen for comfort. Initially, patients may only require supplemental oxygen with exertion but as their disease progresses, the majority of patients will be on supplemental oxygen even at rest. Oxygen therapy can help some patients maintain limited function; however, it may not improve symptoms in some patients.

6 Both the influenza and pneumococcal vaccines should be recommended in all elderly patients because these infections have a significant effect on patients with IPF, given their poor respiratory function. Therefore, vaccinations to help prevent infections should be strongly recommended for patients with IPF.

7 It is thought that gastro-oesophageal reflux is associated with idiopathic pulmonary fibrosis and may contribute to cough in IPF. Gastro-oesophageal reflux is very common amongst patients with IPF and there is some evidence to suggest that treating reflux can slow progression of IPF. However, there is not enough evidence to support treating all patients with anti-gastro-oesophageal medications. Options to treat gastro-oesophageal reflux include PPIs (such as pantoprazole and esomeprazole) or H2 antagonists (such as ranitidine).

8 Azathioprine is an immunosuppressant that inhibits purine synthesis, reducing DNA synthesis and reducing the immune response. It is commonly used in autoimmune conditions and post renal transplants. Side-effects to be mindful of include bone marrow suppression and nausea and vomiting. Corticosteroids reduce systemic inflammatory response; thus in pulmonary fibrosis, corticosteroids help to reduce inflammation within the lung parenchyma. However, systemic corticosteroid therapy is associated with a number of side-effects including osteoporosis, cataracts and glaucoma, peptic ulcer disease, hyperglycaemia, adrenal suppression, mood/personality changes and increased risk of infections. However, the combined therapy of steroids and azathioprine is no longer recommended for idiopathic pulmonary fibrosis as it was found to increase overall mortality and adverse effects. Glucocorticosteroids (such as prednisolone) are still frequently used for exacerbations of IPF but there is no strong evidence to support this. Prednisolone therapy is also recommended for other causes of interstitial lung disease such as sarcoidosis or hypersensitivity pneumonitis.

9 Nintedanib is a tyrosine kinase receptor blocker that inhibits multiple fibrogenic growth factors, reducing overall fibroblast function. It has been shown to reduce the rate of decline of pulmonary function in patients with IPF and it reduces their exacerbation risk. Common side-effects include diarrhoea, nausea and vomiting and deranged LFTs.

10 Pirfenidone is an antifibrotic agent that inhibits collagen synthesis and blocks fibroblast proliferation. It appears to slow progression of IPF for those with mild–moderate disease. Common side-effects include rash and GI system disturbances. There are ongoing clinical trials looking at different medications for IPF, as well as the use of pirfenidone in patients with advanced disease.

11 Idiopathic pulmonary fibrosis is the second most common indication for lung transplantation in adults after COPD. Due to the poor prognosis associated with IPF, it is recommended that patients should be evaluated and referred early for potential lung transplant, prior to the development of end-stage disease. The decision for referral for transplantation should take into account the patient's age, comorbidities and baseline function/physiological reserve. In this patient's case, given their age and limited mobility, they are unlikely to be a lung transplant candidate.

12 Palliative care teams can provide strategies to help patients with symptom control at all stages of the disease. Options include the use of opioids to help with refractory dyspnoea and persistent cough. Non-pharmacological methods such as relaxation exercises and the use of a fan for facial cooling may help as well. For patients with a component of anxiety contributing to dyspnoea, anxiolytics such as midazolam or lorazepam may be utilised to help with symptoms. As the disease progresses, the patient may prefer to be admitted to an inpatient palliative care unit or a nursing home that can provide hospice care for end of life.

CASE 88: Lung transplantation

History

- A 52-year-old female has been referred by her respiratory physician for **consideration of a lung transplantation** [1].
- She has a past medical **history of idiopathic pulmonary fibrosis** [2] and eczema.
- She has **never smoked and does not drink alcohol** [3].

- Despite previously maintaining an active lifestyle, she has an **exercise tolerance of 20 metres** [4], limited by her dyspnoea, and has **home oxygen on 2L at baseline** [4]. Her respiratory symptoms have been **rapidly progressing over the last 6 months** [4].

[1] Lung transplantation is a treatment option for patients with advanced lung disease which has progressed despite medical or surgical management. Lung transplantation offers improved quality of life and long-term survival for patients. There are strict selection criteria developed by the International Society of Heart and Lung Transplantation for patients who are eligible to undergo transplantation. This is due to the limited number of organ donors, immensity of undergoing transplantation, and nature of the procedure, with significant risks associated. Selection criteria include:
- severe disease unresponsive or ineffective to medical therapy
- risk of death from lung disease without transplantation is >50% within 2 years
- the likelihood of surviving at least 90 days after lung transplantation is >80%
- absence of non-pulmonary medical comorbidities that are life-limiting in the first 5 years after transplantation
- satisfactory psychosocial profile and support system.

There are five types of lung transplantations, each with their own advantages and disadvantages: bilateral lung, single lung, split lung bilateral lobar, living donor lobar and combined heart-lung transplantation. Bilateral lung transplantation is most common.

[2] The conditions of advanced lung disease that can be concerned for transplantation include COPD (despite smoking cessation, maximal medical management, pulmonary rehabilitation and supplemental oxygen), IPF, interstitial lung disease (associated with sarcoidosis and rheumatic disease), CF, pulmonary vascular disease associated with New York Heart Association functional class III or IV.

[3] There are contraindications to lung transplantation that are divided into absolute and relative. Some absolute contraindications include untreated/uncontrolled infection (pulmonary and non-pulmonary), active TB infection, malignancy in the last 2 years, significant extrapulmonary organ dysfunction, coronary artery disease, chest wall or spinal deformity, active smoker, drug or alcohol dependency. Some relative contraindications include age >65 years with other relative contraindications, BMI >30kg/m², severe or progressive malnutrition, severe osteoporosis, HIV infection, and untreated/active hepatitis B or C infection.

[4] Exercise tolerance, home oxygen requirements and rate of disease progression are all key factors that are assessed when considering patients for lung transplantation.

Examination

- On examination, the patient had **2L of oxygen via nasal prongs** *in situ* [1].
- She had a **BMI** [2] **of 24kg/m²**.
- Hand examination did not reveal any **stigmata of infective endocarditis** [3]. There were no signs of pale palmar creases or pale conjunctiva.
- She had moist mucous membranes, with a **JVP at 3cm** [4].

- On examination of the chest, there were **no chest deformities or kyphosis** [5].
- There was **no midline sternotomy scar** [6].
- Her apex beat was not displaced, and the heart sounds were dual. On **auscultation there were fine crepitations bilaterally** [7], more on the right compared to the left lung.
- Examination of the abdomen was unremarkable, with no evidence of pitting oedema.

1 Thorough examination will provide clues of potentially undiagnosed comorbidities. General inspection will provide information on the patient's work of breathing and baseline function. Continuous use of oxygen is an indicator of severity of a patient's baseline respiratory function.

2 BMI is important for patients who are being considered for transplantation. Having low BMI may indicate malnutrition and BMI >30kg/m^2 is a relative contraindication for transplantation.

3 Hand exam can reveal features of infective endocarditis which will require treatment prior to consideration of transplantation. Signs include Osler nodes, Janeway lesions and splinter haemorrhages. Other signs on hand exam

can also show features of iron deficiency (koilonychia) and anaemia (palmar crease pallor).

4 Mucous membranes and JVP are used to assess a patient's fluid status. Elevated JVP >3cm suggests fluid overload, which could be suggestive of cardiac or renal failure.

5 Chest and spinal deformities are relative contraindications for lung transplantation.

6 Sternotomy scar suggests previous thoracic surgery, which is a relative contraindication.

7 Chest findings of bilateral crepitations are consistent with idiopathic pulmonary fibrosis.

Investigations

- Prior to transplantation, the patient underwent a range of **pathology tests** [1] including full blood count, UEC, liver function, **coagulation profile** [2], iron studies, **HbA1c and random glucose** [3], and **BNP** [4].

- **Serology and tests for prior or current infection** [5] are also required.
- She was also referred for **cardiac function tests** [6], **respiratory function tests** [7], **assessment of bone health** [8] and **malignancy screening** [9].

1 Basic blood tests are performed to assess patients for anaemia, signs of active infection, renal function and liver function.

2 Coagulation profile will be required prior to undergoing surgical procedures. Abnormalities can also identify bleeding and clotting disorders that are unknown to the patient that may compromise transplantation.

3 HbA1c and glucose are tested to diagnose diabetes in patients without a history. For patients with known diabetes, HbA1c provides information of glycaemic control over a 3-month period.

4 Elevation of BNP >1000 is suggestive of presence of congestive cardiac function.

5 Infection screening in patients is crucial as they will require immunosuppression post transplantation. Infections that require screening include CMV, EBV, hepatitis B and C, HIV, HSV, VZV and TB.

6 Cardiac testing includes baseline ECG, echocardiogram and, for patients above the age of 45, consideration of cardiac catheterisation for diagnosis of coronary artery disease, cardiac abnormality and anaesthetic risk evaluation.

7 Respiratory function test is performed to determine the degree of lung dysfunction and eligibility for transplantation. Tests include spirometry, assessment of lung volumes, DLCO, 6-minute walk test and ABG.

8 Severe systemic osteoporosis is a contraindication for transplantation and hence measurement of bone health is required through a DEXA scan.

9 Malignancy can shorten a patient's life expectancy. In early stages, patients may be asymptomatic. Malignancy screening is required, including colonoscopy within the last 10 years if patients are over the age of 50 years, mammogram and Pap smears in the last 12 months for women and prostate-specific antigen (PSA) for men.

Management

Immediate

Following successful lung transplantation, the patient was commenced on **immunosuppressive therapy** [1] including **prednisolone** [2], **tacrolimus** [3] and **mycophenolate mofetil** [4].

Short-term

She was also prescribed **co-trimoxazole for prevention of P. jirovecii pneumonia** [5] and **valganciclovir for CMV infection** [6].

Long-term

Following transplantation the patient underwent **repeat spirometry and surveillance transbronchial biopsies** [7].

---

1 Immunosuppression following any transplantation is required to prevent both acute and chronic graft rejection. Typically, a combination of agents are used for maintenance immunosuppression including glucocorticoid (prednisolone), a calcineurin inhibitor (ciclosporin, tacrolimus) and nucleotide-blocking agent (azathioprine, mycophenolate mofetil). mTOR inhibitors (everolimus and sirolimus) are alternative agents to nucleotide-blocking agents. Immunosuppression overall is individually tailored to each patient with the aim of using the lowest doses possible to prevent rejection. As time goes on from the initial time of transplantation, the risk of rejection reduces and the intensity of immunosuppression decreases over the first months.

2 Glucocorticoids are always included in ongoing immunosuppression for lung transplantation. Higher pulse doses can be used during periods of acute rejection. There are many side-effects associated with long-term use of glucocorticoids, not limited to increased risk of infection, hypertension, steroid-induced diabetes, mood changes and agitation, glaucoma, osteoporosis and easy bruising.

3 Calcineurin inhibitors include ciclosporin and tacrolimus. The choice between the two agents is dependent on the transplant physician; however, tacrolimus is more commonly used. Tacrolimus is an oral medication which has a narrow therapeutic window. Tacrolimus levels are closely monitored, and the recommended therapeutic dose varies at different stages and for different types of organ transplant. Tacrolimus is metabolised by the CYP 3A4 pathway and has the potential for numerous drug–drug interactions. One of the most common side-effects is renal dysfunction.

4 Nucleotide-blocking agents include mycophenolate mofetil and azathioprine. The choice between the two agents is dependent on the transplant physician. Mycophenolate side-effects include myelosuppression, and regular monitoring of FBC is required. Other side-effects include GI discomfort, nausea and diarrhoea.

5 In patients on long-term suppression, opportunistic bacterial infections can occur. Co-trimoxazole (sulfamethoxazole/trimethoprim) is prescribed for the prevention of P. jirovecii pneumonia (PJP). The standard dosing is 1 double strength (180/600mg) tablet daily, three times a week. Patients with renal impairment may requiring dosing adjustment.

6 Behind bacterial pneumonia, CMV infection is the second most common infection in lung transplant recipients. Antiviral prophylaxis is prescribed to patients with asymptomatic CMV viraemia to prevent progression to invasive disease. CMV disease can present with fever, malaise, leucopenia and thrombocytopenia. CMV can also spread into tissues causing pneumonitis, enteritis and hepatitis. CMV disease is treated with oral valganciclovir or IV ganciclovir. Ongoing monitoring with once- to twice-weekly levels of CMV is used to monitor treatment response.

7 Acute rejection is most likely to occur in the first 6 months and is a concern for all transplant patients, with many patients requiring treatment for acute rejection in the first 12 months after transplantation. Risk factors for acute rejection include HLA mismatching, younger age and immunosuppression regimen. Clinical symptoms include dyspnoea and cough; however, not all patients exhibit symptoms. Patients with symptoms undergo basic investigations including basic bloods, chest imaging (CXR, HRCT chest) and spirometry to assess lung function. Further investigation with bronchoscopy with lavage and biopsy may be required. Some other causes of symptoms aside from acute rejection include infection and airway stenosis. Treatment of acute rejection includes high dose glucocorticoids and ongoing monitoring.

CASE 89: Pleural effusion

History

- An 83-year-old female, previously living independently at home, presented to the ED with a one-week history of **dyspnoea** [1], **dry cough** [2] and fatigue.
- She **denies any haemoptysis** [3].
- She has been diagnosed with **right middle and lower lobe community-acquired pneumonia** [4].
- On presentation she was mildly confused, with oxygen saturations of 89% on air. This is on a background history of hypertension,

hypercholesterolaemia and osteoarthritis. **Despite IV antibiotic treatment for 2 days, the patient remains tachypnoeic and has ongoing oxygen requirements** [5].

- She reports feeling fatigued and is unable to mobilise due to her dyspnoea. Further investigation reveals a **right-sided pleural effusion** [6].
- She has never smoked and **denies any recent travel, loss of weight or swelling in her legs** [7].

[1] Dyspnoea (shortness of breath) is a very common presentation to GPs and the ED. A thorough history, including the nature of onset of symptoms, is vital in differentiating between the potential causes of dyspnoea. Acute causes include acute myocardial infarction, acute pulmonary oedema, anaphylaxis and exacerbation of airways disease (infectious and non-infectious). A more insidious history would be more suggestive of interstitial lung disease, malignancy and pleural effusion.

[2] The presence of cough is important to identify. Further history should be taken regarding the nature of the cough: productive vs. non-productive will provide clues to the underlying aetiology of the dyspnoea. Some patients with underlying airways disease may have a long-standing chronic cough. In these patients, it is necessary to ask whether or not the nature of the cough has changed, and if there are any changes in baseline sputum production, including quantity and colour.

[3] Haemoptysis is a critical symptom to elicit. Most notably it may be an indicator for lung malignancy. Causes of haemoptysis can be considered under three broad categories: infection, tumour and vascular. Infectious causes include TB, bronchitis, bronchiectasis, lung abscesses and aspergilloma. Vascular causes include pulmonary embolism and AV malformations.

[4] Community-acquired pneumonia is a common reason for admission into hospital, particularly in elderly patients. Not all patients with community-acquired pneumonia require admission, and treatment is guided on severity scores such as CORB65 and SMARTCOP. Mild community-acquired pneumonia can be treated with oral antibiotics. A CORB 65 score of 3 requires admission for IV antibiotics.

[5] No improvement of symptoms despite 2 days of IV antibiotics, and with ongoing haemodynamic instability, warrants further investigations. Further imaging in this patient revealed evidence of a right-sided pleural effusion.

[6] There are many causes of pleural effusion. Based on Light's criteria (laboratory findings of pleural fluid), the causes are separated into transudative and exudative causes. Transudative pleural effusion describes fluid leaking into the pleural space due to elevated pressure from the vasculature. These conditions include congestive cardiac failure, liver cirrhosis, nephrotic syndrome and hypoalbuminaemia. Exudative effusions are due to obstruction of the blood vessels secondary to infection (pneumonia, TB), malignancy, connective tissue disease (RA, lupus) and drugs (methotrexate, nitrofurantoin).

[7] Further history can help reduce differential diagnoses of dyspnoea. Recent long-haul travel can give rise to thrombotic embolism, loss of weight is suggestive of a malignancy and swelling of the legs may be due to cardiac failure.

Examination

- On examination, the patient is **hypoxic** [1], saturating at 89% on air, requiring 2L via nasal prongs to maintain oxygen saturations of 95%.
- She is sitting upright in the bed with **no increase in work of breathing** [2] at rest, speaking only in words.
- On examination of her hands there is **no evidence of nicotine staining and clubbing** [3].
- There are **no signs of arthropathy** [4].
- Her JVP is not elevated, and the **trachea is within the midline** [5].
- There is **reduced chest expansion** [6] on the right and **stony dull percussion** [7] over the mid- to lower zone on the right.
- There is **reduced vocal fremitus** [8].
- On auscultation, there are **reduced breath sounds** [9] on the right.
- Examination of the lower limbs **does not reveal peripheral oedema** [10].

1 Hypoxia is a sign of haemodynamic instability and reduced oxygen perfusion. There are many causes of hypoxia, such as hypoventilation, ventilation–perfusion mismatch, right to left shunt and reduced inspired oxygen tension. Normal oxygen saturation is O_2 levels >95%.

2 Increased work of breathing indicates respiratory distress and respiratory failure. Patients with persistent tachypnoea are at risk of tiring. Early assessment with blood gases to accurately assess oxygenation and metabolic state will help guide the need for early intubation, if appropriate.

3 There are a number of causes of clubbing. Specifically, the lung causes of clubbing include lung abscess, bronchiectasis, CF, effusions and malignancy.

4 Hand examination may provide clues regarding the cause of pleural effusions. Pleural effusions can be related to connective tissue diseases such as RA.

5 Trachea in patients with pleural effusions are typically midline. Rarely when there is a large effusion, there can be deviation to the opposite side to the effusion.

6 Chest expansion will typically be reduced.

7 Percussion is classically reported as stony dull percussion. Other causes of dull percussion include collapse, consolidation, elevated hemidiaphragm and lower lobe lobectomy.

8 Vocal fremitus is reduced over the area of the effusion. Due to the dense nature of fluid, sound is not conducted as well and 'ninety-nine' will be 'muffled'.

9 Breath sounds as a result will be reduced. Just above the pleural effusion, the presence of bronchial breath sounds can be appreciated.

10 The presence of peripheral oedema can be due to congestive cardiac failure, or in hypoalbuminaemic states.

Investigations

- Investigations for pleural effusion will include pathology of **FBC, UEC, LFT, albumin, lactate dehydrogenase (LDH)** [1] and **arterial blood gas** [2].
- Additional laboratory tests such as **rheumatoid factor and autoimmune antibodies** [3] can be considered.
- A **chest X-ray** [4] can provide information regarding location and size of the pleural effusion.
- Further imaging may be required with **CT chest** [5].
- The diagnostic investigation would be a **pleural tap, which can also provide therapeutic benefit** [6].

1 Basic bloods can be helpful in determining the cause of the effusion. Elevated white cell count and neutrophilia can indicate presence of an infection. Elevated creatinine on UEC can be suggestive of renal dysfunction. Uraemia itself can also be a cause of an effusion. Derangement of the LFT can be suggestive of cirrhosis. Hypoalbuminaemia can be a cause of pleural effusion or suggestive of other underlying pathology such as malignancy. An LDH is important to perform as this is part of Light's criteria (which will be outlined in Note 6).

2 Arterial blood gases are useful to assess the metabolic state of the patient. Patients with increased work of breathing (respiratory distress) and evidence of respiratory acidosis will benefit from early discussion with critical care teams to consider non-invasive ventilation or intubation.

3 Other associated conditions of connective tissue disease can be further investigated with RF and autoimmune antibodies.

4 Chest X-ray is an important and easily accessible test to help support the examination findings. X-ray will localise and provide information regarding size and possible loculations which would be suggestive of a more complex effusion.

5 CT chest can provide a more defined view of the effusion and whether there are loculations.

6 A pleural tap should be performed under radiological guidance. Complications of the procedure include bleeding, pneumothorax and infection. Pleural fluid should be sent to the laboratory and LDH, protein, pH should be performed. Light's criteria for exudate:
- Pleural fluid protein: serum protein >0.5
- Pleural fluid LDH: serum LDH >0.6
- Pleural fluid LDH >⅔ upper limit of normal serum value.

Management

Management of pleural effusions is divided into non-malignant and malignant causes.

Asymptomatic patients do not require treatment. **Non-malignant pleural effusions are based on treating the underlying cause** [1].

If patients are symptomatic (mainly dyspnoea) of the effusion, then **repeat therapeutic drainage can be performed** [2].

In patients with malignant pleural effusion, **pleurodesis can be considered** [3].

1 Patients who are asymptomatic do not require further treatment. Treatment of non-malignant pleural effusions is directed to the underlying cause.

2 Persistent dyspnoea is the main symptom indication for repeat therapeutic thoracentesis when the effusion is slow to reaccumulate. If patients are reaccumulating too quickly (within a month) then recurrent pleural taps can be difficult for the patient to tolerate.

One of the risks associated with thoracentesis is re-expansion pulmonary oedema. To avoid this, limiting the amount of pleural fluid removed and close monitoring of the patient is important. Any chest pain or hypoxia warrants urgent reassessment. Another significant complication is drainage-related pneumothorax.

3 Pleurodesis is performed by thoracic surgical teams to remove the pleural space, to prevent reaccumulation of pleural effusions. Materials such as sterile talc, bleomycin or zinc sulphate can be used. These agents cause inflammation and subsequent fibrosis into the pleural space. Complications of pleurodesis include pain and transient hypoxia.

CASE 90: Pneumothorax

History

- A **23-year-old** [1] **tall thin male** [2] walks into the ED complaining of chest pain and shortness of breath.
- He denies any **history of trauma** [3].
- He stated that the pain came on all of a **sudden** [4] over the right side of his chest.
- He feels as though the pain is **worse when he tries to take a deep breath** [5].
- He has no associated cough and was **previously well** [6].

- He has **no recent history of plane travel or immobilisation** [7].
- He has an 8 pack year **smoking history** [8].
- He has no history of any **previous lung disease such as COPD, asthma or malignancy** [9].
- He also has no **history of any connective tissue disorders** [10].
- He has not had any **recent medical procedure** [11].

[1] Pneumothoraces can occur in patients of all ages. In the elderly, they are more likely to be secondary to respiratory disease such as COPD, while in the young they are more likely to be primary. Primary spontaneous pneumothoraces are a result of a rupture of a pleural bleb which is usually apical. Either lung can be affected.

[2] Pneumothoraces are more common in males, particularly in young tall males, with a male to female ratio of 6:1.

[3] Traumatic pneumothoraces can be due to both penetrating or non-penetrating chest injuries.

[4] A pneumothorax commonly leads to an acute onset of severe chest pain. However, acute severe chest pain is also associated with a number of other conditions that should not be missed, including acute aortic dissection, pulmonary embolism or mediastinitis such as a ruptured oesophagus. Acute coronary syndromes can also result in severe central chest discomfort. Other musculoskeletal causes, such as costochondritis, or GI causes such as GORD, can also present with chest pain.

[5] Pleuritic chest pain is pain that is sharp and localised to a certain area of the chest, which is aggravated by inspiration or coughing. This is due to inflammation of the pleura leading to pain as detected via parietal pain fibres and therefore, worsens when there is movement of the pleura. Pleuritic chest pain can be due to pleural disease such as pneumothorax, pleural infection secondary to Coxsackie virus, or in connective tissue disease leading to pleural inflammation, such as SLE or RA. It can also be as a result of conditions affecting the peripheral lung itself, such as pneumonia or pulmonary embolism.

[6] Primary spontaneous pneumothoraces in young individuals commonly occur without any known underlying lung disease. Additionally, recent infective symptoms such as fevers and sore throat in addition to pleuritic pain could indicate other causes of the pain, such as Coxsackie infection.

[7] Pulmonary embolism is a major differential for pleuritic chest pain and breathlessness. Risk factors for pulmonary embolism include immobilisation, malignancy, recent surgery, oestrogen-containing contraception and genetic conditions that predispose to thrombophilia.

[8] Smoking is an independent risk factor for primary spontaneous pneumothorax, even without having a history of emphysema.

[9] Underlying lung diseases, such as COPD, interstitial lung disease, TB, CF, lung malignancy and necrotising pneumonia, are all risk factors for secondary spontaneous pneumonia.

[10] Connective tissue disorders such as Marfan's syndrome or Ehler–Danlos syndrome, as well as RA, ankylosing spondylitis and scleroderma, are all associated with spontaneous pneumothoraces.

[11] Medical procedures such as central line insertion, pacemaker insertion and transbronchial biopsy all carry the risk of pneumothorax and it is usually routine after a number of these procedures for patients to have chest X-rays to rule out a pneumothorax. Recent mechanical ventilation also increases the risk of having a pneumothorax.

Examination

- On general inspection, the patient has a slight grimace due to the pain but does not appear to be in **significant respiratory compromise** [1]. He is able to respond to you and is not tachypnoeic.
- **His pulse is 84bpm and regular, his blood pressure is 133/73mmHg and his respiratory rate is 18 breaths per minute** [2].
- He is **afebrile** [3] with a temperature of 36.7°C. He is currently saturating at 93% oxygen saturations without supplemental oxygen.
- On examination of chest and neck, his **trachea is midline and not deviated to either side** [4].

- He has **decreased chest expansion** [5] on the right side in comparison to the left.
- On percussion, he has **increased resonance** [6] on the right side of his chest.
- On auscultation, he has **reduced air entry** [7] into the right side.
- He was also found to have **reduced vocal resonance** [8] on the right side.

[1] The end of the bed assessment is always very useful before directly examining any patient and can help determine the urgency of management.

[2] By looking at this patient's observations, you are quickly able to conclude that he does not have any signs of respiratory failure or cardiovascular compromise. You can then move on to conduct a more thorough assessment without having to commence resuscitation.

[3] While the absence of a fever does not rule out an infective cause, it can help reduce your clinical suspicion for it.

[4] The trachea indicates upper mediastinal position which is determined by intrathoracic pressure. Unequal intrathoracic pressure within the chest wall leads to tracheal deviation, with the mediastinum shifting towards the side with higher negative pressure. In the case of a tension pneumothorax, there is increased pressure on the affected side of the lung due to the hole in the lung acting as a one-way valve, leading to tracheal deviation to the opposite side. A tension pneumothorax is a medical emergency as it results in significant respiratory and circulatory compromise. Other conditions that may lead to tracheal deviation away from the affected side include pleural effusions and large pulmonary masses. On the other hand, atelectasis, previous pneumonectomy and pleural fibrosis can lead to tracheal deviation towards the affected side.

[5] Pneumothoraces lead to reduced chest expansion on the affected side, as the lung on the affected side is not inflating as well as on the healthy side, due to the presence of air in the pleural space.

[6] The resonance during percussion can be used to help distinguish what is present under the skin surface. Duller notes indicate the presence of fluid or a solid mass, while more resonant notes indicate structures containing air. A hyper-resonant percussion note over the lung is indicative of either a hyperinflated lung from advanced COPD or a pneumothorax.

[7] There is reduced air entry on the affected side in patients with pneumothoraces secondary to the collapsed lung.

[8] Listening for vocal resonance involves listening to transmitted sounds from the larynx via the lung tissue to the chest wall. The presence of air or fluid within the pleural space can act as a buffer for the transmitted sounds, resulting in a reduced vocal resonance.

Investigations

- The patient has had a set of bloods on arrival at the ED. On the FBE, the patient has a normal haemoglobin, white blood cell count and platelet count. The patient **does not have an elevated CRP** [1].
- He also has normal electrolytes and renal function. His **coagulation screen was also normal** [2].
- He has **an ECG** [3] that shows a sinus rhythm with normal conduction.
- The patient had a **plain chest X-ray** [4].
- This shows a **clear visible pleural edge on the right side with no lung markings seen distal** [5] to this marking and **evidence of a collapsed lung** [6].
- His **mediastinum is midline on the X-ray** [7].
- At the **level of the hilum, the chest wall is 3cm away from the lung edge** [8].
- The emergency physician decides to perform a **bedside ultrasound** [9] on the patient.
- There is an **absence of lung sliding seen** [10], with M-mode resulting in a pattern of parallel horizontal lines and there are **'A-lines' seen on imaging** [11].
- As the patient already has a pneumothorax identified on chest X-ray, the emergency physician decides not to order a **chest CT** [12].

[1] A relatively normal set of bloods is not unexpected in a patient of this age, but the normal white cell count and CRP also helps reassure us that it is unlikely to be an infective process that explains his symptoms.

[2] The patient may require a procedure for management of a pneumothorax and this will be done regardless in an emergency situation. However, a coagulation disorder may increase the risks of any such procedures.

[3] ECGs are findings non-specific in patients with pneumothoraces. It is not uncommon for patients to be in sinus tachycardia, usually as a result of the pain or difficulty breathing. The presence of a significant rhythm disturbance, such as a bradycardia, may indicate significant hypoxaemia or impending cardiovascular collapse due to a tension pneumothorax.

[4] A plain chest X-ray is the primary useful first investigation for a pneumothorax. Usually it is performed during maximal inspiration, but comparison with expiratory films can be used to further detect any pneumothoraces missed in inspiration.

[5] The pleural edge is radio-opaque and therefore seen as a thick white line, with the air appearing radiolucent distal to it.

[6] The lung is collapsed due to the disruption of the usual negative pressure state in the pleural space as a result of the presence of air.

[7] There should not be mediastinal shift in a simple pneumothorax. The presence of mediastinal shift is a medical emergency as it can quickly lead to cardiovascular compromise.

[8] The size of the pneumothorax forms a key part of the decision regarding its management. This will be covered in the Management section.

[9] A bedside ultrasound is increasingly being used to diagnose pneumothoraces, particularly as part of a focused assessment with sonography for trauma (FAST) scan in trauma settings.

[10] In a pneumothorax, due to the presence of air between the parietal and visceral pleura, it is not possible to visualise the visceral pleura. Therefore, the movement of the pleural line cannot be seen and in M-mode will show a static 'barcode' image. However, while the presence of lung sliding effectively rules out pneumothorax in the area, the absence of it does not confirm pneumothorax.

[11] A-lines are due to reverberation artefact and are seen as horizontal, equally spaced lines on ultrasound, corresponding to the distance between the parietal pleura and the skin. The presence of A-lines indicates the presence of a pneumothorax. On the other hand, B-lines are hyperechoic vertical lines extending from the pleura downwards. They can be present in normal lungs and the absence of these 'comet-tail artifacts' also supports the likelihood of a pneumothorax being present.

[12] Thoracic CT scans are considered the gold standard for detecting and estimating the size of pneumothoraces. They also allow us to investigate the underlying lung disease in the case of secondary spontaneous pneumothorax, such as any underlying bullae in patients with emphysema as well as any cystic lesions. In cases of trauma, patients may not be able to sit upright for a chest X-ray, increasing the risk of missing pneumothoraces. These patients may require mechanical ventilation and it is important to identify and manage any pneumothoraces, as the positive pressure can predispose a simple pneumothorax to develop into a tension pneumothorax.

Management

The management of pneumothoraces depends on their size and whether there is any evidence of cardiovascular compromise, as well as any history of lung disease.

Immediate

This patient's pneumothorax is **large** [1] and therefore, not suitable to be **managed conservatively** [2]. As he is **stable** [3], he should undergo **simple aspiration** [4] of the pneumothorax. If patients are unstable or fail to improve with simple aspiration, they should have a **thoracostomy via a chest tube** [5] and attached to an **underwater seal** [6]. If urgent chest tube thoracostomy is delayed, they should have **needle decompression** [7] of the pleural space.

Short-term

Patients with chest drains are usually admitted to hospital for observation and monitoring. The drain is monitored to check for **'bubbling'** [8] and **'swinging'** [9]. Once all the air is expelled and the lung is re-expanded, these patients can be safely discharged home with instructions to **desist from flying for 1–2 weeks** [10] and to never go **deep sea diving** [11]. These patients should also be advised to **cease smoking** [12].

Long-term

Patients with a primary spontaneous pneumothorax have a **significant risk of recurrence** [13]. Patients with recurrent pneumothoraces should have a **definitive procedure** [14] to prevent further recurrences. The most common procedure performed would be a **video-assisted thoracic surgery (VATS)** [15], but certain patients may have a **chemical pleurodesis** [16].

---

[1] A pneumothorax is considered small if there is <2cm visible rim of air between the chest wall and the lung rim on a chest X-ray at the hilum and it occupies less than half of the hemithorax. These patients are usually not breathless and if stable, are managed conservatively with high-flow oxygen. A large pneumothorax has >2cm rim of air between the chest wall and the lung rim visible on chest X-ray at the level of the hilum and occupies more than half of the affected hemithorax.

[2] These patients are usually observed for around 6 hours with a repeat chest X-ray. If the repeat chest X-ray shows improvement or does not show progression of the pneumothorax and the patient remains stable, then these patients can be discharged home with instructions to return to the ED if they have worsening chest pain or breathlessness. These patients should be reviewed in a few weeks with a repeat chest X-ray. Conservatively managed, small pneumothoraces tend to resolve over the next 3–6 weeks and these patients should be followed up with a repeat chest X-ray to ensure that the pneumothorax is continuing to resolve. If the pneumothorax is still present, these patients may require a procedure to resolve it.

[3] A patient is considered stable if they are normotensive, have a normal heart rate and respiratory rate and have oxygen saturations >90%.

[4] A large pneumothorax would take significant time to resolve if managed conservatively and have increased risks of complications to the collapsed lung, such as infection. Aspiration is a relatively straightforward procedure that helps remove air from the pleural space and allows for the lung to re-expand. Simple aspiration is done using a needle (~18G) attached to a catheter and a three-way stopcock into the chest – usually at the 4th or 5th intercostal space on the anterior axillary or mid-axillary line. Once in the pleural space, the catheter should be advanced and the needle should be withdrawn. The air can then be aspirated using a 50ml syringe up to a total of 2.5L or until resistance is felt (which demonstrates re-expansion of the lung). Once the appropriate amount of air has been withdrawn, patients should have a chest X-ray to ensure reduction of the pneumothorax and rule out any other complications of the chest drain insertion. If the procedure is successful, the patient can be discharged for follow-up as per the management for small pneumothoraces.

[5] Chest drain insertion is the primary management for unstable patients with pneumothoraces. It can be a painful procedure so patients can be given pre-procedural analgesia. The procedure is done using an aseptic technique to minimise infection risk. Local anaesthetic is initially injected to reduce pain. The choice of insertion site is dependent on the doctor, but a common location is the 4th or 5th intercostal space in the anterior axillary or mid-axillary line. For simple spontaneous pneumothoraces, an 8–14Fr small-bore catheter is adequate. There are two possible techniques for the insertion of chest drains. The standard technique involves making a small incision in the skin and using a clamp to

bluntly dissect to create a tunnel into the subcostal space; a chest drain is then inserted. The other option is to use the Seldinger technique by inserting an introducer needle first, then inserting a guidewire and dilating through to the pleural space before passing the chest drain in and removing the guidewire and dilator. Whichever method is used, the drain must be secured at the skin using sutures and dressings. The patient should then have a CXR to confirm tube position.

6 The underwater seal acts as a one-way valve system that allows air to leave the chest, but not re-enter. This is because when the patient breathes out, the intrathoracic pressure rises above the atmospheric pressure and air is released through the tube. However, when the patient breathes in, despite intrathoracic pressure decreasing, the water in the tube stops air from re-entering the pleural space. It is also essential that the underwater seal of the chest drain is placed below the level of the chest to prevent water from rising up the drain into the pleural space.

7 An emergency needle decompression is performed using a long 10–14G needle inserted above the rib at the 2nd intercostal space in the mid-clavicular line. In an emergency situation, this can be done prior to any imaging. The length of the needle required is dependent on the body habitus of the patient, but it should ideally be at least >4.5cm. While an emergency needle decompression can stabilise the patient, these patients should still have a thoracostomy chest drain inserted for ongoing management. While needle decompression is often a life-saving procedure, it is important to remember that it is associated with potential complications such as bleeding and causing a pneumothorax.

8 Bubbling of the drain indicates that air is continuing to leak out of the pneumothorax into the drain. Usually, this would occur over the first 24 hours and should stop once the lung is expanded. If there is no further air leak and the lung is fully expanded on chest X-ray, the chest drain can be clamped for 6–12 hours with a repeat chest X-ray to assess for recurrence of the pneumothorax. If there is no further recurrence, then the drain can be removed and the patient can be discharged home. There is a small risk of a potential tension pneumothorax as a result of clamping the chest drain and if patients develop signs of haemodynamic instability, the chest drain should be unclamped urgently. If there is recurrence of the pneumothorax when the drain is clamped, then it should be unclamped and patients should continue to be monitored, with consideration for suctioning. A prolonged air leak occurs when the chest drain continues to bubble for more than 5 days. These patients will likely require a definitive procedure such as a blebectomy or pleurodesis.

9 Swinging occurs when the water level rises with inspiration and falls with expiration as a result of a change in intrathoracic pressure. If the drain is swinging, it is likely to be in the correct position. However, a drain that is not swinging is likely to be displaced or blocked, and patients should have a chest X-ray to confirm the position.

10 The atmospheric pressure is lower during flying and this means that any pneumothoraces that are not fully healed prior to flying have a risk of expanding. This can result in a tension pneumothorax. The optimal time period to avoid flying is not clear, but recommendations range from 1–3 weeks.

11 Similar to flying, there are significant changes to atmospheric pressure when deep sea diving, with atmospheric pressure increasing as the diver descends. Patients with pneumothoraces are at increased risk of recurrence due to the likely presence of other blebs and bullae, and the change in atmospheric pressure leads to a risk of expansion and further rupture of these blebs, causing a recurrence of the pneumothorax. Additionally, as the diver ascends, the pneumothorax will expand (as the atmospheric pressure reduces), leading to a risk of a tension pneumothorax.

12 Smoking is associated with an increased risk of pneumothorax recurrence, in addition to its numerous other harmful health effects. Therefore, patients should be counselled and encouraged to quit smoking.

13 The reported risk of recurrence varies across studies and is likely determined by a number of patient factors and severity of initial pneumothorax. Nevertheless, the overall recurrence risk is 30–60% for these patients.

14 In addition to recurrence of a primary spontaneous pneumothorax, other indications for a definitive procedure include prolonged air leak, patients who participate in a high risk occupation or hobbies, such as pilots or divers, and individuals who have another reason to have thoracoscopy.

15 Video-assisted thoracic surgery (VATS) has largely replaced open thoracotomy for the management of spontaneous pneumothorax. While open thoracotomy is associated with reduced rate of recurrence, it is also associated with increased rates of complications such as bleeding and pain. Patients with pneumothoraces can have pleurodesis during VATS and/or have closure of the bleb or bulla, with the decision usually being based on the surgeon's practice. The pleurodesis is often performed with mechanical abrasion using dry gauze, but could be performed with talc, particularly in high risk patients.

16 Chemical pleurodesis is usually only performed on patients who are not able to undergo a VATS procedure, as it is associated with higher risk of recurrence. These patients have a chemical irritant injected into the pleural space. Chemical irritants that can be used include talc and tetracyclines.

CASE 91: ANCA-associated vasculitis

History

- A **65-year-old** [1] man presents with a **rash** [2] over his lower limbs appearing as **reddish / purplish spots** [3] .
- He has been feeling unwell for **1–2 months** [4] and has more recently developed **arthralgias** [5] and **a dry cough** [6] .
- He denies any **haemoptysis** [7] but has had some **sinusitis and blood-stained nasal discharge** [8] .

- He denies any other **cardiac or respiratory symptoms** [9] , **gastrointestinal symptoms** [10] or any **neurological** [11] or **ocular** [12] changes.
- He has no history of **other health problems** [13] including no previous **asthma or atopy** [14] and does not take any **regular medications** [15] .

1 ANCA are antineutrophil cytoplasmic antibodies. ANCA-associated vasculitides are rare diseases but important to recognise due to their potential for irreversible organ damage and death, that may be preventable with early detection and initiation of appropriate treatment. Granulomatosis with polyangiitis (GPA; previously known as Wegener's granulomatosis) most commonly affects middle-aged to older people, while eosinophilic granulomatosis with polyangiitis (EGPA; previously known as Churg–Strauss syndrome) is more common in men in their younger to middle-aged years. Microscopic polyangiitis (MPA) is the rarest of the ANCA-associated vasculitides and has a peak incidence between the ages of 30 and 50.

2 Cutaneous manifestations are common in many forms of vasculitis. Palpable purpura is the hallmark of small vessel vasculitides (such as ANCA-associated vasculitis, Henoch–Schönlein purpura, cryoglobulinaemic vasculitis and hypersensitivity vasculitis), while medium vessel vasculitides (such as polyarteritis nodosum) are more typically associated with nodular lesions or livedo reticularis. Large vessel vasculitides (such as giant cell arteritis and Takayasu arteritis) infrequently cause cutaneous features.

3 Inflammation and bleeding of the small cutaneous blood vessels produces raised, red or purple spots which are non-blanching (i.e. do not disappear with pressure). These lesions can coalesce and can be complicated by skin breakdown and ulcer formation in more severe cases. While this appearance is characteristic for small vessel vasculitis it does not differentiate between the broad range of potential causes.

4 Constitutional symptoms such as fever, malaise, anorexia and weight loss are common (albeit non-specific) and may precede symptoms of specific organ involvement by weeks to months.

5 Arthralgias and arthritis occur in up to two-thirds of patients with ANCA-associated vasculitis. They may be migratory in nature and are generally not associated with erosions.

6 Pulmonary involvement is common in ANCA-associated vasculitis, and manifestations range from nodules or cavitating lesions which may be fairly asymptomatic, to diffuse infiltrates or alveolar haemorrhage which tend to present acutely and can result in respiratory failure.

7 It is important to enquire about a history of haemoptysis as this may be an indicator of pulmonary haemorrhage. This is a severe manifestation of ANCA-associated vasculitis with high mortality rates and necessitates urgent treatment.

8 Upper airway involvement is one of the characteristic features of GPA and occurs in over 70% with this form of ANCA-associated vasculitis. Sinusitis with nasal obstruction, discharge or epistaxis are common features. Cartilaginous inflammation affecting the nose, ears and upper airways is also a significant feature. Such involvement is associated with a risk of cartilage erosion and destruction, resulting in complications such as subglottic stenosis, nasal septal perforation and saddle nose deformity.

9 Enquire about symptoms such as chest pain, palpitations and dyspnoea in addition to gathering information about cough and haemoptysis. These may be indicators of other disease features such as serositis, or cardiac involvement. EGPA in particular has a predilection for cardiac muscle and may result in an eosinophilic cardiomyopathy.

10 GI symptoms are less common in ANCA-associated vasculitis, although EGPA can be associated with an eosinophilic gastroenteritis. GI involvement tends to be more prominent in other forms of vasculitis such as polyarteritis nodosum and Henoch–Schönlein purpura. Abdominal pain related to mesenteric vasculitis typically presents as pain that is worse after eating and can be associated with GI bleeding.

11 Neurological involvement is most commonly a peripheral neuropathy or mononeuritis multiplex (including involvement of cranial nerves). Cerebral vasculitis is reported but is a rare occurrence.

12 Ocular manifestations of ANCA-associated vasculitis (particularly GPA) include episcleritis, conjunctivitis, uveitis and retinal vasculitis. Patients can also develop an inflammatory retro-orbital pseudo-tumour which can cause proptosis and extra-ocular muscle dysfunction. It is therefore important to screen for symptoms such as red eye, ocular pain, diplopia and reduced visual acuity as part of the clinical assessment.

13 In a patient presenting with symptoms suggestive of vasculitis, such as a vasculitic rash, a broad range of possible differential diagnoses need to be considered. Broadly these can be separated into primary vasculitides (generally classified according to vessel size – large, medium and small vessel vasculitides) and those occurring secondary to another medical condition. The most common causes of secondary vasculitis are infections, malignancy, autoimmune disease and drugs. Symptoms, signs and risk factors for possible underlying secondary causes should be explored as part of the clinical assessment and initial investigations.

14 EGPA is a form of ANCA-associated vasculitis linked with atopic disease, in particular asthma, allergic rhinitis or sinusitis. Commonly these conditions predate the vasculitic phase of the illness.

15 A multitude of medications have been associated with secondary vasculitis, including vasculitis with a positive ANCA test. These drugs include certain antibiotics (e.g. ciprofloxacin and minocycline), uric acid-lowering drugs (e.g. allopurinol) and antithyroid drugs (e.g. propylthiouracil). Illicit drugs and chemicals used in their preparation can also trigger vasculitis. Onset of symptoms in relation to any new medications or drug use should therefore be explored.

Examination

- The patient is **afebrile** [1] and has normal **haemodynamic** [2] and **respiratory** [3] vital signs.
- There is a **palpable** [4] **purpuric rash** [5] over the lower limbs extending to the knees.
- There are no other **skin lesions** [6] and no **splinter haemorrhages** [7].
- Mild **pitting oedema** [8] to the mid-shins is apparent.
- There is no appreciable **synovitis** [9] clinically.

- Examination of the **eyes, ears, nose and throat** [10] reveals some **paranasal sinus tenderness** [11].
- The **chest is clear** [12] to auscultate and there are no **murmurs** [13].
- There is no **lymphadenopathy or hepatosplenomegaly** [14].
- **Neurological exam** [15] is normal.

1 A fever may be a feature of active ANCA-associated vasculitis, but is not universal and should also prompt consideration of other differential diagnoses that can be associated with secondary vasculitis, such as infection and haematological malignancy.

2 Take seriously any abnormalities of heart rate or blood pressure, as these may be an indicator of cardiac or renal involvement, or significant blood loss (e.g. pulmonary haemorrhage), which may not initially present with overt symptoms, but can be associated with rapid clinical deterioration.

3 In the context of ANCA-associated vasculitis, increased respiratory rate and/or a reduction in oxygen saturation should prompt immediate consideration of pulmonary haemorrhage, which requires urgent confirmation and treatment. These patients should undergo chest imaging and be closely monitored for deterioration.

4 Purpura that can be felt is known as 'palpable purpura' and occurs due to the inflammation of blood vessels that defines a vasculitic process.

5 Purpura refers to the skin or mucosal discolouration arising from bleeding from small blood vessels and has a distinctive appearance. Petechiae are small purpuric lesions up to 2mm across. Other than vasculitis, purpura can also be found in platelet and coagulation disorders, which should be checked for on a full blood count (± blood film) and coagulation studies.

6 While purpura is the most common skin manifestation of ANCA-associated vasculitis, other lesions can also occur, including urticarial and nodular rashes, or occasionally erythema nodosum, pyoderma gangrenosum or neutrophilic dermatoses. These generally have fairly distinctive appearances and may be confirmed on skin biopsy.

7 Splinter haemorrhages are traditionally associated with infective endocarditis but may also be a feature of a primary vasculitic process due to micro-embolic phenomena or immune-mediated injury to vessel walls.

8 Peripheral oedema should prompt consideration of possible renal involvement with glomerulonephritis and renal vasculitis. In such cases proteinuria and hypoalbuminaemia can result in oedema. Most often, however, renal disease is clinically silent in the early stages and therefore requires screening of blood and urine to detect abnormalities.

9 Clinical signs of synovitis such as joint line tenderness, effusions and bogginess may be present in patients who have an inflammatory arthritis as a manifestation of their ANCA-associated vasculitis.

10 Numerous abnormalities of the eyes, sinuses and upper airways can occur in ANCA-associated vasculitis. While a screening examination may detect gross abnormalities such as changes in visual acuity or nasal septal deviation, patients with symptoms in these domains should be referred to ENT or Ophthalmology for formal review.

11 Tenderness to palpation over the frontal and maxillary sinuses is a simple but fairly crude means of assessing for sinusitis. Endoscopic assessment and imaging (usually with CT) provide more detailed assessment and should be performed if suspected.

12 Abnormalities on auscultation such as crackles or reduced air entry should be followed up with chest imaging to detect abnormalities such as pulmonary infiltrates, alveolar haemorrhage or pleural effusions (resulting from serositis).

13 The presence of a new murmur should prompt consideration of secondary vasculitis due to infective endocarditis, which can mimic the clinical presentation of ANCA-associated vasculitis and even produce a positive ANCA test in some patients.

14 Lymphadenopathy and hepatosplenomegaly may be indicators of vasculitis occurring secondary to another condition, such as underlying malignancy. Lymphadenopathy may also be a feature of ANCA-associated vasculitis, especially EGPA.

15 Neurological examination is usually targeted to symptoms such as weakness, numbness or paraesthesias identified by the patient, with the aim of characterising any objective neurological signs, localising the likely level of pathology and directing further investigations (e.g. imaging and nerve conduction studies).

Investigations

- A full blood count shows a **haemoglobin of 102g/L** [1] and **normal platelet count** [2].
- The **eosinophil count** [3] is also normal.
- **Coagulation studies** [4] are normal other than an **elevated fibrinogen** [5].
- **Inflammatory markers are markedly elevated** [6] with a CRP of 95 and ESR of 92.
- The **serum creatinine is 95µmol/L** [7] (eGFR of 80ml/min/1.73m²).
- Liver function tests are normal; however, there is a **low albumin of 24g/L** [8].
- A urine dipstick shows **+++ protein and red cells** [9].

- Microscopy reveals **glomerular red cells** [10] and the **protein–creatinine ratio** [11] is **1200mg/g** [12].
- There are no abnormalities on plain **chest X-ray** [13].
- A **'vasculitic screen'** [14] of blood tests is sent, including **infective serology** [15] and a **range of antibodies** [16] including an **ANCA** [17].
- This returns a **positive cANCA** [18] with an **elevated PR3 titre** [19].
- **Anti-GBM antibodies** [20] are negative.
- A renal **biopsy** [21] is performed with findings of a **necrotising** [22] **pauci-immune** [23] **crescentic glomerulonephritis** [24].

1 Anaemia is most commonly due to inflammation in the context of active vasculitis, but should also prompt consideration of bleeding (especially pulmonary haemorrhage), and rarer causes such as haemolysis. A comparison to baseline haemoglobin measures is helpful if available, and consideration should be given to performing haematinics, a haemolysis screen and investigation for occult bleeding.

2 The platelet count may be elevated as an acute phase reactant. A low platelet count in the context of a purpuric rash should prompt consideration of thrombocytopenic purpura.

3 A peripheral eosinophilia is characteristic of EGPA and along with a history of asthma may precede the development

of vasculitis. Eosinophilic infiltration is important in the pathophysiology of EGPA and seen on biopsy of affected organs. Eosinophilia can also occur in other forms of ANCA-associated vasculitis but is usually less pronounced.

4 Coagulation studies are important, to screen for coagulation disorders which can also produce a purpuric-appearing rash.

5 Fibrinogen is an acute phase protein so is commonly elevated in the setting of active inflammatory disease of any aetiology.

6 Inflammatory markers such as CRP and ESR are commonly increased in active ANCA-associated vasculitis and can be used to help monitor response to therapy and assist with the identification of disease flares.

7 Renal involvement in the early stages is commonly asymptomatic and even a creatinine rise may not occur until a significant proportion of kidney function has been impaired. Renal function which deteriorates over hours to days may signify rapidly progressive glomerulonephritis which is the most acute and severe presentation of renal involvement.

8 Hypoalbuminaemia in ANCA-associated vasculitis may occur due to albumin being a negative acute phase reactant, but may also be a feature of renal protein loss.

9 A urine dipstick followed by formal urine assessment should be performed as part of the initial work-up of any patient with suspected vasculitis. Protein and red cells in the urine should flag the possibility of renal involvement.

10 Formal urine microscopy and red cell morphology should be performed to characterise haematuria. Dysmorphic red cells suggest glomerular origin, while isomorphic red cells are more consistent with lower tract bleeding.

11 Proteinuria can be quantified using the protein–creatinine ratio on a spot urine test. If there is uncertainty a formal 24-hour urine collection for protein can also be performed.

12 Proteinuria in ANCA-associated vasculitis is usually sub-nephrotic. When expressed as mg/g the protein–creatinine ratio approximates the number of grams of protein excreted per day.

13 A chest X-ray should generally be performed as part of the work-up in all patients with suspected ANCA-associated vasculitis. Characteristic changes include multifocal infiltrates or nodules, cavitating lesions or diffuse opacities with alveolar haemorrhage. CT chest is often performed to better characterise any abnormalities.

14 A 'vasculitic screen' refers to a panel of blood tests commonly performed in patients presenting with features of vasculitis, to screen for a range of possible causes. In reality there is no one specific 'set' of tests that should be ordered, but rather investigations should be ordered and interpreted based on the clinical picture and particular differential diagnoses in an individual patient.

15 Investigations for potential secondary infective causes of vasculitis usually include as a minimum blood cultures, hepatitis serology and HIV serology. Screening for chronic viral infections and latent TB is also important due to the risk of reactivation with immunosuppression used to treat ANCA-associated vasculitis.

16 Antibodies such as an ANA, double-stranded DNA, rheumatoid factor and ANCA are often ordered; however, they need to be interpreted with caution. All antibody tests are subject to false positives, and results should be interpreted in conjunction with the history, examination and other investigation results.

17 A positive ANCA refers to the detection of antibodies directed against antigens present within primary granules of neutrophils and monocytes. They can be detected using immunofluorescence, or specific ANCAs can be measured using enzyme-linked immunosorbent assay (ELISA). Confusingly, a small proportion of patients with ANCA-associated vasculitis may be ANCA-negative.

18 Immunofluorescence may form a cytoplasmic staining pattern (c-ANCA) which corresponds with a positive PR3 titre on ELISA, or a perinuclear staining pattern (p-ANCA) which corresponds to a positive MPO titre on ELISA. Sometimes one of the immunofluorescence or ELISA tests may be positive in isolation. In general, the ELISA is considered to be more specific.

19 Confirmation of the presence and titre of either PR3 or MPO has specific disease associations. Positive PR3 (c-ANCA) is most commonly associated with GPA (positive in 80–90% of cases). Positive MPO (p-ANCA), however, is more common in EGPA and MPA. Both types of ANCA, however, can be positive in all forms of ANCA-associated vasculitis, so these associations are not definitive.

20 Antibodies against the glomerular basement membrane (anti-GBM) is a feature of Goodpasture's syndrome, which like ANCA-associated vasculitis can produce a pulmonary-renal syndrome. Some patients have both ANCA and anti-GBM positivity and these patients often have aggressive disease with poorer prognosis.

21 Biopsy forms the cornerstone of diagnosis of ANCA-associated vasculitis and should be pursued in the majority of cases. Common sources of tissue from affected organs that can yield diagnostic results include the lung, kidney and sinuses. Necrotising granulomatous inflammation is the hallmark pathological feature of GPA. Pathological changes in EGPA also classically show a necrotising granulomatous vasculitis, with additional eosinophilic tissue infiltration. Granulomas are typically absent in MPA, which may distinguish it on biopsy from other forms of ANCA-associated vasculitis.

22 Glomerular inflammation with necrotising lesions is typical of ANCA-associated vasculitis. The acute lesion targets the glomeruli and other vessels in the kidney, with vessel wall necrosis resulting in activation of coagulation pathways and formation of fibrin within the necrotic areas. Granulomas are not commonly seen in the kidneys.

23 ANCA-associated vasculitis is distinguished on immunofluorescence by the absence of immunoglobulin staining, hence the term 'pauci-immune', in contrast to other forms of small vessel vasculitis where immune complex deposition is a key feature (such as IgA deposition in Henoch–Schönlein purpura).

24 Crescent formation accompanying necrotising lesions is common in ANCA-associated vasculitis. Crescents form due to proliferation of epithelial cells and monocytes along with capillary wall rupture and fibrin deposition in Bowman's space.

Management

Short-term

Confirm **organ involvement** [1] and await the results of **diagnostic investigations** [2]. Start treatment based on the **clinical urgency** [3]. Commence **high dose steroids** [4]. Involve **relevant specialties** [5] including Rheumatology, ENT and Nephrology. Complete **induction immunosuppression** [6] with combination of steroids and either **cyclophosphamide** [7] or **rituximab** [8] and monitor for **response** [9] and **treatment side-effects** [10]. Aim for **complete remission** [11] and switch to **maintenance therapy** [12] along with **weaning of the steroid dose** [13].

Long-term

Continue to **reduce immunosuppression** [14] and monitor for **disease relapse** [15] and longer-term **complications of the disease and its treatment** [16].

[1] Vasculitis is often multisystem and can target different organs in different patients. Some involved systems are readily clinically apparent due to symptoms and signs, while others are only detected on investigation. Identifying which organs are involved and the severity guides the urgency and aggression of treatment.

[2] The other major goal of investigation is to identify a diagnosis for the vasculitic process. Establishing the diagnosis is not always straightforward and the clinical picture, test results and response to therapy may all form part of the diagnostic assessment.

[3] Often investigations (e.g. antibodies, biopsy results) take time to return. It may be necessary therefore to commence treatment based on suspicion of the diagnosis prior to confirmation. This is especially the case where organ or life-threatening manifestations are present, and treatment may begin concurrently with the diagnostic work-up.

[4] Immunosuppression is the mainstay of therapy for ANCA-associated vasculitis, with high dose prednisolone (sometimes IV pulse methylprednisolone) used initially to achieve rapid disease control. As with other patients receiving high dose steroids, they should be monitored for hyperglycaemia, screened for latent infection, have their bone health assessed and be commenced on co-trimoxazole for pneumocystis prophylaxis.

[5] Multisystem conditions such as vasculitis often require a multidisciplinary approach to assessment and management. Generally, a rheumatologist is involved in managing patients with multi-organ disease in conjunction with other specialists depending on predominant manifestations, such as renal, respiratory, ENT and ophthalmology.

[6] Immunosuppressive therapy in ANCA-associated vasculitis is divided into induction and maintenance phases. Induction immunosuppression is designed to achieve initial remission. In addition to steroids, the most common agents used for induction are cyclophosphamide or rituximab. Plasma exchange is also added to medical therapy in select cases with poor prognostic factors. Milder disease forms without organ-threatening involvement may be treated with less aggressive immunosuppression.

[7] Cyclophosphamide is an alkylating agent which can be used either intravenously (generally preferred) or orally. Prescription should be by a specialised unit experienced with cyclophosphamide. Early side-effects include nausea, bone marrow suppression, infection and haemorrhagic cystitis. Late side-effects may include bladder cancer and gonadal toxicity resulting in reduced fertility.

[8] Rituximab is a chimeric anti-CD20 monoclonal antibody which is likely to be as effective as cyclophosphamide in inducing remission in ANCA-associated vasculitis. It causes rapid B-cell depletion which usually lasts 6–12 months.

[9] Response is usually seen within a few days of commencing therapy and can be monitored based on the patient's clinical features, biochemical markers and improved imaging parameters. The ANCA titre may reduce or become undetectable in patients who have had a good response to induction immunosuppression.

[10] Inform the patient and treating doctors of potential side-effects of therapy. This includes the broad range of steroid-associated side-effects, the risk of infection, infusion reactions and complications specific to cyclophosphamide, as detailed above.

[11] Remission is achieved in around 90% with initial treatment, although relapses are not infrequent. An incomplete response may require a longer course or alternative therapy. Persistent abnormalities require differentiation between active vasculitis and irreversible damage that has been sustained.

[12] When the patient has achieved remission and completed induction therapy they are typically switched to maintenance therapy. Options include azathioprine, methotrexate, rituximab and mycophenolate (less effective). Choice depends on disease severity, side-effect profile, contraindications and access/cost.

13 Steroids are generally continued for many months, but the dose gradually tapered.

14 Maintenance therapy is usually continued for at least 12–18 months. If remission is sustained, then consideration can be given to weaning immunosuppression completely. In patients with recurrent relapses, lifelong maintenance therapy may be appropriate.

15 Relapse can occur at any time and is more common in those who are PR3 positive and have lung or upper respiratory tract involvement. A rising ANCA titre may also be a sign of impending relapse but is not a completely reliable disease marker. Treatment of relapses depends on severity and may range from an increase in steroid dose and maintenance immunosuppression to complete re-induction therapy.

16 Disease-related complications requiring long-term management vary depending on affected organs and may include renal impairment, nasal deformity, subglottic stenosis, neurological damage and respiratory insufficiency. Complications of treatment are common, and in the long term, attention to infection risk, malignancy screening (e.g. bladder cancer screening for those with previous cyclophosphamide exposure), bone health and cardiovascular risk are an essential part of management.

CASE 92: Ankylosing spondylitis

History

- A **26-year-old male** [1] presents with **low back pain** [2] which has gradually worsened since his **early twenties** [3].
- The pain is severe **first thing in the morning** [4] and associated with **significant stiffness** [5] which **improves with movement** [6] as the day progresses.
- He does not have any **neck pain** [7].
- He has also developed left-sided **groin pain** [8] over the last few months, without any other **peripheral joint** [9] symptoms.

- He has had episodes of **plantar fasciitis** [10] in the past.
- He does not report any **constitutional symptoms** [11].
- He has never had **psoriasis** [12], **bowel dysfunction** [13] or **inflammatory eye disease** [14].
- On enquiry about **family history** [15], he recalls an uncle with back problems that resulted in a **stooped posture** [16].

[1] Ankylosing spondylitis has a peak age of onset between the ages of 20 and 30, and males are significantly more likely to be affected compared with females.

[2] Back pain is the most common symptom of ankylosing spondylitis and can localise to the low back, buttocks and posterior thighs. Alternating buttock pain may be a specific feature suggestive of inflammatory back pain.

[3] The onset of symptoms in ankylosing spondylitis is often insidious, and delayed diagnosis is unfortunately quite common. It is not unusual for years to have passed between symptom onset and eventual diagnosis.

[4] Pain often occurs overnight (and may wake patients up) and is characteristically worst first thing in the morning or after periods of prolonged rest.

[5] Associated spinal stiffness, especially in the morning, is also commonly reported in patients with ankylosing spondylitis. Stiffness which improves with movement should be differentiated from the fixed limitations in spinal mobility that occur because of irreversible bony changes such as ankylosis (fusion of bone).

[6] This description is consistent with an inflammatory (in contrast to mechanical) pattern of pain. Inflammatory back pain is a key symptom that points towards possible ankylosing spondylitis. A high degree of suspicion for ankylosing spondylitis is appropriate in young patients (age of onset <40) who have chronic back pain (duration >3 months) with an inflammatory quality (pain after rest which improves with exercise).

[7] All levels of the axial spine can be affected by ankylosing spondylitis – the usual pattern is of initial sacroiliac and lower

spine involvement which progresses cranially as the disease advances.

[8] Groin pain should raise suspicion of hip disease in ankylosing spondylitis. The hips are the most common peripheral joint involved in ankylosing spondylitis (occurring in around 30% of patients).

[9] Peripheral joint involvement occurs in up to half of patients with ankylosing spondylitis and an asymmetric large joint oligoarthritis (e.g. hips, shoulders, knee, ankles) is characteristic. In a proportion of patients (around 20%), peripheral joint symptoms may precede the onset of axial symptoms.

[10] Ankylosing spondylitis and other spondyloarthropathies are associated with enthesitis, which refers to inflammation at the site of tendon, ligament, fascia or joint capsule insertion into bone. Enthesitis affecting the plantar fascia can occur at its insertion into the calcaneum or metatarsals. A common presentation of plantar fasciitis is sharp pain in the heel upon stepping/walking after a period of rest (e.g. first thing in the morning).

[11] Systemic symptoms such as fever, sweats and weight loss are red flag symptoms in patients with back pain. While such symptoms can potentially be attributed to inflammatory back pain, they should prompt exclusion of other not-to-be-missed diagnoses such as infection, malignancy and fracture. This is particularly the case if symptoms occur in an older age group or in patients with relevant risk factors.

[12] Ankylosing spondylitis belongs to a broader group of conditions known collectively as spondyloarthropathies. The other diseases classified under the umbrella term of spondyloarthritis are psoriatic arthritis, IBD-associated

arthritis and reactive arthritis. Spondyloarthritis can also be divided into axial (involving the spine and sacroiliac joints) or peripheral (involving peripheral joints) or both. There is significant overlap between these conditions and shared clinical features including enthesitis, dactylitis, uveitis, psoriasis and subclinical bowel inflammation. Symptoms and signs suggestive of these associated conditions should be sought as part of the assessment of a patient with a suspected spondyloarthropathy.

13 Enquire about symptoms such as abdominal pain, diarrhoea and blood/mucus in the stool which may indicate IBD, which is comorbid in around 5–10% of patients with ankylosing spondylitis. Asymptomatic intestinal ulcerations and colonic inflammation are present in a much higher proportion of patients, reflecting their overlapping pathophysiological basis.

14 Uveitis is the most common extra-articular manifestation associated with ankylosing spondylitis. Typically, uveitis is anterior, unilateral and recurrent and its presence and activity does not correlate with articular disease. Symptoms include pain, redness and visual impairment, and require prompt assessment by an ophthalmologist and treatment with topical and systemic therapies.

15 Familial clustering is seen with spondyloarthropathies due to a strong genetic component contributing to disease development. The most commonly recognised genetic association is HLA-B27.

16 Untreated, ankylosing spondylitis may lead to progressive bony changes that restrict spinal mobility and produce loss of the lumbar lordosis, pronounced thoracic kyphosis and fixed flexion of the cervical spine, resulting in a stooped posture.

Examination

- On **inspection** [1] of the back there are **no obvious abnormalities** [2].
- There is no **midline tenderness** [3] or **sacroiliac joint tenderness** [4].
- The patient has normal **cervical spine** [5] movement and **occiput to wall distance** [6] is 0cm.
- **Thoracic rotation** [7] is normal, and his **chest expansion** [8] is 6cm.
- Lumbar spine **lateral flexion is reduced** [9].

- A **modified Schober's test** [10] is **4cm** [11].
- There is **discomfort on left hip movement** [12] at the extremes of motion, but other peripheral joints examine normally.
- There is no **heel tenderness** [13], **dactylitis** [14] or **psoriatic skin or nail changes** [15].
- **Lower limb neurological exam** [16] is normal.
- There are **no murmurs** [17] or **crackles** [18] on auscultation of the heart and lungs.

1 Examination of the back follows the same framework of inspection, palpation, movement and special tests that applies to joint examination in general.

2 The pathognomonic postural changes and spinal deformity associated with ankylosing spondylitis are advanced features. Ideally, the diagnosis is made well prior to these changes being evident on examination.

3 Assess for bony tenderness along the length of the spine. Severe focal spinal tenderness is not typical of ankylosing spondylitis and should prompt consideration of fracture, spondylodiscitis or malignancy, particularly if other 'red flag' features are present.

4 There are a number of techniques to assess for sacroiliac joint tenderness, including by compression of the pelvis or by applying pressure through a flexed knee with the hip abducted and externally rotated. While these may generate sacroiliac joint pain in patients with sacroiliitis, these tests are poorly sensitive.

5 Test cervical spine movements including extension (lost early in ankylosing spondylitis), flexion (typically more preserved), lateral flexion and rotation. Pain, stiffness and

reduced range of motion may be a feature of both active spinal inflammation and/or secondary bony changes resulting in restricted movement.

6 The occiput to wall test is commonly performed to assess progression of disease, as it reflects loss of lumbar and cervical lordosis with increasing thoracic kyphosis. The patient stands with their back and heels against the wall and the horizontal distance is measured from the occiput to the wall with the patient facing straight ahead.

7 Perform thoracic rotation, ensuring the pelvis is stabilised so rotation is occurring through the thoracic portion of the spine.

8 Chest expansion measures the range of the costovertebral joints and is usually measured at the level of the xiphoid. Normal chest expansion is >5cm.

9 Assess lateral flexion of the lumbar spine, ensuring the patient does not lean forwards. The distance bent is normally >10cm (with the tips of the fingers reaching the distal knee crease) and tends to be lost early in ankylosing spondylitis.

10 The modified Schober's test assesses the degree of lumbar flexion. The patient stands with their feet together and the point of the lumbosacral junction is identified (between the posterior superior iliac spines) along with a point 10cm above the lumbosacral junction. The patient bends forward maximally without bending the knees and the increase between the two points is measured.

11 A normal Schober's test is >5cm. A distance of 4cm is considered a mild reduction and <2cm is considered severe.

12 This may be in keeping with hip joint involvement as part of this patient's ankylosing spondylitis. Hip disease is important to identify because it is associated with higher degrees of disability and worse prognosis overall.

13 The enthesis is a key target of inflammation in patients with spondyloarthritis. Enthesitis can be diagnosed clinically due to tenderness or swelling at the site of bony insertion, and can also be confirmed on imaging such as ultrasound or MRI. Heel tenderness can occur at the insertion of either the Achilles tendon or plantar fascia into the calcaneus. Other sites of enthesitis include the quadriceps tendon and infrapatellar ligament insertions into the patella, common flexor and extensor tendon insertions into the humeral epicondyles, supraspinatus insertion into the humeral greater tuberosity, costo-sternal junctions and various muscle insertions into the pelvis.

14 Dactylitis is the 'sausage'-like appearance of a digit due to a combination of soft tissue oedema, tenosynovitis and joint inflammation. Dactylitis occurs in around 10% of patients with ankylosing spondylitis but is most commonly seen in other forms of spondyloarthritis, such as psoriatic arthritis and reactive arthritis.

15 Examine the skin carefully for the presence of psoriasis and examine the nails for pitting or ridging. Common sites of skin psoriasis are the umbilicus, gluteal cleft, elbow/knees, behind the ears and scalp. The presence of psoriasis may suggest a diagnosis of psoriatic arthritis which can present variably. The most common presentation is of an asymmetric oligoarthritis (often with dactylitis). Other presentations may include a symmetrical polyarthritis mimicking rheumatoid arthritis, spondylitis with or without peripheral involvement (therefore looking similar to ankylosing spondylitis), predominant DIPJ involvement or arthritis mutilans (a destructive form of arthritis resulting in deformity and osteolysis of the digits).

16 Significant neurological complications, such as cauda equina syndrome or cord impingement, can occur with advanced disease.

17 Ankylosing spondylitis can be associated with cardiovascular manifestations such as aortitis and aortic valve disease (especially regurgitation). Extension of this inflammatory process and subsequent fibrosis into the interventricular septum can result in conduction abnormalities. These manifestations tend to occur later in the disease course.

18 Pulmonary fibrosis occurs in a small percentage of patients with ankylosing spondylitis and is typically apical. It tends to occur late, is associated with long duration of disease and is usually asymptomatic. Pulmonary involvement in ankylosing spondylitis can also arise due to restrictive lung disease secondary to costovertebral rigidity.

Investigations

- The patient has a normal **full blood count** [1] and **renal function** [2].
- There is **mild elevation of the CRP and ESR** [3] (CRP 25 and ESR 30).
- The patient is **seronegative** [4] but **HLA-B27** [5] is **positive** [6].
- Plain **X-rays** [7] of the **sacroiliac joints** [8] demonstrate **New York criteria** [9] **bilateral Grade 2 sacroiliitis** [10].
- X-rays of the **spine** [11] show **squaring of the vertebral bodies** [12] and occasional **syndesmophytes** [13].
- X-ray of the hips shows mild **concentric joint space narrowing** [14] on the left side.

1 An FBE is often normal in ankylosing spondylitis but can show features consistent with chronic inflammation, such as a normocytic normochromic anaemia.

2 Renal function is usually intact. While there is the textbook-quoted complication of secondary amyloidosis that can affect the kidneys and cause proteinuria due to uncontrolled inflammation in ankylosing spondylitis, this is exceptionally rare. Renal function is most relevant in practice due to the common use of long-term NSAIDs.

3 Markers of inflammation are non-specific and in ankylosing spondylitis they are less consistently elevated compared with other inflammatory rheumatic diseases. Only around half of patients have significant CRP or ESR elevation with active disease, so the absence of raised inflammatory markers should not negate a story suggestive of inflammatory back pain. Patients who have concomitant peripheral arthritis are more likely to have raised inflammatory markers.

4 'Seronegative' refers to the absence of antibodies associated with other forms of inflammatory arthritis such as rheumatoid factor and anti-CCP. Seronegativity is typical of the spondyloarthropathies.

5 HLA-B27 positivity is strongly associated with ankylosing spondylitis. It is an allele of the MHC Class I molecule which is responsible for antigen presentation to CD8 T cells. The exact role of HLA-B27 in the pathophysiology of ankylosing spondylitis and other forms of spondyloarthritis is not fully understood.

6 A positive HLA-B27 is a useful but non-diagnostic test in the work-up of someone with a suspected spondyloarthropathy. HLA-B27 is positive in 95% of patients with ankylosing spondylitis and in 50–75% of patients with other forms of spondyloarthritis. The presence of HLA-B27 confers a 5–8% risk of ankylosing spondylitis in that individual, which increases to 20% if a first-degree relative is affected. However, the population rates of HLA-B27 are around 8–12% in Caucasians (lower in Asians and African-Americans) and therefore the vast majority of patients with HLA-B27 do not go on to develop a spondyloarthropathy. A positive result therefore has to be interpreted in the context of the clinical picture and other investigation results.

7 Plain X-rays are the first-line imaging of patients with suspected ankylosing spondylitis, looking for characteristic changes of the sacroiliac joints and vertebral bodies. However, it can take years before typical radiographic changes occur. MRI is increasingly used in patients who do not have radiographic changes but a suggestive history for inflammatory back pain. MRI is more sensitive for inflammatory changes which include active inflammatory lesions (e.g. bone marrow oedema, synovitis) and chronic changes (e.g. sclerosis, erosions). Patients with MRI (but not radiographic) changes and symptoms suggestive of ankylosing spondylitis are labelled non-radiographic axial spondyloarthritis, which is treated along a similar pathway to those with ankylosing spondylitis.

8 For the best views, X-rays specifically assessing the sacroiliac joints should be requested. Features of sacroiliitis progress from sclerosis and erosions or irregularity of the joint margins to the more advanced changes of joint space narrowing and ankylosis.

9 The New York criteria are used to grade sacroiliitis changes on X-ray. Grade 0 is normal appearance of the sacroiliac joints, Grade 1 is suspicious changes with some blurring of the joint margins, Grade 2 is minimal sclerosis with some erosions, Grade 3 is definite sclerosis and more severe erosions with or without partial ankylosis, and Grade 4 is complete ankylosis of the joint.

10 The presence of definite radiographic sacroiliitis (defined as bilateral Grade 2 or unilateral Grade 3 or 4 changes) along with inflammatory back pain is considered diagnostic for ankylosing spondylitis according to original classification criteria. More recently broader definitions of axial spondyloarthropathy have been developed to encompass patients with MRI sacroiliitis (without X-ray changes), or the absence of imaging changes but typical spondyloarthritis features with HLA-B27.

11 Radiographic changes of ankylosing spondylitis affecting the spine are best seen on lateral films of the thoracolumbar spine.

12 Squaring of the vertebral bodies is an early sign in ankylosing spondylitis and occurs due to enthesitis affecting the annulus fibrosus at the corners of the vertebral bodies anteriorly. This causes reactive sclerosis, producing the appearance of 'shiny corners' on imaging, as well as local bone resorption and erosive change affecting the vertebral corners, leading to a squared appearance.

13 Vertebral syndesmophytes are the next radiographic change to develop and tend to first occur around the thoracolumbar junction. Syndesmophytes are vertical projections which eventually join together to form 'flowing' syndesmophytes. In late stages the ascending progression of syndesmophytes joining vertebral bodies, calcification of the anterior longitudinal ligament, loss of lumbar lordosis and ankylosis leads to the characteristic 'bamboo spine' appearance of advanced ankylosing spondylitis.

14 As with other forms of inflammatory arthritis, X-rays may show uniform joint space narrowing of affected peripheral joints. Axial migration of the femoral head and osteophytosis can occur in more advanced stages.

Management

Short-term

Provide **education** [1] about the diagnosis and commence an **exercise programme** [2] which includes **stretching** [3]. Start a **regular NSAID** [4], considering **possible side-effects** [5]. Refer to a **rheumatologist** [6] for consideration of **immunosuppression** [7] such as **TNF-alpha inhibitors** [8] and **IL-17 inhibitors** [9].

Long-term

Continue to monitor **disease activity and progression** [10] and balance the benefits of treatment with **side-effects** [11]. Provide lifestyle advice around **weight maintenance** [12] and assess and manage other **cardiovascular risk factors** [13]. Screen for and manage common **comorbidities** [14] such as **chronic pain** [15], **osteoporosis** [16] and **depression** [17].

[1] Patients should be counselled about the diagnosis and the importance of both non-pharmacological and pharmacological strategies in managing their condition.

[2] There is evidence in ankylosing spondylitis to support strengthening and aerobic exercise programmes including water-based exercises. Activities which focus on core strengthening, such as Pilates and yoga, are also recommended. Patients should be advised against contact or high impact sport, however, especially if they have advanced disease. Cycling may also be less preferable due to the flexed position of the spine.

[3] Patients should be encouraged to undertake a daily stretching programme to maintain spinal flexibility and help manage pain. Many patients will benefit from formal physiotherapy input, particularly in the early stages.

[4] NSAIDs are first-line treatment in ankylosing spondylitis and their symptomatic benefit is well established. Daily therapy (as opposed to PRN use) may also be associated with reduced X-ray progression independent of symptom benefit; however, data is conflicting.

[5] Consider potential risks of long-term NSAID use, including renal, GI and cardiovascular side-effects, and where appropriate implement risk reduction measures (e.g. prescribing a COX-2 selective NSAID or a concomitant proton pump inhibitor to reduce GI side-effects).

[6] Ankylosing spondylitis usually requires specialist assessment and management in the first instance. The role of the rheumatologist includes diagnosis, particularly when symptoms and/or investigations are less definitive, and escalation of management with access to biologic therapies.

[7] Traditional disease-modifying antirheumatic drugs (DMARDs) do not have efficacy in axial spondyloarthritis. Some agents (in particular sulfasalazine and methotrexate) may be effective for peripheral arthritis if present. Steroids also do not have a prominent role – their use is reserved for severe disease flares or delivered locally to affected joints via intra-articular injection. If patients have persistent axial inflammatory symptoms despite a trial of NSAIDs and physiotherapy, escalation to a biologic is usually indicated.

[8] TNF-alpha inhibitors (e.g. infliximab, adalimumab, etanercept) were the first biologics shown to be effective in ankylosing spondylitis, with a good symptomatic response in around two-thirds of patients. TNF-alpha inhibitors are also thought to retard radiographic progression. They are also effective for peripheral arthritis, dactylitis and enthesitis.

[9] IL-23 activates Th17 cells to produce IL-17, a pro-inflammatory cytokine which has a key role in the synovitis and enthesitis associated with spondyloarthritis. Agents such as secukinumab (an IL-17A monoclonal antibody) have been shown to have comparable responses to TNF-alpha inhibitors in patients with axial spondyloarthritis.

[10] At each clinic visit patients are assessed using a combination of reported symptoms (e.g. pain, stiffness, function), examination findings (e.g. spinal mobility) and inflammatory markers (although these do not typically correlate well with axial disease activity). The activity of peripheral symptoms (synovitis, enthesitis, dactylitis) and extra-articular manifestations (psoriasis, uveitis, IBD) should also be reviewed if part of the patient's clinical picture.

[11] Ankylosing spondylitis tends to affect younger patients who often have fewer medical issues and therefore tolerate treatment well. Side-effects of NSAIDs are well described, and the main risk of biologic therapies is infection. In patients who have had well-controlled disease for a prolonged period, a trial of tapering treatment and close monitoring for relapse may be discussed.

[12] In addition to the well-known general health risks, being overweight or obese in ankylosing spondylitis is associated with higher levels of disease activity, poorer spinal mobility and physical functioning and poorer response to therapy. Patients should be educated about these associations and attempts at weight loss supported.

[13] Patients with ankylosing spondylitis are at increased risk of ischaemic heart disease. In addition to weight management, patients should also have other modifiable risk factors addressed, including smoking cessation, diabetes, blood pressure and lipid management.

14 Screening for commonly associated comorbidities, such as cardiovascular risk factors, osteoporosis and depression, is a key part of the long-term management of patients with ankylosing spondylitis. Many of these comorbidities contribute independently to key patient outcomes such as quality of life, functional capacity and work disability.

15 As with many rheumatological conditions, ankylosing spondylitis can be complicated by development of chronic pain. Factors include difficult to control inflammatory disease, sustained spinal damage resulting in mechanical pain, and comorbid fibromyalgia. Those with chronic pain may benefit from multidisciplinary input including pain psychology, physical therapy and additional analgesic agents.

16 Ankylosing spondylitis is associated with a lifetime risk of fracture of >10% and patients are particularly prone to vertebral fractures. Patients who present with new, different or worsening back pain usually require imaging to exclude a complicating fracture. It should be noted that bone density assessments of the spine are often falsely elevated in patients with ankylosing spondylitis, due to the presence of syndesmophytes.

17 Significantly higher rates of depression are reported among patients with ankylosing spondylitis compared to the general population. Comorbid mental health issues are important to identify, as they can contribute to symptoms such as pain and fatigue, impact overall quality of life and functioning and reduce adherence to therapy.

CASE 93: Giant cell arteritis

History

- A **74-year-old** [1] **Caucasian** [2] **female** [3] presents with a **right-sided headache** [4] that began **3–4 weeks ago** [5] associated with **tenderness of her scalp** [6].
- She has been unusually **fatigued** [7] and also experienced new **pain and stiffness** [8] of the shoulder and neck region [9], particularly **upon waking** [10], but with no **weakness** [11] or symptoms in her **peripheral joints** [12].
- She does not report any **jaw claudication** [13] or **visual symptoms** [14]. She has a past history of **type 2 diabetes and hypertension** [15].

[1] Giant cell arteritis (GCA), also known as temporal arteritis, is a disease of the elderly, with a mean age of diagnosis of 72 years old. Increased age is the greatest risk factor and the disease is extremely rare in those under the age of 50. The other major type of large vessel vasculitis is Takayasu's arteritis, which typically presents in younger patients, has a strong female predominance and is more common in those of Asian descent.

[2] The highest rates of GCA occur in those of northern European descent. The condition is unusual in those of Middle Eastern or Asian background.

[3] GCA is more common in women, with a female to male ratio of 2:1.

[4] Headache is the most common symptom of GCA and often the presenting complaint. It occurs in around 70% of cases and may fluctuate in severity. While a unilateral temporal headache is classic, any type of headache can occur and hence GCA should be considered as a potential differential diagnosis in any elderly patient presenting with a new headache. It is important, however, to also work patients up for other potential causes of headache, including enquiring about symptoms and risk factors for other red flag diagnoses such as meningitis, an intracranial bleed or malignancy.

[5] A subacute (rather than sudden) onset of symptoms is typical for GCA. Symptoms are often present for several weeks, and may fluctuate, before patients seek medical review and the diagnosis of GCA is considered.

[6] Tenderness over the temporal area or sensitivity of the scalp may occur in GCA. One way of enquiring about this symptom is asking whether the patient notices any discomfort when combing or running their hands through their hair.

[7] Constitutional symptoms such as fatigue, fever and unintentional weight loss occur in up to half of patients with GCA. In some cases, they may be the only symptoms present, leading to difficulties with diagnosis, given their non-specific nature and the need to consider other differentials such as infection, malignancy or other systemic illness.

[8] Pain and stiffness of the shoulder girdle (more common) and/or hip girdle are typical symptoms suggestive of polymyalgia rheumatica (PMR), which sits on the same disease spectrum as GCA but is much more common. PMR occurs in around 50% of patients with GCA, while GCA develops in around 15% of those with PMR.

[9] The pathology in PMR is focused on peri-articular structures around the shoulders and hips such as tendons or bursae, with synovitis being less prominent (but may still occur).

[10] The pain and stiffness of PMR follow a typical inflammatory pattern, with symptoms worse in the morning, lasting sometimes for hours, or after periods of rest, with some improvement with movement or as the day progresses. Compared to GCA, treatment of PMR requires much lower doses of prednisolone (10–15mg) to achieve symptom resolution and disease control.

[11] PMR may cause limited range of motion due to pain but should not cause true muscle weakness. If weakness out of proportion to the patient's pain is present, other differential diagnoses should be considered, such as a myopathy.

[12] It is increasingly being recognised that peripheral joint involvement can occur in PMR, but its presence should also prompt investigation for other diagnoses such as rheumatoid arthritis (which can have a 'polymyalgic' onset). Often these patients will not be as exquisitely sensitive to prednisolone as in true PMR.

[13] Jaw claudication due to ischaemia of the masseter or temporalis muscles is considered the most specific symptom of GCA, but only occurs in up to half of cases. Careful clarification of jaw 'pain' is important, to determine if it

represents true claudication, i.e. pain or fatigue that worsens the longer a patient chews and then is relieved with rest. This pattern of claudication can be likened to angina in the setting of myocardial ischaemia. Tongue claudication can also occur in GCA.

14 Visual loss is the much-feared complication of GCA – it is sudden, painless and rarely reversible once it has occurred. It may be the presenting feature of GCA. Possible presentations of visual involvement may include amaurosis fugax (which occurs due to transient ischaemia of the retina), diplopia (due to ischaemic damage to the oculomotor system) or other less specific symptoms arising from optic nerve ischaemia secondary to inflammation of the ophthalmic artery.

15 Patients with GCA are typically elderly and therefore often have other comorbidities which can complicate treatment, particularly those conditions that are worsened with steroid exposure, such as diabetes, hypertension and osteoporosis.

Examination

- The patient has a **temperature of 37.6°C** [1].
- The **temporal artery** [2] is **slightly prominent** [3] and **tender** [4] on palpation.
- The **temporal artery pulse** [5] is **less prominent** [6] on the right.
- **Ocular examination** [7] including **fundoscopy** [8] is normal, with no evidence of **optic neuropathy** [9].

- The patient has normal **pulses** [10] and **equal blood pressure bilaterally** [11] at 130/80mmHg.
- There are no **bruits** [12].
- There is no **peripheral synovitis** [13] and full range of **shoulder and hip movements** [14].
- On auscultation of the heart there are no **murmurs** [15].

1 A fever may occur in up to 50% of patients with GCA. While these are usually low grade, a smaller proportion of patients may present with high temperatures. GCA should be considered as a possible diagnosis in older patients with pyrexia of unknown origin. Clearly exclusion of other causes of fever, particularly infection and malignancy, is a priority in these patients, prior to attributing symptoms to GCA, especially given that the mainstay of GCA treatment is immunosuppression.

2 The superficial temporal artery arises from the external carotid artery, after division of the maxillary artery. Despite the name 'temporal arteritis', GCA can affect any large vessel including other extracranial arteries of the head and neck, as well as the thoracic aorta and its major branches. The intracranial arteries are seldom involved. Certain symptoms arise according to which arteries are more involved; for example, occipital arteritis may produce a posterior headache, rather than the typical temporal headache.

3 A prominent, thickened or enlarged temporal artery is suggestive of GCA when present, but in clinical practice is generally an uncommon finding.

4 Tenderness specifically over the temporal artery, or over the scalp more generally, may be a sign of cranial artery inflammation in GCA.

5 The superficial temporal artery runs behind the neck of the mandible, upwards near the auricle, then over the zygomatic process where it further divides. The temporal artery pulse is most easily palpated in front of the ear, anterior to the tragus and up along the temple area.

6 It is normal for the temporal artery pulse to be palpable. Absence of the pulse, particularly on the same side as a patient's symptoms, should increase clinical suspicion of GCA.

7 Visual acuity should be documented in each eye. Eye movements should be assessed to identify ischaemic damage to the oculomotor system, which is a rare occurrence in GCA. Visual field defects may be extensive.

8 Fundoscopy is key in the assessment of visual symptoms in GCA. Anterior ischaemic optic neuropathy is the underlying mechanism of visual loss in 80% of cases. Usually this is due to occlusion of the posterior ciliary artery (a branch of the ophthalmic artery) which provides the major blood supply to the retina. Central retinal artery occlusion and posterior ischaemic optic neuropathy are less common mechanisms.

9 GCA-associated anterior ischaemic optic neuropathy appears as white-coloured optic disc oedema with later disc cupping and a pale disc rim. Cotton wool spots may signify focal areas of ischaemia, and central retinal artery occlusion can also be seen. The differential diagnosis for ischaemic optic neuritis includes hypoperfusion and thrombo-embolism.

10 Assessment of peripheral pulses should be performed in patients with suspected or confirmed GCA, as reduction or asymmetry could be an indication of otherwise asymptomatic extracranial large artery involvement.

11 Blood pressure should be checked on both arms as a difference may be a sign of disease affecting the large arteries, such as the subclavian supplying the upper limbs. In general, a consistent difference in BP between arms of >10mmHg may be significant.

12 Vascular bruits can be heard due to arterial wall vibration resulting from abnormal arterial blood flow, such as occurs with a stenosed vessel. Carotid bruits are auscultated either side of the midline in the anterior neck, while subclavian bruits are heard in the supraclavicular fossa.

13 Peripheral synovitis or inflammation of peri-articular structures can occur in PMR. There is also a rare associated condition known as remitting seronegative symmetrical synovitis with pitting oedema (RS3PE) which presents as swelling of the distal extremities.

14 Limited range of motion due to stiffness of the shoulders, neck and/or hips suggests PMR in association with GCA. This is often most evident when the patient is examined earlier in the day or after a period of rest. As mentioned previously, muscle power should be preserved, other than that which is limited by pain.

15 On cardiac auscultation the presence of a decrescendo diastolic murmur loudest at the left sternal edge in expiration is suggestive of aortic regurgitation, which may be a signal of the impending development of an ascending aortic aneurysm.

Investigations

- Laboratory studies show **elevated inflammatory markers** [1] with an **ESR of 102** [2].
- There is a **mild anaemia** [3] and **mildly deranged liver function tests** [4].
- The patient proceeds to a **bilateral** [5] **temporal artery biopsy** [6] which occurs 3 days after **commencing prednisolone** [7].
- The biopsy returns **positive** [8].

- There is **destruction of the internal elastic lamina** [9], **intimal proliferation** [10] and **granulomatous inflammation** [11] but no **giant cells** [12] are seen.
- The patient has a baseline **chest X-ray** [13] which is unremarkable.
- **Further imaging** [14] is not performed at this time.

1 The ESR and CRP are almost always elevated in patients with GCA. They are driven by the production of pro-inflammatory cytokines such as interleukin 6. They tend to rise and fall in parallel, but on occasion one may be more abnormal than the other. GCA with normal inflammatory markers only occurs in around 3% of cases.

2 A high ESR is one of the hallmarks of a GCA (or PMR) diagnosis. In particular, an ESR >100 is particularly suggestive. Other causes of a markedly elevated ESR are bacterial infection (including chronic or occult infection), multiple myeloma or other malignancies. Pregnancy, chronic kidney disease, obesity and anaemia can contribute to elevation of the ESR. Furthermore, the normal range for ESR increases with age – a rule for the normal maximum value of ESR is age divided by two (men) or age plus ten divided by two (women). The trend of the ESR (e.g. elevation from baseline) is therefore important to consider if available.

3 Like in many other inflammatory rheumatological diseases, a normocytic normochromic anaemia is a common marker of chronic disease and inflammation. Usually the anaemia is mild and improves with control of the underlying inflammatory process.

4 Biochemical abnormalities of liver function are not uncommon in GCA. Up to half of patients have elevation of their ALP, and a smaller proportion have elevated transaminases. The aetiology of these abnormalities is unclear, and they tend to resolve with treatment of GCA.

5 In most cases performing a bilateral temporal artery biopsy is preferred over unilateral, as it is associated with increased diagnostic yield. This is because of the presence of skip lesions, meaning areas of normal vessel are interspersed within inflamed sections of the artery. For this reason, obtaining as long a segment of the artery as possible is also helpful in decreasing the likelihood of false negatives.

6 A temporal artery biopsy is the primary modality for confirming a diagnosis of GCA. It can be performed under either general or local anaesthetic. It is a relatively safe procedure with the main uncommon risks being of wound infection or breakdown, bleeding and nerve damage.

7 In a patient with suspected GCA, treatment should not be delayed while awaiting a biopsy, due to the potentially catastrophic complication of visual loss if left untreated. The yield of a temporal artery biopsy remains reasonable up to several weeks after commencing prednisolone. Ideally, however, a biopsy should be performed within 2 weeks (or as soon as possible) from commencing steroids.

8 Despite being the gold standard for GCA diagnosis, a temporal artery biopsy only returns positive in around two-thirds of cases. Therefore, a positive or negative result needs to be interpreted in the context of the pre-test probability for GCA, based on clinical features, inflammatory markers and response to prednisolone. False negative biopsies may occur due to sampling error (skip lesions) or sparing of the temporal arteries (e.g. disease involving other vessels). It should be noted that GCA presenting without typical cranial symptoms (e.g. fever of unknown origin) may still return a positive biopsy.

9 Disruption of the internal elastic lamina is an important finding in GCA and may persist even after a prolonged period of steroid therapy. However, it is not specific for GCA and may also be seen in atherosclerosis and advanced age.

10 Intimal proliferation results in vessel narrowing which can lead to ischaemic symptoms.

11 Granulomatous inflammation composed of mononuclear cell infiltrate and activated macrophages is typical for GCA. Usually the most marked immune cell infiltrate occurs in the media, but the entire vessel wall can be affected.

12 Although 'giant cell' arteritis is named after the characteristic multinucleated giant cell, this finding is not uniformly present and should not be relied upon for diagnosis.

13 Chest X-ray can be used as a screening test for aortic aneurysms (looking for a widened mediastinum), which are more commonly a late complication of disease, usually occurring several years after diagnosis.

14 Imaging techniques targeting the large vessels have an emerging role in GCA. European rheumatology experts have recently proposed imaging guidelines for patients with GCA, but these have not necessarily been adopted worldwide. In patients with suspected aortic arch or major branch disease, CT or MR angiography can identify both structural changes (dilation or stenosis) and to some degree active inflammation (vessel wall oedema, fat stranding). PET-CT scans can indicate inflammatory activity in the large vessels (not the temporal arteries) but not structural changes, and sensitivity is reduced by steroid therapy. Doppler ultrasound of superficial arteries (including the temporal arteries) is being increasingly used, particularly in Europe, to assist with the diagnosis or exclusion of GCA, but requires the availability of experienced operators. In addition to being part of the diagnostic work-up, the role of large vessel imaging in monitoring disease activity over time is another area of current interest. Serial imaging may be performed to monitor patients with extracranial large vessel disease, but the choice of imaging modality, frequency of scanning and interpretation of findings and how they should influence treatment decisions are still unclear.

Management

Short-term

Commence **oral prednisolone** [1] straight away, **prior to the biopsy** [2], at a dose of **50mg daily** [3]. Consider the role of **aspirin** [4]. Screen for **hyperglycaemia** [5], **latent infection** [6], **osteoporosis** [7] and other comorbidities relevant to **prolonged steroid use** [8]. Consider prescribing a **proton pump inhibitor** [9] for gastric protection and **co-trimoxazole** [10] for *Pneumocystis jirovecii* prophylaxis. **Educate** [11] the patient about the **symptoms of GCA** [12], **treatment and side-effects** [13].

Long-term

Review the patient at **regular intervals** [14]. Slowly **taper the prednisolone dose** [15] according to **clinical response** [16] and **inflammatory markers** [17]. Introduce a **steroid-sparing agent** [18] if necessary. Screen for **large vessel complications** [19]. Monitor for and manage **steroid-related toxicity** [20], particularly **cardiovascular risk factors** [21] and **bone health** [22].

1 Prednisolone remains the mainstay of treatment for GCA and symptoms usually respond fairly rapidly (within days) after steroid commencement. Where available, the IL-6 receptor alpha inhibitor tocilizumab can also be used in conjunction with steroids to improve response rates and reduce cumulative steroid exposure. Phase 3 randomised controlled data supports this approach, with the main barrier to use being access and cost, which is dependent on country and health system.

2 When GCA is suspected treatment should not be delayed, due to the high stakes involved with potential visual loss. Once visual loss occurs it is rarely reversible, but new onset visual loss is extremely rare once treatment with steroids has begun.

3 Generally, patients with suspected GCA are commenced on oral prednisolone 40–60mg daily (up to 1mg/kg). Sometimes very high doses of IV methylprednisolone are used over 3 days if visual symptoms have occurred, to preserve as much vision as possible, and minimise the chance of the other eye becoming involved (around a 25–50% risk if steroids are not commenced).

4 The use of aspirin in GCA is controversial due to mixed data supporting its use. The decision to use aspirin is often clinician- and patient-dependent. The possible risks of therapy (e.g. bleeding risk, GI ulcers) and the patient's overall cardiovascular risk profile need to be considered.

5 This patient already has diabetes and will require more intensive blood glucose monitoring while on high dose steroids. Typically, steroid-induced hyperglycaemia peaks 4–6 hours post prednisolone dose, hence checking blood glucose around 2 hours after lunch should be part of the monitoring regimen. Often fasting glucose will be normal.

6 High dose steroids can result in the reactivation of latent infections such as hepatitis B, hence it is routine to screen patients. The tests requested should include hepatitis B surface antigen (sAg), surface antibody (sAb) and core antibody (cAb) to differentiate between patients with active hepatitis B, chronic hepatitis B or previous vaccination. Clinicians will often screen for other organisms, such as strongyloides and tuberculosis using blood tests, depending on individual patient risk.

7 Osteoporosis is a significant risk of steroid use and should be considered from the outset. Assess the patient's fracture risk including a DEXA scan for bone mineral density, identify previous low trauma fractures (including vertebral crush fractures) and address reversible osteoporosis risk factors.

8 The main causes of death in patients with GCA relate to long-term steroid treatment rather than the disease itself. Steroids, unfortunately, remain the most effective and accessible treatment, however.

9 High dose prednisolone is a risk factor for peptic ulcer disease. Consider prescribing an agent for gastroprotection, particularly in patients with additional risk factors (e.g. aspirin use, previous peptic ulcer).

10 Usual recommendations for *Pneumocystis jirovecii* pneumonia (PJP) prophylaxis are in patients receiving prednisolone doses >20mg daily for >3–4 weeks. This is not universally adopted in patients with GCA, however, due to low rates of PJP in this population.

11 Patients need to be aware of the potential catastrophic consequences of untreated GCA (visual loss) and the importance of treatment and regular follow-up.

12 Inform patients about symptoms that could represent active GCA that should prompt review, e.g. headaches, visual change, jaw claudication and constitutional symptoms.

13 Patients are often reluctant to take high dose or prolonged steroid therapy due to concerns about side-effects, so it is important to educate patients about the benefit vs. risk balance and strategies that will be employed to minimise steroid toxicity.

14 Patients require regular review to adjust treatment and assess for clinical features of active disease, treatment-related toxicity and large vessel complications.

15 Prednisolone is typically tapered over 12–18 months. The rate of steroid taper may follow set protocols or be adjusted based on the level of diagnostic uncertainty (e.g. in the setting of a negative biopsy but some degree of clinical suspicion) or unacceptable steroid side-effects.

16 Clinical response is assessed based on the presence or absence of typical symptoms and signs of GCA, as have previously been discussed in this case study.

17 Inflammatory markers usually fall then normalise with therapy. If this does not occur considerations should include refractory vasculitis (including extracranial large vessel involvement), or coexisting infection or malignancy.

18 While some patients achieve disease control and successfully wean and cease steroids without disease recurrence, many patients experience flares with the reduction of steroid dose, especially once doses drop below 15mg daily. In these cases, introduction of a steroid-sparing agent is usually tried. This may be a traditional disease-modifying antirheumatic drug (DMARD) agent such as methotrexate, or if available, the IL-6 inhibitor tocilizumab has also been proven in a phase three randomised controlled trial to be an effective therapy for relapsing disease.

19 Large vessel complications such as arterial aneurysms are often late complications of GCA and can occur independent of disease activity. There is variability in screening practices ranging from clinical assessment only, to regular chest radiographs or more sensitive imaging modalities such as CT or MR angiography. As previously mentioned, recent European guidelines suggest the use of CT or MR angiography at baseline and with follow-up scans periodically to screen for these complications, but not all countries have adopted these suggestions and the frequency of scans and preferred imaging modality remain undecided.

20 There are a broad range of steroid-associated side-effects of which clinicians should be aware. These include a cushingoid appearance, infection and poor wound healing, peptic ulcer disease, osteoporosis, avascular necrosis, steroid myopathy, adrenal suppression, obesity, steroid-induced diabetes, hypertension, dyslipidaemia, insomnia, mood disturbance and cataracts. The principles of screening and management of steroid-related side-effects can be applied to many other rheumatic diseases where patients receive high dose or prolonged steroids.

21 GCA is associated with an increased risk of cardiovascular events, due to both the disease itself and high dose prednisolone use. Blood pressure, blood glucose, lipids and weight should therefore be assessed at regular intervals and optimised with both lifestyle and pharmacological measures.

22 Consider vitamin D and/or calcium supplementation. Many patients should also receive anti-resorptive therapy with a bisphosphonate or denosumab, and this is generally recommended in patients with established osteoporosis (T score <–2.5 or previous low trauma fracture) or osteopenia (T score between –1.5 and –2.5).

CASE 94: Gout

History

- A **62-year-old male** [1] presents with a **hot, swollen and painful** [2] right **knee** [3], which started **overnight** [4].
- He can **barely touch the skin** [5] without significant discomfort.
- He denies any preceding **trauma** [6] or **previous joint symptoms** [7].
- He has **otherwise been well** [8] and denies **fevers** [9] or any **recent infections** [10].

- His past history includes **type 2 diabetes** [11] with complicating **diabetic nephropathy** [12] and **hypertension** [13].
- He drinks **3 to 4 pints of beer daily** [14].
- He remembers his **father having gout episodes** [15] in the past, especially after **eating mussels** [16].

[1] Gout is significantly more common in males than females. This is because oestrogen has a uricosuric effect, thereby promoting the renal excretion of uric acid. Consequently, women experience a rise in serum urate post menopause, and primary gout almost never occurs in premenopausal females. Family history and ethnicity are other relevant demographic risk factors for gout.

[2] Key aspects of a joint pain history include time of onset, distribution of joint involvement and differentiating inflammatory from mechanical pain. Warmth and swelling are obvious features pointing towards an inflammatory cause in this case.

[3] The most common site for gout is the first metatarsophalangeal joint (MTPJ) (podagra); however, knees, ankles, feet, elbows, wrists and hands are also common sites. The first presentation of gout most commonly affects a single joint (in 80% of cases), with polyarticular involvement more common with subsequent flares.

[4] The acute onset of this inflammatory monoarthritis should prompt consideration of septic arthritis (consider risk factors for infection, portals of microbial entry), crystal arthritis (gout, pseudogout), haemarthrosis (consider anticoagulation, bleeding disorders) or traumatic injury. Acute gout typically has an onset over hours, with rapid escalation to maximum intensity, and often starts at night.

[5] Severe pain and sensitivity to touch is a characteristic feature of gout, with the classic association of a patient unable to tolerate even a bedsheet touching their painful joint.

[6] The absence of trauma to the knee makes haemarthrosis or injury less likely differential diagnoses. It should be noted, though, that patients on anticoagulation or with a bleeding

disorder such as haemophilia can develop haemarthroses spontaneously. Local trauma is also a possible precipitant for a flare of gout.

[7] Enquiring about prior joint symptoms may identify previous undiagnosed episodes of gout (especially first MTPJ involvement) or point towards an alternative form of inflammatory arthritis (e.g. inflammatory back pain or psoriasis might point to a spondyloarthropathy). In addition, pre-existing joint damage (from injury or another type of arthritis) is a risk factor for gout in that particular joint.

[8] Recent illness can predispose to gout via a number of mechanisms including increased cell turnover, medication changes, dehydration and renal impairment.

[9] The clinical approach to an inflammatory monoarthritis should include enquiry about symptoms that could suggest septic arthritis. These include infective symptoms such as fevers, sweats and rigors, and other constitutional symptoms. Although severe gout can produce systemic symptoms, they are generally milder in intensity compared to infection, and fevers are generally low grade.

[10] A history of recent infection (e.g. cellulitis) should increase suspicion for a septic joint due to microbial seeding. Other potential portals of entry to consider include skin breaks or recent dental work. Immunosuppressed patients are also at higher risk of septic arthritis and may present in less typical fashion. Enquiring about recent infection is also relevant for the possibility of reactive arthritis, which can present as a monoarthritis (often lower limb large joint) and usually occurs 2–6 weeks post GI or urogenital infection.

[11] Patients with the metabolic syndrome (characterised by insulin resistance, hypertension, obesity and dyslipidaemia) are at higher risk for gout, with an odds ratio of about 3.

12 Gout is a clinical consequence of hyperuricaemia, which in 90% of cases is attributable to decreased renal excretion of uric acid (as opposed to increased uric acid production). The balance of uric acid in the human body depends on uric acid formation (from breakdown of purines, either consumed in diet or synthesised by the liver) and uric acid excretion (two-thirds renally excreted and one-third via the bowel). Chronic kidney disease of any cause affects this renal excretion and is therefore an important risk factor for gout.

13 Hypertension is relevant for gout not only as part of the predisposing metabolic syndrome, but also due to the impact antihypertensives can have on uric acid excretion. Thiazide and loop diuretics inhibit renal tubular secretion of uric acid, and therefore reduce the amount of uric acid excreted by the kidneys, predisposing to hyperuricaemia. Other drugs which increase serum uric acid levels include calcineurin inhibitors (tacrolimus, ciclosporin), antibiotics (especially antituberculous agents) and low dose aspirin.

14 Alcohol intake is an established dietary trigger for gout, as it inhibits renal tubular secretion of uric acid, predisposing to hyperuricaemia. Of the different varieties of alcohol, beer is the worst for gout, as it also has a high purine load.

15 A positive family history for gout may occur due to shared risk factors (e.g. obesity, diet) but in a small proportion of cases can reflect genetic abnormalities. Hereditary cases may involve genetic polymorphisms associated with reduced renal uric acid secretion, or inborn errors of metabolism related to the uric acid synthetic pathway.

16 Dietary factors are possible triggers for acute gout episodes and can contribute to some degree to hyperuricemia. Shellfish (such as mussels!), organ meats and tomatoes are examples of foods that may raise uric acid levels. Importantly, intake of fructose (found in fruit juices and soft drinks) has also been significantly linked to hyperuricaemia.

Examination

- The patient has **stable vital signs** [1] other than **mild hypertension** [2] at 145/92mmHg.
- He has a **BMI of 31** [3].
- Inspection of the right knee reveals a **swollen** [4] and **erythematous** [5] joint.
- There is an obvious **joint effusion** [6] on palpation and marked **tenderness** [7].
- Movement of the right knee show **severely reduced range of motion** [8] secondary to pain.

- He is **unable to bear weight** [9].
- Examination of the **other joints** [10] is unremarkable, including the **hands and feet** [11].
- There are also no abnormalities of any **peri-articular structures** [12].
- There are no visible **tophi** [13] in any **typical sites** [14] and **no other extra-articular abnormalities** [15] are noted on general examination.

1 Usually a patient with gout will have normal vital signs. A low grade fever can be a feature, particularly when severe or polyarticular, but should obviously also prompt consideration of infection. Other vital sign derangements such as haemodynamic instability or abnormalities of respiratory parameters are not attributable to gout and warrant further investigation.

2 This patient has mild hypertension in keeping with his past history. If this was consistent on repeat measurements, escalation of his antihypertensive therapy would be indicated, in addition to reinforcement of non-pharmacological measures. In the setting of a diagnosis of gout, losartan can be a good choice of antihypertensive, as unlike other commonly used drugs such as thiazide diuretics, losartan has been associated with a reduction in serum urate levels via a uricosuric effect.

3 This man's BMI of 31kg/m² puts him in the obese category. It is important to identify cardiovascular risk factors in patients with gout, as hyperuricaemia is a marker of vascular risk, and modifiable cardiovascular risk factors should be addressed as part of the patient's management.

4 Features of inflammation, such as joint swelling, pain, warmth and erythema, occur due to cytokine and inflammatory mediator release during the acute gout attack. This is due to the phagocytosis of uric acid crystals in the joint, which activates an intracellular complex called an inflammasome. This complex stimulates large amounts of the pro-inflammatory cytokine interleukin 1-beta (IL-1B) which is a key driver of inflammation in gout.

5 Erythema is a non-specific sign of inflammation which can be seen overlying the affected joint in gout. Its presence does not help differentiate gout from septic arthritis. It can also be difficult sometimes to distinguish cellulitis from gout, in the presence of erythema, particularly when it affects the feet and is less able to be clearly localised to a single joint.

6 An effusion occurs as a consequence of local inflammation in the joint in acute gout. It can be quite large (sometimes >100ml) and cause a significant amount of pain in its own right due to pressure effect within the joint capsule.

7 Patients with gout are often diffusely tender around the affected joint, not just limited to the joint line. The presence of 'exquisite' tenderness even to light touch is a commonly described feature of acute gout.

8 Reduced range of motion may occur due to both pain and swelling, particularly if there is a large joint effusion. Like the other features of an inflamed joint, however, this does not distinguish from other pathologies. In particular, a septic joint is characteristically highly irritable on movement, with markedly reduced range of motion.

9 Given that gout often affects lower limb weight-bearing joints such as the foot, ankle or knee, an acute attack can significantly compromise a patient's mobility. This may be a factor that leads a patient to be admitted to hospital with a gout flare, as opposed to being managed in the community.

10 An examination of other joints should always be performed in a patient presenting with arthritis, as there may be helpful signs of disease unnoticed or unreported by the patient. Almost any joint can be affected by gout; however, involvement of the shoulders, hips, sternoclavicular joints and spine is unusual, and if it occurs, is generally in patients with longer-standing, poorly controlled disease.

11 Hands and feet are particularly prone to gout, because distal joints generally have lower temperature (further from the core) which reduces the solubility of uric acid. Other factors that affect uric acid solubility and can therefore influence the risk of an acute flare include changes in urate concentration (e.g. drugs, renal impairment), dehydration and acidaemia.

12 Gout not only affects the joints but can also affect peri-articular structures such as tendons and bursae, such as causing olecranon bursitis.

13 Tophi are deposits of uric acid crystals surrounded by granulomatous inflammation. Typically, they are a consequence of repeated attacks of acute gout and persistently high levels of uric acid. Sometimes they can be the first sign that a patient has gout. They are an important complication to identify, because they are associated with chronic joint pain and erosive damage and can become infected. They may have a yellowish colour. They are not usually tender. The best way to reduce the burden of tophi is to aggressively lower uric acid levels in the blood. In occasional cases surgical removal (tophectomy) is performed, particularly if there is associated pain, functional disturbance or infection.

14 In a patient with gout, a careful review of common sites of tophi should be performed. These sites are the surface of the fingers/hands, ulnar surface of the forearms, the elbows (tophi can occur within the olecranon bursa), pinna of the ears, on the Achilles tendons and around the first MTPJs.

15 Patients with gout often have a fairly normal extra-articular examination, and acute gout does not usually cause disruption in other organ systems. The main role of a general examination is to identify features of competing differential diagnoses and signs of gout-related comorbidities, such as renal disease and cardiovascular disease.

Investigations

- Basic bloods show a **normal FBE** [1], a moderately **elevated creatinine of 120µmol/L**[2], and an **elevated CRP of 95 and ESR of 38** [3].
- A **serum uric acid** [4] returned **elevated at 0.51mmol/L** [5].
- A plain **X-ray** [6] of the right knee has no **erosions** [7].
- No **additional imaging** [8] is performed.

- A **joint aspirate** [9] of the right knee is performed.
- The initial results show a **white cell count** [10] of 32 000/mm³, with a **negative Gram stain** [11].
- **Crystal analysis** [12] shows **needle-shaped** [13] crystals which are **negatively birefringent** [14], including **intracellular** [15] crystals.

1 A full blood count may be normal or have a raised white cell count or other non-specific features of inflammation.

2 Reduced renal function is an important risk factor for gout. It would also be important to compare this patient's current reading with his baseline creatinine to detect any superimposed acute kidney injury. Gout can also be a cause of renal complications and impairment due to the formation of urate stones and chronic urate nephropathy. Noting the degree of renal impairment also influences choices of acute gout treatment.

3 The CRP and ESR are commonly elevated in an acute gout attack, usually to a moderate degree. Marked elevations of CRP (in the hundreds) can be seen with severe or polyarticular flares but should prompt thorough assessment to exclude infection.

4 Serum uric acid levels are not diagnostic for gout, but demonstrating hyperuricaemia (a precursor for clinical gout) may still be useful as part of the overall clinical picture. The uric acid level is also important in established gout, as levels form a target for treatment. Serum urate usually needs to reach levels >0.42mmol/L before crystals form. Importantly, however, during acute attacks the uric acid level may paradoxically drop, and therefore is not always a reliable marker of hyperuricaemia at the time of a flare.

5 Hyperuricaemia is defined as >0.42mmol/L in men or >0.36mmol/L in women and occurs in 5–8% of the population. Importantly, hyperuricaemia is often asymptomatic – in fact most patients with an elevated uric acid do not develop clinical gout. The higher the level of uric acid, however, the greater the risk and those with a serum urate >0.6mmol/L have a 5-year prevalence of gout of around 30%. Patients with asymptomatic hyperuricaemia do not require uric acid-lowering therapy as there is no proven benefit at this time. However, it does warrant screening and management of cardiovascular risk factors due to the independent association of hyperuricaemia with cardiovascular disease.

6 In a patient with gout, a plain X-ray may be normal, show soft tissue swelling with acute attacks, or demonstrate erosive changes with more advanced disease. Usually the joint space is well preserved and there is no juxta-articular osteoporosis. Sometimes tophi can also be seen, associated with local joint destruction. In patients with pseudogout, due to calcium pyrophosphate crystals, linear calcific deposition parallel to subchondral bone may be seen, particularly in the knee or triangular cartilage of the wrist.

7 Gouty erosions are typically punched out or rat-bitten in appearance, with sclerotic margins and overhanging edges. They can occur some distance from the joint itself. They can be distinguished from the erosions of rheumatoid arthritis, which tend to be shallower, closer to the joint line and spare the DIPJs – a commonly involved site in gout.

8 While X-ray is the most commonly used imaging in gout at present, other modalities have an emerging role. Ultrasound may show a 'double contour' sign and can also demonstrate erosions. Dual-energy CT is another scan which is able to visualise urate crystal deposition by assigning different colours to materials of different chemical composition. It is most useful in situations where the diagnosis is uncertain and joint aspiration is difficult (e.g. small joint disease, spinal inflammatory arthritis).

9 Joint aspiration provides the definitive diagnosis of gout and is therefore indicated in a patient with a new presentation of suspected gout, or in patients with a known history of gout where there is diagnostic uncertainty as to the cause of an acute presentation.

10 A cell count can normally be obtained quickly on a joint aspirate sample, and therefore provides usefully early diagnostic information. In order to prevent clotting of the sample and allow an accurate cell count, part of the synovial fluid sample should be sent to the lab in an EDTA tube (the same one used for an FBE). As a rule of thumb, a white cell count of 2000–20000/mm³ suggests inflammatory pathology (e.g. rheumatoid arthritis), while >50000–100000/mm³ (with a high proportion of polymorphonuclear neutrophils) is septic until proven otherwise. Crystal arthritis can produce a wide range of cell counts in the inflammatory range, but rarely >100000/mm³.

11 Gram stain is positive in around 30–50% of cases of septic arthritis, so cannot be relied upon to exclude infection if there is clinical suspicion.

12 Crystal arthropathies that can be diagnosed on crystal analysis are gout (monosodium urate crystals) and pseudogout (calcium pyrophosphate crystals). Another form of crystal arthritis, basic calcium phosphate disease, can produce acute and sometimes destructive arthritis, but these crystals cannot be seen on polarising microscopy.

13 Uric acid crystals are typically needle-shaped. In contrast, the calcium pyrophosphate crystals of pseudogout have a polygonal or rhomboid shape.

14 Birefringence refers to the appearance of the crystals under polarising microscopy. Uric acid crystals are negatively birefringent and appear yellow in colour when parallel to the polariser. In contrast, pseudogout crystals are weakly positively birefringent.

15 The presence of crystals in synovial fluid is not always associated with acute inflammatory crystal arthritis. A more specific finding is the presence of intracellular crystals (which are crystals that have been phagocytosed by macrophages) – this finding is completely specific for the presence of gout. It should also be remembered that gout can coexist with other joint diseases, and a diagnosis of gout does not necessarily exclude competing diagnoses.

Management

Short-term

Options for acute management are an **NSAID** [1], **colchicine** [2] or **prednisolone** [3] which can be used **alone or in combination** [4], usually for **3–7 days** [5]. Choice is largely based on **side-effect profile** [6]. Consider **intra-articular steroids** [7] as well. Identify and correct **possible precipitants** [8] of the acute attack. Do not stop **uric acid-lowering therapy** [9] if patients are taking this regularly.

Long-term

Educate [10] the patient about the condition and its management. Advise about **dietary factors** [11] and review the patient's **medication list** [12]. Screen for and manage **cardiovascular risk factors** [13]. Commence **uric acid-lowering therapy** [14] if the patient meets **indications** [15], with **allopurinol** [16], considering the alternative **febuxostat** [17] if **intolerant** [18]. Identify any **cautions** [19] with therapy and emphasise the importance of **adherence** [20]. Continue a **prophylactic** **agent** [21] while adjusting the dose of allopurinol. **Follow up** [22] the patient regularly, with the plan to **increase the dose** [23] of uric acid-lowering therapy until **target uric acid level** [24] is achieved. A **uricosuric agent** [25] can be tried if refractory.

1 All NSAIDs including COX-2 inhibitors can be effective for acute gout. Typically they are used at high doses and are most effective when initiated soon after symptom onset.

2 Colchicine is also effective, particularly in early acute gout. GI side-effects are the main limiting factor, but doses of 1–3 tablets daily (≤1.5mg per day) are normally well tolerated.

3 Prednisolone is generally a second-line option when NSAIDs or colchicine are ineffective or contraindicated (typically with renal impairment). Usually doses of 15–25mg daily are adequate.

4 For more severe or polyarticular attacks, or where a single agent is ineffective, using a combination of acute therapies can be more effective.

5 Usually 3–7 days of treatment are adequate to resolve acute gout. Even without treatment acute gout will often be self-limiting. For more refractory cases a longer tapering course of acute therapy may be required to prevent relapse.

6 The main determinant of which agent(s) to use for acute gout attacks is their side-effect profiles. For example, patients with renal impairment should avoid NSAIDs; colchicine is also avoided or used in low doses in those with advanced renal failure; and systemic steroids are less preferable in patients with diabetes or active infection.

7 In patients with only a small number of affected joints or joints refractory to systemic therapy, intra-articular administration of steroids is an alternative that can be used alone or in combination with systemic therapy. Joint infection should be excluded prior.

8 Precipitants of the acute gout attack should be identified and managed where feasible. These include acute illness, new medications, dehydration, acute kidney impairment and poor compliance to gout therapy.

9 Patients who are on established uric acid-lowering therapy should NOT have this agent stopped during an acute attack, as this may worsen the acute flare.

10 Education is an extremely important part of gout management and should include an explanation of the diagnosis and its possible complications, the difference between acute and preventive medications, dietary and lifestyle factors and treatment adherence.

11 General recommendations are to avoid excess high purine foods (such as organ meats and shellfish), reduce fructose intake (particularly soft drinks and fruit juices) and minimise alcohol (especially beer). Keeping well hydrated is also advisable.

12 Unfortunately, the use of agents which increase gout risk are often necessary (e.g. diuretics in a patient with heart failure). Sometimes alternatives may be feasible, such as switching antihypertensive agents. Some drugs like losartan and fenofibrate may reduce uric acid levels and may therefore be a preferable choice if a drug of its class is otherwise indicated. These agents are not routinely started for the purpose of gout alone.

13 The presence of hyperuricaemia and gout is a marker of increased cardiovascular risk. Screening and aggressive management of cardiovascular risk factors and the metabolic syndrome are therefore a key part of an overall gout management plan.

14 First-line uric acid-lowering therapy is with a xanthine oxidase inhibitor (allopurinol or febuxostat). Traditionally, initiation of uric acid-lowering therapy was delayed for a few weeks after an acute attack, due to concern of worsening flares. This is no longer standard practice and it is acceptable to commence uric acid-lowering treatment at the time of an acute flare, alongside the treatment for acute gout.

15 Indications for uric acid-lowering therapy are repeated gout attacks (at least two per year), tophi or erosions, uric acid nephrolithiasis or urate nephropathy and underlying chronic kidney disease. However, recently it has been suggested that urate-lowering therapy be considered and discussed with the patient at the very first presentation of the disease.

16 Allopurinol is a competitive inhibitor of xanthine oxidase which blocks urate production. It is the first-line and most used uric acid-lowering agent. Starting doses are usually 50–100mg daily (depending on renal function) and doses need to be up-titrated slowly over the following months. Sometimes doses of 800–900mg per day are required to achieve adequate effect.

17 Febuxostat is an alternative newer xanthine oxidase inhibitor which is generally reserved for patients who do not tolerate allopurinol. The starting dose is 40mg daily and can be increased to 80mg daily if necessary.

18 Allopurinol can be associated with rashes, myelosuppression and GI upset. The most severe reaction is allopurinol hypersensitivity syndrome which is associated with fever, rash (including Stevens–Johnson syndrome), liver dysfunction, interstitial nephritis, eosinophilia and vasculitis. Serious cutaneous adverse events are strongly associated with the HLA-B*5801 haplotype, which is particularly prevalent in Asians. Specifically those of Han Chinese, Thai and Korean background should be screened for HLA-B*5801 carriage prior to starting allopurinol.

19 Allopurinol is contraindicated if associated with previous hypersensitivity syndrome. Febuxostat should be cautioned in patients with previous cardiovascular history, due to a possible association with adverse cardiac outcomes. Both xanthine oxidase inhibitors should be avoided with other purine drugs such as azathioprine or 6-mercaptopurine, due to potentiation of toxicity.

20 Poor adherence is one of the most common reasons for failure of uric acid-lowering therapy, and stopping/starting allopurinol may precipitate acute gout flares.

21 Starting uric acid-lowering therapy is associated with risk of precipitating a gout flare. Flare prophylaxis with an NSAID, low dose colchicine or low dose prednisolone is therefore advised at the time uric acid-lowering therapy is initiated. This should be continued for a few months after titration is completed (usually six months in total).

22 Regular follow-up of patients with gout is required, to monitor symptoms and uric acid levels, ensure adherence and manage complications. This is normally coordinated via the GP, sometimes in conjunction with a general physician or rheumatologist.

23 Typically, the dose of allopurinol is increased every few weeks in 50–100mg increments until target uric acid levels are reached.

24 The target level of uric acid in patients with gout is <0.36mmol/L, or for patients with tophaceous or erosive disease <0.3mmol/L, to promote dissolution of the tophi.

25 Uricosuric therapies promote excretion of uric acid via the kidneys. They are no longer in common use; however, agents such as probenecid may be tried in refractory cases.

CASE 95: Non-specific low back pain

History

- A **62-year-old** [1] man who works as a **labourer** [2] presents with **acute** [3] **low back pain** [4] following **repeated heavy lifting at work** [5].
- He describes severe pain across his lower back that is **worse with movement** [6].
- The pain **does not radiate** [7], it does **not wake him at night** [8], and he has no associated **weakness or numbness** [9] in his lower limbs, nor **bowel or bladder disturbance** [10].
- He is **constitutionally well** [11] and has no other indicators of **red flag conditions** [12].
- He has **no significant medical history** [13] and takes **no regular medications** [14].
- He is **struggling to cope** [15] with the pain and is highly concerned about the **cause of his symptoms** [16] and the impact it will have on his job and family.

[1] Back pain is more commonly reported in older people and occurs at approximately the same rates in both women and men.

[2] Heavy physical work, frequent bending, twisting or lifting and prolonged static postures may all increase the risk of back pain. Exercise and sports participation, however, is thought to have a protective effect and should therefore not be discouraged.

[3] The time classification for low back pain is somewhat arbitrarily set as acute (<4 weeks), subacute (4–12 weeks) and chronic (>12 weeks).

[4] Back pain is an incredibly common problem, affecting the majority of people at some point in their life, and is the leading global cause of years lost due to disability.

[5] Work-related back injuries can be associated with certain factors that predispose to poorer prognosis. Heavy physical work demands, job dissatisfaction and the presence of compensation claims have all been associated with chronic back pain and poorer long-term outcomes.

[6] Pain that is worse with movement fits with a mechanical pattern of pain. Inflammatory characteristics include pain that is worse in the morning, with morning stiffness for more than an hour, and pain that is worse with rest and better with movement. These features should prompt consideration of an axial spondyloarthropathy, especially in younger age groups.

[7] It is important to identify radicular pain (sometimes referred to as 'sciatica'), as additional investigation and management options may be of benefit. Radicular pain is typically described as radiating into one (or sometimes both) legs along the course of a spinal nerve root. The patient may describe intermittent sharp, shooting or deep aching pain that can be associated with paraesthesias or other

neuropathic sensations. It can be triggered by increased intra-abdominal pressure (e.g. coughing, straining). It occurs due to compression or irritation of a nerve root (usually lumbosacral) which most commonly occurs secondary to intervertebral disc disease or degenerative changes in the spine.

[8] Nocturnal pain is a symptom that should be taken seriously as it is a feature of several not-to-be-missed diagnoses including spinal infection, cancer, fracture and inflammatory back pain (e.g. ankylosing spondylitis).

[9] Patients with back pain should be assessed for neurological symptoms in their lower limbs which may suggest nerve root compression or, in the most serious of cases, spinal cord or cauda equina compression which are medical/surgical emergencies.

[10] Bowel or bladder issues including urinary retention or incontinence, faecal incontinence or overflow and saddle anaesthesia are all symptoms concerning for cauda equina syndrome, which requires urgent imaging and referral to a spinal surgeon. The cauda equina is the tail of nerve roots that continue along the spinal canal and emerge at their associated vertebral level after the termination of the spinal cord at around level L1–2.

[11] Constitutional symptoms such as fevers, sweats and weight loss are considered 'red flag' symptoms in the assessment of back pain, as they suggest more sinister underlying pathology, in particular infection (e.g. osteomyelitis, epidural abscess, infective discitis) or malignancy (primary or metastatic tumour deposits).

[12] 'Red flag' diagnoses are serious conditions that require urgent investigation and/or management. Exclusion of these red flag conditions is a key priority in the assessment of patients with back pain. The main red flag causes of back pain are infection, malignancy, fracture, neurological compression

(e.g. cauda equina syndrome, spinal cord syndromes) and inflammatory arthritis (e.g. ankylosing spondylitis). A proportion of the medical history in patients with back pain should therefore be dedicated to assessing the likelihood of these diagnoses (based on symptom history, medical comorbidities and risk factors) in order to determine whether further investigation is required. Patients aged <25 or >50 years may be more likely to have a red flag diagnosis.

13 Enquire about relevant past medical history including malignancy (due to the risk of recurrence or metastasis), osteoporosis and fracture risk (e.g. increased age, postmenopausal status, falls or trauma) and recent infections or predisposing factors (e.g. immunosuppressed state, recent travel, IV drug use).

14 Review the patient's medication list, paying particular attention to steroids (osteoporosis and infection risk), other immunosuppressive agents (infection risk), anticoagulants

(risk of retroperitoneal bleeding) and analgesic agents being used by the patient for their pain (with the use of long-term or high dose opioids being of particular concern).

15 In patients with back pain, there are several factors known as 'yellow flags' which have been linked to the development of chronic pain and worse outcomes. Some of these relate to patient beliefs and behaviours, such as high levels of psychological or psychosocial stress, passive coping strategies, avoidance behaviours, negative attitudes towards pain and preference for passive rather than active therapies.

16 A specific cause for back pain can only be identified in around 10% of cases and only a small proportion of patients (<5%) have serious underlying pathology. The priority of the clinical assessment is to exclude these serious causes and then focus on management and functional improvement rather than a specific diagnosis.

Examination

- The patient is **afebrile** [1] with normal vital signs.
- He has a **BMI of 30** [2].
- **Inspection of the back** [3] is unremarkable.
- There is no **focal midline tenderness** [4], but there is **pain on palpation across the whole lumbar region** [5].
- Lumbar spine **movements are limited** [6] in all directions due to triggering of pain.

- The **lower limb neurological examination** [7] is normal including **tone** [8], **reflexes** [9], **power** [10] and **sensation** [11].
- **Straight leg raise** [12] is normal.
- There is intact **saddle sensation and normal anal tone** [13].
- The patient is **able to mobilise slowly** [14] despite intermittent spasms of pain.

1 Identification of a fever should prompt consideration and exclusion of red flag diagnoses as previously discussed.

2 Overweight or obesity predisposes to lumbar spine osteoarthritis which is a common contributing factor in patients with low back pain.

3 Look for the presence of abnormal posture or curvatures of the spine that may be a cause or consequence of mechanical back issues. Lack of lumbar lordosis (i.e. a flattened lower back) is often associated with low back pain. Evidence of trauma or previous surgery is usually readily identifiable.

4 Focal tenderness in an area of the spine may indicate localised pathology at that site but this is neither sensitive nor specific. Midline tenderness reproducible at a specific level may occur with particular red flag diagnoses such as a crush fracture, discitis or bony tumour.

5 More commonly patients have diffuse tenderness across the affected region which may be associated with muscle spasm. Anatomy of the back involves complexly oriented muscle layers, a multitude of joints, overlapping innervation and relatively small cortical representation, which makes

pain localisation extremely difficult. Superimposed pain amplification can further complicate the picture.

6 Major movements of the lumbar spine are flexion, extension and lateral flexion, with rotation more predominantly occurring at the thoracic spine.

7 Performing a lower limb neurological exam is a core component in the assessment of a patient with back pain. Upper motor neurone signs are less common, but suggest pathology originating in the spinal cord (or pathology in the brain occurring unrelated to back pain). Lower motor neurone signs occur with cauda equina syndrome or other nerve root compression syndromes. Familiarity with dermatomes and myotomes is essential in order to localise nerve root involvement based on the physical examination. The most commonly affected nerve roots in patients with back pain or radicular symptoms are L4, L5 and S1.

8 Abnormal tone usually indicates serious neurological compromise in a patient with back pain. Increased tone suggests an upper motor neurone lesion, while reduced tone can occur with cauda equina syndrome.

9 Hyperreflexia suggests upper motor neurone pathology. Hyporeflexia can help localise nerve root pathology, remembering that the knee reflex is mediated by L3/4 nerve roots and the ankle reflex by S1.

10 Generalised weakness of one or both lower limbs should prompt concern for spinal cord pathology and warrants urgent imaging. Weakness that is more focal in nature and follows a myotomal pattern may help localise symptoms to a particular nerve root. Useful associations to remember include: weak knee extension occurring with L4 pathology, weak big toe extension with L5 pathology and weak plantarflexion with S1 pathology. Walking on heels (L5) and walking on toes (S1) are therefore useful screening tests.

11 Performing a sensory examination is most useful in identifying dermatomal sensory abnormalities which can help localise nerve root pathology.

12 The straight leg raise is a provocation test that may be positive in patients with nerve root impingement. The patient lies supine and the examiner passively lifts the patient's straightened leg on one side. Back pain and/or radicular symptoms elicited by elevation of the leg (usually between 30° and 70°) is suggestive of nerve root irritation. The crossed leg raise, where pain is elicited on the side opposite to the leg being elevated, may also be positive and is thought to be a more specific test for nerve root impingement. These tests in general, however, have fairly poor diagnostic sensitivity and specificity and should be interpreted in the context of the patient's symptoms and other findings on examination.

13 Perform assessment of saddle sensation and anal tone in circumstances where there is suspicion of cauda equina compression. The presence of these abnormalities is extremely concerning and should prompt urgent imaging (ideally an MRI of the spine) and referral to a spinal surgical unit.

14 Assessment of gait and mobility gives an indication of the functional impairment related to the patient's pain, which may help guide the intensity of treatment.

Investigations

- Following the patient's **thorough clinical assessment** [1], a diagnosis of **non-specific back pain** [2] is made.
- No **blood tests** [3] are considered necessary at this stage.
- The patient requests **imaging of his back** [4] because he is concerned about work-related **'wear and tear'** [5].

- However, after being provided with some **education and opportunity for discussion** [6] about the **indications for imaging** [7] with modalities such as **X-ray** [8], **CT scanning** [9] and **MRI scanning** [10], the patient is agreeable to not proceed with **further investigations** [11] at present.

1 A thorough clinical history and examination is the most important step in the work-up of a patient presenting with back pain and allows for diagnostic triaging into the following groups: non-specific low back pain (vast majority), radicular syndrome (e.g. nerve root pathology including spinal canal stenosis), suspected serious pathology (red flag diagnoses) and those with non-musculoskeletal causes of back pain which are usually associated with additional symptoms or signs (e.g. pyelonephritis, aortic aneurysm, pancreatitis, peptic ulcer disease).

2 Non-specific low back pain is the diagnostic category of exclusion after consideration of radicular syndromes, red flag diagnoses and non-musculoskeletal causes. Non-specific back pain has a presumed musculoskeletal basis, but there are no specific features or clinical tests that can confidently identify a specific structure as being the source of pain.

3 Blood tests are not indicated in patients with non-specific back pain. They are useful, however, when other causes are being considered. For example, elevated inflammatory markers which are otherwise unexplained may point towards infection or malignancy as a possible diagnosis. Testing for kidney and liver function may also be relevant if pharmacological agents are being prescribed for pain.

4 Imaging should not be routinely performed in patients with non-specific back pain, as the correlation between radiological abnormalities and patient symptoms is poor. Consequently, common findings on imaging will not change patient management and can lead to unhelpful preoccupation with non-significant abnormalities.

5 Rates of degenerative change in the spine on imaging are high, including in asymptomatic patients, and so the identification of such changes is not clinically useful. It is estimated that in asymptomatic patients up to half of middle-aged and almost all elderly patients will have radiological degenerative features, such as disc bulges and tears. Even in patients with neurological compromise on imaging, the correlation of radiological findings with clinical symptoms and signs is notoriously poor.

6 Patients are often concerned about the potential for serious pathology causing their back pain and therefore request further investigation such as imaging. It is therefore important to educate and reassure patients regarding the natural history of non-specific back pain, and the rationale for not proceeding to further investigation.

7 Imaging is indicated in only a small proportion of patients with back pain. Urgent imaging is required for suspected infection, cancer, cauda equina syndrome or in the setting of other major neurological deficits. In patients with a lower index of suspicion for serious pathology, or symptoms of radiculopathy or spinal canal stenosis, a trial of conservative management is reasonable in the first instance, with subsequent imaging only performed if symptoms do not show improvement.

8 Plain X-ray is the first-line imaging modality for patients with a suspected vertebral fracture. If the X-ray is negative and clinical suspicion persists then an MRI may be subsequently performed.

9 There is a fairly limited role for CT in patients with back pain and in general, guidelines recommend proceeding straight to MRI when serious causes are suspected, as most pathology is better delineated with MRI compared to CT. There may be a role for CT scanning, however, in patients in whom MRI imaging is contraindicated (e.g. non-compatible metalware or pacemaker) or unavailable.

10 MRI is the preferred modality for most suspected spinal pathology when imaging is indicated, and in particular is the best modality for detecting and characterising malignancy, infection (e.g. osteomyelitis, abscesses) and neurological compromise (e.g. nerve root or spinal cord impingement).

11 In the first instance non-specific back pain should be managed conservatively and no routine investigations are required. Patients should, however, be warned of concerning symptoms (e.g. fevers, neurological lower limb symptoms, bowel or bladder dysfunction) and have their progress monitored. The diagnosis and need for further investigation can then be reassessed if any new clinical information emerges with time.

Management

Short-term

Reassure and educate [1] the patient about the **favourable prognosis** [2] of non-specific back pain. Encourage **self-management strategies** [3], **return to work** [4] and **gentle escalation of physical activity** [5]. If **non-pharmacological strategies** [6] are insufficient, **pharmacological therapy** [7] such as **short-term NSAIDs** [8] can also be initiated. Most patients can be managed in a **primary care setting** [9]. Schedule a **follow-up appointment** [10] to ensure symptoms are improving as expected.

Long-term

Pain that persists may require more **complex and intensive support** [11]. This may include **psychological therapies** [12], **structured exercise programmes** [13] and, in difficult cases, an **interdisciplinary rehabilitation** [14] programme. **Opioids** [15] ideally should not be prescribed due to **side-effects** [16] and **dependence risk** [17]. Interventions such as **cortisone injections** [18] and **surgery** [19] have specific indications which do not apply to non-specific back pain.

1 The majority of patients with acute non-specific back pain require only simple advice and reassurance to allow the natural history of recovery to take place. Patients should be advised of the benign nature of non-specific low back pain and the extremely low chance of serious underlying pathology.

2 Reassure patients with acute non-specific back pain of the favourable prognosis; >90% of patients have a rapid improvement within the first 6 weeks and will continue to improve for several months thereafter.

3 Patients should be encouraged to adopt a positive and proactive approach to managing their pain and avoid catastrophising and maladaptive coping strategies. Self-management strategies include the use of heat packs for symptom relief, avoidance of prolonged sitting, activity

modification and pacing in order to promote continued functioning despite pain while recovery is underway.

4 Encourage patients to return to work, in a graded fashion and with duty modifications if required. The longer a patient is off work due to their back pain, the lower the chances of them successfully returning in the longer term. The patient's own expectation of return to work is one of the most important predictors of work disability outcomes.

5 Patients should be told to minimise bed rest and stay as active as possible, including continuing to perform their activities of daily living. Bed rest has been shown to decrease functional recovery and increase levels of pain, while staying active increases recovery rates and function.

6 Additional non-pharmacological strategies such as massage, spinal manipulation and acupuncture can also be tried, depending on patient preference. Such therapies have low to moderate quality evidence of small benefit.

7 Pharmacological therapy is second-line and should be used in conjunction with ongoing non-pharmacological measures. Previously paracetamol was recommended as the first-line medication, but due to limited evidence of benefit over placebo, this is no longer the case. NSAIDs are now the preferred first-line choice of analgesic in the absence of contraindications. Skeletal muscle relaxants can also be considered in the acute phase.

8 NSAIDs have moderate quality evidence supporting their efficacy; however, the absolute benefit is modest. As with any medication, their prescription has to balance potential benefits with risks, and should be continued at the lowest effective dose for the shortest possible length of time.

9 Most patients with back pain can be successfully managed in primary care. If there is diagnostic uncertainty (e.g. possible inflammatory back pain) a referral for a specialist opinion may be warranted. Some patients may benefit from early referral to allied health practitioners such as physiotherapy, to support their recovery.

10 Follow-up should be scheduled at around 1–2 weeks. Most patients by this time will be on a trajectory to recovery and further reassurance and education may be all that is required. Patients should be encouraged to participate in regular physical activity to reduce the risk of subsequent flares of back pain. In patients who are failing to improve, reassessment for red flags, exploration of yellow flags and escalation of therapy may be needed.

11 More intensive support may be required in patients with complex pain precipitants or barriers to recovery. Such patients require a biopsychosocial approach to their pain, including management of distress and disability, medical comorbidities and comorbid depression or anxiety if present.

12 Psychological therapies, in particular referral for cognitive behavioural therapy, are recommended in high risk patients or those with refractory back pain.

13 A structured exercise programme is a core recommendation for patients with persistent back pain, and referral to a physiotherapist is recommended.

14 A multidisciplinary rehabilitation programme is advised in patients who are at high risk for poor outcomes or those who progress to chronic back pain. Such programmes combine physical and psychological therapies and have been shown to result in moderate improvement in pain in the short term, although longer-term effects may be smaller.

15 The adverse effects of opioid analgesia use are being increasingly recognised, and they should only be prescribed when other medications are contraindicated, ineffective or not tolerated. Their use requires careful risk–benefit assessment and is strongly discouraged in the setting of chronic back pain. As with any medications, opioids should be used at the lowest possible dose, and their prescription regularly reviewed for evidence of benefit, and ceased in the absence of improvement.

16 Commonly recognised side-effects of opioid use include GI effects such as constipation and nausea, and CNS effects such as sedation (which can affect driving, decision-making and work participation). Less commonly recognised but important side-effects also include potentiation of sleep apnoea, increased risk of falls (particularly in the elderly) and possible interactions with immune function. In addition to these side-effects, there is a phenomenon known as 'opioid-induced hyperalgesia' which paradoxically amplifies pain through sensitisation of the nervous system.

17 Dependence on and tolerance to opioid medications can develop, resulting in a cycle of dose escalation (with associated increased risk of toxicity) without corresponding increases in analgesic benefit. Psychological dependence can also develop, together resulting in significant difficulties when attempting to reduce doses in the longer term.

18 Cortisone injections have not been shown to be of benefit in patients with non-specific back pain. They may have a role in severe or refractory radiculopathy, where immediate reductions in pain are seen in some patients, although benefits are short-term. Limited evidence suggests no benefit of epidural steroid injections for spinal stenosis.

19 Currently there is no evidence to support surgery in patients with non-specific low back pain. There may be a role for surgery in patients with radiculopathy (with congruent symptoms/signs and imaging findings) or spinal canal stenosis where conservative management has failed. Nevertheless, long-term outcomes with surgery remain comparable to non-operative management in many cases, and the presence of yellow flags predicts poorer outcome to surgery, so patients should be carefully selected, and realistic expectations of improvement established.

CASE 96: Osteoarthritis

History

- A **61-year-old** [1] **female** [2] presents with a **several year history** [3] of gradually worsening **bilateral knee pain** [4].
- The pain is **brought on by walking but relieved by rest** [5] and she has **difficulty managing stairs** [6].
- The pain does not **wake her up at night** [7], but she does find it takes a **few minutes to get going after a period of rest** [8].
- She previously played **competitive netball** [9] but had to **give up her previously active lifestyle** [10] due to pain, and consequently has become significantly **overweight** [11].
- She also reports some mild pain in the **small joints of her hands** [12] towards the end of the day, and intermittent pain in the **right groin** [13].
- Her **mother and older sister** [14] have both previously been diagnosed with arthritis due to **'cartilage wear and tear'** [15].

[1] Older age is the biggest risk factor for primary osteoarthritis (OA). Onset is typically over the age of 50 and prevalence increases with age. Symptomatic OA under the age of 40 should prompt heightened consideration of a secondary cause (such as previous joint damage or a predisposing systemic disease, e.g. haemochromatosis, acromegaly).

[2] Female gender is another non-modifiable risk factor for OA and is associated with around double the risk of developing the disease.

[3] Osteoarthritis is a progressive disease which worsens over months to years and is one of the most common causes of chronic joint pain (defined as present for at least six weeks). Inflammatory arthritis (e.g. rheumatoid), crystal arthritis (e.g. gout, pseudogout), chronic joint infections (e.g. mycobacterial, fungal) and joint tumours may also produce chronic arthritis but typically will be clinically distinguishable due to their inflammatory quality or associated systemic symptoms.

[4] Weight-bearing joints such as the knees are commonly affected by OA. Other non-inflammatory processes that may similarly present with chronic mechanical knee pain include conditions such as ligamentous or meniscal damage, chondromalacia patellae, bursitis and patellofemoral pain syndrome. Note many of these additional pathologies can occur (and may be more common) with comorbid OA.

[5] This pattern of joint pain is characteristic of mechanical joint pain. In contrast, inflammatory joint pain is typically worse after rest and improves with movement and is associated with prominent stiffness, including more than an hour of stiffness in the morning upon waking. Patients with inflammatory joint pain may have systemic symptoms such as fever, sweats and loss of weight. Differentiating mechanical from inflammatory symptoms is one of the most important aspects of a joint pain history.

[6] Difficulty with stairs and other knee-bending activities raises the possibility of patellofemoral compartment involvement as part of this patient's knee OA, which typically produces anterior knee pain with exacerbating movements. The other two knee joint compartments affected by OA are the medial tibiofemoral compartment (the most common initial site of involvement) and the lateral tibiofemoral compartment (less commonly affected).

[7] While nocturnal pain can be a feature of advanced OA, it should be considered a 'red flag' symptom that prompts consideration of serious diagnoses such as bone or joint infection, malignancy or fracture, particularly if there are risk factors for these conditions. It can also be a feature of inflammatory arthritis.

[8] This phenomenon of stiffness and pain after immobility is referred to as joint 'gelling', and typically lasts <15 minutes in the setting of OA. This is in contrast to true inflammatory joint stiffness, which is more prolonged.

[9] Biomechanical factors are a risk factor for OA. This includes previous joint injury or overuse (e.g. through sport or occupation), as well as patients with abnormal joint structure (e.g. congenital joint dysplasia) or abnormal joint movement (e.g. hypermobility syndromes). It should be noted, however, that regular low impact exercise is protective, as mechanical loading is required to maintain cartilage integrity.

[10] It is important to appreciate the functional impact of OA on the patient, as this affects patient management. Exploring psychosocial aspects is also significant due to associations of

OA with chronic pain, depression and reduced quality of life. Acknowledging and addressing these factors forms part of a holistic approach to any patient with chronic arthritis and pain.

11 Overweight and obesity is the most important modifiable risk factor for OA, particularly of the knees. It is likely due to a combination of biomechanical factors and the metabolic effects of adipose tissue; hence the association is not only seen with weight-bearing joints, but also other joints affected by OA, such as the hands.

12 Classically, OA affects multiple joints with a typical joint distribution including the spine, hips, knees, hands and feet. Primary OA is less common in the wrists and shoulders. Features of OA of the hands include involvement of the distal and proximal interphalangeal joints, often with bony swelling (Heberden's and Bouchard's nodes, respectively), and carpometacarpal joint disease, which produces squaring of the thumb. Metacarpophalangeal involvement is unusual and should prompt consideration of alternative pathology,

including crystal arthropathy, rheumatoid arthritis and haemochromatosis.

13 Groin pain is often a feature of hip joint pathology. This is significant in this case, not only because it may represent involvement of the hip joint, but also due to the fact that pain generated at the hip may radiate to the knee and be mistaken as knee pain.

14 Genetics plays an important role in the development of OA and may account for up to 60–70% of the risk of developing disease, particularly involvement of the cervical and lumbar spine and the hands.

15 Osteoarthritis is a disease of the whole joint, including the bone, ligaments, muscles and cartilage. This involves a complex interplay of biomechanical factors, genetics, local inflammation and cellular processes. This interplay of factors is not completely understood. The end result is destruction of articular cartilage and loss of the cartilage matrix integrity, with secondary bony changes leading to sclerosis and osteophyte formation.

Examination

- The patient is overweight with a **BMI of 34**[1] but otherwise looks **systemically well**[2].
- She walked normally into the room without any **gait aids**[3].
- Inspection of the knees reveals a mild **varus deformity**[4] and mild **quadriceps wasting**[5] bilaterally.
- There is some **bony swelling**[6] over the joint, but no warmth or detectable **joint effusion**[7] on palpation.
- There are no specific areas of **focal tenderness**[8] and no **Baker's cyst**[9] posteriorly.

- Upon moving the knee joint, there is relatively preserved **range of motion**[10], but some **pain elicited at the extremes**[11].
- Palpable **crepitus**[12] is appreciable on movement.
- **Ligamentous and meniscal tests**[13] were normal.
- Examination of the **hips**[14], **ankles and feet**[15] and **spine**[16] was normal.
- **Heberden's and Bouchard's nodes**[17] were seen on examination of the hands, while the **wrists, elbows and shoulders**[18] examined normally.
- A brief examination of **other organ systems**[19] was unremarkable.

1 Obesity is the major modifiable risk factor for OA; therefore it is important to quantify this on examination, counsel the patient and monitor their weight over time.

2 Unlike some patients with an active inflammatory arthritis, patients with OA do not look systemically unwell as a direct consequence of their joint disease.

3 Assessment of gait and use of gait aids helps to judge the functional impact of lower limb arthritis and screen for biomechanical issues. Patients may have an antalgic gait due to pain on weight-bearing. Hip OA may be associated with a Trendelenburg gait (characterised by the trunk leaning to the affected side and pelvic rotation or drop on the other side). Muscle bulk, limb alignment and foot abnormalities (e.g. flat arches) are other factors identified on gait examination that may be a relevant contributing factor or consequence of OA.

4 Varus (bow-leg) and valgus (knock-knee) deformity can both cause knee OA and occur as a result of OA. Varus deformity is associated with medial joint compartment narrowing (the more commonly affected compartment) and valgus deformity with lateral joint compartment narrowing.

5 The quadriceps muscles are composed of the rectus femoris and vastus lateralis, intermedius and medialis. Weakness and wasting of this muscle group is a hallmark of knee OA, as well as being an important determinant of functional performance.

6 Bony swelling in OA occurs due to the development of bony osteophytes, which are irregular and disorganised bone growths that form around the lips of the joint margin. This type of firm swelling should be distinguishable from the bogginess associated with inflammatory arthritis, which produces a spongier feel at the joint line.

7 Joint effusions arise as a result of excess synovial fluid production due to inflammation of the synovial lining. They are classically a feature of inflammatory arthritis, but small to moderate effusions can also occur as a secondary phenomenon in osteoarthritic joints. There are two characteristic examination tests to detect a knee joint effusion; these are the patellar tap sign which allows detection of larger effusions, and the bulge sign which is more sensitive for smaller effusions.

8 Tenderness along the joint line may be a feature of OA. At the knee, this may be felt around the tibiofemoral and/or patellofemoral joint compartments. Specific areas of tenderness may also occur with other knee pathology, such as tenderness distal to the knee over the medial tibia with pes anserine bursitis, or lateral tenderness over the femoral condyle with iliotibial band syndrome.

9 A Baker's cyst typically presents as posterior knee swelling and occurs as a herniation of the knee joint synovium between the heads of the gastrocnemius. It commonly occurs in patients with underlying joint pathology, such as OA. Baker's cysts are often asymptomatic, but can cause pain or tightness, and in some cases rupture into the calf muscle, leading to swelling, redness and pain which can mimic deep vein thrombosis.

10 Reduced range of motion and deformities can occur with advanced OA due to structural deterioration and asymmetric loss of joint space. Normal range of motion at the knee is 0–5° of extension (straight leg) and 135° of flexion (fully bent).

11 Pain may be elicited at the extremes of joint movement in OA and on weight-bearing. Pain arises from both intra- and peri-articular sources, including the periosteum and subchondral bone, capsular distension with effusions, local inflammation of the synovium, bursae or tendons, ligament degeneration and muscle spasm. Pain does not, however, arise from the articular cartilage itself, which is avascular and aneural.

12 Crepitus is the crackling or grating sensation that can be heard or felt on movement of an affected joint. It is frequently seen in OA on passive range of motion, due to the irregularity of opposing cartilage surfaces.

13 There are a number of described tests to examine for ligamentous and meniscal pathology. These include varus/valgus stress of collateral ligaments, anterior/posterior drawer tests for cruciate ligaments and McMurray's test for meniscal tears. These tests have suboptimal sensitivity and specificity, however, and generally are applied to acute tears, rather than patients with chronic degenerative pathology.

14 Osteoarthritis of the hips typically presents with groin pain (84% of cases) and/or buttock pain (76% of cases). Anterior or posterior thigh pain, and pain around the knee are other common sites where hip OA pain is felt. Importantly, lateral hip pain is less associated with hip OA, and is suggestive of other pathology, such as trochanteric bursitis.

15 The most common distal lower limb joints involved in OA are the first MTPJ, which can produce a hallux valgus appearance, and the subtalar joints, which result in painful inversion/eversion and foot pain on walking.

16 Osteoarthritis of the spine typically affects the lumbar and cervical regions and is a common contributor to chronic neck and back pain. Degenerative spinal disease results in pain and reduced range of motion, and can be complicated by nerve impingement.

17 Heberden's and Bouchard's nodes are the bony swellings which result from osteophytosis at the distal (Heberden's) and proximal (Bouchard's) interphalangeal joints.

18 The wrists, elbows and shoulders are unusual locations of primary OA. They are more likely to be involved in patients with pre-existing damage to these joints, such as those with comorbid inflammatory arthritis, or due to previous trauma or injury.

19 Primary OA is not associated with any specific abnormalities in other organ systems. However, it is prudent to perform a brief screen, to pick up causes of secondary OA or detect systemic abnormalities suggestive of alternative joint pathology.

Investigations

- **Minimal further investigation** [1] is conducted, given the suggestive clinical features for OA on history and examination.
- Routine blood tests recently performed including an **FBE** [2], and **renal and liver function tests** [3] were normal.
- Inflammatory markers including **CRP and ESR** [4] were also normal.

- A **plain radiograph** [5] with **weight-bearing views** [6] of the knees bilaterally showed mild **medial joint space narrowing** [7] as well as one or two small **osteophytes** [8] and mild **subchondral sclerosis** [9] without any **bony cysts** [10].
- No further imaging such as **MRI scanning** [11] was performed in this instance.

1 The diagnosis of osteoarthritis is largely based on the presence of suggestive clinical features, and further investigation is often not required. Indications for further investigation include diagnostic uncertainty (e.g. possibility of inflammatory pathology) or where results may inform choice of management.

2 Full blood count and other basic blood tests are expected to be normal in OA, and if abnormalities are detected, this should prompt assessment for alternative causes.

3 Renal and liver function tests are relevant for the selection of analgesic agents which may form part of this patient's OA management. For example, NSAIDs should be avoided in patients with renal impairment, and liver dysfunction would prompt avoidance or dose reduction of agents such as paracetamol.

4 Inflammatory markers are useful to help differentiate mechanical and inflammatory joint disease and support the findings of an accurate joint history and examination. CRP and ESR are expected to be normal in OA.

5 Plain radiographs are the first-line imaging modality in patients with OA. X-rays are not completely reliable as a diagnostic tool, however, and moderate changes are needed before X-ray abnormalities develop. There is also poor correlation between a patient's symptoms and the presence or severity of changes on X-ray. For example, >50% of adults above the age of 65 have radiographic evidence of OA, but less than a quarter report any symptoms. The hallmark findings of OA on X-ray are captured in the acronym 'LOSS', standing for loss of joint space, osteophyte formation, subchondral sclerosis and subchondral cysts.

6 Weight-bearing views are typically performed to assess radiographic OA changes of the knee, as this gives the most accurate representation of structural alignment and joint space narrowing in the functionally relevant position.

7 Joint space narrowing reflects the cartilage loss of OA, which is often asymmetrical (eccentric), in contrast to inflammatory processes which tend to produce a more concentric loss of joint space. The degree of joint space loss in OA predicts disease progression. Joint space narrowing with knee OA is more commonly seen medially, while with OA of the hip it is seen more prominently at the superior joint margin. It should be noted that cartilage itself is not seen on X-ray.

8 Osteophytes are bony spurs that occur at the joint margins. They reflect an attempt at new bone formation as a response to cartilage loss. Osteophytes should be distinguished from enthesophytes, which are bony growths at the site of ligament or tendon attachments and are a feature of spondyloarthropathies such as ankylosing spondylitis or psoriatic arthritis.

9 Subchondral sclerosis (whitening in the area under the cartilage) is seen due to thickening of the subchondral bone, which occurs as part of the bone remodelling process in response to cartilage loss.

10 Corticated bony cysts may be seen in the subchondral bone in regions of OA. They are a less common radiographic feature compared to other findings.

11 While MRI imaging detects earlier cartilage changes and bone marrow oedema in OA, its role in routine clinical care of OA is not established. However, in patients who present with atypical features, highly inflammatory features, or where there is diagnostic uncertainty, MRI is generally the preferred modality for joint imaging.

Management

Short-term

Provide **education** [1] to the patient about the diagnosis of OA and principles of **self-management** [2]. Discuss **weight loss** [3] strategies and recommend regular **physical exercise** [4]. Consider referral to **physiotherapy or occupational therapy** [5] to assist with physical functioning. Patients may wish to explore **complementary therapy** [6] in addition to standard care. Management can usually be coordinated in **primary care** [7], sometimes with a specialist **referral to Rheumatology** [8] in complex cases.

Long-term

If non-pharmacological strategies are insufficient, commence first-line **analgesia** [9] such as **paracetamol** [10] and/or **NSAID** [11] after consideration of **side-effects and safety** [12]. **Duloxetine** [13] is sometimes used. Avoidance of **opioids** [14] is preferable. **Topical preparations** [15] can also be used on painful areas. Some patients may wish to try **glucosamine or chondroitin** [16] preparations. **Intra-articular injections** [17] of corticosteroids and/or hyaluronic acid may be offered in some specific cases. Severe or refractory cases require surgical referral for consideration of a **joint replacement** [18].

1 It is important to provide patients with a basic understanding of their arthritis, including modifiable risk factors (particularly weight) and the general management approach. Education of this nature may allow greater monitoring and self-management of their condition, and thus improved outcomes including pain, function and quality of life.

2 Self-management is an important concept in patients with chronic disease, designed to promote day-to-day patient responsibility and adaptability around their condition. Self-management strategies in OA may include appropriate initiation of additional analgesia during flares, use of heat/cold to modify symptoms and pacing daily activities.

3 Strong evidence supports weight loss, particularly in knee OA, and even modest losses can produce clinically important improvements in pain and function. A reasonable goal may be a loss of 5–10% of body weight. Referral to a dietitian and/or exercise physiologist may help patients with weight loss strategies.

4 Appropriate exercise therapy improves strength, fitness and mobility in OA, with resultant benefits in pain and function. Aerobic exercises and resistance training, including hydrotherapy, have been shown to be safe and effective. Quadriceps strengthening is particularly important for knee OA. Some patients will benefit from a tailored and supported exercise programme to individualise exercises and maintain motivation.

5 Physiotherapists can help patients with OA perform appropriate exercises correctly and provide advice about mobility aids such as a single point stick (used in the opposite hand). Occupational therapists provide patients with strategies and assistive devices to help manage despite functional limitations.

6 Patients may choose to engage with a diverse range of complementary therapies, from physical therapies like massage and acupuncture, through vitamin or herbal supplements, to hypnotherapy and laser therapy. Most of these therapies have low level evidence at best, generated from poor quality trials.

7 Given its frequency, most OA is managed by GPs. Because of the chronic nature of the condition, regular follow-up in primary care is beneficial to promote weight optimisation, encourage self-management, monitor pain, disability and quality of life, titrate analgesia and refer for consideration of surgery when appropriate.

8 Rheumatologists are sometimes referred patients with OA. Their role is often in the diagnostic stage if there is uncertainty about the presence of inflammatory disease and to guide strategies that may delay or prevent the need for surgery.

9 Symptom-directed analgesia is the mainstay of pharmacological management in OA. There are at this stage no disease-modifying medical therapies available.

10 Paracetamol was previously regarded as first-line analgesia for patients with OA; however, more recent evidence suggests little superiority over placebo. Nevertheless, given its relatively favourable safety profile, a trial of regular paracetamol is reasonable, especially in the elderly or those in whom other agents are contraindicated.

11 NSAIDs are generally more effective than paracetamol for pain in OA. The main limitations of NSAIDs are potential adverse effects, especially with routine use.

12 Consideration should be given to GI, renal and cardiovascular toxicity prior to commencing NSAIDs. Cyclo-oxygenase-2 selective NSAIDs and/or concomitant proton pump inhibitor use may reduce GI ulcer risk.

13 For pain that is refractory to paracetamol and/or NSAIDs, opioids are no longer recommended, given their significant adverse event profile. Although duloxetine is not approved in the UK for OA, studies have shown that it significantly improved pain compared with placebo. More research is still underway regarding use of antidepressants on OA and this may be reflected in future NICE guidelines.

14 Opioids may provide short-term pain reduction compared with placebo in OA. However, they should ideally only be prescribed as a last resort, for short-term use, and in low doses. There is a significant risk of adverse effects (such as constipation, nausea and sedation) and the potential for the development of tolerance, dependence, misuse, hyperalgesia, falls and fatal overdoses with long-term use. Newer agents such as tramadol and tapentadol have opioid activity and additional noradrenaline and/or serotonin uptake inhibition. Similar principles of use apply to these agents, as with pure opioids, since adverse effects can be significant, particularly in the elderly.

15 Randomised trials have demonstrated the efficacy of topical NSAIDs and capsaicin, especially for knee OA. Local application means fewer systemic side-effects; however, skin irritation can occur.

16 Glucosamine and chondroitin are glycosaminoglycan derivatives which form the building blocks of articular cartilage. There is mixed evidence as to the efficacy of these agents in OA, but they are generally considered safe. If patients are keen, it is reasonable to trial these medications, with continuation only if benefit is obtained.

17 Intra-articular injections of corticosteroid and/or hyaluronic acid are sometimes performed in patients with OA, especially when surgical intervention is contraindicated. Although lacking a strong evidence base, short-term benefit is seen in a subset of patients, and therefore the procedure can be offered for painful joints refractory to other management strategies, after discussion of the relative benefits and risks (including introduction of infection, bleeding, cartilage atrophy, and potentially accelerated progression of OA).

18 Joint replacement is the mainstay surgical intervention for advanced OA, most commonly performed for the hip or knee. Most patients report improved pain and function post joint replacement surgery. Surgery is associated with several risks, however (including anaesthetic risks, infection, venous thrombosis, prosthesis malfunction, nerve damage and wound complications), and therefore is reserved for patients with severe clinical symptoms due to OA despite maximally tolerated non-pharmacological and pharmacological management. Other surgical procedures (e.g. joint fusion, osteotomy) may be considered in selected cases.

CASE 97: Polymyositis

History

- A **39-year-old female** [1] presents with a **2-week history** [2] of progressive **weakness and myalgias** [3] affecting her **arms and legs** [4].
- She is normally **fit and active** [5] but is now **tiring easily** [6] and feels **breathless on exertion** [7].
- She also reports **painful hands** [8] and her **fingers changing colour** [9] in the cold weather but no **rash** [10] or other **symptoms of a connective tissue disease** [11].
- She has not had difficulty with **speech or swallowing** [12].
- She has otherwise **been in good health recently** [13] and does not take any **regular medications** [14].
- She has no relevant **family history** [15].

[1] Polymyositis is one of three conditions described under the umbrella term of 'idiopathic inflammatory myopathies'. It has a peak age of onset between the ages of 30 and 60 and women are 2–3 times more likely to be affected than men. Of the other idiopathic inflammatory myopathies, dermatomyositis affects a similar demographic, while inclusion body myositis is more typically a disease of older patients (usually aged over 50) and occurs more frequently in men.

[2] The onset of symptoms in patients with polymyositis is variable. Patients usually present acutely or subacutely; however, symptoms may initially fluctuate episodically or in some cases gradually progress.

[3] Weakness is the most common feature of polymyositis and is associated with muscle pain in around half of patients. While these symptoms suggest pathology at the level of the muscle, there is a broad range of differential diagnoses to be considered, including inflammatory myositis, infectious myositis, rhabdomyolysis, metabolic or endocrine derangements, drugs or toxins and congenital myopathies. Weakness should also prompt consideration of neuromuscular and neurological causes, particularly in the absence of an elevated creatine kinase (CK) or other objective evidence of muscle disease.

[4] Symmetrical and proximal limb muscle weakness is the typical distribution for polymyositis (and dermatomyositis). The pelvic and shoulder girdles are the sites most commonly affected. In contrast, inclusion body myositis has a predilection for the knee extensors and finger flexors.

[5] A young, fit and active patient has significant reserve and therefore even a mild degree of weakness should be taken seriously as it likely suggests significant pathology. Any recent changes in physical activity or preceding heavy exercise is also relevant history, as this may be a trigger for rhabdomyolysis.

[6] Enquire about the reasons for this patient's easy fatigability. Possibilities may be exercise limitation due to pain, weakness or breathlessness, generalised lethargy, or a combination of factors. Quantifying exercise tolerance is useful in judging the severity and impact of disease and as a baseline for monitoring over time.

[7] Exertional dyspnoea is a concerning feature in this patient and one which warrants urgent attention. It may signify respiratory muscle weakness with the risk of respiratory failure, cardiac muscle involvement, interstitial lung disease or pulmonary hypertension. Other cardiorespiratory symptoms such as coughing, palpitations, orthopnoea and peripheral oedema should be sought.

[8] The nature of these 'painful hands' should be explored further. Ask about symptoms suggestive of an inflammatory arthritis, such as joint pain worse in the morning and better with movement, with associated stiffness. Pain may also result from ischaemia (as occurs with Raynaud's phenomenon) or a painful peripheral neuropathy.

[9] This change in colour in the cold weather is suspicious for Raynaud's phenomenon and should be clarified further. Raynaud's phenomenon occurs due to peripheral digital ischaemia from vasospasm of the digital arteries and arterioles. It may be primary or occur secondary to other diseases, such as connective tissue diseases. It is characterised by three phases; pallor, cyanosis and then erythema due to reactive hyperaemia.

[10] A number of rashes may occur with an inflammatory myositis. Dermatomyositis has pathognomonic cutaneous features, and idiopathic inflammatory myopathies can also occur as an overlap syndrome with lupus or scleroderma, which can be associated with their own characteristic skin changes.

11 The umbrella term 'connective tissue disease' encompasses a range of related multisystem disorders. The connective tissue diseases are rheumatoid arthritis, SLE, polymyositis and dermatomyositis, scleroderma, Sjögren's syndrome, mixed connective tissue disease and undifferentiated connective tissue disease. Although labelled as distinct entities, there is often a significant degree of overlap, and myositis in particular can occur as a feature overlapping with any of the other connective tissue diseases. For this reason, a thorough history should include asking about symptoms of all these possibly associated diseases, e.g. joint pains, rash, sicca symptoms, mouth ulcers, alopecia, pleuritic chest pain, respiratory symptoms, Raynaud's, reflux, and so forth.

12 It is important to identify symptoms that may suggest muscle involvement beyond the limbs alone. These include truncal weakness, facial weakness, abnormalities of speech or swallow, respiratory weakness and cardiac dysfunction. If not identified early, such involvement can lead to severe consequences (e.g. heart failure, respiratory failure, aspiration), and therefore these patients should be monitored very closely.

13 Relevant illnesses include anything that may predispose to secondary causes of muscle dysfunction (e.g. electrolyte derangement), infections which can induce myositis (e.g. influenza, enteroviruses, toxoplasmosis), malignancy (due to associations of myositis with paraneoplastic syndromes) or prodromal extramuscular symptoms that may be part of a systemic disease with muscular involvement (e.g. vasculitis).

14 A family history of muscle disease may point to rare hereditary syndromes such as metabolic myopathies, mitochondrial myopathies and muscular dystrophies.

15 A drug history may identify agents associated with muscle disease. Statins in particular can cause a wide range of muscle pathology, ranging from simple myalgias (pain without CK elevation) to myositis (CK elevation), rhabdomyolysis (CK elevation with myoglobinuria or renal impairment) or necrotising myopathy (an immune-mediated myopathy that does not improve with cessation of statin and requires treatment with immunosuppression). Remember to ask about non-prescription medications (e.g. herbal preparations) and illicit drug use (e.g. cocaine, heroin) which can also cause muscle toxicity.

Examination

- The patient is **afebrile** [1] and **respiratory vital signs** [2] are normal.
- **Muscle power is graded at 4+** [3] in the **proximal upper and lower limbs** [4] but **normal elsewhere** [5].
- There is no **rash** [6] on close examination of the **knuckles** [7], **eyelids** [8] and **other sites** [9]; however, there is some **thickening, roughness and fissuring** [10] of the hands, especially over the lateral aspect of her fingers.
- There is **mild synovitis** [11] of the wrist and hand joints.
- Examination of the respiratory system identifies **fine bibasal crackles** [12] and **normal chest expansion** [13].
- There are no signs of **pulmonary hypertension** [14].

1 Fever can be a systemic feature of inflammatory myositis, particularly subtypes with more acute onset and rapid progression.

2 Traditional respiratory vital signs such as respiratory rate and oxygen saturation on air may be abnormal with severe compromise but are not sensitive indicators. Patients with respiratory muscle weakness or interstitial lung disease will not become hypoxic until the condition is advanced and therefore other measures such as a blood gas, spirometry and imaging are required to detect abnormalities in a timely fashion.

3 Muscle power is most commonly graded using the modified MRC scale for manual muscle testing. Those examining should be familiar with the grading system, which ranges from 5 (representing normal muscle power) to 0, where there is no muscle contraction. 4+ power represents definite but slight weakness. Although useful for tracking weakness, there clearly may be inter-rater variability with a grading system of this nature.

4 Assessment of muscle power of the limbs in patients with polymyositis typically finds a pattern of proximal muscle weakness; more so than distal weakness.

5 Neck weakness (e.g. poor head control), truncal weakness (e.g. difficulty sitting up without limb support) or bulbar weakness (e.g. nasal speech, weak cough) may occur and be a feature of more diffuse or severe muscle involvement.

6 Clinically, dermatomyositis is differentiated from polymyositis by the presence of one or more characteristic cutaneous features. Underlying immune mechanisms, antibody associations and biopsy findings may also distinguish between the two forms of myositis.

7 Gottron's sign is pathognomonic for dermatomyositis. This rash appears as violaceous roughened papules or macules, most typically over the extensor MCPJs, but can also occur over the PIPJs, elbows or knees.

8 A purplish or lilac rash over the eyelids, with or without associated swelling, is known as a heliotrope rash and is another classic cutaneous sign of dermatomyositis.

9 Look for additional cutaneous signs suggesting dermatomyositis, including a shawl sign (a macular rash in the sun-exposed upper back and V-line of the chest), a more generalised photosensitive rash (e.g. affecting the face, neck and arms) and holster sign (a rash affecting the thigh over the site a gun holster would sit). Vascular changes such as nailfold erythema or dilated capillaries, and active Raynaud's phenomenon should also be noted and can occur in association with inflammatory myositis.

10 This appearance is suggestive of 'mechanic's hands' which refers to painful, roughened erythematous and hyperkeratotic fissuring or cracking of the palmar and lateral aspects of the fingers. This finding is associated with the "anti-synthetase syndrome", which is a subset of inflammatory myositis often associated with more acute onset, interstitial lung disease and particular antibodies to aminoacyl-transfer RNA synthetases, the most well-known of which is Jo-1.

11 Signs of active synovitis on joint examination include joint line tenderness, bogginess, effusions and stress tenderness. Arthralgias (pain) or arthritis (pain and swelling) occur in around half of patients with polymyositis.

12 Interstitial lung disease associated with connective tissue diseases is most commonly basal predominant, bilateral and results in the characteristic mid- to late fine inspiratory crackles typically associated with pulmonary fibrosis.

13 Chest expansion may be reduced with advanced fibrotic disease, or in the setting of respiratory muscle weakness. Look for accessory muscle use as an additional indicator of respiratory muscle weakness. Normal chest expansion is >5cm.

14 A focused cardiac examination assessing for signs of pulmonary hypertension is an important part of assessing patients with a suspected or confirmed connective tissue disease. Primary pulmonary hypertension may arise, particularly in association with scleroderma and mixed connective tissue disease. Patients with interstitial lung disease can develop secondary pulmonary hypertension as the disease progresses. Signs of pulmonary hypertension include a loud P2, right ventricular heave, tricuspid regurgitation and in more advanced stages, signs of right heart failure.

Investigations

- Blood tests show an **elevated CK of 2300** [1].
- There is a **mild transaminitis** [2] on liver function tests.
- **Renal function** [3] is normal.
- **Inflammatory markers** [4] are mildly elevated, with a CRP of 28 and ESR of 36.
- The **ANA is positive** [5] at a titre of **1:640** [6].
- The ENA panel returns positive for the **Jo-1 antibody** [7], with the other **myositis-specific antibodies** [8] returning negative.

- **Electromyography (EMG)** [9] is consistent with myositis and **MRI of the thighs** [10] shows **diffuse inflammatory changes** [11] bilaterally.
- A **targeted muscle biopsy** [12] is performed and shows **lymphocytic infiltrate** [13] and **muscle fibre injury** [14] consistent with polymyositis.
- A chest X-ray shows basal **reticular and ground-glass changes** [15] and high resolution CT confirms a pattern consistent with **non-specific interstitial pneumonia** [16].
- Lung function testing shows a **restrictive deficit** [17].

1 Muscle-related enzymes such as creatine kinase (CK) and lactate dehydrogenase (LDH) are elevated in most cases of inflammatory myositis and fluctuate with disease activity. In rare cases extramuscular features may be present in the absence of clinical muscle disease (amyopathic dermatomyositis). CK may also appear disproportionately low in relation to disease activity in those with significant muscle atrophy.

2 Patients with myositis may falsely appear to have abnormal liver function test because the transaminases (AST and ALT) are also muscle-related enzymes. Recognising this may prevent unnecessary investigation into deranged liver

function tests, or conversely prompt testing of the CK in patients with an unexplained transaminitis.

3 Renal involvement is not typical for patients with polymyositis or dermatomyositis; however, given the possibility of overlap connective tissue disease syndromes, patients should be screened with renal function and a urine test for proteinuria and glomerular red cells. In rare cases active polymyositis can be complicated by rhabdomyolysis, which is another occasion when assessment of renal function and testing for urinary myoglobin may be helpful.

4 Similar to other connective tissue diseases, inflammatory markers may be elevated in line with disease activity in patients with polymyositis.

5 The ANA is positive in most patients (around 80%) with polymyositis.

6 The titre of the ANA refers to the greatest dilution of serum at which the pattern of immunofluorescence is still seen. In general, titres >1:160 are significant but need to be interpreted in the clinical context, as the ANA can be positive in otherwise healthy individuals.

7 Anti-Jo-1 antibodies are the most common type of anti-synthetase antibody. These antibodies are found in around 15–20% of patients with polymyositis. Interstitial lung disease is much more common in these patients, which confers a poorer prognosis.

8 An increasing number of antibodies associated particularly with inflammatory myositis have been identified and are being routinely tested to help classify patients into specific phenotypic subsets. Some of these antibodies are known as 'myositis-associated antibodies' and are primarily found in overlap forms of myositis. These antibodies include anti-PM-Scl (typically found in overlap myositis with scleroderma) and anti-U1-RNP (associated with mixed connective tissue disease), among others. There is also a group of 'myositis-specific antibodies' which are thought to be more specific for polymyositis and dermatomyositis and are usually mutually exclusive. These antibodies have certain phenotypic associations. For example, anti-Jo-1 antibodies are associated with 'anti-synthetase syndrome', anti-SRP antibodies are associated with a necrotising form of myositis, anti-TIF1 gamma antibodies are linked with cancer-associated inflammatory myositis, and anti-MDA5 antibodies with amyopathic dermatomyositis, cutaneous ulcers and rapidly progressive interstitial lung disease.

9 Electromyography (EMG) and nerve conduction studies (NCS) can be performed to help differentiate between weakness of different causes (e.g. neurological, neuromuscular or muscular). EMG findings in polymyositis may include short duration, polyphasic potentials of low amplitude with evidence of membrane irritability.

10 Generally imaging is targeted to an area of muscle which is symptomatically involved, to maximise the likelihood of identifying affected muscles, which can then be specifically targeted with a biopsy. The quadriceps are often involved and accessible for biopsy, hence the thighs are often imaged when looking for inflammatory myositis.

11 MRI of the muscles can identify muscle oedema, which indicates inflammation as well as showing anatomical detail and atrophy. The findings are not specific, however, and can also be seen in rhabdomyolysis and genetic myopathies.

12 Muscle biopsy is the gold standard for the diagnosis of idiopathic inflammatory myositis. Targeting the biopsy to a site involved on MRI and performing the biopsy prior to commencement of treatment increases the yield. In patients with dermatomyositis a skin biopsy may be an alternative means of confirming the diagnosis; however, the disadvantage of this is that muscle symptoms cannot be definitively attributed to dermatomyositis. Skin biopsy changes consistent with dermatomyositis are an interface dermatitis with epidermal atrophy and perivascular lymphocytic infiltrate. Biopsy findings in cutaneous lupus can appear very similar.

13 Lymphocytic infiltrate, predominantly within the fascicle, is typical of polymyositis. There is a predominance of CD8 cytotoxic T cells. This is in contrast to dermatomyositis, where B cells and CD4 helper T cells are more commonly involved, reflecting the different underlying pathophysiology between these two conditions.

14 The pathology of polymyositis involves diffuse myofibril damage. In comparison, dermatomyositis is characterised by immune-mediated injury to both the myofibres and capillaries, with preferential targeting of perifascicular myofibres.

15 These chest X-ray changes are consistent with the clinical findings that suggest interstitial lung disease, which is a common extramuscular manifestation in patients with a polymyositis or dermatomyositis.

16 Non-specific interstitial pneumonia refers to a pattern of interstitial lung disease characterised by ground-glass opacities and reticulonodular changes. It is one of the more common patterns seen in association with connective tissue diseases.

17 Like other causes of interstitial lung disease, a restrictive deficit (reduced forced vital capacity with preserved forced expiratory ratio) and reduced gas diffusion coefficient would be expected and assists with determining the severity of lung disease.

Management

Short-term

Refer to **rheumatology** [1] and other **relevant specialties** [2] as guided by the presence of extramuscular manifestations. Commence **high dose steroids** [3] after **initial diagnostic work-up** [4]. Consider risks associated with weakness, such as **aspiration** [5], **falls** [6] and **respiratory failure** [7]. Monitor **for initial response** [8] to steroids. Screen for possible underlying **malignancy** [9].

Long-term

Wean prednisolone [10] slowly, usually over a period of 9–12 months. Consider adding other **immunosuppressive agents** [11] or commencing **intravenous immunoglobulin** [12] (IVIg) to facilitate steroid dose reduction. Monitor for and manage **steroid-related complications** [13]. Consider enrolment in a **physical therapy or rehabilitation programme** [14]. Ensure the patient has **regular follow-up** [15] assessing disease control and complications.

[1] Patients with polymyositis should usually be managed by a rheumatologist, or other specialist with experience in inflammatory myopathies, as these are rare conditions that often require specialised treatment.

[2] Patients with connective tissue diseases often have multisystem involvement which requires assessment and coordinated management by various specialties. In cases of inflammatory myositis associated with interstitial lung disease, for example, lung-specific monitoring (e.g. lung function tests, serial imaging, functional tests) and management (e.g. home oxygen, lung transplantation) may be best achieved in conjunction with the Respiratory unit. Similarly, input from Dermatology may assist with refractory cutaneous manifestations of dermatomyositis.

[3] Immunosuppression is the mainstay of treatment for polymyositis (and dermatomyositis) and initial treatment is with high dose oral corticosteroids, usually at a dose of around 1mg/kg. Sometimes pulse intravenous methylprednisolone is used for patients who present with severe manifestations (e.g. dysphagia, respiratory weakness) or have a poor response to oral steroids.

[4] Depending on the severity of the manifestations and index of suspicion for the diagnosis, treatment with steroids may commence prior to all the diagnostic information being available (for example, results of antibodies or biopsies may take several days to return). Ideally, however, the muscle biopsy should be completed prior to initiation of high dose steroids to maximise the diagnostic yield.

[5] In patients with bulbar weakness a speech therapy assessment and dietary modifications may be necessary to minimise aspiration risk, in addition to treatment of the underlying immune process.

[6] Falls risk reduction measures should be implemented in the acute phase in patients with significant weakness. Assessment and management by physiotherapists and occupational therapists should be considered.

[7] Patients with possible respiratory muscle involvement should be monitored with regular bedside spirometry to detect deterioration as early as possible. Patients with deteriorating parameters may need to be transferred to a high dependency or intensive care setting, as they may require non-invasive ventilation or occasionally even intubation. In these severe situations early aggressive immunosuppression, such as with pulse steroids and additional agents, is usually indicated.

[8] Response to steroids is signified by improved clinical parameters (e.g. improving muscle power and myalgias) and biochemical markers (e.g. falling CK and inflammatory markers). It can take up to 2–4 weeks for significant improvement to be realised. If patients fail to respond to initial treatment with steroids, alternative diagnoses should be excluded and treatment escalated.

[9] Polymyositis and dermatomyositis can occur as paraneoplastic phenomena and an underlying malignancy should be considered in every patient. Screening practices vary widely and should include at least age-appropriate cancer screening tests (e.g. mammogram, Pap test, faecal occult blood test) with consideration of additional investigations (e.g. CT CAP, endoscopy, PET-CT scan) as guided by symptoms, signs, antibody status (e.g. high risk of malignancy with TIF-1 gamma antibodies and low risk with anti-synthetase antibodies) or other cancer risk factors. Cancer is detected in around 15–30% with dermatomyositis and 10–15% with polymyositis overall, and most are detected within 1 year of the diagnosis of myositis. The most common underlying cancers are adenocarcinomas, but all types of malignancy have been reported.

[10] Steroids are usually tapered slowly over 9–12 months and patients carefully monitored for disease flares which are a common occurrence, particularly with polymyositis.

[11] Other immunosuppressive drugs are used for refractory disease or as a steroid-sparing agent. Options include hydroxychloroquine, methotrexate, azathioprine,

mycophenolate, cyclophosphamide and rituximab; choice depends on the severity of a patient's disease and involved organs, comorbidities and patient preference.

12 IVIg may be used alongside steroids for induction and maintenance of remission in inflammatory myositis and is often a good option in patients with infective complications that limit use of other immunosuppressive agents. IVIg also has some efficacy for extramuscular manifestations such as skin disease and lung disease.

13 Active surveillance and management of steroid-related toxicity should be undertaken, particularly in relation to bone health and metabolic/cardiovascular risk factors.

14 Once treatment is commenced and patients responding, physical rehabilitation should also be encouraged to maximise functional recovery. This is particularly important given that steroid therapy and hospitalisation can contribute to muscle deconditioning.

15 Regular follow-up should be scheduled; initially more frequently as disease control is established and then stretched out once remission is achieved. Monitoring for disease activity (e.g. symptoms, muscle power, muscle enzymes) and treatment complications should form part of each visit. Manifestations in other organ systems (such as interstitial lung disease) will also require specific monitoring and management.

CASE 98: Rheumatoid arthritis

History

- A **38-year-old woman** [1] presents with a **2-month history** [2] of worsening **painful joints** [3] in her **hands and feet** [4].
- The pain is **worse in the morning** [5] and associated with **marked stiffness** [6] and **difficulty using her hands** [7].
- She has recently **lost 3kg of weight unintentionally** [8].
- She denies any **respiratory** [9], **cardiac** [10], **ocular** [11] or **skin** [12] symptoms.
- She had no **preceding illnesses** [13] and is **usually well** [14]; however, she is a **current smoker** [15].
- Her **sister** [16] was diagnosed with rheumatoid arthritis about 1 year ago.
- She lives at home with her **husband** [17].

[1] Rheumatoid arthritis (RA) is around 2–3 times more frequent in women compared to men. It commonly presents between the ages of 30 and 50 but can occur at any age.

[2] Rheumatoid arthritis often has a subacute onset. Inflammatory arthritis symptoms lasting >6 weeks are suggestive and form one component of current classification criteria, in addition to pattern of joint involvement, serology and acute phase reactants.

[3] A clinical approach to joint pain should include eliciting the time course (acute, subacute or chronic), pattern of joint involvement (distribution, symmetry and number of joints, i.e. mono-, oligo- or polyarthritis) and distinguish mechanical vs. inflammatory pain.

[4] A symmetrical small joint polyarthritis is a classic presentation for RA. Less typical presentations include a sudden-onset widespread arthritis, a large joint mono- or oligoarthritis, polymyalgic symptoms or a systemic illness with prominent constitutional symptoms and extra-articular features (rare).

[5] Distinguishing mechanical from inflammatory pain is a core skill of the rheumatological assessment. Diurnal variation in symptoms – with pain that is worse in the morning or after periods of rest and better later in the day or with movement – is classic. This distinction is made more difficult in the presence of comorbid osteoarthritis, which can lead to mixed inflammatory and mechanical symptoms, or in patients with superimposed fibromyalgia.

[6] Joint stiffness is a key feature on history, suggesting an inflammatory basis. Specifically, the duration of early morning stiffness is informative, with morning stiffness lasting more than one hour being highly suggestive of inflammatory arthritis.

[7] It is important to establish functional impact of symptoms as part of an overall assessment in patients with joint disease. Function may be impaired by active joint inflammation, but also as a consequence of secondary irreversible joint damage. Questions may include enquiring about mobility including the use of gait aids, ability to perform personal care and household tasks, and impact of symptoms on work, relationships and hobbies.

[8] Constitutional symptoms such as unintentional weight loss are common in poorly controlled RA and mediated by cytokines such as tumour necrosis factor. In patients with established RA, weight loss should prompt a close review of disease activity, as well as consideration of other differential diagnoses including infection (increased risk with immunosuppression), malignancy (increased risk with RA) and thyroid dysfunction (due to the predisposition towards comorbid autoimmunity).

[9] Pulmonary manifestations of RA include interstitial lung disease, serositis and pulmonary rheumatoid nodules. Symptoms such as pleuritic chest pain, dyspnoea or dry cough may be clues to respiratory involvement.

[10] Pericarditis is the most common cardiac manifestation of RA. Rheumatoid arthritis is also an independent risk factor for coronary artery disease.

[11] Episcleritis and scleritis are recognised extra-articular features. Sicca symptoms (dry eyes and mouth) may also occur with secondary Sjögren's syndrome.

[12] There are a number of possible mucocutaneous manifestations including rheumatoid nodules, cutaneous vasculitis and mouth ulcers. Rarely, neutrophilic dermatoses such as Sweet's syndrome or pyoderma gangrenosum can also occur.

13 Recent infective symptoms are relevant, as a polyarthritis mimicking RA can result from infections such as parvovirus B19, hepatitis, and arboviruses such as dengue fever and chikungunya. Such infections can sometimes be associated with a positive rheumatoid factor. Viral-associated arthritis is normally self-limited, but a small proportion of patients may develop a chronic course.

14 Establishing a patient's comorbidities has significant implications for the management of RA. Considerations should include chronic infections (e.g. hepatitis, latent TB), malignancy (past or current), kidney or liver dysfunction, lung disease (especially fibrosis), cardiac failure and peptic ulcer disease.

15 Smoking and periodontal disease are some of the well-described environmental risk factors for RA. In particular, smoking is associated with antibodies against citrullinated proteins and may be synergistic with genetic risk factors such as the shared epitope. Furthermore, in people with established RA, ongoing smoking may reduce the efficacy of pharmacological therapies.

16 Genetics is thought to account for around 50–65% of the risk of developing RA. Multiple genetic risk factors have been identified, but the most well-recognised is the 'shared epitope', a common 5-amino-acid motif found on the HLA-DR beta chain. Possessing HLA-DR4, for example, confers a 4 to 5-fold risk of disease.

17 In young females with RA it is important to address family planning at an early stage, as this may influence choice of treatment. Some medications (such as methotrexate and leflunomide) are unsafe in pregnancy and patients should be warned about the need for reliable contraception if prescribed these treatments. Patients also need to be counselled about pregnancy planning and the importance of adequate disease control prior to conceiving. Family planning should also be discussed with men with RA; for example, the use of sulfasalazine is associated with reversible oligospermia and hence has a potential impact on fertility.

Examination

- The patient has an **antalgic gait** [1].
- On **inspection** [2] of the **hands** [3] there is **swelling** [4] of multiple joints.
- There are no obvious **deformities** [5].
- The **skin** [6] and **nails** [7] are normal.
- On **palpation** [8] there is widespread **joint line tenderness** [9] and **bogginess** [10] which **spares the distal interphalangeal joints** [11].

- Examination of **other joints** [12] is **normal** [13] other than a **positive metatarsophalangeal squeeze** [14].
- There are no **extra-articular signs** [15] including no apparent **rheumatoid nodules** [16], **pulmonary crackles** [17] or **splenomegaly** [18].

1 Observing gait is a simple way of screening for lower limb joint involvement.

2 An accurate inspection of the hands may significantly help refine the differential diagnosis. Important features to note include the distribution of joint involvement, any typical deformities, skin abnormalities and nail changes.

3 The hands are a common site where abnormal signs can be detected. There are five classic causes of a symmetrical deforming polyarthritis of the hands: these are osteoarthritis, rheumatoid arthritis, systemic lupus erythematosus (SLE), psoriatic arthritis and gout. Scleroderma can mimic these changes as well, due to contractures secondary to skin tightness.

4 Joint swelling may be due to bony enlargement, synovial thickening or joint effusions. Palpation helps further delineate the type of swelling.

5 Characteristic deformities of rheumatoid arthritis are ulnar deviation and volar subluxation of the MCPJs, swan neck deformity (extended PIPJ and flexed DIPJ), boutonnière deformity (flexed PIPJ and extended DIPJ) and Z deformity of the thumb. Psoriatic arthritis can have a rheumatoid-like pattern and be difficult to distinguish. A Jaccoud's arthropathy can occur in SLE and also looks identical to rheumatoid arthritis; it is differentiated by reversibility of the deformities. Importantly, fixed deformities in RA are usually a sign of irreversible joint damage; the aim is to detect and treat disease early, before such deformities develop.

6 Skin should be carefully inspected for features that may suggest alternative diagnoses, e.g. psoriatic rash (psoriatic arthritis), Gottron's papules (dermatomyositis), tophi (gout), sclerodactyly (scleroderma) or calcinosis (scleroderma). Non-specific features, such as palmar crease pallor, Raynaud's phenomenon and muscle wasting, should also be noted.

7 The nails may provide clues pointing towards psoriasis (pitting and ridging), vasculitis (splinter haemorrhages) or other connective tissue diseases (dilated nailfold capillaries).

8 Joint palpation helps establish the level of disease activity by identifying signs of active synovitis. These signs include joint line tenderness, bogginess, joint effusions and stress tenderness.

9 It is important to accurately identify the joint line when assessing each individual joint. Normal joints in the hand have an easily defined joint line. An inability to feel the joint line may indicate active inflammation due to thickening of the synovium or accumulation of fluid in the joint (effusion).

10 Bogginess refers to a doughy texture of the synovial membrane due to the thickening that occurs with joint inflammation. In healthy individuals the synovial membrane, composed of macrophage-like and fibroblast-like cells, is very thin. In rheumatoid arthritis, immune dysregulation triggers cell infiltration and activation, vascular proliferation, release of pro-inflammatory cytokines and subsequent synovial hyperplasia.

11 DIPJ sparing is a useful clinical clue to differentiate causes of arthritis affecting the hands. Classically, RA and SLE spare the DIPJs, while psoriatic arthritis, gout and OA tend to involve the DIPJs.

12 The distribution of joint involvement in RA includes the hands (MCPJs and PIPJs, sparing the DIPJs), wrists, elbows, shoulders, temporomandibular joint, cervical spine (sparing the lumbar spine), hips, knees, ankles and feet.

13 Often RA initially affects the small joints of the hands and feet, and then subsequently progresses proximally to involve other joints.

14 A positive metatarsophalangeal squeeze test is associated with local joint inflammation and can be a simple technique to identify synovitis in the feet. However, it is not a completely sensitive or specific test.

15 Extra-articular manifestations occur in up to 40% of patients with RA and are much more common in patients who are seropositive. They may be a marker of disease severity, and adequate immunosuppressive therapy is associated with reduced incidence. A thorough examination, especially including the skin, cardiac and respiratory systems, and palpation for the spleen and lymph nodes should be performed.

16 Rheumatoid nodules are associated with seropositive disease. They feel soft and mobile and commonly occur on pressure points (such as the elbows) but can occur anywhere upon or within the body (such as in the lungs). No treatment is specifically required for rheumatoid nodules, unless they are symptomatic or interfering with joint function. Interestingly, nodulosis can also rarely be a side-effect of methotrexate therapy.

17 Fine crackles may be a sign of interstitial lung disease. The lungs are a relatively common location for extra-articular manifestations of RA. The presence of crackles should prompt further investigation, including a chest X-ray (and likely high-resolution CT of the chest), oxygen saturation, lung function tests, as well as assessment for other potential causes (e.g. infection, occupational exposures), ideally with a respiratory physician involved.

18 Unexplained splenomegaly and neutropenia with RA forms the classic triad of Felty's syndrome. Typically, this manifestation occurs in severe, long-standing, seropositive disease. Due to the earlier commencement of effective treatments for RA, Felty's syndrome is seen much less commonly these days. Felty's syndrome is also a diagnosis of exclusion – it is imperative to exclude other causes of splenomegaly and neutropenia, such as haematological malignancy.

Investigations

- Initial blood tests show a **normocytic anaemia** [1], **mild thrombocytosis** [2], normal **renal function** [3] and normal **liver function** [4] other than **reduced albumin** [5].
- The **CRP and ESR** [6] are moderately elevated.
- **Antibody tests** [7] confirm the patient is **seropositive** [8], with a **positive rheumatoid factor** **(RF)** [9], **positive anti-cyclic citrullinated peptide (anti-CCP)** [10], and negative **antinuclear antibody (ANA)** [11].
- Plain **X-rays** [12] are performed of the **hands and feet** [13] which show **periarticular osteopenia** [14] without **joint space narrowing** [15] or **erosions** [16].

1 A normocytic normochromic anaemia of chronic disease is not uncommon in rheumatoid arthritis and tends to correlate with general disease activity.

2 An elevated platelet count may also be a non-specific feature of active inflammatory disease. The white cell count may also be elevated but may be hard to interpret in the setting of prednisolone use. Corticosteroids, particularly moderate to high doses, promote the demargination of neutrophils, which leads to an elevation of peripheral neutrophil and white cell count.

3 Renal impairment is very uncommon as an extra-articular manifestation of RA but is relevant in determining appropriate treatment. For example, NSAIDs would be avoided in the setting of renal impairment, and drugs such as

methotrexate can accumulate and cause toxicity in a patient with chronic kidney disease.

4 Liver function should also be reviewed prior to treatment decisions, as many drug options can cause liver function derangement or may be contraindicated in the setting of liver cirrhosis.

5 Hypoalbuminaemia is another non-specific marker of disease activity that may provide a clue to inadequately controlled inflammatory disease. Liver and kidney disease and poor nutrition should also be considered as possible contributors.

6 The CRP and ESR are probably the most useful blood tests in assessing and monitoring disease activity in rheumatoid arthritis. They tend to fluctuate in sync, and there is some evidence their elevation may predict relevant disease outcomes.

7 Antibody tests should be interpreted with caution and always in light of the clinical picture. The presence of typical antibodies in rheumatoid arthritis is neither necessary nor sufficient for making the diagnosis.

8 Around 70% of patients with rheumatoid arthritis are 'seropositive', i.e. they have detectable rheumatoid factor and/or anti-CCP antibodies. Seropositivity is associated with poorer outcomes, including more frequent extra-articular complications and greater joint damage. These antibodies are predominantly a diagnostic and prognostic tool; and there is usually no role for serial monitoring of antibodies over the course of disease.

9 Rheumatoid factor is an autoantibody directed against the Fc portion of human IgG. It has a sensitivity of around 70% and a specificity of 80%. Low titre RF is less specific than higher titres, and may be found in normal people, chronic infection, malignancies and other connective tissue diseases. Exceptions to this are primary Sjögren's syndrome and cryoglobulinaemia, which can be associated with very high titres of RF.

10 Anti-CCP antibodies have a sensitivity of around 70% and a specificity of 95% for RA. They are antibodies directed against antigens containing citrulline, which is a post-translational modification that can occur to proteins.

11 A positive ANA is a non-specific finding which can be found in up to a third of patients (usually in lower titres) with RA. Rheumatoid arthritis can also overlap with ANA-associated connective tissue diseases such as SLE, Sjögren's syndrome and scleroderma.

12 Plain X-rays are mainly used to assess for disease-related damage and so are commonly normal at baseline if RA is diagnosed shortly after symptom onset. X-rays may demonstrate a range of changes including juxta-articular osteopenia, peri-articular soft tissue swelling, joint space narrowing, erosions and more marked deformity later. Other forms of imaging such as ultrasound and MRI are better for assessing subclinical or early disease activity, and may be more sensitive for erosions; however, their exact place in routine practice is still being defined.

13 Common sites for radiographic erosions of the hands and feet are at the second and third MCPJs, the ulnar styloid and the lateral aspect of the fifth metatarsal head.

14 Periarticular osteopenia is often an earlier radiographic feature of inflammatory arthritis.

15 Joint space narrowing is typically symmetrical, in contrast to OA.

16 Erosions are the hallmark radiological finding of RA and are associated with prolonged inflammation, although they may appear as early as a few months post disease onset. Erosions typically occur at the bare areas at the margin of the joints (marginal erosions). They are thought to occur due to synovial cytokines including TNF-alpha, IL-6 and RANKL which promotes osteoclast differentiation and invasion.

Management

Short-term

Provide **patient education** [1] and establish **treatment goals** [2]. Refer the patient to a **Rheumatologist** [3]. Counsel about **smoking cessation** [4] and taking **regular exercise** [5]. Commence **disease-modifying** [6] therapy **early** [7]. Prescribe short-term **steroids** [8] and initiate **methotrexate** [9], with the option for additional **synthetic DMARDs** [10] and/or **escalation** [11] to a **biologic DMARD** [12] or **targeted synthetic DMARD** [13] in order to obtain **low disease activity** [14]. **NSAIDs** [15] may be used for additional **symptom relief** [16].

Long-term

Regularly review [17] the patient's **disease activity** [18]. Manage **side-effects of treatment** [19] and comorbidities such as **cardiovascular risk factors** [20] and **osteoporosis** [21]. Ensure **immunisations** [22] are up to date. Consider referral to **allied health** [23]. In select cases **surgery** [24] may be required.

1 As with any chronic disease, a discussion should be had with the patient about the diagnosis, management and prognosis. With modern treatments and early intervention, most patients with RA can avoid long-term damage and loss of function.

2 Treatment goals from a medical perspective are to reduce inflammation, prevent damage and reduce long-term rheumatoid arthritis-associated complications, while minimising the side-effects of treatment. Patient-centred goals such as symptom reduction, preservation of function and quality of life are also important to consider alongside.

3 In general, management of patients with RA should be in conjunction with a Rheumatologist.

4 Smoking should be strongly discouraged, due to its association with poorer treatment response, higher disease activity and increased cardiovascular risk.

5 Regular exercise of moderate intensity is associated with better physical functioning as well as psychological wellbeing. Patients should be reassured that exercise is not harmful for their joints.

6 Disease-modifying antirheumatic drugs (DMARDs) in rheumatoid arthritis act within the immune system to reduce joint inflammation and prevent joint damage. They are categorised as conventional synthetic DMARDs (csDMARDs), targeted synthetic DMARDs (tsDMARDs) and biologic DMARDS (bDMARDs).

7 The aim should be to start DMARD therapy early (within 12 weeks of symptom onset) prior to irreversible joint damage, to give the best chance of good long-term outcomes.

8 Steroids (oral, intramuscular, intravenous or intra-articular) can be used in the short term for more rapid disease and symptom control. They have significant side-effects, however, therefore other DMARDs are preferred for long-term use.

9 Methotrexate is the anchor drug of rheumatoid arthritis therapy. In the absence of contraindications, it should be prescribed first-line due to its good efficacy, low cost and generally good tolerability. It should be prescribed with folic acid (not taken on the same day as the methotrexate) to offset side-effects.

10 Synthetic DMARDs work in a variety of ways to non-specifically reduce inflammation and immune activation. Several drugs fall into this category, including glucocorticoids, methotrexate, leflunomide, hydroxychloroquine and sulfasalazine.

11 If synthetic DMARDs alone or in combination are unable to achieve adequate disease control, then treatment should be escalated to include either a biologic DMARD or a targeted synthetic DMARD. All of these agents have comparable efficacy.

12 Biologic DMARDs target specific immune pathways in order to reduce inflammation in rheumatoid arthritis. They are delivered intravenously or subcutaneously. Mechanisms of action include TNF-alpha inhibition (infliximab, adalimumab, etanercept, golimumab, certolizumab), CTLA-4 fusion protein reducing T-cell activity (abatacept), IL6 inhibition (tocilizumab) or anti-CD20 targeting B cells (rituximab).

13 In recent years targeted synthetic DMARDs such as the JAK-inhibitors (e.g. tofacitinib, baricitinib) have become another treatment option, as an alternative to biologic DMARDs in patients with persistent disease activity despite synthetic DMARD therapy. Unlike biologic DMARDs they are available in oral formulations.

14 Treatment should be escalated with the aim of maintaining a patient in low disease activity or remission to prevent disease progression and maintain symptom control.

15 NSAIDs have an anti-inflammatory effect that can reduce pain and swelling; however, they do not reduce joint damage, hence are not 'disease-modifying' agents.

16 Analgesia used for symptom relief (e.g. paracetamol) may help in the short term or in patients with end-stage joint damage, but does not reduce further joint damage or impact the disease course, and hence should not be used in preference to DMARDs.

17 Patients should be medically reviewed at intervals determined by clinical need. Specialist reviews may be every few weeks when the disease is poorly controlled and may extend to 6–12-monthly in stable patients.

18 Disease activity is monitored using a combination of patient-reported symptoms such as pain and stiffness, examination findings such as tender and swollen joint counts, and laboratory parameters such as inflammatory markers (CRP and ESR).

19 Some side-effects are common to many treatments used in RA, including the risk of infection, GI upset and biochemical derangement. Many drugs require regular monitoring of bloods such as FBE, UEC and LFT. Individual drugs may also have unique potential side-effects, of which the prescriber and patient should also be aware.

20 Rheumatoid arthritis is associated with accelerated atherosclerosis and is an independent risk factor for cardiovascular events. Achievement of a low disease activity state and management of modifiable cardiovascular risk factors is therefore warranted in all patients.

21 Osteoporosis rates are higher among those with RA due to both the disease itself, as well as the use of glucocorticoids. Patients should have other osteoporosis risk factors assessed and managed and bone densitometry performed at intervals determined by their overall risk. If anti-resorptive therapy is indicated, there is evidence that denosumab (RANK-ligand inhibitor) may retard rheumatoid erosions. Bisphosphonates are also commonly used for glucocorticoid-induced osteoporosis.

22 Immunosuppressive therapy predisposes patients to develop infections, hence all patients should be encouraged to be up to date with influenza and pneumococcal vaccines. Live vaccines are generally contraindicated if on immunosuppression.

23 Patients with limitations to movement and function may benefit from specific allied health intervention, such as physiotherapists, exercise physiologists, occupational therapists, podiatrists and hand therapists. Some patients may benefit from dietitian input to help with maintaining a healthy weight, or psychology as part of an integrated approach to pain management.

24 Joint surgery is an option in selected patients. Most commonly, joint replacements are performed as a result of secondary OA. Joint fusions and joint realignment surgery may have a role in severe cases.

CASE 99:   Scleroderma

History

- A **45-year-old** [1] **female** [2] presents with **pain in both of her hands** [3], which have also developed a **swollen appearance** [4].
- This has been associated with recent worsening of her **long-standing** [5] **Raynaud's phenomenon** [6] and the development of a slow-healing **fingertip ulcer** [7].
- She reports symptoms of **gastro-oesophageal reflux** [8] and **postprandial bloating** [9] but no history to suggest **GI bleeding** [10].

- She denies any **muscle pain and weakness** [11] or **mucocutaneous symptoms** [12].
- Recently her **exercise tolerance has decreased** [13], but she has no other specific **cardiac or respiratory symptoms** [14].
- Her past history includes **hypothyroidism** [15] on thyroxine replacement.
- She has no **significant family history** [16] and **works in an office** [17].

1 The peak incidence of scleroderma is between the ages of 40 and 60 but it can present at any age.

2 Scleroderma is more common in women (3:1 male to female ratio) but men tend to have more severe disease and a poorer overall prognosis.

3 Attempt to localise the pain (i.e. joints vs. soft tissues) and determine if there are features suggestive of inflammatory joint disease (stiffness, pain worse in the morning or after rest and improved with movement). Pain in scleroderma may be due to arthralgias or myalgias which may or may not be associated with overt inflammation (arthritis or myositis) and can also occur at peripheral sites due to vascular ischaemia.

4 In the earlier stages, skin involvement in scleroderma may be more inflammatory, with soft tissue swelling and oedema. This can be associated with pruritus, particularly in patients with diffuse skin disease. This should be differentiated from swelling due to synovitis, which can also be a manifestation of scleroderma.

5 The presence of long-standing Raynaud's phenomenon prior to the onset of scleroderma is more in keeping with the limited form of the disease, while recent-onset Raynaud's and more rapidly progressive disease tend to be a feature of diffuse scleroderma.

6 Confirm the patient has true Raynaud's phenomenon, which is characterised by biphasic or triphasic colour changes (white, blue, red). Features suggestive of secondary rather than primary Raynaud's phenomenon include a later age of onset, male gender, asymmetric attacks, thumb involvement and severe ischaemia complicated by ulcers or necrosis.

7 Digital complications in scleroderma include fingertip ulcers, pitting of the terminal digits, loss of fingertip pulp (producing the appearance of pseudo-clubbing), overt tissue necrosis or gangrene and infective sequelae which can be both superficial (e.g. cellulitis) and deep (e.g. osteomyelitis). Amputation can be a consequence of severe disease.

8 Gastro-oesophageal reflux is the most common of a wide range of GI features that can occur in scleroderma. These manifestations occur due to hypomotility of the oesophagus and incompetence of the sphincter and are present in most patients with scleroderma, but only around half are symptomatic. Complications include oesophagitis, aspiration and stricturing. Patients may also report dysphagia and regurgitation of food as a result of oesophageal dysmotility.

9 Gut dysmotility extends along the length of the GI tract. Poor gastric emptying can lead to bloating and postprandial fullness; constipation and overflow diarrhoea can occur, and poor bowel motility can be complicated by bacterial overgrowth syndromes.

10 GI bleeding can occur due to ulcers secondary to reflux, gut telangiectasias and gastric antral vascular ectasia, which is a rarer complication that has the endoscopic appearance of longitudinal stripes of red vessels known as 'watermelon stomach'. Bleeding from these various causes may be occult, or present more dramatically with acute haemorrhage.

11 Muscle involvement in scleroderma may be inflammatory (similar to polymyositis) with pain, elevated inflammatory markers and an elevated CK. Often this is associated with overlap forms of connective tissue disease and particular antibody profiles (e.g. PMScl positivity). A non-inflammatory myopathy can also occur due to increased collagen deposits within the muscle. This is usually mild, with minimal CK rise and does not normally require any specific treatment.

12 Features of scleroderma can also occur in overlap or mixed connective tissue diseases. Hence it is useful to enquire about symptoms seen in other connective tissue diseases, such as rashes (e.g. in SLE, dermatomyositis), mouth ulcers (SLE) and alopecia (SLE).

13 Enquire about the factors limiting exercise, in particular dyspnoea and other cardiac and respiratory symptoms which may be indicators of interstitial lung disease or pulmonary hypertension, which are significant organ manifestations associated with scleroderma. As mentioned, patients with scleroderma are also at risk of GI bleeding which can lead to iron deficiency and anaemia, they can have muscle and joint involvement and have higher rates of hypothyroidism, all of which can also contribute to fatigue and reduced exercise tolerance.

14 Chest pain, dyspnoea (especially exertional), syncope, peripheral oedema and cough are relevant symptoms that may point towards heart or lung involvement in scleroderma. Pulmonary hypertension occurs in around 10% of patients and is slightly more common in limited scleroderma. Clinically significant interstitial lung disease occurs in around 30–40% of patients and is slightly more common in diffuse disease. Pericarditis (with effusions and rarely tamponade) and myocarditis can also occur.

15 Other conditions that are recognised to occur in association with scleroderma include hypothyroidism and primary biliary cirrhosis.

16 Rare familial cases have been reported, but overall the aetiology of scleroderma is poorly understood and thought to be multifactorial, with a number of possible genetic and environmental components.

17 Some environmental toxins, such as silica and vinyl chloride, have been associated with scleroderma or scleroderma-like symptoms.

Examination

- The patient has a **blood pressure of 130/80mmHg** [1] and otherwise normal **vital signs** [2].
- There is **skin thickening** [3] and **puffiness of the fingers** [4] with associated **difficulty making a fist** [5].
- There are no apparent **skin changes elsewhere** [6].
- A **dry fingertip ulcer** [7] is seen on the second digit.

- There is no **joint line swelling** [8] or **tendon friction rubs** [9].
- **Dilated nailfold capillaries** [10] are present, as are several **telangiectasias** [11] over the face and chest.
- There is no evidence of **calcinosis** [12].
- The patient has a **mouth aperture of 4cm** [13].
- The **chest is clear** [14] and there is no appreciable **loud P2 or right ventricular heave** [15].

1 Monitoring blood pressure is vital in scleroderma, as hypertension is a feature of the potentially organ- and life-threatening manifestation scleroderma renal crisis. Untreated, accelerated hypertension proceeds to renal failure and in some cases microangiopathic haemolysis. The underlying renal pathology is of endothelial injury, intimal proliferation and arteriolar narrowing. Risk factors include recent-onset diffuse disease, RNA polymerase III antibody positivity and steroid use, particularly doses >15mg daily. ACE inhibitors are the mainstay of therapy for scleroderma renal crisis and significantly improve prognosis.

2 Other abnormalities of circulatory and respiratory vital signs suggest severe cardiac or respiratory involvement, such as pulmonary hypertension, interstitial lung disease, myocarditis or pericardial tamponade. These require urgent assessment and management.

3 Sclerodactyly is a hallmark of scleroderma and changes may include tightness, thickening, swelling and induration of the skin. As with other manifestations of scleroderma, the pathophysiology is based around a combination of

immunological dysfunction and inflammation, pathological vascular changes and tissue fibrosis. The differential diagnoses for thickening of the skin include other rare conditions such as morphoea (a localised form of scleroderma), eosinophilic fasciitis (which may be differentiated on biopsy), scleroedema (another rare condition which can be associated with diabetes), scleromyxoedema (sometimes associated with a paraproteinaemia) and nephrogenic systemic fibrosis (associated with gadolinium exposure in patients with renal impairment).

4 The fingers, hands and face tend to be the earliest sites of skin involvement in scleroderma. Puffiness, arthralgias and soft tissue swelling tend to be earlier features than sclerodactyly.

5 Sclerodactyly can lead to joint contractures, reduced range of movement and tapering of the digits. When severe, this can result in marked functional limitation. Sometimes contractures may be confused for a deforming polyarthropathy such as RA; however, closer inspection will reveal sclerodactyly as the underlying cause.

6 The distinction between limited and diffuse scleroderma is based on the extent of skin involvement. Limited scleroderma has skin disease affecting distal to the elbows and knees and the face only. Typically, limited skin disease has a more indolent onset and progresses slowly. In contrast, diffuse skin disease additionally affects proximal limbs and the trunk and tends to have a more rapid onset and progression. Limited scleroderma is more common than diffuse (4:1). Although the skin disease in diffuse scleroderma is more severe, other organ manifestations such as pulmonary hypertension, interstitial lung disease, renal crisis, GI disease and myositis can all occur in either form, albeit at slightly differing frequencies.

7 Ulcers occur in around half of patients with scleroderma as a complication of Raynaud's phenomenon, with progressive pathological changes in the small vessels leading to digital ischaemia. Common sites are the fingertips, malleoli, heels and toes. Sclerodactyly further predisposes to ulcers (particularly at sites of trauma) and poor wound healing. Ulcers tend to heal slowly, predisposing to complicating infection, which further compromises healing.

8 Palpate the joint lines to determine if there is any synovitis, or whether swelling is more generally related to scleroderma skin changes. The presence of synovitis should prompt investigation for overlap with RA (check rheumatoid factor and anti-CCP and perform X-rays for erosive change) and influences the choice of treatment (low dose steroids and methotrexate are often used for true inflammatory joint disease).

9 Tendon friction rubs are much more common in diffuse scleroderma and are important to identify because they are a marker of poorer prognosis.

10 Abnormal nailfold capillaries are a typical feature of scleroderma, and in patients with isolated Raynaud's phenomenon can predict the later development of scleroderma. Specific patterns can be identified when formal nailfold video-capillaroscopy is performed – enlarged or giant capillaries, haemorrhages, capillary loss and disorganisation of capillary architecture are all features than can be seen in scleroderma.

11 Telangiectasias are dilated vessels which are most commonly found on the hands, face and chest. They blanch with pressure.

12 Calcinosis refers to calcific deposits which occur in the subcutaneous tissues. They usually appear as white or yellowish nodules or plaques that are firm and sit at the surface of the skin. They can become painful and ulcerate, leading to the discharge of the calcium-based material. Calcinosis is notoriously difficult to treat.

13 Skin involvement of the face can lead to a reduction in mouth opening. As a rule of thumb, reduced mouth aperture is suggested if a patient is unable to open their mouth more than the width of their second, third and fourth digits held together horizontally. Limited mouth opening can compromise food intake and oral hygiene.

14 Auscultate the lungs for signs of pulmonary fibrosis, classically Velcro-like inspiratory crackles at the lung bases bilaterally.

15 Examine for clinical features of pulmonary hypertension. In advanced stages signs of right heart failure may occur. Ideally pulmonary hypertension should be detected on screening prior to the development of florid symptoms or signs.

Investigations

- Initial blood tests including an **FBE** [1], **UEC** [2], **LFT** [3] and **inflammatory markers** [4] are normal.
- The **urine** [5] has no protein or red cells.
- **Antibody testing** [6] returns a positive **ANA** [7] with **anti-centromere** [8] staining.
- The **extractible nuclear antigen (ENA)** [9] panel

including **anti-Scl-70** [10] is negative, as is the **RNA polymerase III antibody** [11].
- **X-rays of the hands** [12] are normal. Baseline **pulmonary function tests** [13], a **high resolution CT chest** [14] and a **transthoracic echocardiogram (TTE)** [15] are arranged.

1 Look for anaemia which may reflect occult blood loss (e.g. GI bleeding) or vitamin malabsorption in the case of bacterial overgrowth. Elevation of the WCC may suggest infection (e.g. related to digital ulcers). Cytopenias may be immune-mediated and reflect overlap with other connective tissue disease (e.g. SLE).

2 Renal impairment can occur due to renal vasculopathy, the most extreme presentation being that of scleroderma renal crisis.

3 Primary biliary cirrhosis is associated with scleroderma, and obstructive LFTs should prompt further investigation, including antimitochondrial antibodies.

4 Inflammatory markers are usually normal or only mildly elevated in scleroderma. Patients with inflammatory arthritis or myositis as a manifestation of their scleroderma can, however, have more marked increases in CRP and ESR.

5 Urine is typically normal with scleroderma. Patients with renal vasculopathy may develop proteinuria and haematuria. Unlike other types of connective tissue disease, scleroderma is not associated with glomerulonephritis as the primary renal pathology and therefore active urinary sediment should prompt investigation for other causes.

6 A number of antibodies may be positive in scleroderma, reflecting the contribution of autoimmunity to the disease's underlying pathophysiology. The ANA is highly sensitive for scleroderma, while other antibodies (such as anti-Scl-70) are more specific. Antibodies traditionally associated with other diseases, such as RF, anti-double-stranded DNA (ds-DNA) or ANCA, may also be positive if tested for in patients with scleroderma, and may be associated with increased risk of specific disease manifestations or overlap forms.

7 The ANA is positive in around 95% of patients with scleroderma, making it a very sensitive test (good for excluding if negative), but not specific for scleroderma.

8 Anti-centromere antibodies are not a separate antibody, but rather a staining pattern observed in some patients with a positive ANA. This centromere staining pattern is quite specific for scleroderma, particularly the limited form, where around 70–80% of patients will be positive (compared to around 5% with the diffuse form). There is an association between anti-centromere antibodies and pulmonary hypertension.

9 Certain extractable nuclear antibodies are specific for scleroderma (e.g. anti-Scl-70) or may indicate mixed connective tissue disease (e.g. anti-U1-RNP) or an overlap syndrome (e.g. anti-Ro/La with Sjögren's, anti-PM/Scl with myositis).

10 Anti-Scl-70 (also known as anti-topoisomerase I) is an antibody specific for scleroderma and is found in around 40% of patients with diffuse disease and 15% with limited disease. It has an association with interstitial lung disease.

11 Anti-RNA polymerase III is an antibody that often needs to be requested separately in patients in whom scleroderma is suspected or diagnosed. It is found in around 20% of

patients and is associated with diffuse skin disease and the development of scleroderma renal crisis. There is also a reported association between RNA polymerase III and higher rates of malignancy in patients with scleroderma.

12 Hand X-rays in those with scleroderma may demonstrate calcinosis and resorption of the distal phalangeal tufts, producing a tapered or shortened appearance of the distal phalanx (acro-osteolysis). An erosive arthritis is less typical and usually occurs in patients with features overlapping with RA.

13 Look for a restrictive pattern on lung function (reduced forced vital capacity with preserved forced expiratory ratio) that may indicate interstitial lung disease. Lung volumes and gas transfer may also be reduced. It is important to look closely at the diffusion coefficient as this also drops in patients who have pulmonary hypertension, but in contrast to interstitial lung disease, there is preservation of spirometry and lung volumes. Some patients with scleroderma have both interstitial lung disease and pulmonary hypertension – a clue to this on lung function testing may be a diffusion coefficient that is disproportionately low relative to the restrictive deficit on spirometry.

14 High resolution CT scanning of the lungs is the most sensitive imaging technique to detect interstitial lung disease and in some centres is performed in all patients at baseline. Many patients have mild fibrosis which does not progress to be clinically symptomatic. Extensive changes, however, may be indicative of more aggressive disease. Lung function testing (particularly the forced vital capacity) is a better measure of progression than serial imaging and hence is the preferred means of monitoring.

15 A TTE is a screening test for pulmonary hypertension. It allows for estimation of the pulmonary artery systolic pressure as well as assessment of right ventricular size and function. In around 25% of cases, however, the pulmonary artery systolic pressure cannot be estimated, due to absence of a tricuspid regurgitant jet.

Management

Short-term

Arrange **referral to a Rheumatologist** [1] for assessment and management. Confirm the patient's particular **organ manifestations** [2] and arrange **further investigations** [3] if necessary. Commence **treatment directed at individual disease features** [4]. Educate about **non-pharmacological management** [5] of common manifestations. Prescribe a **proton pump inhibitor** [6] for reflux and a **calcium channel blocker** [7] for Raynaud's phenomenon. Consider the **role of immunosuppression** [8].

Long-term

Monitor and manage progression of **sclerodactyly** [9], **Raynaud's complications** [10] and **GI symptoms** [11]. Check the **blood pressure** [12] at each clinic visit. **Perform annual screening** [13] for interstitial lung disease and pulmonary hypertension and commence **specific therapies** [14] in certain situations. Provide individualised **counselling about prognosis** [15] and in very select cases consider referral for **bone marrow transplantation** [16].

1 Scleroderma is an uncommon and complicated disease to manage and therefore patients should be managed in conjunction with a Rheumatologist. Ideally, patients (particularly those with more complex disease) should be managed by a service that specialises in scleroderma, if available.

2 As with all connective tissue diseases, patients with scleroderma can have a different combination of manifestations with a broad spectrum of severity. It is important to identify and characterise the specific manifestations in any given individual, as this is the main determinant of treatment and prognosis.

3 Further investigations may be directed at better defining disease manifestations and to characterise patient symptoms. For example, patients with severe peripheral ischaemia should have larger vessel disease excluded with an arterial Doppler, and patients with GI symptoms may be considered for endoscopy, gastric emptying studies or breath tests for bacterial overgrowth.

4 There are no proven pharmacological therapies for the overall disease modification in scleroderma and therefore interventions are largely based on targeting organ-specific manifestations.

5 Non-pharmacological strategies are vital in many common manifestations of scleroderma. Patients with Raynaud's should be advised to use gloves and hand warmers and keep their core warm with layers of clothing during winter. For reflux, small meals, raising the head of the bed, avoiding triggering foods and meals close to bedtime can all help with symptom control. Regular moisturising can help with skin symptoms and gentle range of motion exercises may help maintain function.

6 Patients with reflux often need pharmacological therapy in addition to lifestyle measures. Usually a PPI (often twice daily) is first-line, with the option to combine a histamine receptor blocker such as ranitidine. For oesophageal dysmotility or delayed gastric emptying, the addition of a prokinetic agent such as domperidone taken 15–20 minutes before meals can help.

7 Vasodilators can be used in combination with non-pharmacological measures to help prevent or treat digital ischaemia secondary to Raynaud's phenomenon. Usually first-line therapy is with a peripherally acting CCB (such as slow-release nifedipine). Glyceryl trinitrate patches and topical nitrates can also be used. An IV infusion of iloprost, a prostacyclin analogue, can be used in cases of severe ischaemia or impending gangrene.

8 The role for immunosuppression in scleroderma is generally limited to early skin disease and interstitial lung disease, although benefits are only modest. Immunosuppressive agents may also be helpful for patients with inflammatory arthritis or myositis.

9 Patients with early diffuse skin disease may benefit from methotrexate, mycophenolate or cyclophosphamide, although toxicity needs to be balanced against probable small benefits only. Consideration should also be given to the natural history of diffuse skin disease; after initial rapid progression, skin disease generally plateaus and improves slightly over time. Immunosuppression is not generally used for limited skin involvement.

10 Monitor patients with Raynaud's for the development of digital ischaemia, skin ulcers and associated infection. Dressings may be required to assist with healing, and antibiotics should be prescribed if signs of infection develop. Imaging should be performed in patients with chronic ulcers, to exclude underlying osteomyelitis.

11 Enquire about GI symptoms at each clinic review as they can be a significant source of morbidity. Treatment is directed at the particular manifestation. For reflux, if non-pharmacological and combination pharmacological measures fail, fundoplication may be considered. Dietary modification, prokinetic agents and laxatives may be required for poor gut motility. Bacterial overgrowth may require extended courses of antibiotics. GI bleeding may require endoscopic intervention.

12 Blood pressure should be monitored regularly in patients with scleroderma and ACE inhibition is usually the first-line antihypertensive therapy. Patients with scleroderma renal crisis require intensive monitoring of blood pressure and renal function, with rapid up-titration of a short-acting ACE inhibitor such as captopril.

13 Because patients may remain asymptomatic until significant progression has occurred, cardiopulmonary screening with a TTE and pulmonary function tests are usually performed annually in patients with scleroderma.

14 Immunosuppressive therapy such as methotrexate, mycophenolate and cyclophosphamide may provide a small benefit in patients with scleroderma interstitial lung disease. Patients should be monitored and managed in conjunction with a respiratory physician. For pulmonary hypertension, a range of pulmonary vasodilators have proven benefit, including phosphodiesterase 5 inhibitors, prostacyclin analogues and endothelin receptor antagonists. Lung or heart-lung transplantation can be an option in select patients for end-stage disease.

15 Prognosis is quite variable in scleroderma and largely depends on organ involvement and severity. Pulmonary hypertension and interstitial lung disease are the leading causes of mortality.

16 In very select cases there is a role for bone marrow transplantation in scleroderma; however, this is highly specialised and requires careful balance of potential benefits and risks.

CASE 100: Systemic lupus erythematosus

History

- A **25-year-old** [1] **Asian** [2] **female** [3] presents with worsening **small joint pain** [4] and a new **facial rash** [5] which flared after a **trip to the beach on a hot and sunny day** [6].
- She also reports recent multiple **mouth ulcers** [7], increased **hair loss** [8] and very **dry eyes and mouth** [9].
- She has been feeling **generally unwell** [10] with significant **fatigue** [11], but **systems review** [12] is otherwise unremarkable, including no **chest pain or dyspnoea** [13], **gastrointestinal** [14] or **neurological** [15] symptoms.
- She has never had **blood clots or miscarriages** [16].
- She has a history of **Graves' disease** [17] on carbimazole but takes no other **regular medications** [18].
- Her **sister** [19] was diagnosed with SLE around three years ago.

[1] Onset of systemic lupus erythematosus (SLE) is most typically between the ages of 15 and 44. This is an age group where disease-related complications have a major life impact, encompassing physical, psychosocial and reproductive consequences. Premature mortality remains significantly higher in patients with major organ involvement compared to age-matched controls.

[2] Patients of non-Caucasian background, including Asians and African Americans, typically have higher rates of SLE and more severe disease phenotypes including higher rates of lupus nephritis.

[3] Females are much more likely to be affected by SLE, with a 9:1 female to male ratio. It is postulated that hormonal and X-chromosome influences underlie this sex predominance.

[4] Joint pain is common in SLE, affecting 90% of patients. A typical pattern of joint pain in SLE is symmetrical arthralgias of the hands, wrists, knees, ankles and feet. Pain often has inflammatory characteristics (i.e. worse in the morning with associated stiffness and improvement with movement) and can be migratory.

[5] There are a broad range of cutaneous manifestations in SLE. The most commonly seen include the typical malar rash, subacute cutaneous lupus erythematosus (annular-appearing rash which tends to affect the forearms, shoulders, neck and upper torso) and discoid lupus (discrete plaques which commonly affect the face, scalp, neck and upper torso and result in scarring). Less common manifestations include bullous lupus, panniculitis, livedo reticularis, chilblain lupus and urticaria. Cutaneous lupus can occur in the absence of systemic involvement.

[6] Photosensitivity is commonly reported in SLE and both cutaneous and systemic manifestations may worsen with ultraviolet light exposure. This may relate to sun-related cell damage releasing increased autoantigens that are poorly cleared in patients with SLE and provide a stimulus for the dysregulated immune response in these patients and activation of downstream inflammatory pathways.

[7] Mucosal involvement is another common manifestation of active SLE, typically with ulcers affecting the tongue, palate, buccal mucosa and nasal mucosa.

[8] Alopecia is common with active disease and may be scarring or non-scarring. Differential diagnoses include comorbid alopecia areata or hair loss due to drugs or stress.

[9] Dry eyes and mouth are sicca symptoms which are a characteristic manifestation of Sjögren's syndrome. Sjögren's syndrome can occur as a stand-alone connective tissue disease (primary Sjögren's) with or without extraglandular involvement, or can occur in association with another autoimmune disease (secondary Sjögren's). Sjögren's syndrome is associated with SLE in around 15% of cases.

[10] Constitutional symptoms such as fever, weight loss, appetite loss and fatigue are common in patients with SLE and worsen with active disease.

[11] Fatigue is the most common constitutional complaint and is often multifactorial and difficult to manage. In additional to active disease, contributing factors may include poor sleep, depression, thyroid dysfunction, iron deficiency and fibromyalgia.

[12] SLE can affect virtually any organ system in the body and a patient can have organ involvement in any combination and sequence. New disease manifestations can appear any time in the disease course. It is therefore important to screen all the major systems for symptoms that may suggest potential SLE-related involvement.

13 Chest pain, palpitations, dyspnoea or other cardiorespiratory symptoms should prompt consideration of heart or lung involvement in SLE. The most common manifestation is serositis which presents as pleuritic chest pain (sharp pain worse on inspiration). Associated effusions can result in dyspnoea and cardiac and/or respiratory compromise.

14 Gastrointestinal disease is uncommon in SLE. It is seen more frequently in Asian patients. Mesenteric vasculitis, serositis and lupus enteritis are possible manifestations. Abdominal symptoms such as nausea, pain and diarrhoea are in general more likely to be due to other causes, such as medication side-effects or comorbidities.

15 There is a broad array of neuropsychiatric manifestations in SLE which can affect both the central and peripheral nervous systems. These manifestations can be very difficult to diagnose and manage. Possible neurological presentations include seizures, psychosis, transverse myelitis, headache and peripheral neuropathies. Other causes of these presentations require exclusion before attributing them to SLE.

16 Antiphospholipid syndrome (APLS) can occur as a primary entity or in association with rheumatological diseases (of which SLE is the most common). The clinical criteria for APLS include thrombosis of an artery (e.g. stroke, myocardial infarction, peripheral arterial thrombosis) and/or vein (deep vein thrombosis, pulmonary embolus, cerebral sinus thrombosis) and/or pregnancy morbidity (death of a normal foetus after 10 weeks, ≥3 consecutive miscarriages at <10 weeks or premature birth at ≤34 weeks due to pre-eclampsia or placental insufficiency). Patients also need to have at least one positive antiphospholipid antibody (lupus anticoagulant, anticardiolipin antibody, or anti-beta2-glycoprotein-I antibody) which remains positive at least 12 weeks later.

17 SLE is associated with a personal and/or family history of other autoimmune conditions, such as autoimmune thyroid disease.

18 Review medications, particularly checking for those associated with drug-induced SLE, such as minocycline, TNF inhibitors, hydralazine, methyldopa and isoniazid. Manifestations in drug-induced SLE are typically mucocutaneous; serositis, arthritis and cytopenias with renal and neurologic involvement are much less common. ANA, anti-single-stranded DNA and anti-histone antibodies are those typically associated with drug-induced SLE. Symptoms usually resolve within 6 weeks of drug discontinuation.

19 The risk of developing SLE is increased in those with a family history – around 10% of patients have an affected first-degree family member. Although there are some rare monogenic causes of SLE, most cases have a polygenic predisposition, and over 100 genes that individually confer a relatively small increased risk of disease have been identified. Most of these genes are involved in immune responses.

Examination

- The patient is **afebrile** [1] with **stable vital signs** [2].
- There is **tenderness but no swelling** [3] on palpation of the affected joints and no **joint deformity** [4].
- No **Raynaud's phenomenon** [5] is seen.
- There is a **malar rash** [6] over the cheeks and **dry mucous membranes** [7] but no other **mucocutaneous findings** [8].
- The **heart** [9] and **lungs** [10] examine normally although there is **mild pitting oedema** [11] of the bilateral lower limbs, but the **calves are soft and non-tender** [12].
- There is no palpable **lymphadenopathy or hepatosplenomegaly** [13].

1 Fevers can occur in up to half of patients with active disease, but infection always needs to be considered (especially in those on immunosuppression).

2 Cardiac or pulmonary involvement may lead to abnormal haemodynamic or respiratory vital signs. Hypertension may also occur in lupus nephritis. Chronic hypertension, regardless of renal involvement, should be identified and treated due to the increased rates of cardiovascular disease in SLE patients.

3 Arthralgia (pain without swelling) is more common than overt arthritis in SLE and unlike rheumatoid arthritis, joint disease is usually non-erosive. Some patients can have overlap forms of SLE with RA-like inflammatory arthritis with joint swelling and destruction – often these patients are RF and/or anti-CCP antibody positive.

4 Patients with SLE can develop apparent deformities which mimic RA but are reversible and occur in the absence of joint damage or erosions. This form of arthropathy is known as Jaccoud's arthropathy and occurs mainly due to soft tissue abnormalities such as ligamentous laxity and muscular imbalance.

5 Raynaud's phenomenon occurs in up to 50% of patients with SLE but is a non-specific finding that can occur as a primary disease or in association with other autoimmune conditions.

6 The classic 'butterfly' malar rash of SLE is quite specific and appears as erythema and oedema of the cheeks (and forehead) which characteristically spares the nasolabial folds. It is a non-scarring rash. If there is uncertainty about the appearance of the rash, a biopsy can be performed to help differentiate from other causes.

7 Sjögren's syndrome may account for this patient's dry mucous membranes and occurs due to inflammation of the exocrine glands. While dry eyes and mouth are the most classic features of the condition, parotidomegaly, atrophic vaginitis and dry skin can also occur. Blood tests may show a positive ANA, usually in a speckled pattern, anti-Ro (SSA) and/or anti-La (SSB) positivity on the ENA panel, a chronically elevated ESR, a strongly positive RF (high titre) and hypergammaglobulinaemia.

8 Look for ulcers in the nose and mouth, and for any evidence of alopecia which may manifest as diffuse thinning (non-specific), discrete patches of hair loss, broken hairs or scalp rash (e.g. plaques due to discoid lupus which result in scarring and hair loss).

9 Pericarditis, myocarditis and endocarditis are the main cardiac manifestations of SLE. Pericarditis is usually accompanied by pleuritic chest pain, and in some occasions a pericardial rub or signs of a pericardial effusion may be present. When suspected, look for features of pericardial tamponade such as hypotension, elevated JVP, pulsus paradoxus and muffled heart sounds. Myocarditis can

present as heart failure, conduction abnormalities or other arrhythmias. Libman–Sacks endocarditis refers to non-infectious valvular vegetations which can be complicated by valve dysfunction (e.g. regurgitation) or emboli. This manifestation is more common in patients with positive anti-phospholipid antibodies.

10 The most common pulmonary manifestation of SLE is pleuritis with associated pleural effusions, which may result in chest pain and dyspnoea. Acute pneumonitis, interstitial lung disease, diffuse alveolar haemorrhage, pulmonary hypertension and shrinking lung syndrome are all reported in SLE but are rarer manifestations.

11 Pitting oedema may be due to cardiac involvement of SLE (e.g. constrictive pericarditis, pericardial effusion/tamponade, myocarditis or valvular lesions) or renal disease (hypoalbuminaemia in the setting of proteinuria or nephrotic syndrome).

12 Leg swelling in a patient with SLE should also prompt consideration of deep vein thrombosis, given the increased risk of thromboembolism in these patients, particularly if they are positive for antiphospholipid antibodies.

13 Haematological examination findings, such as lymphadenopathy and splenomegaly, can occur in SLE, although infection, malignancy and other rheumatological conditions should be considered in the differential diagnosis when these findings are prominent.

Investigations

- Blood tests show a **mild anaemia** [1] (haemoglobin 104g/L) and **leucopenia** [2] (white cell count 2.7 x 10⁹/L) with **normal platelets** [3] .
- **Creatinine** [4] is normal.
- **Liver function tests** [5] are normal except for an **albumin of 25** (low) [6] .
- The patient has an **ESR of 48** [7] and a **CRP of 10** (both elevated) [8] .

- **Antibody tests** [9] return a **positive ANA** [10] , and an **ENA** [11] panel positive for **anti-Ro** [12] antibodies.
- **Anti-double-stranded DNA (dsDNA) antibodies** [13] are elevated and **C3 and C4 complement levels** [14] are reduced.
- **Antiphospholipid antibodies** [15] are negative.
- **Urinalysis** [16] has **+ blood** [17] and **+++ protein** [18] .

1 Anaemia may be multifactorial in SLE. Assessment should include consideration of general causes such as nutrition (e.g. iron deficiency) and bleeding (e.g. GI), as well as causes secondary to SLE such as autoimmune haemolytic anaemia, aplastic anaemia and anaemia of chronic disease (generally a diagnosis of exclusion).

2 A reduced WCC, particularly a lymphopenia, is common in SLE and can fluctuate with disease activity. Other common differential diagnoses for leucopenia in patients with SLE are intercurrent infection (e.g. viral infections) and medication-induced leucopenia (e.g. immunosuppressive therapies).

3 Thrombocytopenia can occur with active SLE and in some cases a diagnosis of idiopathic thrombocytopenic purpura (ITP) may precede other SLE manifestations. In the presence of thrombocytopenia, it is important to assess for microangiopathy (e.g. haemolysis, schistocytes on blood film), which can be organ- or life-threatening (e.g. with renal involvement) and occurs particularly in association with antiphospholipid antibodies.

4 Renal disease is the most common organ-threatening manifestation in SLE and occurs in around 30–50% of patients. It is crucial to screen for lupus nephritis in those with SLE as it is often asymptomatic in early stages. Importantly the serum creatinine and eGFR may be preserved and abnormalities indicating renal involvement may only be picked up on urine examination. If declining renal function is detected, this requires urgent assessment and usually a renal biopsy with rapid initiation of immunosuppression.

5 Hepatic involvement is less common but does occur in SLE. Derangement of liver function tests may be due to medications used to treat SLE (e.g. azathioprine, methotrexate), other autoimmune conditions (e.g. autoimmune hepatitis), infective hepatitis or other comorbidities (e.g. fatty liver).

6 Hypoalbuminaemia may be responsible for the patient's peripheral oedema. Low albumin may be a negative acute phase reactant in the setting of active inflammatory disease or may indicate more serious organ involvement with lupus nephritis (which can present as nephrotic syndrome) or rarely a protein-losing enteropathy.

7 The ESR commonly fluctuates alongside disease activity in SLE and is a useful marker for monitoring. Persistent ESR elevation despite apparent disease control should prompt consideration of chronic infection (especially in patients who are immunosuppressed) and hypergammaglobulinaemia (may be monoclonal, e.g. myeloma, or polyclonal, e.g. Sjögren's syndrome).

8 Classically the CRP does not rise significantly in active SLE. A high CRP, especially one disproportionate to ESR elevation, should raise concern for intercurrent infection.

9 Antibody tests are helpful for the diagnosis of SLE but alone are not diagnostic. If SLE is suspected clinically, ANA, ENA, anti-dsDNA, antiphospholipid antibodies and complement components (C3, 4) should be sent in the first instance. Interestingly, autoantibodies in SLE can often be detected years before clinically apparent.

10 The ANA is almost universally positive in patients with SLE (i.e. highly sensitive), but importantly is not specific for this diagnosis. Therefore, a negative ANA can be useful in excluding SLE, but a positive ANA is not helpful in confirming the diagnosis and must be interpreted in the context of the clinical findings and other investigations.

11 In patients with a positive ANA, ENA testing identifies the specific nuclear antigen that is the target of an auto-antibody. A range of ENAs can be found in SLE. Those of most significance are anti-Ro/SSA and anti-La/SSB antibodies (associated with secondary Sjögren's syndrome), anti-Smith (the most specific antibody for SLE but only found in around 20% of cases), anti-U1-RNP (associated with mixed connective tissue disease which can involve SLE features) and anti-ribosomal P (very specific for SLE and may have an association with CNS involvement).

12 Positive anti-Ro antibodies in this patient fit with the clinical picture of sicca symptoms suggesting secondary Sjögren's. Anti-Ro is also significant in SLE due to its

associated pregnancy complications which develop due to transplacental passage of maternal antibodies. Pregnant women with anti-Ro antibodies require foetal monitoring during pregnancy for congenital heart block, and neonates need to be monitored for neonatal lupus which presents with a rash, haematological abnormalities and deranged LFTs.

13 Anti-dsDNA antibodies are less sensitive than ANA (found in 60–70% of SLE patients) but more specific (95%) for a diagnosis of SLE. Anti-dsDNA antibodies are also used to help monitor disease activity, as titres generally increase with disease activity. Some patients, however, never have a positive anti-dsDNA despite active disease, and others always have high titres even when clinically the disease is quiescent. It is therefore important to consider serological activity alongside clinical activity when making treatment decisions.

14 The production of autoantibodies in SLE leads to the formation of immune complexes and complement activation and consumption. Complement components such as C3 and C4 therefore reduce in active SLE and are useful markers of disease activity in some patients. Other patients, however, similar to anti-dsDNA, may have persistently normal or abnormal complements regardless of disease activity.

15 Test for antiphospholipid antibodies (lupus anticoagulant, anticardiolipin and beta-2-glycoprotein-I antibodies) which are found in 30–40% of SLE patients and are associated with thrombosis and pregnancy morbidity.

16 Assessment of the urine is key when evaluating a patient for possible SLE and the urine should also be monitored at regular intervals to detect the development of lupus nephritis, which may be otherwise silent until irreversible damage has occurred.

17 Microscopic haematuria should be characterised further with phase microscopy to determine if red cells are dysmorphic (suggestive of glomerular haematuria, as occurs in lupus nephritis) or isomorphic (suggestive of lower tract bleeding).

18 Proteinuria on dipstick should be followed up with formal quantification, most commonly with a spot urine protein–creatinine ratio in the first instance, and sometimes with a confirmatory 24-hour urine collection. If significant proteinuria and/or haematuria is detected, a renal biopsy is usually indicated to determine the presence and class of lupus nephritis, which determines subsequent management.

Management

Short-term

Confirm the **diagnosis of SLE** [1] and characterise **organ manifestations** [2]. Ensure follow-up by a **Rheumatologist** [3]. Commence **hydroxychloroquine** [4] in most patients and **individualise** [5] any **additional immunosuppression** [6]. Aim to **minimise steroid exposure** [7]. Educate about **sun protection** [8] and **smoking cessation** [9] and counsel about **family planning** [10].

Long-term

Monitor disease activity [11], **damage accumulation** [12] and **treatment side-effects** [13] at **regular intervals** [14] and **adjust therapy** [15] accordingly. Institute preventive measures such as **vaccination** [16], **bone protection** [17], **cardiovascular risk reduction** [18] and **cancer screening** [19].

---

1 The diagnosis of SLE is made based on the combination of suggestive clinical features and supporting immunological findings. There is no single diagnostic test and while there are well-known classification criteria for SLE which can be helpful, their primary role is for identifying patients for research purposes and not for clinical diagnosis. SLE encompasses a spectrum of presentations, and patients in whom SLE is the most fitting diagnosis may not always meet traditional criteria.

2 SLE is a highly heterogeneous disease with a diverse range of manifestations. It is therefore key to identify which manifestations are present in an individual patient, as this impacts prognosis and choice of therapy.

3 Patients with SLE should be managed by a Rheumatologist, and if accessible, ideally in a specialised clinic, particularly for those with complex disease. Often other specialists are also involved in management of particular organ manifestations; for example, nephrologists commonly co-manage patients with lupus nephritis. Coordination and communication between specialists are paramount.

4 Hydroxychloroquine is an anchor drug in SLE, and as a general rule should be prescribed in all patients unless there are contraindications. In some patients with milder disease it may be adequate as sole therapy. The main side-effect of concern is the risk of retinopathy with long-term use; hence patients should have regular eye screening.

5 Management of patients with SLE and choice of immunosuppression are individualised according to disease manifestations, severity, patient comorbidities, possible side-effects and medication tolerance, pregnancy plans and patient preference.

6 Immunosuppression regimens for patients with SLE may include corticosteroids for rapid disease control or refractory disease, a range of traditional immunosuppressive agents (methotrexate, azathioprine, mycophenolate, calcineurin inhibitors, cyclophosphamide) and occasionally biologic agents (rituximab, belimumab). In general principles,

milder manifestations such as skin and joint disease can be controlled with hydroxychloroquine and/or methotrexate. More severe manifestations, such as lupus nephritis, haemolysis or severe serositis, require azathioprine or mycophenolate, and life-threatening manifestations, such as severe renal disease or CNS involvement, are treated with cyclophosphamide.

7 Although highly effective for controlling inflammation in SLE, prolonged use of moderate to high dose steroids is associated with significant side-effects and treatment-related morbidity. Steroid-sparing agents should be preferably prescribed where possible.

8 Given the association between ultraviolet exposure and disease activity, patients should be counselled about minimising sun exposure and adopting sun protection techniques such as sunscreen and protective clothing.

9 Smoking is associated with more active SLE and cardiovascular disease, which is a significant cause of mortality in patients with SLE.

10 Family planning, including contraception and pre-conception counselling, is vital in patients with SLE who are often young women of reproductive age, and the topic should be revisited at regular intervals. Considerations include thrombotic risk with hormonal contraception, timing and preparation for pregnancy (aiming for stable disease on medications that are safe in pregnancy), possible SLE-related pregnancy risks (particularly for those with antiphospholipid syndrome and positive Ro antibodies), as well as careful antenatal monitoring (usually in a high-level centre with specialty support).

11 Disease activity is monitored using a combination of clinical features and investigations which may be specific to certain organ involvement (e.g. serum creatinine and urinary protein/blood testing with lupus nephritis, cytopenias with haematological manifestations) or non-organ specific (e.g. ESR, complement levels and anti-dsDNA).

12 Damage refers to irreversible consequences of disease activity or treatment in SLE. Examples include renal failure, cardiovascular events, avascular necrosis and many other potential complications. The accumulation of damage correlates with overall prognosis including survival.

13 The various immunosuppressive agents used in SLE have different side-effect profiles and the treating doctors should be familiar with the specifics of each medication. The main issues to consider (except for hydroxychloroquine) include increased infection risk and the need for regular blood test monitoring to detect derangements of full blood count, renal and liver function.

14 Patients with active disease, severe manifestations or heavy treatment burden are followed up frequently (e.g. 1–3-monthly), while those with stable disease may be suitable for less regular review (e.g. 6- or 12-monthly). Disease flares can be highly unpredictable in SLE, however, and patients should be advised to contact their treating rheumatologist if they develop symptoms of active disease between appointments.

15 Medications and doses are titrated over time based on the balance between efficacy (to control inflammation, reduce symptoms and prevent damage) and toxicity (which can cause side-effects and irreversible damage in their own right).

16 In general, inactivated vaccines are safe and effective in patients with SLE. Patients should be counselled about receiving influenza and pneumococcal vaccines, as well as other routinely recommended immunisations. Live vaccines are the exception and are contraindicated in patients who are immunosuppressed.

17 Osteoporosis is a common complication of SLE itself, glucocorticoid therapy and lifestyle factors (e.g. sun avoidance, reduced physical activity). Fractures are five times more common in patients with SLE than age-matched controls, including a significant burden of fractures in premenopausal women. Bone density screening, optimisation of vitamin D and calcium and in some cases anti-resorptive or anabolic therapy, are required.

18 Aggressive management of cardiovascular risk factors is warranted due to the excessive rates of premature atherosclerosis and cardiovascular events seen in patients with SLE. Control of disease activity, minimisation of steroids, management of hypertension and hyperlipidaemia, smoking cessation, weight optimisation and screening for and managing hyperglycaemia, are all important aspects of the overall care of patients with SLE.

19 Due to a combination of the disease and its treatments, patients with SLE are at slightly higher risk of malignancy and should undertake age-appropriate cancer screening. Particular considerations include cervical cancer screening in women (rates are up to eleven times higher in patients with SLE than the general population) and skin checks (in particular for those on immunosuppressive agents, such as azathioprine, which are associated with non-melanomatous skin cancer).

INDEX OF CONDITIONS